W9-BKK-484

Cardiology Essentials in Clinical Practice

Gabriel A. Adelmann

Cardiology Essentials in Clinical Practice

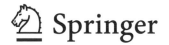 Springer

Gabriel A. Adelmann
The Yorkshire Clinic,
West Yorkshire

ISBN: 978-1-84996-304-6   e-ISBN: 978-1-84996-305-3
DOI: 10.1007/978-1-84996-305-3
Springer Dordrecht Heidelberg London New York

British Library Cataloguing in Publication Data
A catalogue record for this book is available from the British Library

Library of Congress Control Number: 2010932881

© Springer-Verlag London Limited 2011
Apart from any fair dealing for the purposes of research or private study, or criticism or review, as permitted
under the Copyright, Designs and Patents Act 1988, this publication may only be reproduced, stored or
transmitted, in any form or by any means, with the prior permission in writing of the publishers, or in the
case of reprographic reproduction in accordance with the terms of licenses issued by the Copyright Licensing
Agency. Enquiries concerning reproduction outside those terms should be sent to the publishers

The use of registered names, trademarks, etc., in this publication does not imply, even in the absence
of a specific statement, that such names are exempt from the relevant laws and regulations and therefore
free for general use

The publisher makes no representation, express or implied, with regard to the accuracy of the information
contained in this book and cannot accept any legal responsibility or liability for any errors or omissions that
may be made

Cover design: eStudioCalamar, Figueres/Berlin

Printed on acid-free paper

Springer is part of Springer Science+Business Media (www.springer.com)

To my teacher of blessed memory, Naomi Kaplinsky MD

Preface

Being a Cardiology fellow is, no doubt, one of the most daunting commitments one can make as a physician. The time- and stress-intensive work schedule is followed by long hours of study, in an ever-expanding field, making it occasionally quite challenging to master both the classical teachings and their cutting-edge developments. Maybe the most useful tool for making sense of the profusion of guidelines, textbooks, and medical papers, is to draw tables (which show the different entities at a glance, while underscoring both their similarities and their differences) and schematics (true to the adage that a picture is worth a thousand words). It has been the author's intent to provide these tools to those who take an interest in Cardiology, whether as fellows, or as a matter of general medical information. The vast majority of the tables and figures are original, and, in conjunction with the concisely conceived text, aim to provide a comprehensive image of each condition, while duly reviewing the all-important specific details. Every effort has been made to ground the text in the existing practice guidelines, as well as in the latest medical research. Inevitably, however, some of the information will already have been updated by the time the reader uses this book. The relevant medical trials and resources have been outlined both in the text, and in the suggested bibliography, to facilitate following up on the issues of interest.

It is the author's sincere hope that this book should serve as a valuable tool in the quest for a wide-ranging, yet precise knowledge of cardiology.

Acknowledgments

My thanks go, first and foremost, to Professor Naomi Kaplinsky, of blessed memory, who taught me the value of clarity and of focusing on the patient as a whole, while never forgetting the small details. This combination, she thought, was the key to good medical practice.

This book could not have been completed without the help of my dear friend, Dr. Adrian Ionescu MD, FRCP, FESC, whom I have been looking up to ever since our early days in medical college. Not only did he provide the imaging material for this book, but, in fact, he was the first to encourage me to write it.

My thanks go to Professors Samuel Sklarovsky, Alberto Toruncha, Zvi Fisman, and Radu Ciudin, who provided insight, encouragement, and help. Special thanks to Bert Pampelmo, who provided the ECG tracings and meticulous editorial support, and for doing this with a smile.

Bogdan Alexandru Ungureanu has drawn the schematics, with precision, speediness, and, not least, lots of patience for the multiple corrections and adjustments I kept requesting.

I wish to thank Bertha and Sheda Braunhut for their confidence and generosity. If not for them, this project could have never been achieved. Many thanks to my dear friends, David Greer, Diana, Florin and Mihnea Tritean, and Oana, Mircea and Filip Enache who have all become my second family in more ways than one.

Finally, I would like to thank Grant Weston and Cate Rogers from Springer, for believing in this project and making it become a reality.

Contents

Contents

1.1 Diagnostic Tests: Overview

Background: Diagnostic tests use chemical (medication, dyes, radioactive material) and/or physical agents (radiation, ultrasound, magnetic fields) to produce certain reactions in vivo or in vitro. These reactions may be chemical (e.g., blood tests), pharmacological (e.g., HR acceleration under medication), or physical (e.g., X-ray absorption by tissues). The resulting signal (electrical, optical, etc.) differs in its characteristics (intensity, wave morphology, etc.) according to the type of tissue and to the presence or absence of disease. The normal or abnormal signals, recorded and displayed on an electronic or paper support, assess the presence, severity, localization, and reversibility of disease and help optimize therapy. Unfortunately, medical tests are often performed despite there being no reasonable chance of their influencing therapy (e.g., a nuclear scan in a terminal patient will not lead to angiography and revascularization).

A popular *classification* distinguishes *imaging vs. nonimaging tests* (curbs, graphs, figures, etc.). The distinction is more complex than meets the eye, as the nature of diagnostic "images" depends heavily on the technology involved. A good case in point is mitral regurgitation. Imaging by left ventriculography genuinely reflects a volume of blood regurgitating from the LV into the LA. Imaging by color Doppler echocardiography, on the other hand, is reconstituted from digital data, a "pseudo-imaging" process relying on nonimaging data. The risk of error increases with the degree of electronic image processing, often causing discordances between the results of the different tests. It is therefore recommended that "cross-modality follow-up" be avoided where, for instance, an initial echo result is later compared to cardiac CT.

G.A. Adelmann, *Cardiology Essentials in Clinical Practice*,
DOI: 10.1007/978-1-84996-305-3_1, © Springer-Verlag London Limited 2011

Another classification distinguishes *noninvasive vs. invasive* tests: the former are performed first, and the latter, for subsequent confirmation or for interventional purposes. Tests requiring minimal trespassing of the natural barriers (e.g., TEE, tests using IV contrast material) are termed *minimally invasive.* As to the test results, these may be *positive, negative,* or *nondiagnostic.* The latter category is very important, as it can generate confusion. For instance, if an EKG stress test fails to demonstrate ischemia, but the target HR has not been reached, failure to reach the test endpoint (diagnosis of ischemia) should be clearly stated on the diagnosis sheet. Statements such as "No evidence of ischemia was observed at the attained HR" are acceptable only if followed by the unambiguous conclusion, "nondiagnostic test"; otherwise, the patient may decide on his own to discontinue the medical workup. Another possible cause of confusion is that a test yielding normal results is termed *negative,* a counterintuitive manner of expressing an essentially *positive* message.

Appropriate use of a medical test depends on three main, strongly interconnected factors: properly understanding the question the test is meant to answer; using a reliable test; and using the test for an appropriate indication.

1. *Proper understanding of the question the test is meant to answer:* Perhaps the most important point regarding medical tests is that not they, but the physician is required to provide diagnosis and therapeutic answers and decisions. This entails correct acquaintance with the test's rationale, especially in the case of older tests. For instance, EKG stress test shows the functional impact of epicardial coronary stenoses; however, most infarctions are due to thrombosis on shallow, "angiographically noncritical" plaques, i.e., precisely the ones missed by the exercise stress test. Not taking this into account may lead to serious misinterpretation of the "normal" results of a test.

2. *Use of a reliable test.* An ideal medical test should be *safe,* with easily reversible adverse effects (e.g., Aminophylline to neutralize Dipyridamol on a nuclear scan); *cheap* (widely available); *noninvasive* (to minimize complications); and, obviously, *sensitive* and *specific.* In real life, there is a trade-off between test sensitivity and specificity, as both cannot be maximal at the same time. It is equally necessary to avoid false-positive and false-negative diagnoses. Fine-tuning this principle, however, requires taking into account

the potential threat the disease may pose to the individual or to the community. For instance, many mitral regurgitant murmurs are "innocent" and do not require an echocardiogram; in other words, auscultatory detection of a mitral systolic murmur (viewed here as a "test") has low specificity for heart disease. (It can be caused by many other factors, e.g., sympathetic stimulation, anemia, enhanced audibility due to a thin thoracic wall, etc.) However, if the patient has morphologic features suggestive of Marfan's disease, the relevant characteristic of the systolic murmur "test" is not its low specificity, but its high sensitivity for MR. (Most cases of MR do display a systolic murmur.) As MR is of great potential concern in Marfan patients, an echocardiogram is strongly indicated.

The actual significance of a positive/negative test result is discussed in Table 1.1.

Based on these characteristics, certain test-related parameters can be calculated (Table 1.2). For clinical practice, PPV and NPV are perhaps the most important, since they make it possible to conclude, in face of a positive or negative test, whether the patient actually has the disease or not. For instance, a normal stress test has a high negative predictive value for the diagnosis of ischemia and allows ruling out this diagnosis, in patients in whom it was entertained.

"The number of patients indeed suffering from the disease" is obtained, at the time of preclinical test validation, using the current gold-standard test. If the gold standard is also safe, cheap, noninvasive, and accurate, there is little reason to attempt replacing it by a new test. However, gold-standard tests tend to be expensive and/or invasive, prompting the search for alternative tests, validated against the gold standard.

3. *Using the test for an appropriate indication*

> **A medical test is as useful as its indication is appropriate**
>
> Indication appropriateness means that:
>
> - The test result can modify the patient's management (treatable disease, available treatment, appropriate candidate for treatment)
> - Bayes' principle is respected, i.e., the patient has an intermediary pretest probability of disease

Table 1.1 Positive and negative test results

Setting	Significance	Correct result?	Consequence (1)	Consequence (2): treatment
"True positive"	Positive result, disease present	Yes	Correct diagnosis	Appropriately started
"True negative"	Negative result, disease absent	Yes	Correct diagnosis	Appropriately withheld
False positive	Positive result, but disease absent	No	Incorrect diagnosis: "false alarm"	Inappropriately started
False negative	Negative result, but disease present	No	Incorrect diagnosis: diagnosis missed	Inappropriately withheld

Table 1.2 Characteristics of medical tests

Parameter	Definition	Significance
Sensitivity	True positives/all patients, where "all patients" = true positives + false negatives	Of 100 people with the disease, how many have a positive test
Specificity	True negatives/all patients, where "all patients" = true negatives + false negatives	Of 100 healthy subjects, how many have a negative test
Positive predictive value (PPV)	True positive/all positives, where "all positives" = true positives + false positives	Of 100 individuals with a positive test, how many really have the disease
Negative predictive value (NPV)	True negative/total negatives, where "all negatives" = true negatives + false negatives	Of 100 individuals with a negative test, how many are really disease-free

Sensitivity, specificity, PPV, NPV: an analogy

Consider you are at a shooting booth, at the County Fair. Some of the clay ducks are filled with coins. Your chances of hitting the jackpot depend not only on how good a shot you are, but also on how frequent the winning targets are. Being a good shot is the equivalent of having good sensitivity and specificity at shooting targets (you will hit "most of the targets, and almost nothing but the targets"), but this accounts for little if the "prevalence" of winning targets is low (and conversely, if all the targets are winners, even if you are a poor marksman, you will still win the jackpot, provided you are able to shoot at least one target).

Bayes' principle: The prevalence of the disease in a community influences the predictive value of any medical test, irrespective of its sensitivity and specificity. For a disease prevalence of 100% (all the members of the community have the disease), the PPV of a test, however unrefined (were one to be carried out), is 100%: not only those with a positive test, but also those with a negative test have the disease! In real life, tests help establish diagnoses when there is neither a very high nor a very low pretest probability of disease (in the first case, treatment is warranted, and in the second, the diagnosis can be safely ruled out). In other words, a test is useful in patients with a moderate probability of disease (Bayes' principle); the PPV/NPV quoted for any medical test are based on this assumption, and ignoring this key point will lead to misdiagnosis.

Transposing these considerations to the medical field, a stress test is as useless in an obese 50-year-old diabetic male complaining of typical angina as it is in a 20-year-old with stabbing chest pain that worsens on positional changes. Clearly, the former patient requires angiography, and the latter, reassurance. Bayes' principle must be interpreted with great attention to the question at hand. For instance, when assessing the effectiveness of treatment for a given disease, a stress test is often performed. The point here is not that the pretest probability is 100% (disease known to be present); what we are asking now is: "How probable is it that the disease should require a change in treatment?" and if the probability of *this* being the case is intermediate, the test is warranted, and Bayes' principle is respected. *The pretest probability of disease,* a key aspect with Bayes' principle, is assessed statistically, based on age, gender, race, lifestyle, and genetic endowment. The medical test reclassifies the intermediate pretest probability as either low or high; this is the *posttest* probability of disease. Depending on the specificity and sensitivity of the test and on the degree of clinical suspicion, therapy is now instituted, or a more precise test is performed. For instance, a 45-year-old male with mild HTN and atypical chest pain has an intermediate probability of coronary disease, and an EKG stress test is recommended. Supposing the stress test is positive, one can opt either for conservative therapy, for a more precise stress test (echocardiographic or nuclear), or for coronarography. A negative test in this setting largely rules out ischemia, but in case of a high degree of clinical suspicion, further testing may be chosen nevertheless (in these cases, in fact, stress echo, nuclear scan, or even coronarography should be chosen to start with). The age- and gender-adjusted statistical probability for a given disease is based on observational studies in the population. For instance, most of our knowledge relating to coronary disease was obtained by the *Framingham study,* focusing on the natural medical history of more than 5,000 inhabitants and their offspring in a Massachusetts town. This study has been going on continuously since 1948, second- and third-generation cohorts being added to the initial cohort.

An important question arises at this point, namely, how to define "intermediate risk" for a disease or another. Semantically, it would make sense to think it means a 50% risk over a specific follow-up time (2, 5, 10 years). However, due to the extremely high importance of such diagnoses, the threshold for designating risk as "intermediate" is usually set at much lower thresholds (for instance, intermediate risk of CAD is defined at a 1-5% threshold) Therefore, in clinical practice, the majority of subjects undergoing a diagnostic test will have normal results (Up to 90% of those with intermediate pretest probability are in fact healthy, with low posttest disease probability.)

1.2　Diagnostic Tests in Cardiology

These include the following: *chemical analysis of the serum,* to detect *risk factors* for heart disease (dyslipidemia, diabetes, homocysteine, inflammatory markers, etc.) or *evidence of myocardial lesions* (troponin, CK, BNP, myosine); *analysis of the cardiac electrical signals* (EKG and related techniques), to detect ischemia, ventricular hypertrophy, rhythm and conduction disturbances, LV aneurysm, or pericardial lesions; *X-ray techniques,* based on differential absorption of X-rays

by the organs. These techniques include *chest X-ray, invasive angiography* (using contrast material), *cardiac CT and angio-CT*; and *ultrasound (sonographic) techniques,* based on differential reflection of ultrasound by the different types of tissue, offering both imaging and nonimaging data. The echocardiogram is usually performed in a noninvasive or minimally invasive manner (TEE, TTE) but can be carried out invasively as well (IVUS; intracardiac echocardiogram). Due to its wide availability and to the extensive range of information it provides, echocardiography is a staple of clinical cardiology; *scintigraphic (nuclear) techniques,* based on differential absorption of radioactive substances into the myocytes, widely used for the diagnosis of ischemia and for assessing the reversibility of ischemic myocardial damage; *MRI* (based on the differential vibration of hydrogen ions in the tissues exposed to a magnetic field); *invasive monitoring* of pressure in the blood vessels and heart cavities, by catheter-based techniques; and *myocardial biopsy,* usually from the RV (more accessible than the LV).

1.2.1　Serum Analysis

Serum analysis is discussed in the relevant chapters. In addition to the "usual" blood tests, integration of genetic information in patient management is slowly making its way into clinical practice. The initial "direct candidate gene" approach has been abandoned, in favor of genome-wide association scans (GWAS), to identify individual or clusters of disease-associated alleles. Some prominent examples include genetic assessment of the risk for CAD/MI (9p21), and AF (4q25), or prediction of response to pharmacotherapy such as Warfarin (CYP2C9/VKORC1).

1.2.2　The Electrocardiogram

The electrocardiogram (EKG) records the currents resulting from cyclical variation of electrolyte concentration on both sides of the myocyte membrane, along the phases of the cardiac cycle. EKG analyzes the patterns of depolarization and repolarization associated to different types of heart disease. Additionally, there is a well-defined correlation between the phases of the electrical and of the mechanical activity of the heart (systole, diastole). This allows EKG to serve as a landmark against which different physiological events are timed, as to their place in the cardiac cycle. Thus, above and beyond its intrinsic diagnostic value, EKG is invaluable in timing short-lived echocardiographic events and in gating SPECT images (see below).

The spread of the electrical impulse from the sinus node to the rest of the myocardium is reviewed in Table 1.3.

Repolarization progresses through the myocytes in a reverse sequence as compared to depolarization; the first regions to depolarize also repolarize the first. The conduction system plays no role in the progression of repolarization. Repolarization translates on the EKG as the T wave, occasionally followed by a U wave. As to the *mechanical correlate of the EKG waves,* systole lasts from the onset of Q wave (or, in its absence, from the onset of the R wave), approximately until the

middle of the T wave, while diastole lasts from the middle of the T wave until the onset of the Q (R) wave (Fig. 1.1).

There is only partial superposition between electrical de/repolarization and mechanical systole/diastole.

Electrical de/repolarization spreads gradually over the entire myocardium, with apex-to-base LV activation. The IVS and the LV free wall are activated simultaneously. At each moment, different territories are at different points of depolarization/systole or of repolarization/diastole. The EKG tracing is a vectorial sum of these processes, hence the partial "dissociation" between the electrical and the mechanical events.

Table 1.3 The normal EKG: waves and segments

Name	Function	Situation and description	EKG
Sinus node (SN)	Impulse generation	In RA, next to SVC ostium; fires at 60–100 impulses/min. SN has sympathetic and parasympathetic innervation. Vascularized by RCA (ischemia can cause arrhythmia and heart block)	P wave
Intraatrial (internodal) tracts	Impulse conduction SN → AVN	In the atrial myocardium	PQ Interval
Atrioventricular node (AVN)	Delays impulse transmission to the ventricles	Decelerates impulse progression by approximately 0.1 s, allowing completion of atrial systole before ventricular systole; functional block important in rapid atrial rhythms (AF, flutter, etc.) Vascularized by RCA (85%) or by LCx	PQ interval
His bundle	Conduction	Upper IVS, in direct continuation with AVN	PQ
Left bundle	Conduction	Left side of IVS; short, thick bundle, splits into anterior and posterior hemibundle	PQ
Left anterior hemibundle	Conduction	Spreads depolarization to the anterior portion of the LV	PQ
Left posterior hemibundle	Conduction	Spreads depolarization to the posterior portion of the LV	PQ
Left middle hemibundle[a]	Conduction	Spreads depolarization between the portions covered by the other two hemibundles	PQ
Right bundle	Conduction	Right of IVS; no hemibundles; spreads depolarization to RV	PQ
Purkinje network	Conduction	Final ramifications of the bundles; carries depolarization to the myocytes	QRS complex
Myocytes	Excitation, contraction	Excitation/contraction coupling	QRS complex

[a]Present in 60% of individuals

Fig. 1.1 The normal EKG. The *arrows* are pointing to the P, QRS, and T waves, respectively

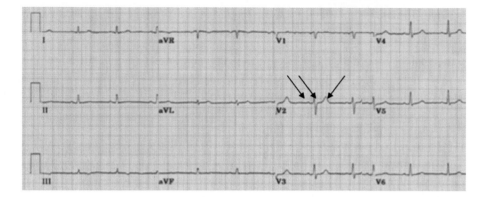

The main elements of interest on the EKG include the following: frequency and regularity of the cardiac electrical activity; sinus or nonsinus rhythm; AV dissociation; conduction disturbances; electrical wave amplitude and morphology; and the electrical axis of the heart. The latter is defined as the vectorial sum of the "local" de/repolarization processes and indicates the direction of de/repolarization propagation through the myocardium. The normal electrical axis points from the right shoulder towards the left nipple, oriented from −30° to +90° (on a clock dial, between 2:00 and 6:00 o'clock). Orientation to the left of −30° or to the right of +90° is considered left/right deviation. *The importance of EKG* in the diagnosis of the different cardiac conditions is briefly reviewed in Table 1.4.

Practical aspects: Out of the numerous permutations possible for a total of ten electrodes (one for each limb, and six for the chest), only a few pairs are of practical importance. Different pairs of electrodes visualize different LV segments, each segment being visualized by several sets of derivations (Chap. 2). Older machines record the derivations sequentially, while newer ones stock information relative to the same cardiac cycles, so that all derivations depict the same electrical event. At the usual paper speed (25 mm/s), each horizontal 1 mm segment = 0.04 s; thus, a 5-mm block corresponds to 0.20 s (200 ms). Wave amplitude is also measured (on the vertical axis, every 1 mm = 1 mV). There are several widely used EKG modalities, including resting EKG; EKG stress test; EKG monitoring; and EPS. The main limitations of resting EKG include the very short time span of cardiac activity being displayed and the absence of information relative to the physiologic response to stress. This information is supplied by EKG monitoring and by stress testing, respectively. The indications and contraindications of stress testing are discussed in detail

Table 1.4 Using the EKG in clinical practice[a]

Type of disease	EKG helps diagnose
IHD	Ischemia: presence, severity, extension, acute or chronic nature (in select cases), response to therapy, complications (arrhythmia, postinfarction pericarditis, etc.)
HF	LVH, arrhythmia
VHD	LA dilatation (MS); LVH (AS, AI); arrhythmia
Arrhythmia and heart block	Prolonged QT, Brugada, WPW syndrome, etc.; type, severity, paroxysmal or chronic nature, response to treatment
Peric. disease	Diagnosis of pericarditis
Cardiac trauma	Complications (ischemia, arrhythmia)
Congenital heart disease	Diagnosis of the disease and of its complications: chamber dilatation or hypertrophy, arrhythmia, etc.
Diseases of the great arteries	Aortic dissection (extension to the coronaries); supravalvular aortic stenosis (LVH); PE (Chap.10)

[a]The supporting role of EKG in cardiac imaging (nuclear scan, echocardiography) is discussed together with the corresponding techniques

in the relevant chapters. Briefly, *EKG stress testing* is indicated for the diagnosis and follow-up of myocardial ischemia or for the diagnosis of certain types of arrhythmia and for assessing their clinical impact (tolerability). As discussed in Chap. 2, EKG stress test provides a wealth of information beyond the EKG changes, which is incorporated in the final analysis. Importantly, EKG monitoring is carried out in *any* type of stress test, where it serves for the diagnosis of arrhythmia and/or for image gating (with SPECT imaging). The different protocols are reviewed in Chap. 2. Stress test can be performed using either a treadmill or a stress bicycle. The stress test is terminated when a clinical or EKG endpoint is reached, in case of complications, or if the patient cannot continue the physical exertion (mainly due to fatigue or leg pain). The most notable adverse events during stress testing include myocardial ischemia, arrhythmia, syncope, and worsening of heart failure. The stress EKG (even in its "resting component") is slightly different from the resting EKG, due to the difference in electrode placing (all of the electrodes are on the chest) and to the erect position of the patient, unlike the supine position used with classical EKG. Caution is therefore needed when comparing a "classical" EKG to a stress tracing. *The cardiopulmonary stress test* is a combination between a classical stress test and chemical analysis of the expired gasses, yielding the maximal oxygen consumption capacity, (VO_2 Max), also known as "aerobic capacity." This represents the maximum capacity of the patient's body to carry and use oxygen during exercise and is measured in liters of O_2/min or in mLO_2/kg body mass/min. Normal values: in males, 3.5 L/min (45 mg/kg/min); in females, 2 L/min (38 mg/kg/min). A decrease <12–14 mL/kg/min is a severe prognostic criterion in HF and an indication for transplant, in suitable patients. The test also helps distinguish pulmonary from cardiac causes of effort dyspnea and evaluate the efficacy of cardiovascular rehabilitation in HF patients. Practically, the test is carried out as a modified stress test, with a special device fitted over the patient's nose and mouth; this device only allows breathing through the mouth and stores the expired air in a special tank, preventing its remixing with the room air. O_2 and CO_2 contents of the expired air are measured, and VO_2Max is calculated.

EKG monitoring overcomes the shortcoming of classic EKG of offering only short-span information. Self-limiting episodes of heart disease classically consist of arrhythmia, but modern technology allows monitoring short-lived ischemic episodes as well. Commonly used EKG monitoring techniques include the following: in-hospital monitoring (in the ICU, or ambulatory monitoring, also called telemetry); Holter monitoring; loop recorders; and self-monitoring. The EKG monitoring data are electronically stored, allowing analysis and comparison to subsequent events. ICU EKG monitoring is specifically aimed to diagnose arrhythmia, and thus, one or two derivations are sufficient; however, if the nature of the arrhythmia (ventricular or atrial) is not readily apparent, it is possible to record additional derivations. Typically, ICU patients have a few resting EKG tracings daily, in parallel with EKG monitoring. Diagnosis of ischemia on the EKG monitor generally requires confirmation by a standard tracing. Over-interpretation of the monitor tracing may lead to false diagnosis of MI; any impression of significant ST segment shifts must be confirmed by routine 12-lead EKG. *The Holter test* provides a long-duration EKG recording (up to 3 days or more, as compared to the 10–15 s of a resting EKG), substantially facilitating the diagnosis of short-lived arrhythmic or ischemic episodes. However, the suspected event may fail to occur during the study, yielding false-negative results. A Holter report typically mentions the most bradycardic and the most tachycardic HR recorded and the nature, number, time of occurrence, and duration of arrhythmic episodes. Correlation with a symptom diary kept by the patient is very important. Many lessons have been learned from Holter tracings about normal heart physiology (HR variability, common occurrence of APBs and VPBs in normal subjects, etc.) If a false-negative Holter result is suspected, the test can be repeated, or *self-monitoring* using patient-activated recording devices, as well as *implantable loop recorders* (Chap. 6) may be used.

The electrophysiological test (EPS) is carried out with catheter-borne electrodes introduced directly into the heart cavities. The electrodes are positioned under fluoroscopy (rarely, intracardiac echo) guidance. The rationale is that numerous arrhythmias are due to areas of inhomogeneity in the propagation of depolarization, the coexistence of depolarized and nondepolarized areas generating pathologic currents and arrhythmia. Inhomogeneity can be caused by areas with excessively high or low conduction capacity (abnormal conduction tracts, scar, etc.); these areas can be identified by EPS and subsequently destroyed by catheter ablation. EPS is also useful for diagnosis of heart block and is a preliminary component of pacemaker and ICD implantation. EPS will be discussed in more detail in Chap. 6.

1.2.3 X-Ray Techniques Used in Cardiology

X-ray techniques used in cardiology include chest X-ray, CT, and invasive contrast angiography (cardiac catheterization). Tissue penetration by X-rays is inversely correlated with the metal content (e.g., calcium in bones and iron in blood); conversely, muscle and air allow unhindered X-ray passage. Radiographic techniques are cheap, accessible, and generally harmless, although angio-CT does deliver potentially oncogenic amounts of radiation.

1.2.3.1 Chest X-Ray

The classical X-ray image is a *summation image,* superposing 3D information on a 2D plane. In affluent countries, X-ray films have been superseded by electronic data storage technologies. Chest X-rays are usually performed with the radiation source behind the patient (postero-anterior, or PA images). However, with bedridden patients, the film is placed under the patient's back, and the X-rays are administered in the opposite direction, i.e., antero-posterior (AP). On AP images, the heart appears larger, occasionally creating the false impression of cardiac dilatation. This problem is generally minor. The main sources of misdiagnosis with chest X-rays include the following: *using a suboptimal radiation regimen,* with suboptimal visualization of the intrathoracic structures; *performing the X-ray in expiration,* which causes poor visualization of the pleural recesses (obscuring small pleural effusions) and changes the position of the heart in the thorax; and *incorrect patient positioning* (creating false asymmetry between the two sides of the thorax). The heart is visualized together with the pericardium, as a triangular summation image. Pathological changes of interest to the cardiologist include cardiomegaly; pulmonary congestion; pericardial and pleural effusion; and changes in the intrathoracic vessels. Alongside the heart, the chest X-ray also visualizes parts of the skeleton, the large vessels of the thorax (aorta, SVC, PA), the diaphragm, the upper abdomen, and, in women, the breast shadows. Incidental pathological findings in these organs need confirmation by a dedicated X-ray study using a proper radiation regimen.

1.2.3.2 Computer Tomography

Computer tomography (CT) is an X-ray technology displaying "virtual sections," at an average slice thickness of 0.5 mm, an excellent spatial resolution.

(The Greek root, *tomo-,* expresses the concept of "slicing".) The tomographic approach is in contradistinction to the summation principle of classical X-ray studies. Computerized reconstruction techniques can be used to yield a "pseudo-3D" image; this is used, for instance, with angio-CT. Not all CT techniques are of an imaging nature; for instance, assessment of the *intracoronary calcium score* is a nonimaging CT technique. For imaging purposes, spiral (helicoidal) CT is currently the most popular technique. The name alludes to the trajectory of the radiation source within the machine, as it rotates around the patient's body. This technology is especially suited to cardiac CT, as (being very fast) it allows the patient to hold his/her breath during the whole duration of the test, avoiding respiratory changes in cardiac position (a cause of artifact); additionally, it requires a lower dose of contrast. A similar technology is the "multislice CT" technique.

1.2.3.3 Cardiac Catheterization

Arterial Catheterization

Diagnostic

- *Coronary and peripheral artery catheterization* (carotid, renal, femoral artery, etc.), which provides imaging of arterial stenosis and of angioplasty results and complications.
- *Ventricular catheterization,* for diagnosis of ventricular dysfunction (visual assessment of contractility, measurement of LVEDP); of MR; and of aortic and MV area.
- *Aortic catheterization* (during cardiac catheterization), to assess aortic root dilatation, as well as the presence and severity of AI.
- *Invasive BP monitoring* (usually through the radial artery).

Therapeutic

- *Angioplasty*
- *IABP*
- *Other procedures* (e.g., controlled infarction of the IVS in patients with HOCM; injection of angiogenesis factors, etc.); catheter-based aortic valve replacement

Venous Catheterization

Diagnostic

- *Swan–Ganz catheterization,* to measure the pressures in the RA, RV, PA, and the wedge pressure (PCWP). Advancing the catheter tip into a small PA branch allows measuring the PCWP, very close in value to the LA pressure, which is increased in patients with LV dysfunction. (The LA pressure can be measured directly by transseptal access from the RA). Swan–Ganz catheterization also allows measuring the CO (RV and LV output are normally equal). Combined right and left cardiac catheterization allows to evaluate the severity of MS or AS (Chap. 5). Complications of Swan–Ganz catheterization include infection; thrombosis (possible PE); TV lesions (TR); and hemorrhage.
- *Pulmonary arteriography,* the gold-standard test for PE
- *RV catheterization for cardiac biopsy* (routine post-transplant follow-up; less frequently, for diagnosis of infiltrative heart disease).
- *EPS*
- *Peripheral venography,* consisting in IV contrast injection, e.g., for diagnosis of DVT in the lower limb veins. By and large, this test has been superseded by Doppler sonography.

Therapeutic

- *Repair procedures for congenital or acquired heart disease* – ASD occlusion, PTMC (starts as right heart catheterization, and then, by perforation of the interatrial septum, accesses the LA), pulmonary valvuloplasty, etc.
- *Pacemaker or ICD insertion*
- *Peripheral or central venous port insertion;* CVP is most frequently inserted through the jugular or subclavian vein. Multiport CVP allows measuring RA pressures, administering IV medications, and taking blood samples. In ambulatory patients requiring chronic IV therapy, entirely subcutaneous CVP systems are available, including a capsule with a silicone lid, into which a needle can be inserted (through the skin) up to 1,000 times, for administration of medication and/or blood sampling. A typical ambulatory CVP device is the *Portacath.*

The practical steps of left cardiac catheterization include the following: anamnesis regarding allergy to iodine or coexisting renal disease; insertion of a peripheral venous port; preparation of the right femoral (or, as alternatives, the left femoral or the radial) artery; guide-wire, then catheter insertion, under fluoroscopic guidance; cannulation of the coronary ostia; contrast injection and visualization of the coronary arteries from different angles, by moving both the catheterization table and the X-ray source. Standard and, if needed, individualized views are used. After examination of the coronaries, the catheter is withdrawn and then gently pushed into the LV, through the AV. Left ventriculography is contraindicated in critical AS (total obstruction of the LV/aorta communication can cause syncope) and when echo has shown LV thrombus (risk of embolism). Contrast is injected and a few cardiac cycles are observed, to assess global and segmental LV contractility, MR, or the presence of MI complications, such as myocardial rupture. If angiography reveals coronary stenosis amenable to angioplasty, this can be carried out directly. At the conclusion of the procedure, the catheter is withdrawn, and the arterial port of entry (femoral or other) is sealed with biological glue or prolongedly compressed with a special device, to avoid bleeding. The use of bioglue allows early ambulation, whereas mechanical compression requires bed rest for about 12 h. *Catheterization through the radial artery* may be necessary in case of femoral artery disease (malformations or severe atherosclerosis); of inguinal cutaneous infection; and of advanced abdominal aortic atherosclerosis (risk of cholesterol embolism). *The contraindications* of cardiac catheterization (iodine allergy, renal disease, diabetes) can generally be overcome by special pre- and post-test measures (Table 1.5). Of note, angio-CT also requires contrast injection, and thus is not an ideal solution to this problem. Often, without being *contraindicated,* catheterization is simply *not indicated,* as in patients with low pretest probability of stenosis; on suboptimal medical treatment; or if previous angiography already showed coronary anatomy not suitable for intervention. *The main complications* of left catheterization include the following:

- *Hemorrhage: External bleeding* is usually controlled by arterial compression but occasionally requires surgical suture. *Pseudoaneurysm* (bleeding between the femoral artery layers, a potential cause of limb ischemia) is usually controlled by strong

Table 1.5 Contraindications for catheterization

Contraindication	Rationale	Prevention measures
Diabetes	Possible renal damage by the contrast material	Saline infusions, to increase blood volume and dilute contrast; renal-protective (hypoosmotic) contrast material; Acetylcysteine[a]
Renal failure	As above	As above; occasionally, dialysis
Allergy to iodine	Dyspnea, syncope, hypotension	Antiallergic medication (cortisone, NSAID)
Severe decompensated HF	Possible pulmonary overload (contrast is water-based)	Diuretics or even dialysis

[a]See Chap. 2

and prolonged artery compression but may require surgical suture.

- *Lower limb ischemia*
- *Severe angina or arrhythmia,* by temporary ischemia (the contrast-filled coronary artery does not carry oxygen).
- *HF* (high volume of hyperosmotic contrast material)
- *Peripheral embolism* with plaque fragments (the "blue toe syndrome"); this is generally self-limiting.

The *complications of angioplasty* are discussed in Chap. 2. The risks of morbidity and mortality after cardiac catheterization are <2% and <1‰, respectively, in properly selected patients.

The practical steps of right heart catheterization are similar to those of left catheterization (see below). The position of the catheter can be assessed by fluoroscopy; by pressure curve morphology (Fig. 1.2), which changes throughout systole and diastole and in the different parts of the SVC/RA/RV/PA/PA wedge continuum; and by EKG morphology (using an electrode at the tip of the catheter).

The complications of right heart catheterization include the following:

- *Pneumothorax:* mild cases are self-limiting, while more severe ones may need air evacuation, to prevent

pulmonary collapse (when the lung appears as a knob, in the hilus).
- *Hemothorax, hemo-pneumothorax* (the hypertransparence corresponding to the air collection is on top of the radioopaque bloody effusion).
- *Arrhythmia and heart block*
- *RV perforation with hemorrhagic pericardial effusion,* which may lead to tamponade (emergency pericardiocentesis required). Routine chest X-ray is obtained after right catheterization, to ascertain the position of the radioopaque catheter tip and to rule out complications.

1.2.4 MRI

MRI visualizes tissues by exposing them to electromagnetic fields, which cause the water-bound hydrogen ions (protons), normally aligned along multiple axes, to align along the same axis. If this "new order" is deranged by another magnetic field, perpendicular on the first, the protons dealign, but are rapidly "returned to order" by the first field. This dealignment/realignment process is differentiated by the water content of the tissues. Realignment generates electromagnetic waves that express these differences and are processed to produce images of the organs. In some cases, contrast substance is necessary (gadolinium, a noniodine-based compound). Gadolinium behaves differently under electromagnetic fields than do the body tissues and creates a contrast that helps distinguish certain structures, such as the vessel wall from the lumen. MRI holds the promise of enabling "molecular imaging," i.e., selective imaging of target tissue or cells using magnetic nanoparticles.

The adverse effects of MRI include *problems related to ferromagnetic (iron-containing) objects,* which, under the magnetic field, can migrate; become overheated, causing internal burns; function abnormally (pacemaker and ICD de-calibration, credit card demagnetizing, etc.); cause image distortion (e.g., orthopedic implants, tooth fillings); or cause skin irritation (tattoos with ferromagnetic dyes). Ferromagnetic objects can be exterior (jewelry, watches, clips, zippers, credit cards, etc.) or seated inside the body (pacemaker, ICD, vascular clips, implantable pumps, cochlear implants, tooth fillings, bullets, shrapnel, etc.); *claustrophobia and panic attacks;* and *Gadolinium-related problems,*

Fig. 1.2 The correspondence between the RA pressure tracing and other diagnostic tests: (1) Normal RA pressure tracing. The RA and RV systole increase the RA pressure (a, v waves), whereas the descending movement of the TV at the onset of RV systole and the RA emptying into the RV decrease the RA pressure (x, y descents); (2) Pericardial tamponade: both the x and y descents are blunted, as the RA is compressed throughout diastole. The echocardiogram reflects a pandiastolic invagination of the RV (concave white line); (3) Constrictive pericarditis: irtually, all the RV filling occurs in the early part of diastole, causing an exaggerated y descent; MRI reveals pericardial calcification (black "halo" around the heart); (4) When the RA and the RV contractions are simultaneous, rather than sequential, there is a giant a wave in the RA pressure ("cannon a wave"), visible on physical examination as a prominent retrograde wave in the jugular vein. The EKG shows atrioventricular dissociation, as in this patient with complete AV block; (5) Severe TR causes a giant v wave, distinguished clinically from the cannon a wave by its timing in relation to the peripheral pulse. Blood regurgitates in systole in other veins as well, e.g., the hepatic vein, leading to systolic flow reversal (Doppler tracing, *full arrow*, opposed to normal flow, dotted *arrow*)

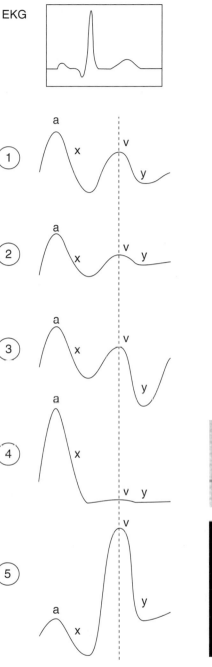

including allergy and, in rare renal patients, systemic nephrogenic fibrosis, a serious syndrome. In renal patients, Gadolinium elimination by dialysis is recommended after MRI. MRI must be used cautiously in pregnant women; however, it is usually considered safe in this setting.

Similar to CT, MRI has a "cine-" and an "angio-" modality. According to the machine settings, MRI can display blood either in black or in white. However, coronary angio-MRI requires use of gadolinium. MRI can be used in practically any field of cardiology. This includes assessment of myocardial ischemia, hibernation, and scar; of VHD and of its impact on the myocardium; of structural myocardial changes (hypertrophy, dilatation, aneurysm, etc.); of ventricular dysfunction; diagnosis of intracardiac tumor and clots; structural and functional evaluation of the pericardium (thickness, effusion, constriction or tamponade); and diagnosis of aortic and great artery pathology. The spatial resolution of cardiac MRI is excellent (1.5 mm). However, the other imaging modalities can, by and large, provide the same information more cheaply and are also available in emergency settings. Therefore, the clinical use of cardiac MRI is usually limited to the diagnosis of cardiac malformations and of ARVC.

1.2.5 Echocardiography

Echocardiography is based on reflection of ultrasound by the cardiac structures and by the circulating blood. The echo transducer contains a piezoelectric crystal, capable of generating sound when stimulated electrically, and electrical signals when stimulated by ultrasound; thus, the transducer functions for both emission and reception of ultrasound. Echocardiography can be noninvasive (TTE, by far the most frequently used), semi- (or minimally-) invasive (TEE, contrast echo), or invasive (IVUS, intracardiac echocardiography). The main limitation of *TTE* is the limited number of available imaging angles, corresponding to the "sonographic windows," usually the intercostal, subcostal, and suprasternal areas. This shortcoming is overcome by *TEE,* which allows transducer rotation at 360° in multiple planes. TEE has the disadvantage of being a semi-invasive procedure and is contraindicated in patients with inflammation or oral, esophageal, and/or gastric tumors. Bleeding or esophageal rupture are rare, but very serious complications. Light sedation (Midazolam) and oropharyngeal anesthesia with lidocaine spray are used. Dentures are removed. If the patient falls asleep, they are awakened, so they can hold their breath, inspire deeply, etc., as needed. The patient is instructed to indicate any significant pain, which may indicate damage to the GI tract and mandate discontinuing the test. EKG monitoring is used both for safety and for better timing of cardiac events. The probe is gently rotated and pushed, to obtain the images. *IVUS and intracardiac ultrasound* are performed in the cath lab (Chap. 2).

Echocardiographic data can be displayed in an imaging or nonimaging fashion. However, some of the "imaging" modalities are not "pictures" of the heart, and, conversely, data reflecting blood flow can be displayed as "images." A classification of echo-derived data taking this distinction into account is presented below.

1.2.5.1 Data Reflecting the Size and Excursion Amplitude of the Heart Structures and of the Blood Vessels

Tissues of different density reflect ultrasound to different degrees. Most of the reflected sound (echo) has the same frequency as the initial ultrasound, emitted by the transducer; however, a small part of the echo wave front has a frequency double or triple the original one, designated as "second and third harmonics." Classical imaging was based on the fundamental harmonic, but currently second harmonic imaging is commonly used. With fundamental harmonic imaging, the deeper the reflecting tissue, the weaker the echo. The opposite holds true with the secondary harmonic, allowing to improve image parameters. Second harmonic imaging is also the technology used with contrast echo.

The Echo Data Display Modalities

The echo data display modalities have evolved along the decades.

A (amplitude) mode was the first clinically usable technology. Data was displayed as a mobile dot on a screen; the tracing could be printed out, as a curve reflecting the excursion of an isolated point in the heart, followed over time. As the point moved toward the transducer, the curve ascended, and as it moved away, it descended.

M (motion) mode echo is the direct successor of A-mode technology and consists in a set of superimposed curves and segments, following the cardiac activity during systole and diastole. The vertical projection corresponds to the amplitude of the excursion (in mm), while the horizontal projection is that of time. M-mode echo can be viewed as the sum of a whole set of A-mode exams, the different sampling points being aligned along an axis. M-mode imaging has a better temporal resolution than B mode and is still used for observation

Table 1.6 M- and B-mode echo: a comparison

Parameter	M mode	B mode	Practical importance
Imaging	No	Yes	B-mode echo allows fast, intuitive global assessment of the heart
Real time	No	Yes	Real-time imaging offers a more intuitive impression of heart structure and function. Non-real-time imaging displays several cardiac cycles on the same image
Temporal resolution	Higher	Lower	Higher temporal resolution enables to observe short-lived phenomena[a] and to identify end-systole and end-diastole, when the width and thickness of cardiac chambers and walls are measured
Spatial resolution	High	High[b]	Both modalities can pinpoint even minute abnormalities

[a]Frame-by-frame examination of the B-mode images does not necessarily solve this problem; B mode harvests less sets of images per unit of time, and if the observed phenomenon lasts less than the interval between two B mode frames, it can be missed

[b]Earlier B-mode imaging systems had lower spatial resolution; current high-frequency transducers and harmonic imaging improve the spatial resolution, making it equivalent to that of M-mode imaging

of very short-lived events and for measuring the cardiac walls, vessels, and cavities at the exact moment of end-diastole. While both these operations can also be performed on B-mode images (frame-by-frame analysis, freeze-frame measurements), the time resolution of M-mode echo is higher (Table 1.6). Practically, an area of interest is identified on the B-mode echo, an interrogation axis is positioned, and the M-mode function is started. A miniature B-mode image is usually displayed in a corner of the screen, for imaging guidance throughout the M-mode study.

Real-time (B = brightness) mode, where "brightness" alludes to the different shades of gray allocated to the reflected echoes. With B mode, the concept of "imaging" reaches its entire intuitive meaning, since, unlike with A or M mode, the data are displayed as actual sections through the heart. B mode is the default contemporary echo-imaging method. The images display the heart in motion, in (almost) "real time," the very short delay corresponding to the "back-and-forth trip" of the ultrasound towards and from the tissues, plus the echo-processing time. The image is a circle sector, with the tip (transducer) upwards; this image can be reverted. Table 1.6 shows a comparison between M- and B-mode echocardiography, and Fig. 1.3 further illustrates the correspondence between these two modalities.

Care must be taken to obtain images resulting from ultrasound that falls perpendicular to the investigated tissues; failing to do so will lead to obtaining foreshortened images and false estimates about the thickness and diameter of cardiac chambers and walls.

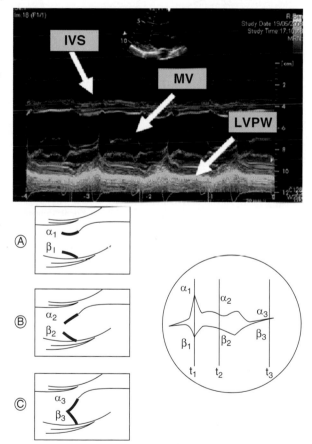

Fig. 1.3 Correspondence between M-mode and 2-D echo. *IVS* interventricular septum; *MV* mitral valve; *LVPW* left ventricular posterior wall. The schematic within the round border follows the excursion of two points, α and β, on the mitral leaflets (for instance, the tips of the leaflets), at three points in time (t_1, t_2, t_3, displayed in rectangular panels A, B, and C, respectively)

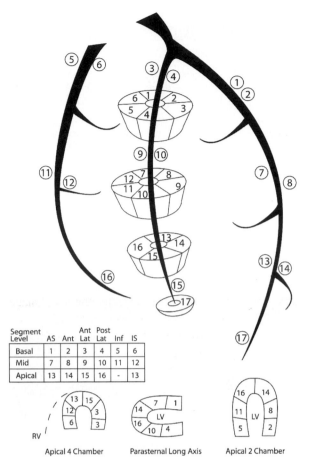

Segment Level	AS	Ant	Ant Lat	Post Lat	Inf	IS
Basal	1	2	3	4	5	6
Mid	7	8	9	10	11	12
Apical	13	14	15	16	-	13

Apical 4 Chamber   Parasternal Long Axis   Apical 2 Chamber

Fig. 1.4 The 17 segments of the LV, viewed from the conventional transversal and longitudinal imaging planes. The longitudinal views are designated according to the echocardiographic terminology. For a comparison to nuclear medicine display and terminology, see Fig. 1.5

According to the coronary supply, the LV is divided into different segments; thus, identifying an abnormality in a given segment (hypokinesis, decreased radiotracer captation, late hyperenhancement on MRI, etc.) allows to pinpoint the culprit coronary artery. If the pathological changes are of sufficient magnitude (severity of abnormality) and extension (number of involved segments), coronarography is warranted; and if significant stenoses are found in the particular artery noninvasively indicated as culprit, revascularization (by PCI or CABG) is indicated. After many years of using different segmentation schematics for the different imaging modalities (a fact considerably complicating cross-modality comparisons), a unified 17-segment model has been adopted (Fig. 1.4). However, due to technology-specific considerations, the visual display of essentially equivalent images is sometimes different (Fig. 1.5). Images may also be displayed in a "condensed" image (bull's eye map), where the LV segments are presented side by side, as if the heart were a funnel, looked at from the inside, from base to apex.

Segments 1, 2, 7, 8, 13, 14 correspond to the LAD; segments 3, 4, 9, 10, 15 correspond to the RCA; and segments 5, 6, 11, 12, 16 correspond to the LCx.

Intravascular (IVUS) and intracardiac ultrasound are invasive varieties of echo imaging. IVUS is performed as an adjunct to, and by means of, cardiac catheterization. The intracoronary transducer allows precise assessment of the morphology and severity of stenoses suboptimally defined by catheterization; of the quality of stent deployment; of in-stent restenosis; and of the complications of angioplasty (coronary

Echocardiography		
4-chamber view	Parasternal long axis	2-chamber view
Nuclear Medicine		
Horizontal long axis	N/A	Vertical long axis

Fig. 1.5 Differences in image display and terminology between echo and nuclear medicine (longitudinal sections)

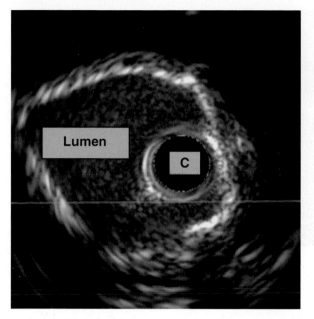

Fig. 1.6 *IVUS* heavy calcification (shaggy circumferential white rim) in the LMCA; *C* catheter

dissection, rupture, etc.). An example of severe coronary calcification detected by IVUS is shown in Fig. 1.6.

Intracardiac ultrasound is rarely performed, mainly to facilitate correct EPS electrode positioning.

Contrast echocardiography uses a suspension of microbubbles, with a protein shell and a gas core. The gas is set free by a microexplosion of the bubble, triggered by ultrasound; since the transducer is placed on the thorax, above the heart, this is where the explosions occur. The emitted gas serves as contrast material. Echo contrast agents have been found safe, despite isolated reports of serious adverse reactions, including a number of fatalities, associated with their use. The technique is most useful for *visualization of the LV endocardial border* in suboptimal studies (approximately 5% of echo studies, mainly in obese or emphysematous patients, but occasionally in normals as well). "Salvage" of these tests avoids obtaining "inconclusive results", with the necessity of subsequent tests. *Myocardial contrast echo* aims to visualize myocardial perfusion and to offer essentially the same information as a nuclear scan, but much cheaper, and accessible at the bedside. Despite decade-long development, this method still serves mostly for research purposes.

Two- vs. Three-Dimensional B-Mode Echo

Just like MRI, CT, or nuclear scan, the classical B-mode imaging is a 2D tomographic image ("slice") through the heart, imaging a 2D plane of interest. (Unlike other imaging modalities, which basically provide transversal, frontal, or sagittal sections, echocardiography can obtain intermediate planes, by transducer rotation.) Currently, the vast majority of echo machines are still 2D, but 3D echo may well become the standard technology of the future. 3D echo is not a hologram, but still a 2D display, using data from multiple imaging planes, integrated into a single image, using the graphic rules of perspective. Early systems were based on analysis of several cardiac cycles, one 2D section at a time, yielding a "hybrid," heavily engineered (and thus error-fraught) image. Modern systems actually *record* echoes in 3D; "real-time image *construction*" has taken the place of "nonreal-time image *reconstruction*." This allows to precisely evaluate LV volume, thickness, and EF; postinfarction scar size; ischemia; presence and mechanism of VHD, etc. Figure 1.7 presents a 3D image of the MV, alongside the 2D images the image was obtained from.

"Dimensionality" In Echocardiography

In geometry, the number of dimensions of a point (the region of interest with A-mode echo), a line (M mode), a surface (2D B mode), and a volume (3D B mode) is 0, 1, 2, and 3, respectively. Correspondingly, A-mode echo is "zero-dimensional," M-mode echo, "one-dimensional," and B mode, either 2- or 3-dimensional. (Real-time 3D echo has occasionally been designated "4D" echo, the fourth dimension being that of time. As, with current technology, all 3D studies are in real-time, this terminology is seldom used. The designations, zero- and one-dimensional, are not used in practice, but are suggested here for better understanding of "dimensionality.")

1.2.5.2 Data Reflecting the Velocity of Blood Flow or of Cardiac Structure Motion

Background

The Doppler phenomenon consists in the change in frequency of a sound wave, when the wave source

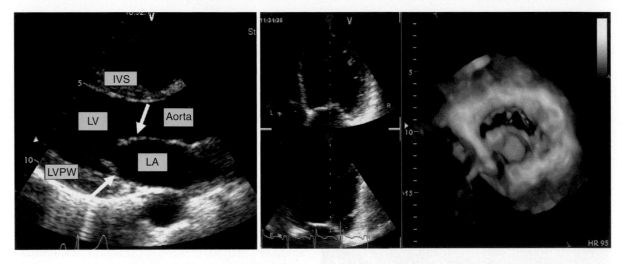

Fig. 1.7 The normal M- and B-mode echocardiogram. *LA* left atrium; *LV* left ventricle; *MV* mitral valve; *IVS* interventricular septum; *LVPW* LV posterior wall. *Left panel:* Parasternal long axis (PLax) view; *Right panel:* counterclockwise from upper left: 4-chamber view of the LV; 2D 2-chamber view of the LV; 3-D image obtained by processing the 2-D images

moves relatively to the observer. The typical everyday example is the increased frequency of an approaching siren, a frequency that subsequently decreases, as the siren is receding. This principle is applicable to the analysis of blood flow, using the blood cells as reflectors, and computing the frequency shift of reflected ultrasound, as compared to the baseline frequency, to yield information about the velocity and direction of flow. (The application to tissue-motion velocity is discussed at the end of the present section.) Doppler data can be displayed in two formats: *nonimaging,* as graphs displaying the variation in time of flow velocity through normal or abnormal passages (e.g., normal or diseased valves), along the phases of systole and diastole, or *(pseudo)-imaging,* where each and every Doppler interrogation point (sample of interest) is allocated a color (shades of red, for flow approaching the transducer; shades of blue, for flow away from the transducer; the shades are brighter for faster flows), and superimposed upon the B-mode echo, to yield "images" of the blood flow. This is referred to as "color Doppler." The correspondence between color and nonimaging and color Doppler display is shown in Fig. 1.8.

Pulsed- and Continuous-Wave Doppler

The blood flow graphs are curves of different shapes, characterized by their situation in the cardiac cycle (systole or diastole); their duration (measured as the horizontal projection of the curve); their velocity (measured as the vertical projection of the curve); and their direction (towards/away from the transducer, reflecting as a curve displayed above/below the zeroline). If *all* the sample blood volumes along the interrogation axis are displayed, the area under the curve is displayed in white (each pixel corresponding to the velocity of one sample of interest at a given moment), while if only the maximum-velocity samples are displayed, the curve is (usually) a line, not a 2D surface. But the "white-filled" and "contour" time-velocity curves differ in yet another important way, as they are measured by two different Doppler methods. *Contour curves* ideally reflect the time-velocity relationship of one single reflector (red blood cell). The vertical projection of each point corresponds to the velocity, and the horizontal projection, to time. Even the most precise Doppler machines actually investigate volumes of interest containing many RBCs (rather than a single one), and thus, the "line" is usually a band (as thick as the flow inhomogeneity between the different reflectors is great). If the sample of interest is at the site of very turbulent flow, with considerable flow inhomogeneity, the band may be as thick as to fill out the entire area under the curve. The modality enabling flow analysis at a given point (usually, a valve, a stenotic area within the ventricles, or an abnormal cardiac communication, such as an ASD or a VSD) is termed "pulsed-wave" Doppler (PWD), a term inspired by the discontinuous emission of ultrasound by the transducer. (The "waiting time" between pulses corresponds to the "return journey" of the reflected ultrasound.)

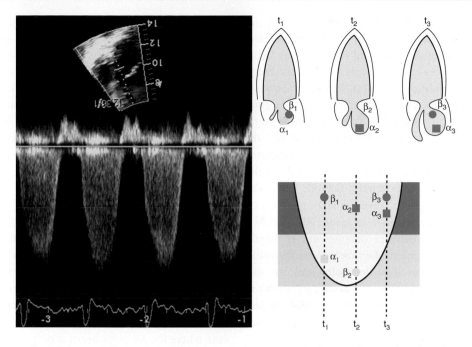

Fig. 1.8 Correspondence between color and continuous-wave Doppler. The three schematic frames follow the position and velocity of two reflectors (sample volumes of blood) within the regurgitant jet, displayed in an imaging or nonimaging manner (*upper and lower strips of left panel*). Higher velocities are displayed in brighter shades (*yellow* vs. *red*). The velocity of the α reflector decreases significantly between t_1 and t_2 and then increases modestly (t_3). The velocity of the β reflector increases significantly between t_1 and t_2 and then decreases significantly (t_3). The small control image (*upper left panel*) was inverted for the purpose of more intuitively showing the correspondence under discussion. In reality, it is displayed with the tip pointing upwards, hence the "upside-down" scale on the right border of the image

PWD is extremely useful for assessing blood flow in a particular area of the heart. This is especially important in case of superimposed lesions (e.g., subaortic and valvular aortic stenosis), when it is not clear which stenosis is responsible for the measured pressure gradient. B-mode image assessment suggests the culprit area, which is then investigated by PWD. Unfortunately, PWD cannot measure high-flow velocities (>2 m/s), frequent with VHD; velocities of this magnitude cause *signal aliasing*, i.e., "wrap-around" of the time-velocity curve on the other side of the zero-line (for instance, for a flow occurring towards the transducer, part of the curve is displayed *below* the zero-line, as if the flow were taking place away from the transducer). With color Doppler, aliasing manifests as interspersing of a flow depicted in red or in blue with shades from the "opposite" color spectrum. *"White-filled" curves* reflect the flow velocities all along the interrogation axis (rather than in a single point, as with PWD). Each pixel in the area under the curve reflects the velocity of some point or other on the interrogation axis, at that moment; again, the vertical projection corresponds to velocity, and the horizontal one, to time. The peak and mean

flow velocity along the axis can thus be measured (the latter, by integral calculus, the software for which is incorporated in the echo machine). This tracing is obtained by continuous emission and reception of ultrasound from the transducer ("continuous-wave Doppler, CWD"). CWD can measure high velocities, up to 5–6 m/s, but cannot localize the point of maximum velocity. Table 1.7 reviews the similarities and differences between PWD and CWD.

Table 1.7 PWD and CWD: a comparison

Characteristic	PWD	CWD
Sample of interest	A point	A line[a]
Typical graph aspect	A line[b]	A surface[b]
The maximum and mean velocity	Refer to the precise point of interest	Refer to the entire interrogation axis
Maximum detected velocity	Approximately 2 m/s	Approximately 6 m/s

[a]This is quite similar to M-mode echocardiography, with the difference that what the latter plots against time is not the velocity, but the spatial excursion of the points under investigation
[b]The additional dimension is represented by time

In clinical practice, both PWD and CWD are used, alongside color Doppler. Blood flow direction and velocity measurement are crucial for assessing VHD, abnormal intra- or extracardiac communications, blood vessels, and LV diastolic function. *Valvular stenosis* is assessed mainly based on nonimaging data; the tighter the stenosis, the higher the flow velocity, and the larger the pressure gradient between the proximal and the distal chamber. In case of multiple or superimposed stenoses, PWD allows to distinguish and individually assess each stenosis. Importantly, B-mode echo may also show telltale signs of severe VHD (calcification and restricted valve excursion in severe AS, flail MV in severe MR, etc). *Valvular insufficiency* is mainly assessed by color Doppler. The more severe the insufficiency, the larger the abnormal color area, and the larger its base ("stem"). Visual assessment allows to semi-quantitate regurgitation as trivial, mild, moderate, or severe. Nonimaging Doppler allows more precise quantitation of regurgitation (Chap. 5).

There are several similarities and differences between the color Doppler aspect of valvular insufficiency and stenosis. *Similarities:* relevant Doppler events may occur both in systole and diastole (e.g., MS/AI manifest in diastole, and MR/AS in systole); blood flow through diseased valves is turbulent and fast and is displayed in bright colors (blue or red/yellow). *The difference* is that *regurgitation* progresses "into the wrong chamber, at the wrong moment" (e.g., MR flow returns, in systole, from LV to LA), while flow through a *stenotic valve* is "in the right chamber at the right moment" but has excessive velocity. (With valvular insufficiency, it is improper to term velocity as "increased," since the flow should not take place at all.) The highest-flow velocities are seen with MR and AS. *Abnormal cardiac communications* are also assessed based on flow velocity; the higher the velocity, the narrower the passage, and thus (as opposed to the case of valvular stenosis), the less severe the condition. An important complication of many such communications is PAH, which can also be evaluated by Doppler (Chap. 5).

Doppler echo is also used to assess *the large blood vessels* (aorta, PA, pulmonary veins, occasionally LMCA ostium; Chap. 11) and *LV diastolic function,* based on the diastolic transmitral flow (Chap. 4).

Tissue Doppler measures the cardiac structure velocity throughout systole and diastole, a velocity of the order of cm/s. This is very similar to M-mode echocardiography, with the exception that the latter does not use Doppler and measures excursion amplitude, not motion velocity. (A hybrid M-mode/ tissue Doppler display is also possible.) Tissue Doppler is helpful for (but not restricted to) evaluation of LV diastolic function and of LV/RV contraction synchronicity, in HF candidates to CRT (Chap. 4). Tissue Doppler is time-consuming and accounts for only a small fraction of the activity of a usual echo lab.

Doppler Echo: Technical Aspects

The main condition for obtaining accurate Doppler data is proper alignment of the (linear) interrogation axis with the central axis of blood flow (a 3D event). Failing to do so will cause recording velocities that are lower than in reality, as only the horizontal projection of the velocity vector will be measured. In the extreme case where the Doppler beam is perpendicular to flow axis, the recorded velocity is zero, regardless of how high it really is. Of note, it is impossible to obtain *higher*-than-real velocities, since the projection of a vector is at most the length of the vector itself. Obtaining good alignment requires extensive experience and is achieved by fine angulation, translation, and rotation of the transducer. Normal flow is laminar, i.e., the different imaginary cylindrical flow "layers" have the same direction and velocity, as if "telescoped" within each other (in reality, the layers adjacent to the vessel wall have smaller velocities, due to the friction forces). Conversely, pathologic flow (e.g., MR) is turbulent, with numerous flow directions and velocities. These jets are often eccentric, i.e., not parallel to the central axis of the valve (just as the valve lesion itself is often asymmetrical), and frequently one is dealing not with one but with several "splayed" jets, each requiring separate Doppler alignment for accurate measurement. Color Doppler, especially with TEE (where the transducer rotation facilitates alignment), is very useful in this context.

Stress Echocardiography

Stress echocardiography is used for diagnosing ischemia and for evaluating its response to therapy. Inducible ischemia manifests as exercise-induced regional LV dysfunction. The universal 17-segment

LV model is used (Fig. 1.4). Stress echo is also useful in VHD, to assess hemodynamic deterioration or PAH exacerbation with exercise. The test is carried out using controlled exercise on a treadmill or stress bicycle, or by infusion of Dobutamine (Chap. 2). After usual (B-mode) image harvesting, optimal-quality (not "foreshortened," not extrasystolic or postextrasystolic), "representative" cardiac cycles are displayed side-by-side, in an endless-loop (non-real time) format, for rest/stress LV function comparison. This allows noticing even subtle changes in regional LV function. Basically, stress echo for diagnosis of ischemia is based on induction of stunning, which can last very briefly. If stress images are taken >90 s after stress, some areas of stunning may have already recovered, missing ischemia (false-negative result). Therefore, it is important to rapidly return the patient from the treadmill to the echo bed. This limitation does not apply to bicycle testing. Subtle EKG changes under echo stress are not unusual; rarely, these may reach the criteria for a positive EKG stress test, even in face of a normal echo stress test. In this case, the echo result dictates the conclusion. (Theoretically, EKG records "subtler" events and earlier stages of ischemia than echo. However, these findings are generally dismissed, as their practical significance is not clear.) *Dobutamine stress test* is used in patients unable to perform physical exercise, as well as in those being assessed for myocardial viability (hibernation). For the latter indication, the end point is demonstration of partial functional recovery of akinetic resting segments exposed to low doses of Dobutamine, followed by renewed functional deterioration at higher doses (Chap. 2). Adverse effects include palpitations (with or without objective arrhythmia, at times severe), restlessness, trembling, BP increases or decreases (the latter do not carry the same severe prognosis as with stress echo). Simply interrupting the infusion is therapeutic, as circulating Dobutamine is rapidly metabolized.

The Clinical Importance of Echocardiography

Echo is a key diagnostic modality, displaying in detail the structure and function of the heart and great vessels and the blood flow through the valves, heart chambers, vessels, and abnormal or man-made interchamber communications. Additionally, IVUS offers information about native and postinterventional coronary anatomy.

Other advantages of echo include its availability in the outpatient clinic, at the bedside, and in the OR; its non-invasive or minimally invasive nature; and its safety in pregnancy.

1.2.6 Nuclear Perfusion Scan (Myocardial Scintigraphy)

Nuclear Perfusion Scan (myocardial scintigraphy) is based on following IV radioactive tracer uptake by the myocytes. Uptake is decreased or absent in ischemic or scarred myocardium. As with stress echo, imaging is carried out both at rest and stress. Nuclear imaging provides tomographic slices, obtained by *temporal* summation of the radiation from the same section through the heart, harvested over many cycles. This is mandated by the low level of radiation emitted by the myocardium. Proper allocation of a certain quantum of radiation to a specific slot in systole or diastole is made possible by simultaneous EKG gating. The images are displayed in endless-loop format. EKG gating and the use of the high-radiation tracer, technetium, make SPECT imaging possible. SPECT displays myocardial perfusion and LV function at the same time; a matched decrease of both improves the diagnostic yield, avoiding false-positive and -negative diagnosis. LVEF can be precisely calculated, and the contribution of specific segments assessed. In addition to the computed assessment, LVEF can be semi-quantitated visually as normal or mildly/moderately/severely decreased. LVEF assessment by nuclear scintigraphy is termed MUGA ("multiple uptake gated angiography").

Only the LV is usually displayed on a nuclear study. (The pericardium and endocardium do not absorb the tracer at all, and the thin-walled RV and atria do so very modestly.) Nuclear scan has a spatial resolution of approximately 1 cm; thus, a nuclear study displays approximately 8–10 sections. The images are tomographic sections, either transversal (perpendicular to the long axis of the heart; circular shape) or longitudinal (parallel to the long axis of the thorax; "U" shape; Fig. 1.4.). The longitudinal plane can be parallel to either the lateral or the anterior wall of the thorax, yielding sagittal and frontal sections. Sections at different levels through the heart are displayed as a series of circles, respectively "U"-shaped images. Resting and stress images are displayed in parallel rows, with the

Fig. 1.9 Thallium redistribution, indicating ischemia in the inferior wall. *Upper row* (stress): filling defect in the inferior wall (*arrows*); *lower row* (rest): normal aspect. Note the "filling in" of the segments indicated by in the upper vs. lower row. Should both rest and stress images have shown a perfusion defect, the diagnosis would have been that of irreversible filling defect (*scar*). A normal patient would have normal images both under stress and at rest

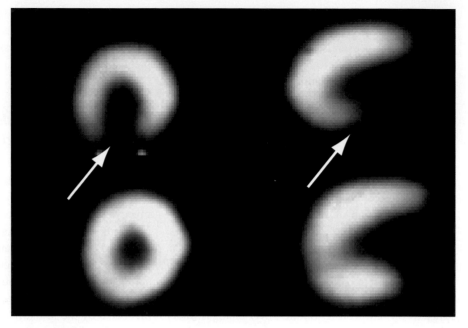

corresponding sections superimposed. These images are displayed in color, by electronic processing, similar to color Doppler. Normal radiotracer uptake is displayed in brighter shades; decreased uptake, in darker shades; and absent uptake, in black ("absence" of that segment from the yellow-colored contour). The universal 17-item LV segmentation is used (see Chap. 2) (Fig. 1.9).

Images can also be presented as a "bull's eye" display, showing, on a single frame, the information from all the individual nuclear scan sections. With transversal sections, for instance, the more apical (lower-diameter) sections are displayed within the contour of the more basal (larger-diameter) ones. The resulting composite image is the equivalent of "looking into the heart" from the MV towards the apex, much as one would look into a funnel. The extension of perfusion defects or scar can be visually assessed, as well as automatically quantitated. The different protocols for nuclear imaging are discussed in Chap. 2. Metabolic imaging (using FDG, fatty acids, or other metabolic tracers usually reserved for PET imaging) is available with new-generation SPECT cameras, yielding information regarding perfusion, ischemia, and viability. Nuclear scan has virtually no *adverse effects,* as the radiotracer doses are minute and decay rapidly. (The images are recorded during this very short life span.) However, Dipyridamole may cause adverse effects (Chap. 2). After the test, the patient can

return to daily routine without endangering themselves or the community. However, nuclear scan is usually avoided in pregnancy. Cardiac nuclear imaging is contraindicated in patients who had iodine 131 therapy or other nuclear imaging procedures within a certain time, depending on the specific agent. The longest such "waiting period" is of 12 weeks, after iodine 131 therapy. Oral intake (except for water) and coffee consumption <4 h are not allowed. Contraindications to dipyridamole and adenosine include allergy to these agents, chronic theophylline therapy (this must be discontinued for 36 h); severe asthma or AV nodal block; and caffeine consumption within 12–24 h.

Safety measures for the medical team include minimizing contact with the patients, wearing a safety badge to record the monthly amount of radiation each member of the staff is exposed to, etc.

The clinical indications for nuclear scan include diagnosis of ischemia and of myocardial hibernation, as well as precise quantitation of LVEF.

PET scan follows the vascular spread and the myocardial uptake of radiotracers. The tracers being taken up by myocytes are similar in structure to glucose and identify areas of abnormally decreased metabolism. Virtually any metabolic process can be investigated. The main cardiologic application of PET is diagnosis of ischemia and, as a gold standard, of myocardial hibernation. However, due

Table 1.8 Echocardiographic and nuclear imaging: a comparison

Characteristic	Echocardiography	Nuclear study
Cost	Low	Higher
Use in emergencies	Yes	No[a]
Availability at the bedside	Yes	No
Safety in pregnancy	Yes	Unclear
Diagnosis of ischemia	Yes[b]	Yes
Diagnosis of hibernation	Yes[c]	Yes[d]
Diagnosis of regional and global LV function (LVEF)	Yes	Yes[e]

[a]See Chap. 2 for the possible use of nuclear scan in the chest pain unit
[b]Stress echo
[c]Dobutamine echo only
[d]Mainly using Thallium; PET is the (seldom used) gold standard for hibernation assessment
[e]By SPECT imaging, ideally using technetium

to the high cost and logistic difficulties, cardiac PET is infrequently used. Hybrid PET-CT or PET-MRI techniques can be used (Chap. 2) (Table 1.8).

1.2.7 Myocardial Biopsy

Myocardial biopsy is routinely used for the follow-up of posttransplant patients and, less commonly, for the diagnosis of cardiac infiltrative disease or for the differential diagnosis between constrictive pericarditis and restrictive CMP. The RV is used, being more easily accessible. The most important complication is RV perforation, with possible tamponade. Traumatic TR can also be seen. As many infiltrative diseases affect the myocardium in a "spotty" fashion, several samples are typically harvested, from different areas of the myocardium.

1.2.8 Other Diagnostic Applications

Catheterization: Coronary angioscopy offers direct visualization of the blood vessels, using a catheter-borne optical device. This is mainly used as a research tool. *Intracoronary Doppler (Doppler flow-wire)* assesses the functional importance of a stenosis. This may be

required with stenoses of borderline angiographic severity, to assess the necessity of angioplasty (see Chap. 2 for further discussion). *NOGA mapping* explores myocardial excitation/contraction coupling (the degree of myocardial shortening produced by an excitation current of a certain intensity). This is achieved with an intraventricular catheter. NOGA is used for research purposes, including detection of stunned or hibernating myocardium, LV aneurysm, aberrant conduction tracts, etc. *Spectroscopic catheter-based plaque interrogation* is a novel method for diagnosis of rupture-prone plaques. The downside is the failure to identify plaque erosion, which accounts for a large percentage of acute coronary thromboses. Additionally, there is no current immediate therapeutic impact to this diagnosis, other than implementation of more stringent primary prevention measures. However, a new generation of plaque-sealing devices ("gently expanding stents"), if clinically validated, could offer the ideal therapeutic counterpart to this diagnostic method.

Echocardiography: Myocardial speckle tracking assesses regional and global LV contractility, based on measurement of systolic myocyte strain. Tracking ensures that one and the same area is being followed throughout the cardiac cycle. Still at its beginnings, this technique holds significant promise and has been found useful in predicting graft rejection in posttransplant patients, for follow-up of patients with heart failure, etc.

Nuclear cardiology: Infarct-avid imaging: new agents are being developed for early diagnosis of infarctions insufficiently substantiated by "classical" tests. These scans can become positive as early as 60 min after chest pain onset, well within the window of opportunity for thrombolysis. *MIBG imaging* visualizes the cardiac sympathetic nerves; even with preserved local LV function, their destruction could be a harbinger of future HF and arrhythmia. *Technetium-NOET imaging* aims to correct the relative inability of Tc imaging to identify hibernating myocardium. *Fatty acid imaging* is based on a physiological principle classically used by PET: ischemic myocytes undergo a "metabolic switch" and transition from their usual source of energy (fatty acids) to glucose. While PET demonstrates *increased* glucose metabolism in ischemic cells, fatty acid mapping shows *suppressed* fatty acid metabolism.

CT: The recently introduced "dynamic volumetric CT" allows cardiac (and cerebral) imaging within only a few minutes.

Bibliography

Guidelines

Hendel RC, Berman DS, Di Carli MF, et al. ACCF/ASNC/ACR/ AHA/ ASE/ SCCT/SCMR/SNM 2009 Appropriate use criteria for cardiac radionuclide imaging: a report of the American College of Cardiology Foundation Appropriate Use Criteria Task Force, The American Society of Nuclear Cardiology, The American College of Radiology, The American Heart Association, The American Society of Echocardiography, The Society of Cardiovascular Computed Tomography, The Society for Cardiovascular Magnetic Resonance, and The Society of Nuclear Medicine. *Circulation.* 2009;119:e561-e587.

Douglas PS, Khandheria B, Stainback RF, Weissman NJ. ACCF/ ASE/ACEP/ AHA/ASNC/SCAI/SCCT/SCMR 2008 Appropriateness criteria for stress echocardiography. *J Am Coll Cardiol.* 2008;51:1127-1147.

Buxton AE, Calkins H, Callans DJ, et al. ACC/AHA/HRS 2006 Key data elements and definitions for electrophysiological studies and procedures: a report of the American College of Cardiology/American Heart Association task force on clinical data standards (ACC/AHA/HRS Writing Committee to develop data standards on electrophysiology). *Circulation.* 2006;114:2534-2570.

Schoenhagen P, Nissen SE, Murat Tuczu E, et al. *IVUS Made Easy.* London: Taylor & Francis, Inc; 2005. ISBN-13: 9781841845951.

Lester SJ, Tajik AJ, Nishimura RA, et al. Unlocking the mysteries of diastolic function: deciphering the Rosetta stone 10 years later. *J Am Coll Cardiol.* 2008;51(7):679-689.

Thomas JD, Popovic ZB. Assessment of left ventricular function by cardiac ultrasound. *J Am Coll Cardiol.* 2006;48:2012-2025.

Peterson GE, Brickner ME, Reimold SC. Transesophageal echocardiography. Clinical indications and applications. *Circulation.* 2003;107:2398.

Poh KK, Levine RA, Solis J, et al. Assessing aortic valve area in aortic stenosis by continuity equation: a novel approach using real-time three-dimensional echocardiography. *Eur Heart J.* 2008;29:2526-2535.

Bharucha T, Roman KS, Anderson RH, et al. Impact of multiplanar review of three-dimensional echocardiographic data on management of congenital heart disease. *Ann Thorac Surg.* 2008;86:875-881.

Miller JM, Rochitte CE, Dewey M, et al. Diagnostic performance of coronary angiography by 64-row CT. *N Engl J Med.* 2008;359:2324-2336.

Jacobson AF, Lombard J, Banerjee G, et al. 123I-mIBG scintigraphy to predict risk for adverse cardiac outcomes in heart failure patients: design of two prospective multicenter international trials. *Nucl Cardiol.* 2009;16(1):113-121. Epub 2009 Jan 20.

Duerden RM, Pointon KS, Habib S. Review of clinical cardiac MRI. *Imaging* 2006; 18, 178-186.

Suggested Reading

Shah MR, Hasselblad V, Stevenson LW, et al. Impact of the pulmonary artery catheter in critically ill patients. Meta-analysis of randomized clinical trials. *JAMA.* 2005;294:1664-1670.

Coronary Artery Disease

2

Contents

2.1 Atherosclerosis

2.1.1 Cardiovascular Disease: Background

Environmental and patient-related risk factors cause atherosclerosis, a diffuse disease affecting virtually all the arterial territories (the noncardiac impact is reviewed in Chap. 11); atherosclerosis may cause ischemia; ischemia may manifest either as stable angina pectoris, or as acute coronary syndrome (ACS); ACS may manifest either as unstable angina, or as acute MI; and finally, acute MI may show ST-elevations (STEMI) or not (NSTEMI). Atherosclerosis will be discussed first, and clinical ischemic syndromes (ACS, stable angina) will be dealt with subsequently. As atherosclerosis and ischemia are strongly linked, there is substantial overlap in regard to diagnosis and therapy. To avoid redundancies while preserving a systematic approach, diagnosis of atherosclerosis and of ischemia will be presented together. In regard to therapy, atherosclerosis treatment (tantamount to risk factor management, assuming revascularization is only carried out in the presence of ischemia) will be presented in Sect. 2.1, while the management of ischemia will be discussed in Sects. 2.1 and 2.3.

2.1.2 Atherosclerosis: Definition and Mechanisms

Atherosclerosis is a continuum of lesions resulting from the deposition of cholesterol in the arterial wall, favored by circulating oxidized LDL cholesterol. In turn, cholesterol deposition triggers an inflammatory reaction resulting in arterial wall thickening and decrease in the vessel

G.A. Adelmann, *Cardiology Essentials in Clinical Practice*,
DOI: 10.1007/978-1-84996-305-3_2, © Springer-Verlag London Limited 2011

internal diameter (lumen narrowing or total occlusion). The latter may be chronic, by gradually increasing cholesterol and inflammatory cells deposits, smooth muscle proliferation, and fibrosis, or acute (thrombosis on the surface of a fissured or ruptured plaque, the most significant complication of atherosclerosis). Atherosclerosis tends to involve a multitude of sites, and is thus a "diffuse" disease; however, in a given artery, it often presents as spotty involvement (although "even" atherosclerotic "lining" of the endothelium is also possible). Veins are usually spared, unless surgically transposed into an arterial bed (e.g., saphenous vein grafts in CABG surgery). Macroscopically, the affected vessels (visualized at surgery or autopsy, or indirectly, by invasive or noninvasive imaging) usually display *atherosclerotic plaques* of different shapes and contours, protruding into the vessel lumen to different degrees. Atherosclerotic plaque starts evolving in the first years of life (Table 2.1). The initial lesion consists of infiltration with macrophages replete with oxidized LDL ("foam cells"), alongside minimal extracellular lipid deposits. The exact trigger of cholesterol deposition is debated; endothelial lesions produced by tobacco smoke or unidentified infective agents might play a role. Atherosclerosis involves a cycle of oxidized LDL cholesterol deposition (partly countered by cholesterol removal as HDL), vessel inflammation, and further endothelial injury. Occasionally, these phenomenons are very rapid, causing the so-called *accelerated atherosclerosis* (substantial plaque growth and smooth muscle proliferation).

The healing process involves fibrosis and calcification, increasing vessel wall rigidity and encroaching on the lumen. By the same token, these plaques are "stable," i.e., not prone to fissure/rupture. It is precisely the less obstructive plaques that tend to rupture and expose the thrombogenic core to blood flow, with platelet activation and platelet thrombus, then fibrin thrombus formation.

In the 1980s, at the onset of the modern era of atherosclerosis science, the degree of vascular lumen decrease was considered to simply reflect the plaque burden: the larger the plaque, the greater the degree of vessel obstruction, it was assumed, with the relationship being a linear one. Later work, however, has disproven this. In the acute setting (ACS), vascular occlusion is due not to the physical burden of the plaque, but to an occluding thrombus, while in the chronic setting, the relationship between plaque burden and percent stenosis is not linear. The blood vessel is a living structure, reacting to the atherosclerotic lesions by *vascular remodeling*, classified as (a) *positive*, i.e., vascular dilatation accommodating the plaque: the lumen is unchanged for a plaque burden ≤40%, i.e., an amount of plaque that would obstruct 40% of the lumen, were the vessel an inert conduit. Thus, wall thickness and *outer* vessel diameter increase, but the *inner* diameter remains unchanged; (b) *negative* (significant lumen decrease despite relatively modest plaque burden).

- Positive remodeling – positive effect (lumen larger than expected, given the plaque burden)
- Negative remodeling – negative effect (lumen smaller than expected, given the plaque burden)

Table 2.1 The phases of atherosclerosis: a clinical perspective

Stage	Approximate patient age	Microscopic structure	Macroscopic aspect	Clinical relevance
Initial lesion	Childhood	Isolated macrophages replete with oxidized LDL ("foam cells")	"Normal" endothelium	Clinically inapparent; ideal time for healthy lifestyle choices
Fatty streak	Teens to early adulthood	More foam cells, minimal extracellular lipid deposits.	Endothelial streak	
Intermediate lesion	>20	Extracellular lipid deposits increase[a]	Atherosclerotic plaque	Clinically inapparent or evident[b] (stable angina); primary or secondary prevention
Atheroma	>30	Core of extracellular lipids[a]	Atherosclerotic plaque	
Fibroatheroma	>30	Core of extracellular lipids,[a] smooth muscle proliferation, fibrosis, calcification	Atherosclerotic plaque	
Fissured plaque	>30	As above; ruptured or fissured fibrous cap	Fissured plaque, occlusive thrombus	ACS or self-limiting event

[a]Alongside intracellular lipids

[b]The first sign of disease is an acute ischemic event or SCD in up to two-thirds of males and in up to half of the females

The impact of atherosclerosis is far more complex than simple physical bulk, as the plaque causes a host of functional processes, globally known as *endothelial dysfunction*. These processes include, but are not limited to, a decrease in NO secretion and an increased release of serotonin, thromboxane A$_2$, and thrombin, causing vasoconstriction or abnormal vasodilatation under vasoactive substances, at the site of the plaque. The prototype of vasospastic angina is Prinzmetal's angina. Atherosclerotic plaques vary widely not only in regard to their bulk, but also in their proneness to rupture and cause thrombosis and MI. In a potentially groundbreaking discovery, Hydrogen Sulfide was found to act as a major physiologic vasodilator and regulator of BP, alongside NO.

Accelerated atherosclerosis consists in substantial plaque growth (smooth muscle proliferation), as a result of initial platelet activation. *Vulnerable plaque*, i.e., fissure- (rupture-) and thrombosis-prone plaque has certain characteristics, discussed under "ACS."

> Stable plaque causes stable angina; unstable (vulnerable) plaque causes unstable angina or MI. Many vulnerable plaques are shallow (non-obstructive).

The clinical impact of atherosclerosis: The main cause of ischemia, potentially affecting any organ system, atherosclerosis is also the main cause of morbidity and mortality worldwide. Some organs are more affected than others, mainly the heart (ischemic heart disease), brain (stroke), and lower limbs (PVD). Ischemic injury in other organs (mesenteric arteries, kidneys, etc.) is common as well.

2.1.3 Risk Factors for Atherosclerosis

Hypertension: see Ch. 3

Lipids: *Cholesterol* is a lipid essential for life. It is a component of cell membranes and a precursor of adrenal and sex hormones, liposoluble vitamins, and bile salts. The main source of cholesterol is endogenous secretion, but alimentary intake is also important. The main dietary sources include cheese, egg yolks, beef, pork, poultry and shrimp. Serum cholesterol levels are more strongly correlated with the total intake of saturated and trans-fats than with the intake of cholesterol as such (The trans-fats occur in trace amounts in natural products, but are much more plentiful in some brands of margarine, shortening, fast food, snacks, and commercial baked goods. They increase LDL and decrease HDL levels). In the circulating blood, cholesterol occurs as the lipid moiety of a lipoprotein compound, which, unlike cholesterol itself, is soluble in the serum. In increasing order of density, the types of lipoproteins include: chylomicrons, very low, intermediate, low and high density lipoprotein (VLDL, IDL, LDL, HDL), all atherogenic, with the exception of HDL, which is antiatherogenic. The strongest focus has been on oxidized *LDL* ("bad cholesterol"), which initiates and maintains the atherosclerotic plaque. The desirable levels of total and LDL cholesterol depend on the past medical history (Table 2.2). LDL is usually calculated based on the formula: LDL = total cholesterol−total HDL−VLDL, with VLDL approximated as 20% of the TG value. This assessment is based on three different measured values, each with their own coefficient of error, and thus itself subject to error. The calculations are not accurate if the TG level is >400 mg/dL (4.5 mmol/L). Therefore, direct LDL

Table 2.2 Total and LDL cholesterol: targets[a]

Medical history	LDL	HDL	Total cholestrol
Primary prevention of atherosclerosis			
≤1 risk factor, not including diabetes	<115 (<3)	Low: ♂, <40 (<1); ♀, <45 (<1.2); satisfactory 40–60 (1–1.5); high >60 (>1.5)	<190 (<5)
≥2 risk factors; diabetes	<100 (<2.5); if feasible[b], <80 (<2)		<175 (<4.5); if feasible, <155 (<4)
Secondary prevention of atherosclerosis			
All patients	<100 (<2.5); in severe cases, consider <80 (<2)[b]	As for primary prevention	<175 (<4.5)

[a]Milligram per deciliter (mmol/L)
[b]The AHA advocates decreases to <70 mg/dL <1.8 mmol/L)

measurement is gaining popularity. It is recommended to test cholesterol every 5 years for people ≥20 years of age. While LDL remains pivotal for risk assessment and setting therapeutical goals, patients with the same LDL level can have a significantly different risk of atherosclerosis, even after adjusting for other factors (e.g., TG level, HDL level). The atherogenic effect of LDL is strongest for small, dense LDL particles, sdLDL; sdLDL increases are more common in CAD patients than increased LDL levels as such.

Serum levels of sdLDL are reflected by the level of *apolipoprotein B*, a ligand enabling LDL uptake by the cells (there is only one apoB molecule per LDL particle, which accounts for the good correlation). Apolipoprotein B is not "dedicated" to LDL, but is present in all the lipoproteins (VLDL, IDL, LDL, chylomicrons). As all of the apoB is in atherogenic lipids, and all atherogenic lipids include apoB, apoB indicates the total atherogenic burden in the circulating blood. It is a better predictor of CAD than LDL, in patients with both normal and increased LDL levels. In the general population, values >150 mg/dL are considered increased, while in high-risk patients (additional risk factors or already present atherosclerosis), levels <90 mg/dL or even <80 mg/dL are optimal. Unfortunately, these measurements are still not part of the standard clinical practice. *Apolipoprotein A* and *the ratio apoB/apoA1* are also better risk indicators than LDL, but they, too, are of restricted availability.

HDL ("good cholesterol") is a protective factor only in cultures where unhealthy lifestyles promote a high prevalence of atherosclerosis. This suggests that smoking, obesity, sedentary life style, and diabetes exert their deleterious influence at least partly by decreasing HDL levels. Moderate hypertriglyceridemia is also frequently associated with low HDL levels and with high levels of sdLDL. The protective action of HDL has been traditionally ascribed to mobilization of cholesterol from the vessel wall (and delivery to the liver, for metabolization), but antiinflammatory, antithrombotic, and anti-apoptotic mechanisms are also probable. The desirable levels of HDL cholesterol are >45 mg/dL, and the optimal ratio of total cholesterol to HDL is <5/L (the lower, the better). The higher the HDL levels, the more effective the cardiovascular protection (Table 2.2). The size of HDL particles is also important, large particles being the most protective.

Lp(a) ("lipoprotein little a") is another component of the LDL spectrum; values >30 mg/dL are high-risk for atherosclerosis. Niacin may be effective in decreasing Lp(a) levels.

Non-HDL cholesterol (the sum of the atherogenic cholesterol fractions, i.e., LDL, IDL, and VLDL) is calculated as the difference between total cholesterol and HDL and may be a better risk indicator than LDL; however, the desirable levels are not clear.

The Importance of LDL and HDL: Comments While several landmark studies and meta-analyses have clearly shown a reduction in cardiovascular morbidity and mortality in both primary (WOSCOPS, AFCAPS/TexCAPS, HPS, PROSPER, ALLHAT-LLT, ASCOT-LLA, CARDS) and secondary prevention (4S, CARE, LIPID, PROVE-IT-TIMI22, TNT, IDEAL), and while there was a strong relationship between event lowering and decreased LDL levels, recent data has raised some

---

LDL: Is It the Chief Villain?

The age-honored affirmative answer to this question may have been influenced by several factors.

- The technology bias: initial focus on LDL and HDL was mainly motivated by the then-available technology, and not because of some scientific proof of their prominence as the most harmful lipids. We might be continuing to follow, in the 2000s, technological limitations of the 1960s.
- Besides, LDL assessment itself is subject to error (LDL is not directly measured, but calculated, with unreliable results at high TG concentrations). Additionally, there appears to exist a seasonal variation to LDL levels (lower levels in the summer).
- LDL reduction reduces the risk of clinical events by 40–50%; thus, in more than half of the patients, some other (possibly also lipid-related) mechanism is operative in atherogenesis.
- The ENHANCE study has not found any significant IMT regression (admittedly a surrogate end-point), despite effective LDL lowering.
- Conversely, the JUPITER trial has shown that substantial benefit is to be gained from statins in people with "normal" LDL levels (but elevated CRP levels).
- Despite a great reduction in cardiovascular events, there is little evidence that LDL level reduction prolongs life expectation in any patients but males <70 with already established CAD.

intriguing questions regarding the true prominence of LDL as the main event-driving factor.

Triglycerides: Unto themselves, TG are not taken up into plaque; however, they are hydrolyzed into atherogenic cholesterol-rich remnant particles. Hypertyriglyceridemia is atherogenic by direct toxicity (IDL, small VLDL particles) and by its associated thrombogenic and HDL-decreasing effects. It is frequently associated with other risk factors, (diabetes mellitus, the metabolic syndrome). Levels >150 mg/dL (>1.7 mmol/L) are considered high-risk, but lowering TG is not a primary goal in atherosclerosis management, as TG increase covariates with other risk factors and may not be an independent risk factor. Despite the yet unclear role of TG in the pathogenesis of cardiovascular disease, many clinicians start a second agent (niacin or a fibrate) beside statins, in patients with high TG or very low HDL levels. Moderate, rather than high TG levels are the most hazardous, as very high levels (a significant risk for pancreatitis) tend to involve larger, less toxic particles. If TG are 200–499 mg/dL, non-HDL-cholesterol (total cholesterol-HDL cholesterol) should be <130 mg/dL, and, if feasible, <100 mg/dL.

Therapy of hyperlipidemia: Underlying conditions such as hypothyroidism or nephrotic syndrome must be corrected, as in these patients treatment for dyslipidemia alone will not be successful. The treatment of hyperlipidemia includes dietary and pharmacological measures, and, exceptionally, plasmapheresis. The duration of therapy is usually lifelong.

Diet: Daily cholesterol intake should not exceed 300 mg in healthy subjects, and 200 mg in those with atherosclerosis or multiple risk factors. Saturated fat (*meat or dairy* products such as fatty meats, butter, fat cheese, cream, etc.) should be avoided. *Seafood* is rich in cholesterol and should be eaten in moderation. *Wholegrain cereal, vegetables and fruit*, as well as ≥1 weekly serving of fish (especially the fatty varieties) should be encouraged. Lean meat and low-fat dairy products are also recommended. An egg daily is allowed, as eggs are an excellent source of nutrients and have a low absolute cholesterol content. *Margarine* does not contain cholesterol, but most of the abundant saturated fat it contains is turned into cholesterol in the patient's body. Generally, the harder (less fluid) a margarine, the higher the amount of saturated fat (highest in baking margarine). *Vegetables and fruit* are lipid-poor and may have several additional beneficial

actions. *Sterols and stanols* from corn, wheat, and soybeans and *sulfites* from onions, leeks, garlic, cabbage, cauliflower, lettuce, broccoli, radishes might decrease LDL; *lignans*, phytoestrogens found in linseed oil, vegetables, sesame seeds, and pumpkin seeds might decrease LDL and TG. *Dietary fiber* is found in vegetables, mainly grain and cereal. Fiber reduces LDL synthesis (and thus the risk of CAD) and decreases the risk of developing the metabolic syndrome or full-blown diabetes. *Tannin* is an antioxidant from cocoa, chocolate, tea, wine, grapes, and pomegranates; it may inhibit, among others, the oxidation of LDL. As different vegetables contain different phytochemicals, it might be advisable to eat vegetables having a variety of colors. At least five three daily servings (handfuls) of vegetables and two pieces of fruit are recommended. Fresh or frozen vegetables are the best source of nutrients, but canned vegetables are also acceptable (provided they do not contain excessive amounts of salt); vegetable or fruit juice does not provide bulk (unless the pulp is also eaten). Overcooking may destroy some of the nutrients, but normal cooking may actually increase nutrient bioavailability, by breaking the cell walls in the vegetable or fruit; thus, cooking may increase threefold the bioavailability of antioxydants. The much-publicized Mediterranean diet is based on reduced intake of saturated fats, moderate alcohol intake, and high intake of fish, vegetables, and fruit. In lower-risk hypercholesterolemic patients, as well as in case of non-severe LDL elevations, an attempt at dietary correction may be made, with repeat assessment after 3 months. In case of insufficient cholesterol lowering, drug therapy is started, generally with a statin.

Pharmacologic treatment: Therapy of hyperlipiodemia currently revolves around LDL management. TG elevations despite LDL control may justify a further attempt at non-HDL choleserol correction, occasionally with Niacin or fibrates. HDL levels are not a therapeutic target, but may mandate better control, to optimize the ratio of total cholesterol to HDL to <5/L. Antihypercholesterolemic drugs include statins, Ezetimibe, fibrates, Niacin, and bile acid resins. Rarely, plasmapheresis is required. *Statins* are first-choice in hypercholesterolemic patients. They reduce cholesterol levels by 30–50%, usually allowing to reach the recommended levels. If necessary, other agents may be added, or the surrogate aim of cholesterol lowering to ≤50% of the initial level may be chosen. Statins inhibit hepatic synthesis of cholesterol and TG, by interfering with the activity of HMG-CoA reductase. The most important *adverse effects* (albeit not the most common ones) include headache, LFT derangement (usually reversible), and rhabdomyolysis. Other adverse effects include URTI-like symptoms; GI upset; rash; dizziness, insomnia; joint and muscle pain; albuminuria, hematuria; edema; chest pain; and anaphylaxis or angioneurotic edema. Statins are *contraindicated* in patients with active liver disease, as well as in pregnant or lactating women. Patients under statin treatment require periodic LFT monitoring (discontinuation considered if transaminase levels exceed three times the upper normal limit). In patients with severe myalgia, statins should be discontinued. If myalgia is non-severe, immediate CK measurement is indicated, and statins should be discontinued if CK is elevated. Cholesterol and TG are measured at one month after treatment onset, then annually. The main statins include Atorvastatin (10–80 mg q.d.); Fluvastatin (20–80 mg q.d.); Pravastatin (10–40 mg q.d.); Simvastatin 10–80 mg q.d.); Rosuvastatin (5–40 mg q.d.); and Lovastatin (10–80 mg q.d.). Statins have significant drug interactions, most importantly with fibrates (the risk of rhabdmomyolysis is relatively increased, but remains low). Grapefruit or its juice may increase the levels of Atorvastatin, Lovastatin, and Simvastatin to dangerous levels. Grapefruit should be avoided or be eaten hours apart from statin administration. A class of drugs typically administered chronically, statins actually start exerting their beneficial activity very quickly. Thus, a high loading dose of statin (Atorvastatin 80 mg), given in the 24 h preceding PCI in the statin-naïve patient may provide protection against periprocedural MI.

The practical use of statins first involves establishing a therapeutic aim (Table 2.2), and starting the drug at a routine dosage, with or without a preliminary waiting period of up to 3 months, for maximum effect of dietary changes (Certainly, the use of statins does not obviate the need for a strict diet.). Statin doses are increased according to LDL follow-up results, obtained every 1–3 months. Generally, dosage is doubled up to the maximum allowed dosage. If this is still not sufficient, Ezetimibe may be added, or a more potent statin may be chosen (e.g., Rosuvastatin instead of Simvastatin).

The groundbreaking Jupiter trial has demonstrated that statins reduce cardiovascular morbidity and mortality even in the presence of apparently normal lipid

---

LDL Is at Target Levels. Is Lipid Management Successfully Concluded?

Not necessarily. Besides awaiting further data regarding the utility and modality of increasing HDL, it is reasonable to

- Measure CRP, and if high, increase statin dosage
- Measure Lp(a) and if high, start niacin
- Measure apoB levels and consider statin dosage increase, to bring apoB to a target level of <90 mg/dl

---

levels, if hsCRP is high. While this trial used Rosuvastatin, the protection is believed to be a class-effect of statins.

Antihyperlipemic therapy in children: The issue of antihyperlipemic therapy in children has been much debated; while early atherosclerosis is the ideal time to initiate primary prevention, there is no experience with life-long anticholesterol therapy. The targets in children are the same as in adults, and dosages depend on age and body weight. Optimal LDL levels are <100 mg/dL (<130 mg/dL acceptable). Therapy (dietary, and, if needed, pharmacologic) is recommended for LDL >190 mg/dL, or, in presence of ≥2 additional risk factors, for LDL >160 mg/dL. In boys, therapy is delayed until age 10, and in girls, until menarche. Healthy life styles should be taught from the earliest age.

Statins: beyond LDL: Statins (mostly the newer-generation agents) also lower TG. Rosuvastatin, for instance, decreases TG levels by up to 30%. Statins also increase HDL, but less than fibrates or Niacin. Non-lipid effects of statins include improvement in the endothelial function; antiinflammatory activity; plaque stabilization; and antithrombotic action. In addition to their cardiological use, statins may reduce the incidence of colon and rectal cancer by up to 50%.

Other agents effective in dyslipidemic patients: *Ezetimibe* (10–20 mg q.d.) inhibits intestinal cholesterol absorbtion (cholesterol secreted into the intestine as biliary salts is normally recycled by reabsorbtion). Ezetimibe is usually recommended as a supplement to statins, when a full dose is not effective or not tolerated. If statins are not tolerated at all, Ezetimibe may be used on its own, but results are generally suboptimal. Similarly to statins, it may cause muscle ache or LFT disturbances, and, additionally, headache and GI upset. Despite an up to 20% LDL level reduction, Ezetimibe does not increase the action of statins in lowering the carotid IMT, a surrogate marker of atherosclerosis evolution. As the results of large trials with this drug will not be available for several years, Ezetimibe use is currently at the physician's discretion. *Bile resins* prevent intestinal recycling of LDL, by increaseing fecal elimination. They have practically no contraindications. The adverse reactions include constipation, diarrhea, flatulence, and inhibition of the intestinal absorbtion of drugs and liposoluble vitamins. Infrequently used since the advent of statins, resins are occasionally required in statin-resistant or -intolerant patients. The main agents include Cholestyramine (2–4 g b.i.d.), Colesevelam (2.5–5 mg b.i.d.), and Cholestypol (1–8 g b.i.d.). *Fibric acid derivatives* activate the peroxisome proliferator-activated receptors (PPARs), to decrease LDL, VLDL and remnant particle levels, decrease hepatic secretion of TG, and increase HDL production. Adverse effects include abdominal pain, nausea, diarrhea, LFT disturbances, eczema, muscular pain and occasional rhabdomyolysis (especially in combination with statins). Gemfibrosil may also cause AF and vision disturbances, and Fenofibrate may cause pancytopenia. Representatives include Bezafibrate (200 mg t.i.d. for the short-acting compound, 400 mg q.d. for the long-acting one); Ciprofibrate (100–200 mg q.d.); Gemfibrosil (600 mg b.i.d., 30 min before meals); and Fenofibrate (200 mg q.d.). The addition of a fibric acid derivative to a statin potentiates the LDL-lowering effect, and has a favorable impact on HDL and TG levels. However, there is increased risk of toxicity, especially to the muscle. The ACCORD study is currently evaluating CVD outcomes in a double-blind manner, comparing Simvastatin + Fenofibrate vs. Simvastatin + placebo. ABT-335 is a derivative of the fibric acid is currently being evaluated as adjunctive antihyperlipemic therapy.

Niacin (vitamin B3, nicotinic acid) blocks fat breakdown in adipose tissue, increasing HDL and reducing total cholesterol, TG, VLDL and LDL levels. It might also be antiinflammatory and inhibit the secretion of leptin (with a major role in atherosclerosis). The dosage is 1–2 g b.i.d. or t.i.d. These doses cause severe flushing and occasional pruritus, rash, dizziness, diarrhea, and abdominal pain. The prostaglandin-mediated flushing can be countered by NSAID or food administration prior to Niacin ingestion, or by a prostaglandin inhibitor (laropiprant) added to

niacin. The niacin/laropiprant combination has recently been approved for use in Europe. Niacin is contraindicated in severe hepatic disease, ulcer, hypotension, and in those with bleeding tendency. *ω-3 fatty acid* (eicosapentaenoic acid, EPA and docosahexaenoic acid, DHA) intake should be derived mainly from fatty fish. In high-risk patients, these agents may decrease risk of lethal arrhythmias, decrease TG levels, decrease plaque growth rate and slightly lower BP. The recommendation for fatty acid replacement therapy should be individualized, with 1 g q.d. recommended in patients with documented CAD, and 2–4 g q.d. in patients in whom TG decrease is desired, although, as mentioned, this is not a formally recognized therapeutic target.

There have been conflicting reports in the literature regarding the effect of fatty oils on atherosclerosis. The differences may stem from the study design and populations or from the type and/or potential dietary source of the compound under study. Thus, beside fish-derived ω-fatty acids, research has also focused on the vegetable-derived α-linolenic acid. While the OMEGA study has found no benefit to ω-3 fatty acid therapy in optimally treated post-MI patients, there are still no definitive conclusions to date.

Plasmapheresis is occasionally necessary in congenital dyslipidemia. It consists in replacement of part of the patient's own plasma with donor plasma (with normal cholesterol levels).

Future therapies for dyslipidemia will probably include a genetic approach, using viral vectors to deliver normal genes to the patient's cells, to compete with, and functionally inactivate, the defective ("hyperlipidemic") genes. In preliminary studies, the cholesteryl ester transfer protein (CETP) inhibitor Anacetrapib was found to reduce LDL and increase HDL levels. Darapladib, an inhibitor of the lipoprotein-associated phospholipase A2 (lp-PLA2), has not been found effective in improving the surrogate-endpoint of IVUS-assessed plaque morphology.

Smoking, a major atherosclerosis risk factor, is the main cause of preventible death worldwide. More than 4,000 compounds have been identified in cigarette smoke (60 being oncogenic). About 30% of CAD-related fatalities are attributable to smoking. Active and passive smoking are equally dangerous and affect all age groups, starting in intrauterine life. Smoking decreases HDL and increases LDL levels. Additionally, nicotine and carbon monoxide cause endothelial damage, setting the stage for atherosclerosis; CO also decreases RBC O_2 transport capacity. In HTN patients, smoking increases the risk of malignant crises. Smoking causes tachycardia, increases myocardial O_2 demand, and may precipitate ischemia. The effect of smoking is cumulative, often over many decades. Lifelong exposure is assessed by multiplying the number of years of smoking by the average number of daily packs; <12 pack-years is considered light smoking, while ≥20 pack-years represent heavy smoking. Cardiovascular morbidity and mortality increase proportionally with exposure to smoke; however, even "light" smoking is a severe hazard. *Smoking cessation*, even after decades-long addiction, significantly reduces cardiovascular risk. One year after smoking cessation, the risk decreases by half, and after 15 years, it equals that of non-smokers. Quitting smoking before the age of 40 prolongs life by an average of 4–5 years. Smoking cessation is feasible, but, unfortunately, rarely achieved, for several reasons: nicotine and certain additives are highly addictive; peer pressure in many age groups and cultures also plays an important role. Unfortunately, defeatism and time shortage preclude proper anti-smoking counseling by the medical personnel (smoking cessation should be discussed at every single encounter with the patient).

The main strategies for smoking cessation are reviewed in Table 2.3. About one-third of people who earnestly attempt to quit smoking are able to achieve this and persist in not smoking on the long run.

The so-called "light" *brands* of cigarettes are generally just as dangerous as the regular ones, as the lower nicotine content is compensated by deeper inhalation and more frequent "puffing," resulting in the same net toxic intake. The smoking simulators used for brand testing detect less smoke intake due to the ventilation orifices at the base of the cigarette; however, these orifices are generally sealed by the smoker's lips, precluding any real advantage. *Non-cigarette smoking*: Classically, *cigar or pipe smoking* was believed less noxious than cigarette smoking, as the inhalation patterns were different. However, most current cigar or pipe smokers are ex-cigarette smokers, carrying over the cigarette-smoking inhalation patterns, and thus the risk is the same. *Hookah* (*shisha, nargileh*) smoking is at least as dangerous as cigarette smoking, as the water filtering typical to this technique removes only some of the toxic compunds. A typical 1-h session of hookah smoking exposes the user to volumes of inhaled smoke many times larger than those from a single cigarette. *Tobacco chewing* mainly causes palate malignancies;

Table 2.3 Strategies for smoking cessation

Method	Remarks
Behavioral approaches	
Abrupt ("cold turkey") cessation	Requires tremendous willpower, but has the best results; up to 90% of patients able to refrain from smoking on the long run use this method
Workshops for smoking cessation	Effective if the patient's motivation is high
Pharmacological approaches	
Nicotine replacement therapy	Commonly used, but only modestly effective
Varenicline,[a] a nicotine receptor blocker	Better than nicotine replacement, but may cause neuropsychiatric disturbances and suicidal behavior
Bupropion,[b] an antidepressant	C/I in diabetics, epilepsy, anorexia nervosa, bulimia, or active brain tumors; may cause suicidal behavior in the young
Anti-nicotine vaccine	Under study
Clonidine	Occasionally used to blunt sympathetic activation associated to smoke cessation.
Hypnosis, acupuncture, self-help approaches, plant extracts (chamomile, kava-kava, etc.)	Inconclusive results

[a]0.5 mg q.d. for 3 days and b.i.d. for an additional 3 days; and 1 mg b.i.d. thereafter, for 3 months
[b]150 mg q.d., then b.i.d. for 2–3 months, while the patient continues to smoke; 10–14 days into the treatment, the craving for smoking should abate, enabling smoking cessation. The second dose is taken a few hours before bed time, as it might cause insomnia. Success rates are up to 25% (around 50%, in some studies).

however, it does create addiction to nicotine, likely to be satisfied at some point by cigarette smoking. *Cigarette holders* are probably as effective as the filter and the ventilation system they contain. The latter might be occluded by the smoker's lips, just like with "light" cigarettes. *Passive smoking* associates a 30% increase in CAD risk. Low weight at birth, SIDS, early-onset atherosclerosis, learning difficulties, and tobacco addiction in adulthood are all more frequent in children exposed to cigarette smoke. Additionally, there is a higher risk of spontaneous abortion in mothers who are smokers.

Diabetes (fasting glucose >125 mg/dL) is a major risk factor for CAD. Hyperglycemia causes endothelial dysfunction (decreased levels of NO); increases production of thromboxane and of free O_2 radicals; stimulates smooth muscle cell proliferation and migration and platelet aggregation; increases LDL and TG levels, and decreases HDL levels; increases coagulability; damages the vasa vasorum and vasa nervorum; and inhibits the development of collateral circulation. These effects cause CAD to be more frequent and more severe (three vessel-disease, diffuse atherosclerosis, increased prevalence of MI, increased MI mortality, increased coronary restenosis rate). Cardiovascular risk increases with the severity of diabetes and decreases with adequate diabetes control, best quantified by the HbA1c levels. Overt diabetes increases the risk of cardiovascular disease two to threefold in men and three to fivefold in women. Additionally, diabetes causes non-atherosclerotic cardiac damage, including CMP and cardiac autonomic system dysfunction. Diabetes may occur either *overtly* or as *pre-diabetes* (fasting glucose 100–125 mg/dL and/or abnormal oral glucose challenge test), both conditions associating insulin resistance, itself a risk factor for atherosclerosis. Diabetes may occur in conjunction with the other components of the metabolic syndrome. Maintenance of euglycemia is key in the treatment of the diabetic patient. The American Diabetes Association recommends a target of HbA1c ≤7%, and of 6.7 mmol/L (120 mg/dL) for fasting glucose levels; the (European)

International Diabetes Federation recommends ≤6.5%, and 6.0 mmol/L (108 mg/dL), respectively, with postprandial glucose levels ≤7.5 mmol/L (135 mg/dL). However, strict glucose control increases the risk of hypoglycemia, especially deleterious to the heart.

Increased body weight (Table 2.4) is a major risk factor for atherosclerosis, both *directly* (the adipose tissue is an endocrine organ, secreting a vast array of peptide and non-peptide substances, a key compound being adiponectin), and *indirectly,* by increasing LDL and TG, and decreasing HDL levels; causing insulin resistance or frank diabetes; and stimulating inflammation. Multivariate adjustment for other risk factors shows that overweight is not an individual risk factor for atherosclerosis, but acts by increasing the prevalence of dyslipidemia and of glucose metabolism disturbances. Management is based on reduced caloric intake and physical exercise. Fat intake must be reduced to less than or equal to one-third of total caloric intake, with saturated and trans-fatty acids ≤7%. These recommendations are not attenuated by the widely-publicized "obesity paradox," a decreased risk for cardiovascular complications in the obese, possibly due to lower systemic vascular resistance and plasma renin activity.

The pharmacological approach to weight loss is reviewed in Table 2.5. Use of these medications remains at the physician's discretion.

Sedentary lifestyle causes weight gain and cardiorespiratory deconditioning. Physical exercise including ≥30 min of moderately vigorous activity daily, ≥5 days weekly is recommended. "Moderately vigorous" exercise is defined as reaching 60–75% of maximal HR in a Bruce protocol, or as "moderate exertion" on a Borg scale.

Homocystein is an essential aminoacid; congenital hyperhomocysteinemia is associated to extensive, severe and premature atherosclerosis. Milder elevations also increase risk, but correction of elevated homocysteine levels seems not to influence cardiovascular endpoints. Therefore, correction of elevated homocysteine levels remains optional, and should be mainly considered in high-risk patients. Levels of 5–15, 16–100,

Table 2.4 Assessment of excess body weight

Condition	Body mass index (kg/m²) Men/women	Waist circumference (cm) Men	Women
Overweight	25–29.9	≥94	≥80
Obesity	≥30	≥102	≥88

Table 2.5 The pharmacological approach to weight loss

Agent	Mechanism	Dose	C/I and adverse effects
Orlistat	Inhibits intestinal lipases, and thus digestion and absorbtion of fats	60–120 mg b.i.d.	GI upset, flatulence, steatorrhea
Sibutramine	Metabolized to compouds that induce early satiety	10 mg q.d., may increase to 15 mg q.d. after 4 weeks	GI upset, dry mouth, dysgueusia, paradoxical hunger, joint or muscle pain, headache, dizziness, seizures, insomnia, flushing, arrhythmia, melena, hematemesis, jaundice, fever and rigors, chest pain, HTN
Rimonabant	Endocannabinoid inverse agonist, reduces hunger	Suspended due to serious side-effects, including severe depression and suicidal ideation	

and >100 μmol/L are considered normal, moderately, and, respectively, severely increased. Homocystein can be decreased by dietary or pharmacological measures. The former include especially leafy vegetables (lettuce, spinach, etc.), folic acid-fortified cereals, and chicken, beef and beef consumption. Effective drugs include folic acid 5 mg q.d., vitamin B6 250 mg q.d., and vitamin B12 0.5 mg q.d (however, see Table 2.19).

Genetic factors (family history): At-risk individuals have a first-degree relative with early-onset CAD (<55 for male, <65 for female relatives); the correlation is less strong, but still present, for second-degree relatives. The earlier the onset and the greater the number of affected relatives, the higher the risk. Family history is as an independent risk factor for atherosclerosis. Several genetic loci have been investigated, for instance, variants in the chromosomal region 9p21. While the exact role of this variant remains to be defined, the magnitude of risk may be comparable to that imparted by hypercholesterolemia. Additionally, the ACE polymorphism may predict, among others, the rate of restenosis after angioplasty. The ability to individually predict the response to given therapies by genetic makeup analysis ("pharmacogenetics") holds promise for the future.

Other factors: *Hypercoagulability* is rarely the sole cause for complicated atherosclerosis, but mutations in factor V (Leyden) or factor II (prothrombin) do cause a somewhat increased risk. *Inflammation* (increased CRP levels) increases the risk of stroke, of CAD, and of severe CAD (ACS). Chronic inflammatory diseases, such as psoriasis, rheumatoid arthritis, periodontitis, or recent respiratory infection have been shown to be independent risk predictors for cardiovascular events (However, patients with rheumatoid arthritis may have

an uncommonly *good* prognosis for CAD, a fact recently attributed to methotrexate therapy). In younger men, the risk of CAD or its complications is proportional with *HR*. Chronic tachycardia has been postulated to promote atherosclerosis, but in women and in the elderly, this is not an independent risk factor. The impact of routine administration of β-blockers or CCB on morbidity and mortality is unclear. While Ivabradine has not been found to improve prognosis in patients with stable angina and LV dysfunction, some benefit was observed in those with HR ≥70 bpm, thus somewhat clarifying the threshold definition for a "fast" HR. *Psychosocial factors* (stress, depression, social isolation) are independent risk factors for atherosclerosis and CAD. These patients also tend to have unhealthier life styles and lower compliance to medical therapy. The risk of atherosclerosis is independently increased in patients with *renal dysfunction,* especially end-stage renal failure. The association is most likely explained by coexisting diffuse severe atherosclerosis and HTN. *Female gender*: Hormonal protection before menopause defers the risk of complicated atherosclerosis, but overall, more women than men succumb to atherosclerosis. Women are underrepresented in most major trials, and thus the treatment is extrapolated from that used in men. Chest pain is often "atypical" in women, precluding timely treatment. *Other possible risk factors* include: elevated myeloperoxidase levels; micro- or macroalbuminuria, defined by the urinary-albumin-to-creatinine ratio (UACR); fibrinogen levels (which tend to covariate with other risk factors, and are reduced mainly by lifestyle changes); pollution (possibly by triggering a systemic inflammatory response); increased PTH levels (studied in elderly males); and low serum levels of vitamin D (associated with more

Table 2.6 The metabolic syndrome

Component[a]	Severity
Central obesity	Waist circumference >102 cm (♂), >88 cm (♀)
Elevated TG	≥1.7 mmol/L (150 mg/dL)
Low HDL	<1.03 mmol/L (40 mg/dL) (♂), <1.29 mmol/L (50 mg/dL) (♀)
HTN[b]	BP ≥135 mmHg (syst.) and/or ≥85 mmHg (diast.)
Increased fasting plasma glucose levels	>5.6 mmol/L (100 mg/dL)

[a]Metabolic syndrome diagnosed in the presence of ≥3 components
[b]Or previously diagnosed, currently treated BP

classic risk factors, such as HTN, diabetes, or obesity, and with high TG levels).

The metabolic syndrome is a combination of atherosclerosis risk factors, including: central obesity (adipose accumulation in the abdomen, rather than in the limbs), HTN, low HDL, raised TG and high blood glucose levels, resulting from insulin resistance (the combination of the two latter characteristics has earned this syndrome the alternative designation of "insulin resistance syndrome".) The metabolic syndrome substantially increases the risk of atherosclerosis and of full-blown diabetes. The concern that the "metabolic syndrome" is not a true entity, but simply reflects the coexistence of highly prevalent individual conditions, appears unfounded, as the presence of one component dramatically raises the probability of finding others. There are several formal definitions of this syndrome. The NCEP-ATP III (National Cholestrol Education Program Adult Treatment Panel III, Table 2.6) definition is the most predictive of cardiovascular complications. The concept of " metabolic syndrome" (for which there is yet no specific therapy as such) advocates active investigation for additional risk factors, in the presence of one such factor. The treament addresses individual risk factors.

Global cardiovascular risk: While established CAD, type 2 diabetes, type 1 diabetes with microalbuminuria, or very severe individual risk factors entail high risk for (further) manifestations of CAD, the prognostic importance of risk factor coexistence or of lesser risk profiles is not immediately apparent. In these patients, CAD risk is best assessed using a prognostic score called, intuitively, "SCORE." This assesses 10-year cardiovascular mortality (fatal atherosclerotic event). Ten-year

risks of <1, 1–4, 5–9, and ≥10% are considered low, moderate, increased, and very increased, respectively. The score is calculated based on age, gender, cholesterol levels, BP, and smoking status; there are separate tables for different country groups (high- and low-risk), according to the prevalence of healthy lifestyles. As many countries transition to healthier lifestyles, the SCORE may overestimate the risk in those populations. Additional tables exist, taking into account the cholesterol: HDL ratio. The SCORE is read off a table. In low-risk patients (10-year risk <5%), the only necessary action is periodic risk reassessment. The risk appears lower in women, but is in fact merely deferred, post-menopausal women having risks similar to those of men. Cardiovascular risk can also be estimated using the Framingham data, by calculating either the Framingham, or the ATP score. The Framingham risk score is calculated based on sex, age (not validated for <35 or >74), total cholesterol, HDL, BP, diabetes, and cigarette smoking. The ATP score differs in that it only refers to systolic BP, and takes into account the presence or absence of antihypertensive therapy. In addition, the Framingham score automatically classifies patients with diabetes and/or PVD as high-risk. The short-term (10-year) risk for developing CAD is considered low at <10% (<5%, according to other authors); intermediate at 10–20%; and high, at ≥20%. The database for total cholesterol being larger than that for LDL, the predictions are more robust than those using LDL. The latter, however, currently remains the primary target of therapy.

Risk Assessment, A Matter of Definition

The widely divergent definitions of "severe risk" as assessed by the Framingham (AHA/ACC) and the SCORE (ESC) scales based on very similar risk factors underscores the need for harmonization of the language and definitions used in the medical community when dealing with a medical condition.

2.1.4 Atherosclerosis: Diagnosis

The diagnosis of atherosclerosis coincides with that of its main complication, ischemia, and is reviewed in the next section.

2.1.5 Atherosclerosis: Treatment

Primary prevention of atherosclerosis consists in risk factor management. The treatment of atherosclerosis as such (secondary prevention, coronary revascularization) is integral part of the treatment of coronary ischemia, and is reviewed in the next section. A "polypill" containing low doses of Atenolol, HCTZ, Ramipril, Simvastatin, and Aspirin has been introduced in some countries, to facilitate compliance and ensure implementation of proven prophylactic therapy in patients at risk for cardiovascular events. Novel drug delivery systems are being actively investigated as well. For instance, recent research has shown the feasibility of drug delivery to the myocardium using drug-laden microspheres, injected directly into the myocardium.

2.2 Ischemia: Overview

2.2.1 Definition and Mechanisms

The main cardiac impact of atherosclerosis is myocardial ischemia, i.e., an absolute or relative decrease in myocardial perfusion. This can be due either to increased metabolic requirements (during stress), or to decreased blood flow through the coronary arteries; occasionally, the two components coexist. Rarely, ischemia is due to decreased O_2 delivery (anemia, methemoglobinemia, etc.), or to coronary compression (*bridging,* a congenital malformation where a portion of the coronary artery has an intramyocardial, rather than subepicardial course, with compression of the artery on each ventricular systole; *congenital coronary anomalies,* where the coronary artery courses between the aorta and the PA, with coronary compression between these two vessels).

The risk factors for ischemia can be classified into: *risk factors for atherosclerosis,* i.e., the histopathological substrate of ischemia; and *risk factors for thrombosis* upon the preexisting support of atherosclerosis. With stable angina, only the first class of risk is operational, whereas the genesis of ACS requires the presence of both classes. The risk factors for thrombosis mainly pertain to *plaque composition* (lipid-rich plaque with a thin fibrous cap is the most prone to rupture); *factors leading to plaque erosion or rupture* (inflammation, hemodynamic trauma, etc.); and, less frequently, *hypercoagulability syndromes.*

Coronary flow can decrease gradually or abruptly. The former scenario involves a gradual increase in plaque dimensions, ultimately increasing coronary resistance to flow; the clinical correlate is *stable angina pectoris.* Acute flow decrease occurs as a result of intracoronary thrombosis, and causes *ACS.* The two mechanisms (obstruction by gradual plaque growth vs. acute thrombotic occlusion) may also coexist, as clots may form on already prominent plaques; however, the less protruding plaques are often the most vulnerable. A comparison of stable angina and ACS is presented at the beginning of Sect. 2.3. Briefly, stable angina is due to increased resistance to flow (due to the mechanical bulk of the plaque or to endothelial dysfunction), while ACS is due to thrombotic occlusion of the coronary artery, with different degrees of distal embolization into the microcirculation, with fragments of thrombus.

The supply/demand imbalance inherent to ischemia is counteracted by several mechanisms, aimed either at increasing blood flow, or at decreasing myocardial consumption. *In the acute setting,* the operative mechanisms include vasodilation and the activation of the endogenous thrombolytic system, while in the *chronic setting,* adaptive mechanisms include: vasodilation (which may increase flow up to fivefold as compared to baseline, but is decreased by the endothelial dysfunction associated to atherosclerosis); vascular remodeling; and the development of collateral circulation. Reduction of O_2 consumption occasionally achieves complete correction of the demand/supply imbalance; however, this comes at the cost of LV dysfunction (Table 2.7).

The main clinical, diagnostic, and therapeutic aspects of myocardial ischemia are reviewed in the present section, while the clinical syndromes (ACS and stable angina) will be reviewed in Sect. 2.3.

2.2.2 Clinical Manifestations

The typical symptom of CAD is retrosternal heaviness (chest discomfort), described as a crushing, squeezing, or constricting sensation in the precordial and substernal areas, often associated with a sense of impending doom. Pain onset may occur at rest or after physical or psychological stress. Pain may be mild or absent, especially in the young (<40), the elderly (>75), and in diabetic or postoperative patients. The pain typically radiates to the left arm, neck, jaw, shoulder, right arm,

Table 2.7 Ischemia-related conditions

Entity	Correction achieved by	Practical importance
Hibernation	Severe hypokinesis[a] (to decrease O_2 requirements)	Myocardial contractility may be regained by revascularization
Preconditioning	Adaptation of myocardium to ischemic conditions	Reduced functional impact of future ischemic episodes
Scarring	Replacement of myocardium with metabolically inert scar tissue	Irreversible functional loss; revascularization is pointless

[a]Hibernation is a chronic state, only reversible by revascularization (PCI or CABG), while stunning is an acute, short-lived condition, reversible spontaneously or under drug therapy. Classification of hibernation as an adaptive mechanism and of stunning as a complication of ischemia might appear arbitrary, as both consist in LV dysfunction resulting from decreased myocardial flow. However, hibernation more appropriately qualifies as an adaptive mechanism and has a different molecular base than stunning.

and epigastrium, often causing confusion with rheumatic or GI problems. Additional symptoms include profuse sweating, dyspnea (occasionally, pulmonary edema), palpitations, confusional state, nausea, vomiting, etc. GI symptoms are especially frequent in patients with inferior MI. The pain may last for a few minutes or more; longer duration (>20 min) is usually, but not always, a sign of ACS, usually MI. The chest discomfort subsides spontaneously or under Nitroglycerin; lack of response to Nitroglycerin of otherwise typical pain pleads in favor of the diagnosis of acute MI. The *physical examination* reveals nonspecific findings, including pallor, tachypnea, tachycardia, evidence of atherosclerosis in other territories (e.g., carotid bruits), evidence of pulmonary congestion (rhales), functional MR, etc. ACS (Sect. 2.3) may present with rhythm and conduction disturbances.

2.2.3 Ischemia Workup

2.2.3.1 Electrocardiography

Electrocardiography (EKG) is the cornerstone of CAD diagnosis, although both false-negative and false-positive diagnoses are frequent. EKG may reflect myocardial ischemia or its complications (rhythm or conduction disturbances, post-MI pericarditis, etc.). EKG signs of ischemia include ST elevations or depressions and T wave inversion, conformational changes, or pseudonormalization. EKG allows localization of the ischemic segment, of the responsible artery and even of the approximate point of stenosis (Table 2.8). EKG is relatively poor at examining the posterobasal and lateral LV walls, leading to underdiagnosis of ischemia in the LCx distribution.

A provocative recent study has found little incremental value to EKG on top of sound clinical assessment for risk stratification of patients with suspected angina. Both resting and stress EKG appeared of no value in this study. This finding, if validated, will serve as a strong reminder that it is mostly the superficial (non-flow limiting) plaques, i.e., the ones usually missed by EKG, that are responsible for acute MI.

EKG stress test: *General remarks*: The EKG stress detects pathologic changes under increased metabolic demands (controlled physical exercise), in patients with a normal rest tracing. Preexisting resting EKG abnormalities (WPW, LVH, or pacemaker rhythm) may render the stress test impossible to interpret, while other conditions (digitalis treatment, electrolyte abnormalities, intraventricular conduction disturbance) reduce the sensitivity and specificity of the test. The average sensitivity and specificity of the EKG stress test are 68 and 77%, respectively (less, in women). While reduced physical capacity is one of the main reasons for obtaining an inconclusive exercise stress test, it is by itself associated to an increased incidence of cardiac and noncardiac events. *Indications*: The indications for EKG stress testing are reviewed in Table 2.9.

Practical aspects: Preliminary interruption of β-blockers and non-dihydropyridine CCB (used for CAD, HTN or arrhythmia) is required for primary diagnosis of ischemia; however, for functional status evaluation (i.e., assessment of the protection provided by medication), discontinuation is not recommended. Exercise follows different protocols, all using a gradual increase in physical stress, but differing in the duration and workload of each stage (Table 2.10). Protocols can be achieved on a bicycle or on a treadmill. In the US, the treadmill is preferred, as large segments of the population do not regularly ride a bike,

Table 2.8 Ischemia location by EKG

Limb leads	Chest leads: V 1	2	3	4	5	6	7–9	3–4R	MI localization	Responsible artery
LAD-dependent MI										
I, aVL									High lateral[a]	LCx or RCA
	■	■							Anteroseptal	Distal LAD or diagonal
	■	■	■						Anterior	Midlad or diagonal
	■	■	■	■					Anterolat.[b]	Proximal or midLAD[c]
			■	■	■				Lateral	Distal LAD or diagonal
RCA or LCx –dependent MI[d]										
II, III, aVF									"Small" inferior	Distal RCA or LCx
	■	■					■		True post. MI[g]	Proximal RCA or LCx
								■	RV MI[g]	Proximal RCA or LCx

[a]L1 and aVL can be involved alone or in combination

[b]Also termed "extensive anterior MI"

[c]If stenosis is proximal to first septal perforator (proximal LAD), fascicular or BBB is typically associated

[d]The culprit artery in these territories depends on coronary dominance (i.e., the artery supplying the PDA); this is the RCA, the LCx, or both in right, left, or co-dominant circulation respectively, accounting for 70, 10, and 20% of the population, respectively.

[e]Mirror-image: increased R wave amplitude and duration and a R/S ratio in V_1 or V_2 >1 (mirroring posterior wall Q waves); ST depression and large, inverted T waves in V_1–V_3 (mirroring posterior wall ST elevations and hyperacute T waves)

[f]Direct image of the posterior MI

[g]Often associated to inferior MI (infero-posterior MI±RV MI). The LV segment lying on the diaphragm is currently designated as "inferobasal," rather than "posterior".

and the estimated peak O_2 (i.e., the maximum achieved exertion) is spuriously low.

Interpretation and comments: The main EKG-related data provided by stress test are reviewed in Table 2.11. The intrinsic advantages of the test (availability, safety, physiological, rather than drug-induced exertion) are undermined by the low sensitivity and specificity of ST segment depressions for ischemia; in addition, the 1-mm cutoff value is arbitrary. Additional EKG-related or EKG-independent factors increasing the diagnostic and prognostic yield are briefly reviewed in Table 2.11. The table also reviews findings pertaining to the severity and prognosis of ischemia (rather than its mere presence); in patients with "very positive" tests, an early invasive therapy might be justified. As classical exercise stress test does not individualize the target HR, beyond age and gender, a subjective rate of perceived exertion (RPE) has been introduced. In both its variants (the Borg scale, ranging from 6 to 20, or the modified Borg scale, ranging from 1 to 10), the patient rates effort severity from "nothing at all" to "very, very hard"; a score >18 (Borg scale) or >9 (modified Borg scale) defines "maximal exertion."

Stress test is interrupted if definitely positive or negative (>80% of THR or 110 bpm under β-blocker therapy; recovery completed, in the absence of diagnostic EKG or clinical changes); if the patient cannot carry on (mostly, due to orthopedic problems or fatigue); and in case of a complication. In case of symptoms or ST depressions <1 mm, the test may be cautiously continued. The test can be continued beyond 100% THR, for assessment of functional status; any EKG changes are interpreted in the clinical context. An inconclusive stress test should be followed by another noninvasive test, such as stress echo or nuclear scan.

Table 2.9 Indications and Contraindications of EKG stress testing

Indications	Contraindications[a,b]	Remarks
Diagnosis of obstructive[c] CAD		
Intermediate pretest probability of obstructive or vasospastic disease, based on symptoms, or (Class II indication) on risk factors, especially diabetes. Test also indicated in patients with occupations potentially affecting public safety (pilots, etc.)	WPW, paced rhythm, LBBB, >1 mm resting ST depression	Complete RBBB, resting ST depression <1 mm (with or without LVH), digitalis effect acceptable, but decrease sensitivity and specificity
Risk assessment and prognosis of known CAD (excluding early post-MI patients)		
Recent marked change in clinical status; unstable angina (low-risk, if asymptomatic for ≥8–12 h; intermediate risk, if asymptomatic for ≥2–3 days[d])	High-risk unstable angina; severe co-morbidity limiting candidacy for revascularization or ability to exercise; periodic follow-up in asymptomatic patients[e]	WPW, paced rhythm, LBBB, <1 mm resting ST depression acceptable, mainly for non-EKG-related endpoints aiding prognosis assessment
Early post-MI patients		
Submaximal test at 4–6 days; symptom-limited test early (2–3 weeks) or late (3–6 weeks) post-MI for risk stratification,[f] evaluation of medical therapy and prescription/evaluation of cardiac rehabilitation	Severe co-morbidity limiting candidacy for revascularization or ability to exercise; periodic follow-up in asymptomatic patients; to assess physiological significance of stenoses detected at catheterization	As above

[a]Situations posing an unacceptable risk, or making the stress test uninterpretable
[b]Additional *absolute contraindications*: severe arrhythmia, HF, or aortic stenosis; aortic dissection; PE; myo-, peri- or endocarditis; significant non-cardiac disease; *Relative contraindications*: milder degrees of arrhythmia or other cardiac or non-cardiac disease; electrolyte disturbance; HTN (resting systolic BP >200 mmHg and/or resting diastolic BP >110 mmHg), HOCM; LMCA stenosis or equivalent; AV block; ventricular ectopy or aneurysm; advanced or complicated pregnancy
[c]EKG stress test does not identify non-flow-limiting plaques, the most prone to cause MI
[d]Possibly 12 h, if asymptomatic and repeat troponin negative
[e]A non-Class I, yet very popular indication
[f]In an era of aggressive early revascularization, this population should decrease dramatically; practically, availability issues make it most relevant to current practice

Table 2.10 Stress test protocols

Protocol	Characteristics[a]	Required fitness[b]	Remarks
Bruce	Large workload increments between stages	High	Widely used, enables cross-center comparisons. Disadvantages: stage IV can be either walked or run, which influences O_2 consumption
Modified Bruce	Lower workload increments	Moderate	May still be excessively demanding for unfit persons
Cornell	Adaptable according to the fitness level	Variable	
Balke	Large workload increments between stages	High	
Naughton	Lower workload increments	Low	
Ramp protocol	Continuous, computer-generated, individualized increases in workload	Average	Individualized workload increase avoids early termination of test

[a]The Bruce protocol stages are 3 min long; with the other protocols, the stages are 2 min long
[b]For successful completion of test protocol

Table 2.11 Exercise stress test EKG data

	EKG data[a]	Non-EKG data
Presence	Positive[b] test: horizontal or downsloping ST segment depression ≥1 mm in ≥2 contiguous leads[c]; ST elevation in ≥2 contiguous leads; ST elevation ≥2 mm not associated with post-MI Q waves.[d] Probability of ischemia increases when changes involve a larger number of leads and/or appear at a lower workload; with ST depressions that are downsloping (as opposed to horizontal) and/or persist >1 min into recovery; with a disturbed ST/HR curve[e]; and possibly, with the magnitude of ST depression	Reproduction of typical symptoms on exercise; BP decrease or failure to rise on exercise
Location	ST depressions generally do not localize ischemia; ST elevations do (ischemia in the territory corresponding to the involved leads)	–
Severity/prognosis	ST elevation not associated with post-MI Q waves indicate severe transmural ischemia; the magnitude of ST depressions correlates not only with the probability, but possibly also with the severity of CAD	Systolic BP decrease or failure to rise on exercise[f]; functional capacity <3–5 METs of workload[g]; HR decrease ≤12 bpm after 1-min recovery (18 bpm, if supine); exercise-induced LBBB; ventricular ectopy[h]; chronotropic insufficiency[i]

[a]T wave dynamics are nonspecific; in the absence of LVH and of VHD, U wave inversion is very suggestive of ischemia
[b]Stress test is positive regardless of the time of exercise-induced changes onset. Normal EKG only represents a negative test if ≥80% of the age-predicted maximum HR has been attained, and recovery was uneventful
[c]ST segment is measured from the isoelectric baseline (PR interval), at 80 ms. past the J point; a cutoff of ≥2 mm depression increases specificity, but decreases sensitivit
[d]If associated to Q waves, ST elevations likely reflect segmental dyskinesia (pathogenesis similar to that of ST elevations in patients with an MI-related LV aneurysm)
[e]Computerized quantitation of ST depression at the end of each stage, to increase the diagnostic yield
[f]Normally, SBP increases >10 mmHg, but is <230 mmHg at peak exercise, and DBP either decreases or increases, but not >120 mmHg. A hypertensive response under exercise may reflect poor control of known underlying HTN or predict HTN onset in the future
[g]That is, patients unable to complete stage II of a standard age- and gender-adjusted Bruce protocol
[h]At stress or on recovery; additionally, >7 PVCs/min. On recovery; PVCs in the recovery stage of the exercise have been found to have a potentially higher predictive value than even exercise-induced arrhythmia, and may warrant further work-up for coronary ischemia
[i]That is, the inability to adequately increase HR on exercise, assessed by the "chronotropic response index": CRI = (peak HR-resting HR)/age-predicted maximum HR- resting HR); normal >0.8 (0.62, under β-blockers)

Integrating the Prognostic Data of the Stress Test: the Duke Score (DTS)

The most popular exercise test-based score, (Duke) grades exercise-induced anginal pain (0=none, 1=non-exercise limiting (assuming the test was not discontinued at the appearance of anginal pain in the first place; 2=exercise-limiting), then calculates (manually, or using a nomogram) an index, DTS=exercise duration (min) – 5× maximal ST deviation – 4× anginal score.

The risk of cardiovascular morbidity and mortality is low, intermediate, or high, for a DTS ≥5, 4 to −10, or ≤10, respectively.

Complications (arrhythmia and acute ischemic events) are infrequent, assuming most high-risk patients are excluded using clinical and laboratory indicators (according to Bayes' principle, stress test should be carried out in intermediate-risk individuals).

2.2.3.2 Echo

Echo demonstrates ischemia-related segmental hypokinesia, identifying the affected artery and assessing the extent of the damage. The degree of LVEF decrease is the main prognostic factor after MI, and is routinely measured. Occasionally, segmental dysfunction is used for diagnosis of MI (Sect. 2.3). Contrast echo serves to better delineate the LV endocardial border, in patients with technically difficult studies. However, myocardial contrast echo, suggested as a potential "one-stop shop" method displaying both perfusion defects and the resulting LV dysfunction is still not widely applied in clinical practice. The 17-segment schematic of the LV, as used in all imaging modalities, is reviewed in Chap. 1.

Stress Echo

Principles: Stress echo (SE) assesses stress-induced myocardial ischemia manifesting as stunning in the territories depending on the involved arteries. Stunning is generally short-lived (thus, SE is safe), and can be identified and quantified as new-onset or exacerbated segmental hypokinesis.

Technique: SE uses either physical exercise on a treadmill or stress bicycle, or Dobutamine-induced tachycardia, based on stepwise increases in the dosage of the IV-administered sympathomimetic agent. The test compares resting and stress regional LV function, imaged from the standard windows (parasternal long- and short axis; apical two- and four-chamber views). A representative resting cardiac cycle (not an extrasystole or a postextrasystolic beat, and not a foreshortened image) is chosen, digitized, and displayed in endless-loop format, side by side with a corresponding stress cycle. Clips must only include ventricular systole, as "snippets" of diastole may be read as false-positive (spurious hypokinesia). Abnormalities must be identified in ≥2 adjacent segments, and, if possible, confirmed from two different views. The basal inferior and basal septal segments are most prone to false-positive readings. With bicycle stress test, images are obtained at rest, before peak and at peak stress, and at recovery; the treadmill protocol uses two sets of images, one at rest, and one immediately (<90 s) after stress, both with the patient in left lateral decubitus. Using a bicycle offers the advantage of recording images at the time of peak effort, avoiding false-negative reads (rapid recovery from stunning); however, accurate imaging may be difficult due to motion artifact (attenuated by having the patient lean forward on the bicycle).

Interpretation: *Table 2.12*

Stress echo tends to be less sensitive than stress scintigraphy, most probably reflecting underdiagnosis of relatively small ischemic myocardial areas. While this may affect the ability of stress echo to establish *the*

Table 2.12 Stress echo

Contractility		
Rest	Peak exercise or high-dose[a] Dobutamine; recovery	
	Improved contractility[a]	WMA[b]
Normal	No ischemia	Inducible ischemia[c]
WMA	Stunning or hibernation[d]	Scar

[a]Low doses of Dobutamine (or low-intensity physical exercise, imaged during a bicycle stress test) may also increase contractility; if this increase is followed by recurrent WMA, the territory is hibernating. Such segments also benefit from revascularization
[b]Akinetic or dyskinetic segments (especially if thinned out and brightly lucent) usually correspond to scar
[c]Paradoxically, both normalization of a previous WMA and WMA onset in a previously normal segment signify myocardial ischemia; however, the clinical settings differ. In a patient with normal resting LV function, the test is performed for the diagnosis of ischemia, whereas in patients with a resting WMA, it is performed to assess the reversibility of the abnormality (i.e., its capacity to recover after revascularization)
[d]That is, less hypokinetic or frankly normalized, if there was a baseline WMA, or hyperkinetic, if baseline contractility was normal

presence of CAD, *the prognosis* of such localized changes is generally benign, and missing candidates for interventional therapy is highly unlikely.

Indications: SE is used (a) *for diagnostic purposes:* when baseline EKG precludes an EKG stress test, or when the suspicion of CAD remains, despite an inconclusive EKG stress test; (b) *for prognostic and management purposes (risk stratification),* to assess the severity (magnitude of LV dysfunction, size of the affected area, reversibility of segmental dysfunction) and localization of ischemic involvement. Stress echo can be used in asymptomatic patients with risk factors for CAD; with suspected stable angina, to establish the diagnosis, prognosis, and optimal management; with low-risk unstable angina; or for post-MI risk stratification if PCI was not performed; (c) *for assessing the functional significance of angiographically documented stenoses.*

The possible *complications* when using physical exercise are those discussed for EKG stress test. The complications of Dobutamine stress test include: *hypotension* (due to activation of the Bezold–Jarisch reflex, i.e., vagal triggering by the myocardial C fibers, activated by increased LV contractility in face of a relatively underfilled LV); and arrhythmia, angina exacerbation, headache, dizziness, nausea, shortness of breath, tremor, or flushing. Of note, the hypotension associated to the Dobutamine stress test does not carry

Table 2.13 Capabilities and shortcomings of rest (R) and stress (S) echo in the diagnosis of MI

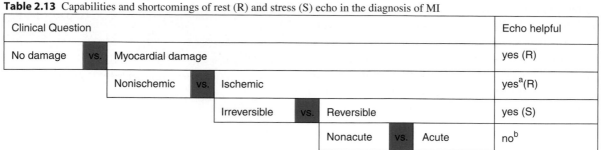

Clinical Question				Echo helpful
No damage	vs. Myocardial damage			yes (R)
	Nonischemic	vs. Ischemic		yes[a] (R)
		Irreversible	vs. Reversible	yes (S)
			Nonacute vs. Acute	no[b]

[a]Ischemic damage usually follows a coronary distribution pattern. This criterion is not 100% specific, as non-ischemic damage, e.g., myocarditis, can occasionally also follow a segmental pattern
[b]Except if a recent normal echo is available, and there was no intervening ischemic episode

the same severe prognosis as with exercise stress test; Dobutamine discontinuation is usually sufficient to abort the symptoms. The capabilities and shortcomings of echo for diagnosis of ischemia are summarized in Table 2.13.

2.2.3.3 Nuclear Scan

Principles: Using a gamma camera, the test detects myocardial uptake of a nuclear tracer injected IV. Uptake depends on the coronary blood flow (affected by atherosclerosis) and on myocardial integrity (affected by ischemia). Ischemia manifests as decreased segmental myocardial radiotracer uptake on a perfusion scan, and as segmental WMA on gated SPECT. Correlating decreases of perfusion and regional function improves the sensitivity and specificity of the nuclear scan. The changes may be obvious at rest or under stress, and their magnitude, location, and temporal evolution offer

important diagnostic clues. Stress may be elicited by exercise on a treadmill or a bicycle, or by administration of pharmacological agents, mainly including vasodilator agents (Dobutamine nuclear scan is possible, but rarely used). The action mechanism of vasodilators differs from that of exercise or Dobutamine (Table 2.14).

Technology: *Radiotracers:* Nuclear scan can be performed using thallium (Tl), technetium (Tc), or both. *Thallium* has a long half-life (approximately 3 days), precluding administration of large doses. This decreases spatial resolution and makes Tl suboptimal for gated SPECT, which requires good endocardial border delineation (segmental LV function is assessed based on the systolic inward progression of the endocardial border). On the positive side, the long half-life of Tl makes possible the phenomenon of *redistribution* (hypo- or non-captating segments "fill in" a number of hours after the initial stress images). The standard waiting period for redistribution is 4 h; this *early redistribution* is indicative of ischemia (perfusion of the ischemic segment is

Table 2.14 Stressor mechanisms in nuclear perfusion scans

	Exercise, Dobutamine	Dipyridamole, Adenosine
Mechanism	Exerting the myocardium supplied by stenotic arteries disturbs the local O_2 supply/demand balance	Selective vasodilatation of the healthy coronaries, as the stenotic ones are already maximally vasodilated
Tracer uptake in the affected segment is less than in the neighboring segments[a]	Yes	Yes
Tracer uptake in the affected segment is less than the local metabolic needs	Yes	Not as a main mechanism[b]
Remarks	"Absolute" ischemia	"Relative" ischemia

[a]The ischemic segment(s) "stand out" as showing low uptake, since the degree of tracer uptake is compared to that of the non-ischemic segments. *All* the segments being ischemic may cause a false-negative read, a hazard substantially diminished by correlation with LV function and with "high-risk findings"
[b]Some degree of steal phenomenon (diversion of blood from the affected territories to the healthy ones) does occur, as demonstrated by the feasibility of vasodilator stress echo (rarely used)

"slow," but not absent). However, up to 40% of segments with absent early redistribution may improve functionally after revascularization – an unacceptable rate of "missed opportunities" for interventional therapy. These patients may be singled out by checking for *late redistribution,* at 24 h. Late redistribution is diagnostic of myocardial hibernation. The logistical burden of next-day imaging may be solved by rest reinjection of Tl later the same day, to boost fill-in of the initially non-captating segments. With Tl imaging, the stress images are obtained first; if they are normal, there is no need for resting imaging. *Technetium* has a much shorter half-life than Tl, i.e., 6 h. This allows injection of higher doses of tracer (since the decay is fast and the total exposure to radiation is still low), ensuring better spatial resolution and making EKG gating possible. Unfortunately, Tc does not redistribute. While this allows to diagnose ischemia (a second radiotracer dose is injected a few hours after the first, followed by repeat imaging), Tc is not ideal for assessment of myocardial hibernation (viability). Segments retaining at stress >60% of the count recorded at rest tend to improve after revascularization. Tc protocols generally use the "rest first" approach, since the higher tracer dosage given with stress would require a longer waiting time for adequate decay before the second dose is given. *Dual isotope imaging* uses resting Tl and stress Tc imaging significantly shortens the protocol (no waiting between rest and stress), while keeping the advantages of gated SPECT (Tc imaging). As Tl and Tc have different energy levels, stress imaging with Tc is not influenced by the still strong Tl-related radiation.

Imaging technology: Unlike echo, where each and every cardiac cycle is individually imaged, with nuclear scan several hundred cycles are summed up electronically (temporal summation), as the radiation emitted per cycle is very faint. The camera continuously records the emitted radiation, and "allocates" each count to the different phases of systole and diastole, based on a simultaneous EKG tracing. Proper count allocation to a specific slot within either systole or diastole requires a regular heart rhythm. These images are displayed either in a static, or (with gated SPECT) in a dynamic, endless-loop format. The sections are either *transversal* (apex-to-base short-axis sections) or *longitudinal*, running from the septum to the lateral wall (vertical long axis, corresponding to the echocardiographic two-chamber view), or from the inferior to the anterior wall (horizontal long axis, corresponding

to the four-chamber view; of note, the RV is normally not visualized by nuclear scan). The LV segmentation and its correspondence to coronary anatomy are discussed in Sect. 2.1.

The radiotracer is injected approximately 1 min before peak stress, so its distribution indeed reflects cardiac function under stress (even if the patient is "resting" in the scanning machine during the actual readings). *Dipyridamole*, if used, is injected at doses of 0.14 mg/kg/min, over 4 min, followed by radiotracer injection after an additional 4 min. Headache, nausea, hypotension, dizziness, flushing, and AV block may ensue, occasionally requiring neutralization with an IV bolus of 50–100 mg Aminophylline. Dipyridamole acts by stimulating *adenosine* release. The latter is also available for IV administration as such (140 µg/kg/min over 4 min). It has the same adverse effects as Dipyridamole, but, due to its very short half-life, adverse effects usually disappear with infusion interruption. *Interpretation*: Ischemic segments may have decreased, absent, or abnormally delayed tracer uptake. The responsible artery or arteries can be inferred from the involved segments. As with echo, two questions are answered: whether ischemia is present, and whether it is reversible (Table 2.15).

High-risk findings (probable severe coronary disease) include increased pulmonary uptake (ischemia-related increased LVEDP) and transient ischemic dilatation (TID) of the LV after stress. The latter may represent true LV ischemic dilatation or diffuse subendocardial ischemia, falsely displacing the perceived endocardial border inward, i.e., increasing the LV diameter. The degree and extent of LV dysfunction are assessed on SPECT scan, by the same semi-quantitative method used for echo assessment. Corroboration of information relative to perfusion and to regional LV function improves diagnostic accuracy. LVEF can be calculated with greater precision than with echo, although, for most clinical applications, the two methods are similarly appropriate. An exception, however, is LV function evaluation in patients before and between courses of cardiotoxic chemotherapy (most commonly, Adriamycin), where scintigraphic evaluation is the norm.

The indications for perfusion scan are, by and large, the same as those for stress echo. A special indication for pharmacologic (rather than exercise) stress test is the presence of LBBB or of pacemaker rhythm, which may create imaging artifacts under exercise.

Table 2.15 Nuclear perfusion scan

Uptake at rest[a]	Uptake after stress[a]	Interpretation	Reversibility after revascularization
Normal	Normal	No ischemia	N/A
Normal	Decreased	Inducible ischemia	Yes
Normal	Decreased at 4 h[b], improved at 24 h[c]	Hibernating myocardium	Yes
Decreased	Decreased	Scar	No
Decreased	Improved	Reverse redistribution, mainly[d] seen in post- MI patients[e]	Occasionally

[a]The terms "decreased" and "improved" are preferred to "normal" or "abnormal," as radiotracer uptake follows a continuum. The highest uptake in the image (brightest spot) is considered "normal" and serves for comparison to the other segments
[b]Myocardial uptake in viable segments generally retains ≥50–60% uptake – the only indicator of viability when using Tc
[c]Can also be checked by Tl reinjection, at rest
[d]Reverse redistribution has been reported (rarely) in normals or in patients with non-ischemic heart disease (e.g., sarcoidosis)
[e]The significance is debated. Explanations include hyperemia in the peri-MI area or myocardial salvage by therapeutic or spontaneous thrombolysis

The complications are those of any stress test. The adverse effects of pharmacological agents and the recommended management were discussed above.

2.2.3.4 Positron Emission Tomography

Positron emission tomography (PET) is based on the phenomenon of positron annihilation, whereby the radiotracer emits protons, a process that can be imaged, to obtain (a) an absolute quantitation of capillary blood flow to the myocardium, using perfusion agents. This is different from the relative quantitation achieved by SPECT, where the brightest spot on the image is considered "normal," and the rest of the image is calibrated accordingly; (b) imaging of the myocardial metabolism, using FDG, a "fake" glucose that is absorbed, but cannot be processed, by the myocytes; (c) identification of fragile atherosclerotic plaque, an application currently of research interest only. Viable myocardium is characterized by preserved myocardial metabolism despite decreased blood flow. PET is the gold standard for demonstration of myocardial viability. Due to the relatively burdensome logistics and to the higher cost, this procedure is used relatively infrequently. A combined approach, using SPECT for myocardial blood flow, solves the main logistical problem, as it is precisely the PET-specific flow tracers that (unlike FDG) have a short shelf-life. Metabolism is then investigated with PET, in this *hybrid SPECT/PET* approach.

2.2.3.5 Cardiac CT

MDCT (multidetector, also called multislice CT) is the gold standard of noninvasive coronary angiography. It has a high negative predictive value, allowing to rule out CAD. Due to its high cost and reduced availability, MDCT cannot yet be recommended as an initial screening agent, but is ideal in patients with ambiguous symptoms and a nonspecific stress test. Of note, the test is radiation-intensive, and concern has been raised about its potential oncogenicity. *Detection of coronary calcification,* a marker of atherosclerosis, using *EBCT (electron-beam CT)* has high sensitivity (90%) but low specificity (54%) for prediction of future CAD and stroke, and is best used as a screening tool. Abnormal results require confirmation by angiography (classic or angio-CT). EBCT is strongly supported by some, but considered by others as not conclusively providing additional information in patients in whom an accurate risk profile has been calculated by simpler methods. The amount of coronary calcium is usually expressed by the Agatston score: a score of zero, <100, 100–399, 400–999, and >1,000 corresponds to absent, mild, moderate, severe, and extensive calcification, respectively. *CT imaging of the myocardium* may be used for assessment of LV aneurysm, thrombus, etc. The "triple scan" approach, i.e., CT to rule out ACS, aortic dissection, and PE, has recently made significant progress both in the image quality and in the amount of administered radiation, which has been significantly diminished with the current techniques.

2.2.3.6 Cardiac MRI

Cardiac MRI can be used in several manners in the diagnosis of CAD: *MRI angiography* is mainly indicated for the diagnosis of congenital coronary anomalies; in the field of atherosclerosis, it currently serves as a research tool, able to define not only myocardial perfusion and coronary anatomy, but plaque morphology as well. This enables angiography, classically a luminogram (delineating the inner vessel border) to assess not only the *extent,* but also the *type* of plaque. Identification of vulnerable plaques may justify aggressive risk factor control. *MRI stress test* is an emerging technique, able to demonstrate both perfusion and regional wall motion abnormalities. Due to its increased cost and limited availability, it is especially recommended in patients with technically difficult echo studies; *MRI myocardial imaging* may demonstrate LV aneurysm, thrombus, etc.

2.2.3.7 Coronary Angiography

Coronary angiography is the current gold standard for coronary anatomy definition, also allowing PCI, if needed. Coronary angiography generally represents the last step of workup (clinical and EKG evaluation, stress testing). Occasionally, however (very high suspicion of coronary disease, ACS, recent cardiac arrest) there is neither time nor justification for preliminary noninvasive testing. Invasive coronarography is a *luminogram,* demonstrating the severity of stenosis, but not the stable or vulnerable nature of the plaque. Even as a luminogram, contrast coronarography is suboptimal, as it represents a summation image, i.e., a 2-D representation of 3-D structures; despite imaging from different angles (standard or nonstandard views), the degree of stenosis occasionally remains ambiguous. In these patients, intravascular ultrasound *(IVUS)* may help assess stenosis severity, plaque

anatomy, and coronary remodeling. IVUS is invaluable for detecting diffuse disease (atherosclerosis, transplant vasculopathy), evenly narrowing the coronary bed and often undetected by classical angiography. The functional significance of "borderline" (50–70%) stenoses is occasionally not clear, i.e., it is not obvious to what extent the perfusion of the dependent myocardium is decreased (Table 2.16). This may be clarified by assessment of vasodilator-induced flow increase, which is impaired by atherosclerosis (endothelial dysfunction).

2.2.3.8 Biological markers

The use of *biological markers* in the diagnosis of CAD is reviewed in Table 2.17.

2.2.3.9 Other Diagnostic Methods

Assessment of the intima-media thickness: (IMT), defined as the span between the intima/lumen and the media/adventitia boders is measured bilaterally by B-mode ultrasound, at the distal 1 cm of the common carotid, at the bifurcation, and at the proximal 1 cm of the internal carotid artery. Values >1.3 mm are an independent risk factor for stroke and (a fact questioned by some) coronary atherosclerosis. High-resolution ultrasound allows plaque characterization (ulceration, thrombosis, etc.), with prognostic relevance for future CVA. IMT is strongly associated with atherosclerosis, and serves as a surrogate endpoint for evaluating the regression or progression of atherosclerotic disease. However, not all the processes of thickening of the intima-media are due to atherosclerosis. *The ankle-brachial index (ABI)* is the ratio between the systolic BP in the brachial and the posterior tibial or dorsalis pedis arteries, measured with a Doppler probe, after release of compression with a sphygmomanometer

Table 2.16 Assessing the functional impact of coronary stenosis

Parameter	Definition	Determinants	Normal Values
Vasodilator reserve	Ratio between baseline and maximally enhanced flow	Epicardial stenosis and microvascular impairment	>3[a]
Fractional flow reserve (FFR)	The ratio between flow velocity immediately distal to the stenosis in the aorta	Epicardial coronary stenosis	1[b]; <0.75 distinctly abnormal

[a]There is substantial individual variability. Normal tissue flow is >2 mL/min×g
[b]Aortic flow propagates to the distal coronary bed "as if the stenosis weren't there." FFR-guided PCI has been recently proven to carry substantial clinical benefits, by reducing the risk of death, MI, or repeat revascularization by 30%, as compared to patients in whom stenting decisions were based on QCA assessment alone

cuff. A ratio <0.9 is an independent risk factor for PVD and for coronary and cerebral complications. The procedure is time- and skill-intensive. It is not sensitive to lower degrees of atherosclerosis, and can yield false-negative results in patients with severe atherosclerosis, due to spuriously increased arterial pressure resulting from increased vessel rigidity. *Opthalmoscopy* has been suggested as a screening tool in asymptomatic patients, as there is a good correlation between retinal and global atherosclerosis. Several *novel technologies* hold promise to revolutionize the diagnosis of coronary ischemia and to improve its timeliness, a critical point overall, but especially relevant in STEMI patients. These include ST-segment shift detection by an intracardiac electrogram monitoring system built into the latest generation of ICD, as well as systems entirely dedicated ST-shift detection, similar to an implantable Holter device, and providing a sound alert in case of significant ST segment shifts.

2.2.4 Evaluation for Cardiovascular Risk Before Noncardiac Surgery

Evaluation for cardiovascular risk before non-cardiac surgery is recommended depending on the severity of risk factors or of preexisting atherosclerosis, as well as according to the type of surgery being contemplated. Patients in need of emergency, life-saving surgery should be operated on as needed, under optimal perioperative surveillance. As a rule of thumb, the indication for preoperative evaluation is stronger if the patient- and surgery-related risk are higher (Table 2.18). In patients with no known heart disease, but present risk factors and a low (or unknown) functional capacity, preoperative evaluation is also reasonable.

The tests to be performed are adapted to the patient's specific problem. An EKG is almost universally obtained, and EKG monitoring is indicated in patients with known CAD. An echo should be obtained in patients with LV

Table 2.17 Biomarkers in the diagnosis of CAD[a]

Marker	Diagnostic value	Prognostic value	Remarks
Troponin	Distinguishes NSTEMI-ACS from UA	NSTEMI-ACS has a poorer prognosis than UA	Mild increases occasionally first detected at 48–72 h, leading to an initial classification as UA[b]
hsCRP[c]	None	Portends poorer prognosis[d]	Reflects the systemic inflammation that triggered ACS and/or inflammation in the vulnerable plaque
BNP	None	As above[d]; prognostic value preserved after adjustment for LVEF or Killip class	Reflects LV dysfunction; useful for differential diagnosis of dyspnea
RFT	None	Portends poorer prognosis[d]	Creatinin[e], CrCl, cystatin C[f]

[a]Novel markers, investigating oxidative stress, coagulation cascade activation, vascular-specific inflammation, etc., are under study
[b]This underscores the importance of clinical diagnosis for management decisions. There are multiple non-ACS (cardiac or non-cardiac) causes for troponin elevation, some of great clinical concern (PE, aortic dissection, etc.). Non-cardiac troponin elevations are frequent with creatinine levels >2.5 mg/dL (μ mol/L). For other comments, see under "STEMI"
[c]High-sensitivity CRP assay
[d]May help management decisions in areas where PCI is not universally available
[e]Creatinin varies with age, gender, muscle mass, and race
[f]Less dependent on the factors that influence creatinine levels; as yet unclear clinical relevance (not superior to formula-adjusted CrCl); normal 0.5 – 1.0 mg/L (may vary among laboratories)

Table 2.18 Patient- and surgery-related risk before non-cardiac surgery

Risk	Surgery-related	Patient-related
High	Vascular surgery	Active heart disease (unstable or severe angina; worsening, decompensated, or new-onset HF; significant arrhythmia; severe AS or severe MS)
Moderate	All procedures not considered either high or low	Established atherosclerosis, including coronary (inactive), as well as patients with ≥3 risk factors for atherosclerosis
Low	Endoscopic procedures; breast; cataract; ambulatory; or superficial surgery	All other patients

dysfunction, overt HF, or VHD. An EKG, TTE or TEE, and an imaging stress test are indicated in accordance with the principles exposed above. Preoperative revascularization (by CABG or by PCI) is recommended in patients with ACS; three-vessel disease; LMCA disease; and two-vessel disease with significant proximal LAD stenosis and decreased LV function. PCI has been shown inferior to CABG in patients with complex coronary lesions (SYNTAX trial), and to optimal medical therapy, in patients with stable CAD (COURAGE trial) or with an occluded infarct-related artery (OAT study). However, according to newly published registry data, LMCA artery stenting appears effective and safe. Bare-metal stents are indicated if the contemplated surgery cannot be deferred >12 months, as this is the minimal duration of dual antiplatelet therapy after DES deployment. Pre-operative revascularization is mostly warranted in patients with significant wall motion abnormalities (≥5 abnormal segments), but this indication, too, is relative, and individualization is required. The recommended treatment is similar to that which would be chosen were it not for the surgical event. Invasive (Swan–Ganz) hemodynamic monitoring requires individual tailoring; by no means is it routinely indicated. The same holds true for prophylactic IV Nitroglycerin. Body temperature and glucose concentration must be maintained normal.

Despite these precautions, *perioperative MI* still occurs in 2–6% of all surgical patients; the actual incidence is strongly influenced by comorbidity and the type and duration of surgery. Up to 50% of cases may go undiagnosed, a very important aspect, as perioperative MI is an independent predictor of 6-month mortality. The clinical manifestations may be obscured by those of the underlying disease, as well as by sedation and analgesia. Diagnosis follows the usual procedures. There are no randomized data regarding therapy, which follows the general rules observed in any MI, with the important caveat that thrombolysis is contraindicated and anticoagulation must be used cautiously, if at all.

2.2.5 Ischemia: Therapy

Myocardial ischemia consists in the imbalance between myocardial demands and coronary flow; thus, therapy will seek to decrease the former and to increase the latter. Myocardial demands are mainly decreased by slowing the HR (other mechanisms are operational with some newer-generation agents used in stable angina; see Sect. 2.3). The bulk of the available therapeutic measures address restoration of decreased blood flow, involving relief of coronary stenosis, spasm, and/or thrombosis. The aims and modalities of CAD treatment are reviewed in Table 2.19. Properly speaking, management of the patient with risk factors only does not belong to the spectrum of ischemia therapy, since what is being prevented is in fact ischemia *onset*. However, as the ultimate purpose of this prevention does refer to myocardial ischemia, these patients are also included in the table.

Myocardial revascularization may be achieved pharmacologically, interventionally (PCI or CABG), or by a combination of the two approaches. The main therapeutic agents and modalities are reviewed below, while the specific indications in the ACS and in the stable angina patient are discussed in Sect. 2.3.

Table 2.19 Therapy of myocardial ischemia: aims and modalities

Condition	Treatment – aims	Treatment – modalities
Risk factors	*Prevent* plaque formation (*primary prevention*)	Risk factor management, including (where appropriate) drug therapy for hyperlipidemia, smoking cessation, weight loss, increased homocystein levels[a]
Stable angina	*Prevent* plaque growth and artery occlusion; *treat* ischemic symptoms	As above, + nitrates, β-/calcium-blockers, Aspirin, elective revascularization, and newer dugs (Sect. 2.3)
ACS	*Prevent* further plaque fissure/rupture and coronary thrombosis; *treat* thrombosis, its symptoms and complications; *Prevent* ACS recurrence and coronary restenosis (*secondary prevention*), rehabilitate patient after ACS	As above, but revascularization or IV thrombolysis are urgent or emergent; oxygen; morphine; IABP

[a]Use of Aspirin in primary prevention is not warranted, even in the presence of risk factors, due to an unfavorable risk/efficacy balance in this setting; however, other data indicate that women aged ≥65 may still benefit from primary prevention with Aspirin 81 mg to 100 mg q.d. Lowering homocystein with folic acid and vitamin B_{12} was not proven beneficial

2.2.5.1 Pharmacological Therapy

General therapeutic agents are reviewed in Table 2.20. *Antiplatelet agents* are reviewed in Table 2.21, followed by a discussion of resistance to Aspirin and Clopidogrel. Newer agents are briefly discussed.

Aspirin resistance manifests as the inability to inhibit platelet aggregation (as assessed by various tests). However, as the target degree of platelet activation is still unclear, assessment of platelet (in)activation for clinical purposes is not recommended. When Aspirin resistance is suspected, Clopidogrel is empirically substituted. Aspirin resistance was believed to be in part due to COX-2 receptor activation (Aspirin is only effective on COX-1 receptors); however, COX-2 inhibitors have been proven deleterious in CAD patients. Aspirin can be ineffective when used concurrently with other NSAID agents, which block its binding site. *Aspirin hypersensitivity* mainly manifests as bronchospasm or skin rash; true anaphylaxis is rare. Aspirin desensitization may be an option, especially in settings where the alternative drug, Clopidogrel, is not available. *Clopidogrel resistance* has also been reported, but is difficult to assess clinically; furthermore, there is no proven correlation between lab test results and clinical outcomes. The association of PPIs with Clopidogrel has recently been proved to not significantly decrease the antiplatelet activity of the latter agent, despite initial reports to the contrary.

In case of significant bleeding under platelet inhibitors, or when emergency major surgery is required, the action of Aspirin or Clopidogrel must be neutralized. This is achieved as shown in Table 2.22.

Agents under development: SCH 530348, the first thrombin receptor antagonist, is being evaluated by the TRACER trial; it is a candidate as an adjunct therapy, to be used together with Clopidogrel.

Antithrombin agents are reviewed in Table 2.23, followed by a brief review of some important issues related to Heparin and LMWH.

Gradual discontinuation of Heparin treatment is empirically recommended, to avoid the rebound phenomenon (a high-risk period for recurrent thrombosis). The main caveat of Heparin is an occasionally very serious syndrome, Heparin-induced thrombocytopenia, seen in 3–5% of patients exposed to UFH, and in <1% of those exposed to LMWH. This syndrome is classified as reviewed in Table 2.24. Platelet counts should be monitored daily in patients treated with UFH. Pseudo-HIT can be caused by platelet aggregation in vitro, in EDTA-containing vials. Repeat platelet counts should be obtained using citrate-containing vials, to avoid false reads.

LMWH: It was noted early on that the anticoagulant potency of UFH is variable from batch to batch, due to the difference in molecular weight and in pharmacological activity between the many component molecules. There arose the question whether isolating some of the molecular components of UFH would make the therapeutic action more predictable. The low-molecular weight fraction of UFH was shown to possess unique pharmacological abilities. Unlike UFH, which binds to both antithrombin III (AT III) and to several coagulation factors (factors IIa (thrombin), Xa, IXa, XIa, and XIIa), very small fragments containing the binding site for factor Xa sequence more or less selectively inhibit the latter. All LMWH have a Factor Xa/thrombin activity ratio >1.5:1 (most commonly, 2–4:1); Fondaparinux does not act on thrombin at all. LMWH have revolutionized anticoagulation: (1) *safety-wise,* as they have a lower incidence of adverse effects and a more predictable anticoagulant activity as compared to Heparin, making over- and under-dosage less likely. The more predictable dose-effect relationship that that of UFH is due to the almost complete absorbtion by the S.C. route; less protein binding; and to the lesser degree of platelet activation; (2) *efficacy-wise,* as they are superior to UFH for several crucial indications: Fondaparinux is preferred to Heparin in STEMI patients not undergoing thrombolysis; Fondaparinux and Enoxaparin are as good as Heparin in patients undergoing thrombolysis; and, although not indicated for primary PCI, they are highly effective in patients being prepared for rescue PCI or for routine post-thrombolysis PCI; and (3) *logistics-wise,* as they may be self-administered in many conditions (not related to ACS), and generally do not require lab monitoring (although the latter is available, as anti-factor Xa level assessment, target: 0.5–1.5 U/mL). On the negative side, LMWH are significantly more expensive than UFH.

In case of significant bleeding under UFH or LMWH, or when emergency major surgery is required, the anticoagulant drugs must be neutralized. For UFH, this is achieved by administration of Protamin (see under "Treatment of hemorrhagic stroke"). With LMWH, Protamin is less active than with UFH, and activated factor VII may be used, but caution is recommended, as this may cause thrombosis.

Table 2.20 The pharmacological treatment of CAD[a]

Agent	Mechanism	Clinical effect	Indications	C/I; adverse effects and their treatment
Agents reserved to ACS therapy				
Oxygen	Ventilation-perfusion mismatch and excessive lung water may cause modest early hypoxemia even in uncomplicated ACS. O_2 may limit ischemic injury and reduce ST elevations	Symptom relief	Absolute: SaO_2 <90%; relative: in all ACS patients[b]	Excess O_2 can cause systemic vasoconstriction or, in COPD patients, respiratory depression
Morphine	Relieves pain, which increases sympathetic activity, favoring plaque fissuring and thrombus propagation; Peripheral vasodilation and the reduction in the work of breathing are helpful in pulmonary edema	Symptom relief, sedation	All patients complaining of chest pain	Vagomimetic effects (countered with IV atropine 0.5–1.5 mg); low HR and BP (countered with IV Dopamine or Dobutamine, or with Naloxone, IV 0.1–0.2 mg, may repeat after 15 min)
Antithrombin agents	Inhibit thrombus growth	Symptom relief	All patients	See Sect. 2.3
Thrombolytics	Dissolve occluding clot	See STEMI		
Agents reserved to stable angina therapy				
Ivabradine[c]	Slows HR by inhibition of the sinus node	Symptom relief	Second-line agent	luminous phenomena (sensations of enhanced brightness); bradycardia, headaches first-degree AV block, VPBs, dizziness, blurred vision
Trimetazidine	Improves myocardial glucose utilization by depressing fatty acid metabolism	Symptom relief	Second-line agent	None notable
Ranolazine	Indirectly prevents the calcium overload contributing to cardiac ischemia	Symptom relief	Second-line agent	May prolong QT and cause LFT alterations
Nicorandil	Peripheral venous dilatation; may reduce death and hospitalization for angina	Symptom relief	The only newer agent with a Class I indication	Flushing, palpitation, weakness, headache, mouth and perianal ulcers, nausea and vomiting
Agents used in all CAD patients[d]				
Nitrates	Vasodilation (a) peripheral (arterial and venous dilation reduces pre- and afterload reduction); (b) epicardial and collateral vessels; (c) of the atherosclerotic coronaries	Symptom relief	Ischemic discomfort; IV in ACS patients with ongoing discomfort; HTN; pulmonary congestion; coronary spasm	BP <90 mmHg or decrease ≥30 mmHg below baseline, HR <50 or >100 bpm), or suspected RV MI; phosphodiesterase inhibitor for erectile dysfunction <24 h[e]

(*continued*)

Table 2.20 (continued)

Agent	Mechanism	Clinical effect	Indications	C/I; adverse effects and their treatment
β-blockers[f]	Decrease myocardial O_2 demand by reducing HR, BP, and myocardial contractility. Prolong diastole (by reducing HR), increasing myocardial perfusion. Reduce the frequency, severity and duration of stable angina episodes; the risk for myocardial necrosis, in unstable angina; MI size, complications and recurrence rate; and the risk of lethal ventricular tachyarrhythmias.	Symptom relief	All patients	HR <60 bpm; systolic BP <100 mmHg, ≥moderate LV failure; PR >0.24 s; 2-d or 3-d degree AV block; active asthma; cocaine-related MI (may exacerbate coronary spasm). Antidote: IV β-adrenergic agonists (i.e., Isoproterenol 1–5 μg/min).
Antiplatelet agents	Inhibit formation of platelet clot	See Table 2.21	All patients	See text
ACE inhibitors	Reduce oxidative stress, improve endothelial function, favorable effect on adhesion molecules and cytokines, inhibit LDL uptake by macrophages, prevent myocardial and perivascular fibrosis and LVH	Reduce mortality, MI, stroke, and HF in patients with cardiovascular disease or high-risk diabetes	All patients	See Chap. 3
ARB	As above	Suboptimal results	in ACEI-intolerant high-risk patients ≥55[g]	See Chap. 3
Statins	See text		All patients	See text

[a] The dosages are discussed in the text

[b] In patients with severe HF or a mechanical complication of STEMI, continuous positive-pressure (C-PAP) breathing or mechanical ventilation may be required

[c] Preliminary data seem to demonstrate the feasibility of Ivabradine treatment as an alternative to Metoprolol in STEMI patients

[d] ACEI or ARB are indicated in patients with HF, diabetes, or HTN. In patients with LV dysfunction (EF <40%) and diabetes or HF, aldosterone antagonists are used on top of ACEI CCB are generally used in stable angina. Their use in ACS is reserved for the occasional patient with Prinzmetal's angina, where they help release coronary spasm

[e] Most of the randomized data date from the pre-thrombolytic era. The utility of IV administration is uncertain; if this route is chosen, IV Atenolol 5–10 mg, followed by PO Atenolol, 100 mg q.d

[f] Forty-eight hours for tadalafil

[g] The ONTARGET trial has found an important decrease of hard cardiovascular endpoint incidence in patients with high-risk cardiovascular disease or diabetes treated with either ACEI or ARB, but combining the two classes increases the rate of adverse events, without added benefit

Table 2.21 Antiplatelet agents

	Mechanism	Adverse effects[a]	Remarks
NSAIDs			
Aspirin[b]	Irreversible inhibition of platelet cyclo-oxygenase, decreasing formation of thromboxane A2 (a stimulant of platelet aggregation)	Gastric irritation	Other NSAID drugs, especially COX-2 inhibitors, are C/I in CAD[c]
Thienopyridines			
Clopidogrel (Plavix)	Inhibit ADP-induced platelet aggregation	GI upset, rash, neutropenia, purpura, dyspnea	Has replaced Ticlopidine
Prasugrel (Ef(f)ient)			Higher efficacy and bleeding rates than with Clopidogrel[d]
Ticlopidine (Ticlid)			Rarely used today
Ticagrelor			Superior to, safer than Clopidogrel in reducing MACE; twice-daily dosing; the only reversible antiplatelet agent
IIb/IIIa inhibitors			
Abciximab (ReoPro)	Binding to the IIb/IIIa platelet receptor, instrumental in platelet aggregation. Blockade of the final pathway of platelet aggregation and, under high shear forces, of the von Willebrand factor as well	Thrombocytopenia, hypersensitivity reactions	An expensive monoclonal antibody
Eptifibatide (Integrilin)		Thrombocytopenia	
Tirofiban (Aggrastat)		Thrombocytopenia	
Phosphodiesterase inhibitors			
Dipyridamole (Persantine)	Countering of platelet aggregation driven by Phosphodiesterase and by other mechanisms; coronary vasodilatation by inhibition of Adenosine degradation	Angina (coronary "steal"); dizziness, hypotension, headache, rash, GI upset, dyspnea, palpitations	No longer used in CAD; diagnostic use in nuclear cardiology
Cilostazol (Pletal)	Countering of platelet aggregation driven by Phosphodiesterase	headache, palpitations, diarrhea, peripheral edema	Unlabeled use as adjunct to Aspirin after coronary stenting[e]

[a]In addition to bleeding, which can be seen with all these agents
[b]Aspirin is the only agent routinely used in stable angina. Triflusal is an antiaggregant related to the salicylate group, with an as yet unclear place in the antiplatelet armamentarium; Clopidogrel is recommended in patients with Aspirin intolerance or resistance
[c]Recent studies suggest that the safest NSAID agent in CHD patients is Naproxen. However, definitive data are still pending
[d]Early Prasugrel treatment might be switched to Clopidogrel after 30 days, as the advantage with Prasugrel is highest early on
[e]This might reduce in-stent restenosis rates

Oral direct thrombin inhibitors have recently reached clinical applicability. Dabigatran, Rivaroxaban and a host of other compounds (Table 2.23) are being assessed in patients with coronary disease. A new agent, provisionally called SCH 530348, the first thrombin *receptor* antagonist, holds the promise of reducing ischemic events without increasing bleeding, in elective PCI patients.

Vitamin K antagonists (VKA) have a relatively modest place in the treatment of CAD. They are to be continued, in addition to antiplatelet therapy, in patients with another indication for their use. In case of LV thrombus, VKA are indicated on a long-time basis (target INR 2–3), as the cause of LV thrombosis is most frequently LV aneurysm, a chronic condition. In high-risk patients in whom Clopidogrel is not

Table 2.22 Reversal of antithrombotic therapy

Agent	Reversal	Remarks
Aspirin, Clopidogrel	Platelet transfusions[a]	Effect persists for 5–10 days, the normal lifespan of platelets; 10–20% of platelets are naturally renewed daily
IIb/IIIa inhibitors[b]	Platelet transfusions	Abciximab: platelet infusion effective, optimal duration not clear; Tirofiban or eptifibatide eliminated renally, effects last 4–8 h. Immediate neutralization more problematic; FFP or plasma cryoprecipitate supplementation useful, as it acts on fibrinogen-dependent platelet aggregation

[a]Recommended dose, $5–7 \times 10^{11}$ platelets in a 70-kg adult; for reference, a typical platelet unit contains $0.6–0.8 \times 10^{11}$ platelets (random platelets), and thus $1–1^1/_2$ units are required for each 10 kg of body weight
[b]IIb/III a inhibitors can also decrease platelet counts without actual hemorrhage; close follow-up is mandatory. Drug discontinuation and platelet supplementation are recommended for platelet counts <10,000/μL. No clear guidelines exist for lesser platelet decreases. Bivalirudin may be equally effective as the IIb/IIIa inhibitor + heparin combination, and can be used in case of uncertainty regarding the origin of the platelet decrease

available and/or not tolerated, Warfarin is added, with a target INR of 2–2.5. The same target is used for Aspirin-resistant patients, in whom Clopidogrel is unavailable or ineffective.

Fibrinolytic Therapy: See Sect. 2.3

2.2.5.2 Interventional Therapy

Interventional therapy includes PCI or CABG. Revascularization may represent (a) *in ACS patients:* an alternative to IV thrombolysis; a rescue procedure after failed IV thrombolysis; or a routine procedure after IV thrombolysis; (b) *in patients with stable angina,* an elective procedure. These different scenarios are discussed in Sect. 2.3.

PCI; Most PCI procedures are performed with stent deployment, to avoid the high restenosis rate of simple PTCA (up to 40% at 6 months). As opposed to the default transfemoral approach, transradial PCI shows significantly fewer bleeding complications and equivalent procedural success. In certain European nations, the transradial approach has become the preferred approach. Simple (stentless) PTCA is reserved as a bridge to subsequent, definitive therapy (e.g., subsequent CABG, in patients presenting with ACS, and in whom rapid restoration of flow of the culprit artery is sought). However, restenosis still occurs in up to 30% of bare-metal stents, especially in small vessels, in patients with suboptimal post-intervention results, long lesions, diabetes, LAD lesions, or untreated stent edge dissection. Drug-eluting stents (DES) have dramatically decreased restenosis rates (by inhibiting neointimal proliferation), but late thrombosis is increased, mandating at least 1 year of dual antiplatelet therapy

(Aspirin + Clopidogrel). The possibility that the lower restenosis rate achieved by DES might be compromised by a higher incidence of late stent thrombosis has polarized the cardiologic community. While these concerns appear to have been alleviated by the substantial amount of data accumulated since the initial reports regarding this issue, some DES may pose more risk than others. Figure 2.1 shows pre-and post-PCI images in the RCA and the LCx arteries.

Other percutaneous techniques: *Covered stents* are approved for coronary perforation and, on a case-by-case basis, for coronary aneurysm therapy. *Atherectomy devices* capitalize on the concept that, while classic PCI procedures simply flatten out and "redistribute" the atherosclerotic plaque, it may be possible to actually remove the latter from the vessel. *Cutting balloon devices* consist of several atherotomy blades, and are currently used in ostial and bifurcation lesions, as well as for in-stent restenosis. *Rotational atherectomy* uses a burr-like device that shaves off the plaque. Despite ensuring a higher procedural success, this approach does not improve outcomes; it is, however, useful before stenting of arteries that are severely calcified, undilatable, chronically totally occluded, as well as with bifurcation lesions. *Directional coronary atherectomy (DCA)* is rarely used today, except for the case of some debulking procedures. *Excimer laser*, at one time thought to improve outcomes due to the effective tissue section and to the minute size of the debris it creates, has not been found to improve outcomes and is rarely used today. *Mechanical thrombectomy devices*, creating a number of high-pressure fluid jets to macerate the thrombus, and able to subsequently absorb the debris, have actually been found to be deleterious in ACS, but newer generations of devices may improve ST segment resolution

Table 2.23 Antithrombin agents

	Mechanism	Adverse effects[a]	Remarks	Advantages	Disadvantages[b]
Indirect thrombin inhibitors					
Unfractioned Heparin (UFH)[c]	Activates AT III, which inactivates coagulation factors, (crucially, factors II=thrombin and X)	HIT, HITT, elevated AST/ALT, osteoporosis, hyperkalemia	Thrombin and Factor Xa inhibition are equally potent	Widely available; monitored by aPTT	Unpredictable anticoagulant potency, due to the non-homogenous molecular mix; risk of HIT
Low-molecular weight Heparin (LMWH)[c,d]	Mostly activates the site of AT III responsible for factor Xa inhibition	HIT, HITT, rash, fever, hematoma at injection site	Factor Xa inhibition 2–4[e] times more potent than thrombin inhibition	Less frequent adverse events, more predictable anticoagulant potency	More expensive than UFH; not optimal for primary PCI; risk of HIT lower than with UFH
Danaparoid	Factor X/factor II inhibition >22: 1	Fever, nausea, constipation	Similar action, different structure than LMWH	Chemically unrelated to Heparin, thus an option in HIT(T)	monitoring in patients with extremes of weight or renal failure; no longer available in the US
Direct thrombin inhibitors					
Argatroban[f]	Reversible binding to active site of thrombin	Hypotension, dyspnea, nausea, vomiting, fever	Alternative to Heparin in HIT or HIT-prone patients	Monitored by aPTT; no dose adjustment in renal failure; effect quickly reversed on discontinuation; relatively cheap	Prolongs INR (monitoring necessary in patients transitioned to Warfarin); adjust dosage in liver failure (hepatic metabolism)
Bivalirudin	Reversible binding to active site of thrombin	Hypotension, nausea, headache, back pain	Class I recommendation in primary PCI	Same efficacy, less bleeding than with Heparin+IIb/IIIa inhibitors, in ≤moderate-risk PCI patients	Adjust dosage in renal failure
Lepirudin	Irreversible binding to active site of thrombin	Abnormal LFT, rash, cough, bronchospasm, dyspnea, fever, anaphylaxis[g]	Reduce dosage in renal failure	monitored by aPTT	Slower action reversal on discontinuation; INR prolongation; dose adjustments in renal failure
Dabigatran	Reversible binding to active site of thrombin	Nausea, GI upset, fever, hypotension, insomnia, peripheral edema, anemia, dizziness, DVT, headache, LFT elevation	The first oral direct thrombin inhibitor	Monitoring possible, but generally not necessary[h]	

[a]All agents can cause bleeding
[b]Other than the specific adverse effects
[c]UFH and LMWH also induce endothelial secretion of tissue factor inhibitor, reducing factor VIIa complex activity
[d]Different brand names; use cautiously, if at all
[e]The exact ratio varies with the different preparations; Fondaparinux has no antithrombin action
[f]Rivaroxaban, an oral factor Xa inhibitor approved for DVT prophylaxis after orthopedic surgery, is being evaluated in ACS patients by the ATLAS ACS TIMI 51 trial. Additional factor Xa antagonists under study include apixaban, edoxaban, and otamixaban
[g]Several lethal cases of anaphylaxis have been reported
[h]INR can be prolonged, but is not useful for monitoring. aPTT relates to drug levels, but is not sufficiently precise for monitoring purposes. Ecarin clotting time (ECT) offers accurate monitoring, but is not widely available; and Thrombin Time (TT offers accurate monitoring, but is not standardized; the therapeutic target: TT/control ratio=10–20)

Table 2.24 Heparin-induced thrombocytopenia

Characteristic	Type I (HIT)	Type II (HITT[a])
Mechanism	Nonimmunologic: direct interaction between heparin and circulating platelets causes platelet aggregation	Immunologic: antibodies to heparin-platelet factor 4 complexes stimulate platelet aggregation and thrombin generation, partly by direct endothelial activation
Incidence[b]	10–20%	1–3%
Onset[c]	First 48–72 h	5–10 days[d]
Diagnosis	Clinical; no lab tests necessary	Several assays available
Clinical course	Benign; Plt count usually does not fall <100,000/mm³, and often normalizes within 4 days despite continued Heparin use	Severe, occasionally fatal[e]; Plt count usually falls to <100,000/mm³ (but usually not <10–20,000/mm³), or by up to 50% of initial level
Complications	Generally absent	Arterial or venous thrombosis in 30–80% of patients: DVT, PE, MI, skin necrosis, limb gangrene
Management	Frequent Plt counts	Immediately discontinue heparin; start anticoagulation with a direct thrombin inhibitor[f]

[a]The last letter in the acronym stands for "thrombosis"
[b]From all Heparin-treated patients
[c]After Heparin therapy onset
[d]The offending antibodies persist up to several months, and on re-exposure to Heparin platelet levels may drop within hours
[e]Ten percent mortality with early recognition, up to 30% otherwise
[f]Both for the treatment of HIT, and for that of the underlying condition requiring anticoagulation

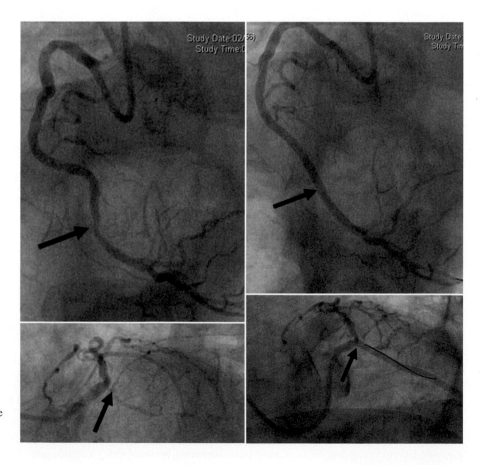

Fig. 2.1 Stenotic and post-PCI coronary arteries. The *arrows* indicate the coronary stenosis in the *left panels,* and the aspect of the same area after dilatation. As, in the illustrated cases, PCI was highly successful, the post-dilatation aspect is virtually undistinguishable from normal anatomy. This illustrates both the utility, and the limitations of the classic luminogram, which demonstrates both stenosis and procedural success, but does not image the endothelial damage caused by either the atherosclerotic plaque, or by the controlled trauma which is PCI. *Upper row:* distal RCA stenosis. *Lower row:* ostial LCx occlusion. Note the apparent absence of the LCx (*left panel*) and the wide patency of the artery after dilation (*right panel*)

and post-procedural myocardial blush. *Brachytherapy* consists in endothelial irradiation, to prevent neointimal proliferation, the main cause of in-stent restenosis. Long-time dual antiplatelet therapy is required subsequently. Brachytherapy is rarely used today.

Not surprisingly, percutaneous technology is in the focus of intense research. There is hope that biodegradable stents, currently under study, might decrease the rate of late stent thrombosis. *Other stents* being developed are designed, among others, to capture circulating endothelial precursor cells that promote vascular healing. *Distal protection devices* (the PercuSurge device, different filters, etc.) are mainly used in degenerated saphenous vein grafts, although newer generations may prove useful in ACS. These devices are all the more important since, to date, there is no medical therapy to counter reperfusion injury (Cyclosporine has been recently suggested to reduce reperfusion injury, a finding requiring further validation).

The success of PCI can be assessed in several ways. The following parameters are assessed post-dilatation: the vessel diameter; the epicardial blood flow; and the coronary capillary flow. *The postintervention vessel diameter* is assessed by the QCA method (quantitative coronary angiography), using a software that detects the luminal border of the vessel and expresses the stenosis as a percentage of the diameter of the healthy adjacent segment (Fig. 2.2).

The postintervention vessel diameter is assessed semiquantitatively using the TIMI flow score, as shown

it Table 2.25; finally, *the postintervention capillary flow* is assessed using the TIMI blush score (a whitish coloration reflecting the presence of the contrast material in the microvasculature; Table 2.26).

The complications of PCI are reviewed in Table 2.27.

In-Stent Complications

- In-stent restenosis with bare-metal stents
- In-stent thrombosis with DES

CABG There are several *CABG techniques,* both in regard to the conduits being used (arterial vs. venous grafts), and in regard to the surgical approach (on- or off-pump CABG). Overall, arterial grafts are preferable, having a >90% 20-year patency, as compared to a 60–70% 10–year patency for SVGs. Interestingly, however, arterial graft patency depends not only on the harvesting technique (not surprisingly, in situ grafts have higher patency rates than free grafts), but also on the target vessel (for instance, the 10-year patency of LIMA grafts is of 95% when used on the LAD, but of 76% only, when used on the RCA). The preferred artery used for CABG is the LIMA, but the RIMA, the radial, and the gastroepiploic artery are also used. A hybrid arterial and venous approach can also be used.

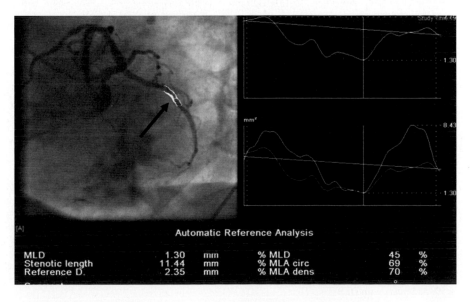

Fig. 2.2 Quantitative coronary analysis (QCA) of a lesion in the LAD

Automatic Reference Analysis					
MLD	1.30	mm	% MLD	45	%
Stenotic length	11.44	mm	% MLA circ	69	%
Reference D.	2.35	mm	% MLA dens	70	%

Table 2.25 The TIMI flow score

| TIMI grade | Antegrade flow | | | Alternative designation |
	Intensity	Completeness	Speed[a]	
0	Nil	N/A	N/A	Coronary occlusion
1	Faint	No	Slow	Penetration without reperfusion
2	Delayed or sluggish	Yes	Slow	Partial reperfusion
3	Normal	Yes	Rapid	Complete reperfusion

[a]Assessed subjectively, or objectively, by the TIMI frame count, i.e., the number of frames it takes the contrast material to reach the distal vasculature. TIMI frame count is of research interest only

Table 2.26 The TIMI Blush Classes

| Grade | Blush | | |
	Intensity	Persistence by next injection	Appearance
0	0 (absent blush)	–	–
1	Present	Yes, strongly	Stain
2	Moderate	Yes, moderately	Stain
3	Intense	Mild or absent	Ground-glass

Bleeding complications in the therapy of ischemia: The main complication of antithrombotic and fibrinolytic therapy is bleeding. Therefore, assessment of the bleeding risk and (where appropriate) of bleeding severity is an essential component of management, both in STEMI and in NSTEMI/UA patients. Risk factors for bleeding include age, female sex, a past history of bleeding, renal failure, and iatrogenic factors, such as the use of IIb/IIIa inhibitors, combined antithrombotic therapy, and the length of antithrombotic therapy.

Table 2.27 Complications of PCI

Complication	Incidence	Remarks
Peri-procedural MI	0.5–1.4%	Defined as enzyme elevation greater than threefold upper limit of normal
Abrupt vessel closure	<1%	Most frequent in acute MI, complex lesions, and poor post-PCI flow in the culprit artery
Athero- and thromboembolism	Variable	Most frequent with ACS, degenerated vein grafts, and rotational atherectomy; may cause no-reflow and MI. may be prevented by distal protection devices and is treated with vasodilators (Adenosine, Nitroprusside, Verapamil)
Coronary perforation	0.1–1.1%	More frequent with atherectomy and excimer laser
Vascular access site complications	Up to 5%	Include requirement for transfusion; pseudoaneurysm; artery occlusion; infection; retroperitoneal bleeding
Contrast-induced nephropathy	3–7%	Diabetes mellitus is a risk factor; prevented with Acetylcysteine, hydration and low-osmolar agents[a]
Allergy to contrast material	1–2%	Anaphylaxis in 0.1–0.2%. Prevented by low-osmolar agents, cortisone on the evening before and on the morning of the procedure, associated with antihistamines
In-stent thrombosis	<1%[b]	With bare metal stents, endothelization at 2–4 weeks avoids this; long-term double antiplatelet therapy is required with DES
In-stent restenosis	Variable[c]	Use DES instead of bare-metal stents

[a]The efficacy of low-osmolar agents has been questioned. IV bicarbonate has been used for prevention of contrast nephropathy, based on relatively scant data. A recent retrospective analysis has found no benefit to this approach.
[b]Under dual antiplatelet therapy; depending on the, length, and complexity of the stenosis, the vessel diameter, the initial procedural success, and the patient's risk factors (age, diabetes, etc.)
[c]<5% at 2 years with DES

Table 2.28 Assessing bleeding severity in patients treated with fibrinolytic and/or antithrombotic therapy

Manifestation			Severity		Manifestation		
			TIMI	GUSTO			
ICH					**ICH**		
Overt bleeding[a]	*and*	Hb drop >5 mg/dL	Major	Severe or life-threat.	Causes hemodynamic compromise	*and*	Requires intervention[b]
	and	Hb drop 3–5 mg/dL	*Minor*	*Moderate*	No hemodynamic compromise	*and*	Requires blood transfusion
	and	Hb drop <3 mg/dL	Minimal	Mild	No hemodynamic compromise	*and*	No blood transfusion required

[a]Including internal bleeding demonstrated by imaging, e.g., CT-detected retroperitoneal hemorrhage
[b]Intervention is virtually always required

Assessment of bleeding severity is reviewed in Table 2.28. A striking divergence between the GUSTO and the TIMI assessments is outlined in italics. Non-TIMI major bleeding (i.e., bleeding clinically judged as significant, but not covered by the TIMI criteria) was recently shown to be just as important as TIMI major bleeding in predicting mortality.

The management of bleeding complications depends on their severity. Thus, minor bleeding requires minimal local measures, while major bleeding requires interruption and neutralization of antiplatelet and anticoagulant therapy, unless manageable by local measures alone (e.g., profuse bleeding localized at the puncture site). ICH may require surgical drainage. The management of intermediate-grade bleeding is individualized.

Hemorrhagic stroke is the most severe manifestation of bleeding. The risk factors for this potentially devastating complication include: age >65, or, in other analyses, >75; low body weight (cutoff value differs in different analyses; weight <65 kg is universally considered a risk factor; in some analyses, the cutoff value in male patients is of 80 kg); HTN (cutoff value differs in different analyses; BP >170/95 mmHg is universally considered a risk factor); using a non-Streptokinase (SK) agent; black race, female gender, prior stroke or Nifedipine use, or excessive anticoagulation (INR ≥4, aPTT ≥24 s). Each element is graded with one point, to establish a score, which is then checked against nomograms, to establish the absolute risk. A 2–3% risk of ICH implies "equipoise" (equal risk/benefit ratio) between IV thrombolysis and primary PCI, while a risk >4% (corresponding to ≥5 risk factors) is considered high, and favors primary PCI.

Diagnosis: Clinically, ICH presents with the usual signs of stroke (Chap. 11), including changes in the level of consciousness, focal neurological signs, headache, nausea, vomiting, seizures, (occasionally, with acute HTN) and, in severe cases, coma and death. While these signs may be seen with either ischemic or hemorrhagic stroke, the latter must be considered present until proven otherwise. A fulminant course, especially in the first 24 h after initiation of treatment, is especially suggestive of hemorrhagic stroke. *Management* of stroke during thrombolytic therapy includes (1) *immediate pre-emptive measures*: discontinuation of fibrinolytic, anticoagulant, and antiplatelet therapy; (2) *CT diagnosis* (hemorrhagic vs. ischemic stroke); (3) *Therapy*: Ischemic stroke – see Chap. 11. Thrombolytic therapy appears safe and effective in catheterization-related stroke. The management *of hemorrhagic stroke* consists in administration of FFP, 2 units; Protamine (1 mg for every 100 U of UFH given in the preceding 4 h); cryoprecipitate 10 units; and platelets 6–8 units. In patients with incipient cerebral herniation, reduction of intracranial pressure is recommended (Chap. 11). HTN control is of the essence. If BP is ≤160/90 mmHg, only follow-up is recommended; for systolic BP 160–180, treatment is individually tailored; and if systolic BP is >180, treatment is required, and should be more aggressive if there is a suspicion of increased intracranial pressure. Control of hyperglycemia (with insulin) and of fever (with Paracetamol) are important in stroke patients. *Prognosis*: the most important predictors of mortality include the Glasgow Coma Scale score, the time from thrombolysis to ICH onset, the ICH volume, and advanced age.

2.3 Ischemia: Clinical Syndromes

2.3.1 Overview

As mentioned, myocardial ischemia can be due either to increased myocardial demands or to decreased perfusion. The latter can be caused by a gradual decrease in the vascular lumen (with a corresponding increase in the resistance to flow, up until complete occlusion and total flow cessation), or to acute lumen occlusion, caused by coronary thrombus. Table 2.29 shows schematically a comparison between the two scenarios. The rest of the present section is dedicated to the discussion of these two scenarios (The reader is also referred to the beginning of Sect. 2.2.).

The Canadian classification of angina pectoris includes four grades of severity (Table 2.30). While grade I usually corresponds to stable angina, and grade IV to NSTEMI/UA, grades II and III can correspond to either.

2.3.2 Acute Coronary Syndrome

2.3.2.1 Background

The concept of ACS revolves around another concept, that of *vulnerable plaque*, with a large lipid core, low density of smooth muscle cells, high concentration of inflammatory cells and a thin fibrous cap. Such plaques are prone to fissuring (superficial damage) or

rupture (involving deeper layers), under the impact of flow-dependent factors (circumferential wall stress) and of macrophage-secreted enzymes that lyse collagen. Exposure of the lipid core to the blood flow results in clot formation. The first to appear is a platelet-rich, not fully occlusive thrombus. This manifests with typical anginal pain and EKG changes, with or without myocardial necrosis (enzyme increase); however, at this stage there are no ST elevations on the EKG. In the absence of myocardial necrosis, the resulting syndrome is termed *unstable angina,* while if the enzyme levels increase, the condition is termed "non-ST elevation MI" (NSTEMI). Despite the similar pathogenesis, NSTEMI has a worse prognosis than unstable angina, justifying separate classification. If thrombus growth is countered by the patient's

Table 2.30 The Canadian Classification of Angina Pectoris

Grade	Angina occurs with	Limitation of everyday activity
I	Strenuous activity only	None
II	Walking or climbing stairs rapidly, in the cold, or under stress; walking >2 blocks on the level, climbing >1 flight of stairs at normal pace	Slight
III	Walking 1–2 blocks on the level, climbing 1 flight of stairs at normal pace	Marked
IV	The slightest activity or at rest	Extreme

Table 2.29 ACS and stable angina: a comparison

	Stable angina	ACS
Timeframe of lumen narrowing	Gradual (decades)	Sudden (minutes)
Pathogenesis	Vessel occlusion by increasing plaque volume	Flow cessation due to clot formation; distal embolization to the microcirculation
Disease mechanism	Ischemia at times of increased O_2 demand[a]	Ischemia typically not related to increased O_2 demand[b]
Adaptive mechanisms	Vasodilation[c]; vascular remodeling, collateral circulation	Vasodilation; spontaneous thrombolysis
Clinical manifestations	Chest pain of various intensities	Severe chest pain
EKG changes	ST and T wave changes; no ST elevations	ST and T wave changes; ST elevations, with STEMI
Enzyme elevation	No	Yes or no

[a]The relationship between O_2 demand and ischemia onset is not linear. Occasionally, certain types of activity are more prone than others to cause ischemia and chest pain, despite no apparent excessive O_2 consumption
[b]Occasionally, physical or psychological stress cause sympathetic discharge increasing O_2 consumption at the same time as plaque destabilization, with thrombus formation
[c]Normal vasodilation can increase blood flow up to fivefold. The vasodilator capacity is decreased by endothelial dysfunction

Table 2.31 Acute coronary syndromes

		ST elevation		
		Yes		No
Biomarker elevation	Yes	STEMI	Usually, with Q wave	NSTEMI
			Rarely, no Q wave	
	No	Aborted STEMI or non-MI ST elevation		UA

own thrombolytic system or by timely administration of antithrombotic therapy or of spontaneous thrombolysis, blood flow is reestablished, and the acute episode remits. In the contrary case, a fibrin-rich, completely occlusive thrombus forms, and the resulting condition is termed "ST elevation MI" (STEMI). These distinctions are reviewed in Table 2.31.

Differentiating the Ischemic Syndromes

- Stable angina and ACS are differentiated clinically.
- Unstable angina and MI are differentiated by laboratory tests (biomarker level).
- STEMI and NSTEMI are differentiated by EKG.

The diagnosis and treatment of ACS are discussed under "MI," below.

2.3.2.2 Myocardial Infarction (MI)

Definition and Diagnosis

MI consists in necrosis of one or several segments of the cardiac muscle, due to acute coronary ischemia. Necrosis is defined as an increase and subsequent fall in cardiac biological markers (troponin is preferred for diagnosis), in the setting of symptoms and EKG changes suggestive of ischemia. MI can span the spectrum between microscopic and extensive, with vast prognostic differences. The largest MIs involve the proximal LAD; however, with preexisting LV dysfunction, even a small MI can have catastrophic consequences. *Diagnosis*: For clinical use, the definition of MI requires the adoption of quantitative criteria. While pain is notoriously difficult to quantitate, the degree of ST segment deviation and biomarker elevation follow a continuum, and require establishing a threshold value beyond which they are considered "positive." The threshold values for ST deviation are reviewed in this section. In regard to biomarkers, even minute

elevations can be detected by current assays. Technically, such elevations correspond to "true" MI s, but their clinical relevance is unclear. Therefore, a threshold for significance has been arbitrarily established, as follows:

- For non-procedure related MI: above the 99th percentile of the upper reference limit (URL) in that population.
- For PCI-related MI: >3× the 99th percentile URL.
- For CABG-related MI: >5× the 99th percentile URL, within ≤72 h of procedure, when associated with new Q waves or new LBBB, or angiographically documented new graft or native coronary artery occlusion, or imaging evidence of new hypokinetic segments.

Occasionally, MI is diagnosed even in the absence of definitive evidence of myocardial necrosis. In victims of *SCD* occurring before there was time to obtain blood samples, or before the biomarker levels could rise, the diagnosis of MI is based on symptoms of ischemia, typical EKG manifestations, or on autopsy findings (fresh coronary thrombus and/or of pathological findings typical for MI). In patients with *angiographic or angioscopic evidence of fresh thrombus*, MI is diagnosed before the biomarker levels had time to rise (short time lag between symptom onset and angiography, or thrombus formation at the time of angiography or angioscopy). MI is often diagnosed retrospectively, by chance or as a result of workup in a patient raising the suspicion of CAD. In clinical practice, it is often necessary to diagnose MI in retrospect. Old MI is diagnosed based on EKG (pathologic Q waves), imaging tests (thin, non-contractile myocardium, lack of radionuclide uptake), or typical pathological findings, at autopsy.

Pathogenesis

MI is caused by acutely decreased coronary blood flow, most frequently due to coronary thrombosis. The other main mechanism is embolism, either (frequently) with fragments from an in situ thrombus, or (less commonly) with fragments from an intracardiac thrombus, a valvular vegetation, tumor, etc (see Table 2.32). Thrombus forms on plaques with a fissured or ruptured fibrous cap, exposing the subendothelial tissue to the blood flow. This exposure triggers platelet and coagulation system activation and formation of platelet, then fibrin clot. Occlusion mainly occurs in coronary segments with minimal (10–40%) stenosis, generally corresponding to vulnerable plaques (large lipid core, inflammation). Vessel occlusion is dynamic, with recurrent obstruction and spontaneous reperfusion, and various degrees of vasospasm. Distal embolization with clot fragments may cause microvascular occlusion and prevent reperfusion despite flow restoration in the infarct-related artery. The amount of myocardial necrosis depends on the size of the vessel involved, but also on the presence or absence of collateral circulation and on the time lag to treatment. Necrosis starts within approximately 20 min of ischemia onset (see MI classification by stage, below) and progresses from the subendocardial to the subepicardial layer, as the former has greater metabolic demands and lower direct and collateral perfusion. In animal models, the onset of ischemic necrosis requires ≥20 min, and complete necrosis of all the myocytes at risk requires ≥2–4 h, while pathological evidence of healed MI (i.e., scar tissue) requires ≥5–6 weeks.

Prevalence and Importance

Acute MI is the leading cause of death in United States and Western Europe, with an overall mortality of >30% (including out-of-hospital fatalities). These high mortality rates are not likely to abate in the foreseeable future, as therapeutic progress is being offset by a worldwide increase in the prevalence of risk factors. Progress in MI therapy has dramatically increased the prevalence of severe HF (as a sequella of extensive MI, previously universally fatal), a key contemporary cause of morbidity. *Classification*: Based on the clinical circumstances, there are several types of MI (Table 2.32); one and the same MI can belong to more than just one "category."

Additional classifications are used: (1) *STEMI vs. NSTEMI* (see above); (2) *Q-wave (transmural) vs. non-Q wave (non-transmural) MI.* Spontaneous non-Q wave MI (Q wave absence not a result of therapy) has a better short-term prognosis (better collateral circulation), but an increased risk for long-term morbidity and mortality (due to the very reason of collateral formation, i.e., more advanced atherosclerosis). The incidence of non-Q wave MI has dramatically increased in the thrombolytic era, with an improved long-term prognosis; (3) *by size,* i.e., by the percentage of the necrosed myocardium: microscopic (focal necrosis), small (1–10%), moderate

Table 2.32 Clinical classification of MI

Type	Operative criterion	Definition: mechanism	Definition: pathogenesis
1	Pathogenesis	Decreased O₂ supply by in situ occlusive thrombosis	Plaque erosion, rupture, fissuring, or dissection
2	Pathogenesis	(1) Increased O₂ demand; (2) Decreased supply not related to occlusive thrombus	(1) Anemia, arrhythmia, HTN; (2) coronary spasm or embolism; hypotension
3	Conjecture based on limited clinical evidence	SCD, presumed to be of cardiac origin[a]	As with types I or II
4a	Iatrogenic	MI related to PCI	Disruption of flow in the artery under treatment, in side branches or in collaterals, by dissection, distal embolization, slow flow or no-reflow phenomenon, and/or microvascular plugging
4b	Iatrogenic	MI related to stent thrombosis	See text
5	Iatrogenic	MI related to CABG[b]	As with PCI

[a]The supporting evidence does not include biomarker elevation
[b]In addition to the mechanisms operational with PCI, CABG may cause myocyte necrosis by trauma from suture needles or manipulation of the heart, reperfusion injury, O₂ free radical toxicity, or the non-reperfusion phenomenon. This injury tends to be diffuse, subendocardial (rather than focal), and is not included in the definition of MI. The corresponding troponin increase is usually below the fivefold threshold required for CABG-related MI. Moreover, new ST–T abnormalities are frequently seen in patients after CABG, even in the absence of myocardial ischemia. In these patients, demonstration of new segmental LV dysfunction is essential in establishing the diagnosis of MI

(10–30%), and large (>30%); (4) *by location*; (5) *by time of diagnosis*: evolving (hours), acute (hours to days), healing (up to 5–6 weeks), and healed MI (>5–6 weeks).

Non-Q Wave vs. Q-Wave MI Prognosis: A Comparison

Prognosis depends on whether the non-Q status is attained spontaneously, or as a result of thrombolysis. Spontaneous non-Q wave MI has a better short-term, and a worse long-term prognosis, whereas thrombolysis-related non-Q wave MI has a better prognosis all around. Improvement in symptom-to-intervention time may diminish the short-term prognosis disparity between Q wave and non-Q wave MI.

Two Classifications of MI, Two Different Implications

- STEMI vs. NSTEMI: therapeutic implication (only STEMI benefits from acute thrombolysis)
- Q-wave vs. non-Q wave MI: prognostic implication (see above)

Diagnosis

Clinical manifestations – The typical *symptom* of MI is severe anginal pain, as reviewed in Sect. 2.2. The pain is similar to that of angina pectoris, but more severe and of longer duration (typically, >20 min), and is not relieved by either rest or Nitroglycerine. Unlike the pain of PE or aortic dissection, which is maximal from the start, MI-related pain increases gradually. Acute severe pain in the back may be caused by either MI or aortic dissection, or, occasionally, by coexistence of the two. Dyspnea (occasionally, pulmonary edema), palpitations, confusional state, nausea, vomiting, and profuse sweating are typical in the MI patient. GI symptoms are especially frequent in patients with inferior MI. Severe MI may present as cardiogenic shock or SCD. *Physical examination* is important for prognosis and to rule out conditions that might masquerade as MI (Table 2.33).

The degree of pulmonary congestion at presentation is classified according to the Killip class system (Table 2.34). The Killip class is influenced by compensatory hyperkinesia in the healthy myocardium; thus,

Table 2.33 Clinical[a] Differential Diagnosis of MI

	Pain	EKG	Troponin	Regional[b] WMA
(Myo)pericarditis	Worse when supine, better when leaning forward[c]	Diffuse ST elevation (no mirror-image, except for aVR and V_1)[d]; PR depressions, peaked T waves, concave (rather than convex) ST elevations	Elevation persists >1 week[e]	Absent in non-MI-related pericarditis
Aortic dissection (not complicated with MI)	Maximal from the beginning, can be migratory	no EKG changes	Elevated in ≤10% of patients with Type A dissection	No
PE	Maximal from the beginning	Sinus tachycardia; ST/T changes mimicking MI[f]	Increased troponin in cases of severe RV strain	WMA mainly involve the RV[g]
GI disorders (reflux, spasm, inflammation, etc.)[h]	Pain does not radiate	Usually normal; EKG manifestations of inferior MI may be seen in acute cholecystitis	No troponin elevation	No

[a]The EKG differential diagnosis is reviewed in a separate table
[b]Wall motion abnormalities
[c]Pericarditis and MI may coexist
[d]Large, "wrap-around" LAD may cause similar changes
[e]Patients with greater cTnI elevations (>1.5 μg/L) tend to have more severe ST elevations, and potentially be more prone to be misdiagnosed as MI
[f]In addition to the S1Q3T3 pattern (S wave in LI, Q wave in LIII, T wave inversion in L III), sinus tachycardia, RBBB, right axis deviation
[g]In massive PE, there may exist a leftward shift in the IVS, with LV compression
[h]Specific tests may be useful esophageal manometry, HIDA scan to rule out cholecystitis); response to antiacids, spasmolytics, etc.

Table 2.34 The Killip classification[a]

Class	Definition	Characteristics	Patients (%)	Mortality rate (%)
I	No HF	No rhales	85	5
II	HF, no pulmonary edema	Rhales <50% of lung fields	13	14
III	Pulmonary edema	Rhales >50% of lung fields	1	32
IV	Cardiogenic shock	Hypotension, peripheral hypoperfusion	1	58

[a]The data are based on the GUSTO-I trial

Table 2.35 The inadequacies of classical EKG terminology In MI

	Terminology	Why the terminology is confusing
Q wave	"Necrosis"	Necrosis is currently defined as biomarker elevation, and not all biomarker elevation associates a Q wave. Moreover, unlike necrosis, Q waves can be transient
ST changes	"Injury current"	The term was coined to suggest a myocardial involvement severity less than with necrosis, but more than with "lesion". However, many MI patients with "injury currents" actually have myocardial necrosis
T wave changes	"Ischemic current"	The term "ischemia" encompasses the notions of "injury" and "necrosis". Patients with T wave abnormalities can span the spectrum from normal to acute (or old) MI

while an advanced class portends a poor prognosis (in the early thrombolytic era, the mortality in cardiogenic shock, i.e., Killip Class IV, was ≥50%), a lower class does not necessarily correspond to a small infarct-related area. Assuming optimal therapy, the Killip score on admission is the best prognostic predictor in MI patients, as it reflects not merely MI size, but also the impact of MI on the specific patient. Even a small MI may lead to advanced Killip classes, in presence of significant previous myocardial compromise.

EKG manifestations reflect ischemia and its complications (arrhythmia, conduction disturbances, reviewed below and in Chap. 6). EKG also provides a gross estimate of MI size (large MI generally involves a greater number of leads or causes LBBB or RBBB). MI affects ventricular depolarization and repolarization, i.e., the QRS complex, the ST segment, and the T wave. While EKG has preserved its central role in MI diagnosis, the classical terminology, coined decades before the biomarker assay era, has become inadequate and confusing (Table 2.35).

The EKG manifestations of acute MI are reviewed in Table 2.36. *EKG monitoring* is mandatory during the patient's stay in the ICU, and especially at the time of thrombolysis and early thereafter.

While any component of the EKG may be permanently affected by previous MI (e.g., "frozen" ST elevations with LV aneurysm, permanently inverted T waves, etc.), the formal diagnosis of old MI is established based on Q waves and/or the amputation of R waves. The changes must be present in ≥2 contiguous leads, and include any of the findings below:

- Q waves ≥30 ms and ≥0.1 mV, in any two contiguous leads (including RV leads), except for $V_1–V_3$.
- Q waves or QS complexes ≥30 ms and ≥0.2 mV, in leads $V_2–V_3$.
- R waves ≥40 ms *and* R/S >1, *and* a concordant positive T wave *and no* conduction defect, all in leads $V_1–V_2$.

Equally important the diagnosis of reinfarction during recovery from the initial MI, before the ST–T changes have entirely normalized. Reinfarction is diagnosed in presence of new ST elevations ≥0.1 mV, in any two contiguous leads, especially in a suggestive clinical setting. New Q waves must be carefully assessed, to establish if they correspond to the initial event or to the recurrent one.

The evolution of the EKG in acute MI is shown in Fig. 2.3.

Table 2.36 EKG manifestations of acute MI

	Finding	Significance	Remarks
Ventricular depolarization			
Q wave	Pathologic Q waves are larger than 25% of the corresponding R wave and/or have a width of ≥40 ms[a]	In MI, Q waves represent a "see-through" image of the myocardial depolarization in the opposite wall of the heart	Classically the hallmark of old MI, Q waves may actually appear within minutes of ischemia onset and can be transient.
R wave	R wave amputation = a decrease in the expected (or previously documented) R wave amplitude, e.g., poor progression of R waves in the anterior chest walls	Decrease in the depolarizing myocardial mass of the affected segment	Occasionally, the R wave is completely obliterated, and the QRS complex becomes a QS complex
S wave	May become obliterated by ST segment elevation	EKG is a summation picture; "smaller" events may be obscured by temporally contiguous "larger" events	S waves have secondary importance in the EKG diagnosis of acute MI
The interval between completion of depolarization and the beginning of repolarization			
ST segment	Elevation[b]/depression	Ischemic subendocardium or subepicardium fail to depolarize normally, and there is a transmyocardial ionic gradient; the normal "electrically inert" (isoelectric) ST segment now records an electrical current	Identification of ST segment elevations as described is an indication for thrombolysis
	Elevation ≥1 mm (for leads V_2–V_4, ≥2 mm in men and ≥1.5 mm in women) in ≥2 contiguous leads,[c] i.e., in groups	Transmural or subepicardial injury[d]: the electrical ST vector points toward the area of subepicardial ischemia	
	Horizontal or downsloping depression >0.5 mm[e] in ≥2 contiguous leads	Subendocardial injury: the electrical ST vector points toward the area of subendocardial ischemia	ST depressions can be the direct image of subendocardial ischemia or a mirror-image of subepicardial ischemia (occasionally invisible as such, i.e., in posterior wall MI)
Ventricular repolarization			
T wave	Upright or inverted	As for the ST segment	(a) Same mechanism as for ST elevation; (b) restoration of normal repolarization vector
	Upright; (a) increased amplitude and width; (b) normal	(a) Subepicardial ischemia (hyperacute stage of MI); (b) old MI	
	Inverted >0.1mV, in ≥2 contiguous leads	(a) Subepicardial ischemia	

(continued)

Table 2.36 (continued)

Intraventricular conduction[f]

Finding	Significance	Remarks
New LBBB	Involvement of a large myocardial mass in the anterior LV wall	LBBB unto itself, in a setting suggestive of MI should lead to thrombolysis in adequate candidates[b]
New RBBB	May represent involvement of a large portion of the anterior LV wall[g]	Complicates interpretations of ST changes in V_1–V_3[g]

[a]As opposed to normal Q waves, occasionally visible in leads I, aVL, V_5 and V_6, and corresponding to septal depolarization

[b]Measured from the J-point, i.e., where QRS ends and ST begins

[c]Often with reciprocal ST depressions in the contralateral leads. A 1- or 2-mm threshold increases specificity, but decreases sensitivity

[d]Abnormalities of the subepicardial action potential and transmural conduction (among other mechanisms) are believed to be involved

[e]Occasionally, the ST shift is slightly less than the required magnitude, in one of the leads

[f]The Sgarbossa score for MI diagnosis in LBBB patients increases specificity but decreases sensitivity, leading to significant underuse of thrombolysis in extensive anterior MI. Criteria for MI include: concordant ST elevation $\geq$1 mm in $\geq$1 lateral (V_5–V_6) or inferior (LII, III, aVF) lead; ST depression $\geq$1 mm in $\geq$1 anterior (V_1–V_3) lead; or discordant ST elevation $\geq$5 mm in $\geq$2 contiguous leads

[g]RBBB associated to independently diagnosed acute anterior MI carries a poorer prognosis. In MI patients, RBBB at presentation carries poorer prognosis than LBBB; however, RBBB is not an *independent* indication for thrombolysis. RBBB may obscure ST–T changes in V_1–V_3; positive (pseudonormalized) T waves in these leads strengthen the suspicion of ischemia

Fig. 2.3 Anterior wall MI.
Top panel – acute phase
(first few hours after onset);
Middle panel – subacute
phase (first few days);
Bottom panel: chronic phase
(beyond the first few days).
Note the gradual descent of
the ST segments and the
appearance of Q waves. In
this patient, there is still some
residual ST elevation,
possibly indicative of LV
aneurysm formation.
In this case, the T waves have
taken a permanent negative
configuration, but they may
also become isoelectric or
revert to the normal positive
configuration

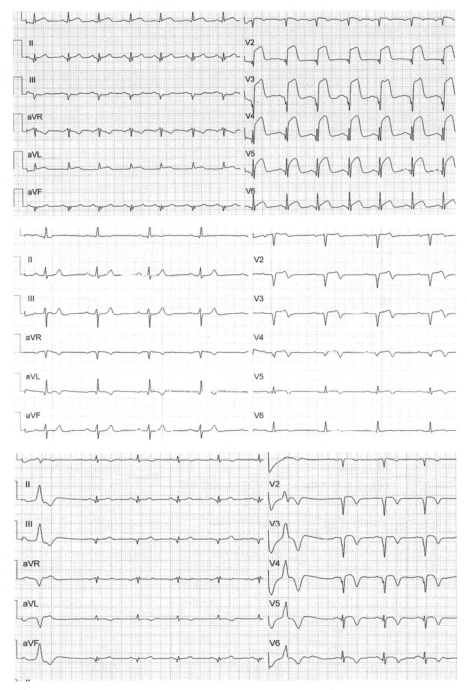

Biomarkers: The clinically useful necrosis markers are troponins T and I, and CK-MB; myoglobin is used less frequently. The dynamic of these markers is reviewed in Table 2.37.

The preferred biomarker is troponin, a complex of proteins important for striated muscle contraction. Both types of troponin can be used for diagnosis, but cTnI is more widely available than cTnT. Troponin may be elevated in a variety of non-MI disorders, either cardiac (CMP; cardiac trauma, occasionally iatrogenic, such as after CPR; arrhythmia and AVB; the Takotsubo syndrome; myocarditis; drug cardiotoxicity); or non-cardiac (aortic dissection, PE, stroke, subarachnoid hemorrhage; renal failure; respiratory failure, sepsis, extreme exertion, rhabdomyolysis, etc.).

Table 2.37 Biomarkers in the diagnosis of MI

Marker	Troponin T[a]	Troponin I[a]	CK-MB	Myoglobin
Initial elevation (hours from occlusion)	3–12	3–12	3–12	1–4
Peak elevation (hours from occlusion)	12–48	24	24	6–7
Normalization (days)	5–14	5–10	2–3	1
Blood samples (initial MI)	At initial evaluation; 6–9 h later; and at 12–24 h, if the initial results are negative, but the suspicion of MI is high[b]			
Blood samples (reinfarction)	On initial suspicion, and 3–6 h later[b]			
Blood samples (PCI[c])	Before or immediately after the procedure; at 6–12 h; and at 18–24 h			

[a]A rising and falling pattern is necessary to distinguish MI-related elevations from background elevations; with presentation >24 h after symptom onset, this pattern is not necessary

[b]The preferred biomarker is troponin. When troponin is used, recurrent MI is diagnosed if there is a ≥20% increase of the value in the second sample

[c]PCI virtually always causes ischemia, but patients with associated biomarker elevation have a worse prognosis

An *imaging test* (most frequently, an *echo*) is routinely obtained, as the degree of LVEF decrease is the main prognostic factor after MI. Additionally, if for whatever reason biomarkers have not been obtained or have already normalized, demonstration of new segmental hypokinesia or akinesia or loss of normal systolic thickening, in a suggestive clinical context, meets the definition for MI. Echo is ideal for triaging in chest pain units, as a normal test has a negative predictive value >95% for acute MI. If acute MI has been ruled out, echo often establishes the correct diagnosis (e.g., PE). Contrast echo improves LV endocardial border delineation in technically difficult studies. Myocardial contrast echo, suggested as a "one-stop shop" method allowing to identify perfusion defects at the same time as the resulting segmental LV dysfunction has not reached the threshold of clinical applicability.

To summarize, in the MI patient, resting echo is useful for: (a) *demonstration of new segmental dysfunction* in a suggestive, but not clear-cut clinical context (anginal pain and EKG changes present, biomarker results not, or not yet available); in the occasional patient in whom the EKG is nondiagnostic (e.g., preexisting BBB), echo allows localization of the affected segments and identification of the culprit artery. Echo also allows to classify ST depressions in V_1–V_2 as direct or mirror-images (anterior vs. posterior hypokinesis); (b) *assessing the impact of MI* and/or thrombolytic therapy on LV function. This initial assessment tends to overestimate the damage, as, in addition to necrosis, it includes areas of stunned myocardium. Re-assessment at 4–6 weeks after discharge is essential, to avoid chronic overmedication and undue psychological trauma to the patient; (c) *assessing MI-related damage reversibility*; thin, non-thickening, dyskinetic areas are irreversibly damaged (scarred); akinetic areas are usually irreversibly damaged, but can occasionally be viable; and hypokinetic areas are often viable. Hibernating myocardium can be distinguished from myocardial scar by means of Dobutamine echo; (d) *assessing the effect of chronic medication* on myocardial remodeling, a chronic sequella of MI.

Radionuclide imaging may diagnose MI even in the absence of biomarker elevations, but can only be performed in a hospital setting, where the much simpler biomarker assays are also available. Moreover, diagnostic data only become available a few hours after radiotracer injection, making nuclear scan useless in patients with suspected MI, in whom therapeutic decisions (including thrombolysis, if appropriate) are urgent. Therefore, in the MI patient, radionuclide imaging is mainly used for the diagnosis of myocardial hibernation. If acute STEMI has been ruled out, and the clinical question regards the presence or absence of ischemia, radionuclide tracer can be injected at presentation, with imaging after few hours. A normal perfusion scan has a very high (>95%) negative predictive value for coronary ischemia. Just like echo, radionuclide imaging provides localization of the ischemic segments; in addition, it demonstrates coronary flow impairment and, by means of SPECT imaging, segmental contractile dysfunction. *MRI* can assess myocardial perfusion, contraction, and viability. However, due to the availability of cheaper and less cumbersome methods, the current role of MRI in the diagnosis of MI or of myocardial viability is restricted. Acute MI reflects on MRI as delayed gadolinium hyperenhancement, i.e., over-captation in the infarcted area approximately 20 min after injection (well within the acceptable window for thrombolysis). In real life, the one important indication for MRI in the diagnosis of coronary ischemia is demonstration of occasional underlying coronary malformations. *CT* scan has capabilities and limitations similar to those of MRI. CT demonstrates fresh MI as a focal area of hypoenhancement (decreased contrast uptake), followed, later on, by focal hyperenhancement. As mentioned, angio-CT is widely used for the diagnosis of coronary atherosclerosis. *Diagnostic coronary angiography* is by definition performed in all patients undergoing PCI or CABG. Routine cardiac catheterization has been proposed as an anatomic risk stratification tool, in all post-MI patients. Thus, the CARESS-in-AMI study has showed substantial advantage for routine early PCI in all high-risk STEMI patients (even if successfully treated with fibrinolytics). If this study receives further confirmation, routine PCI in all non-low risk STEMI patients (just as is undertaken in NSTEMI patients) may become the rule.

Assessment of the Extent of Myocardial Involvement in Acute MI

At comparable levels of collateral circulation, ischemic preconditioning, and preexisting myocardial damage, the size of the involved myocardial segment is proportional with the caliber of the infarct-related artery. *In the acute stage*, the extent of myocardial damage is assessed: (1) *clinically,* by the Killip class; (2) *by EKG, in STEMI* (number of involved leads, severity of ST elevations); (3) *by echo* (magnitude and extension of segmental LV dysfunction; however, necrosis and stunning cannot be distinguished); (4) *using biomarkers,* to obtain a more accurate estimate of the MI size. *In the late stage*, echo, radionuclide studies, or cardiac MRI allow to assess the extent of myocardial involvement, which is the major prognostic factor after MI. The key issue of post-MI damage assessment is discussed under Sect. "2.3.12," below; (5) *Novel approaches:* Eighty-lead EKG mapping, using a special vest and a computer to display the data as color maps permits better visualization of classical EKG "blind spots" (posterior, inferior, right-sided, or high lateral walls).

STEMI

A subgroup of MI patients displays a set of characteristics that merit separate discussion. *The pathogenesis* involves a fully occlusive thrombus; *the prognosis* is generally worse than with non-complete vessel occlusion; *the EKG* displays ST elevations, satisfying certain criteria; and *the treatment* includes IV thrombolysis in appropriate candidates (discussed below). This type of MI is termed "ST-elevation MI" (STEMI). New-onset LBBB has similar clinical characteristics, and is discussed together with STEMI. Occasionally, STEMI is diagnosed retrospectively, based on development of new pathological Q waves. The EKG stages of STEMI evolution are outlined in Table 2.38. Of note, acute MI is *not* the most frequent cause of ST elevation in patients with chest pain (unrelated LVH is more frequent, and unrelated LBBB is just as frequent as acute MI). Additionally, >90% of healthy males have ≥1 mm ST elevations in ≥1 precordial lead.

Conditions that may mimic STEMI on the EKG are reviewed in Table 2.39.

The EKG differential diagnosis between acute MI and acute pericarditis is illustrated in Fig. 2.4.

MI Treatment

Background: MI treatment involves different measures in the acute phase (when the accent falls on early restoration of the coronary blood flow, to minimize necrosis, and in treatment of complications) and in the post-MI patient (where the aim is to prevent late complications and recurrences of the MI). In either setting, the treatment may be pharmacological or interventional, as discussed above. The treatment of STEMI is characterized by the option of IV thrombolysis, which has not been proven beneficial in other types of ACS (NSTEMI, unstable angina); however, an early interventional therapy is the preferred approach in all types of ACS, including STEMI. If this approach is implemented, there is virtually no distinction between the therapies of the different types of ACS, although the actual guidelines may differ in the strength of recommendation of the different approaches. This is justified by the evidence-based approach, i.e., on the available data derived from large-scale trials or metaanalyses; however, the practical impact of these occasional finer points is generally modest. STEMI treatment will be reviewed first, to be followed by a table summarizing the particularities of NSTEMI therapy. Therefore, while in the following discussion, the term STEMI is used, most comments also apply to NSTEMI. Importantly, this

Table 2.38 The EKG Evolution of STEMI

Stage	Q	ST	T	EKG
Hyperacute	No	May be elevated	Increased amplitude and width	
Transmural injury	No	Markedly elevated	Increased amplitude and width	
Necrosis	Yes	Starts normalizing	Inverted[a]	
Necrosis and fibrosis	Yes	No	Inverted[a]	
Fibrosis	Yes	No	Upright	

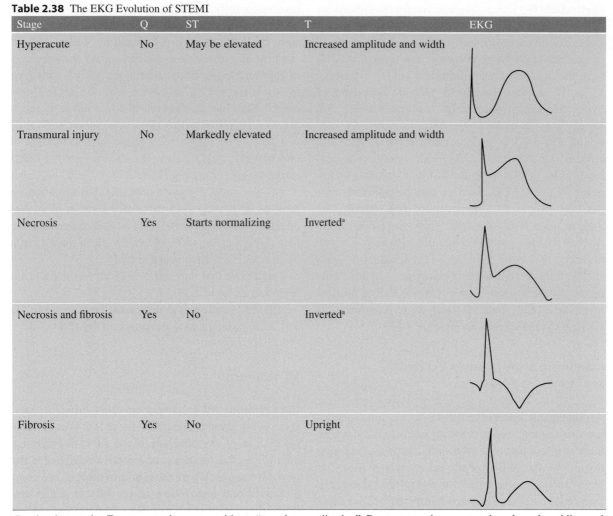

[a]Previously negative T waves may become positive – "pseudonormalization". R waves may be amputated or altogether obliterated, turning the QRS complex into a QS wave

does not include IV thrombolysis, an approach reserved to STEMI patients.

MI Treatment : General Measures *Oxygen* is routinely used, although there are no clear efficacy data, and future placebo-controlled trials are improbable. While O_2 administration in dyspneic patients (especially if hypoxemic) is clearly indicated (occasionally, by orotracheal intubation and mechanical ventilation), the grounds for routine administration in all-comers are less clear; at any rate, O_2 administration in uncomplicated cases should not exceed 6 h. The idea of intracoronary administration of hyperbaric O_2 in STEMI patients undergoing PCI was tested in a small study,

with unconvincing results and a higher incidence of bleeding in the treated arm (due to the cumbersome technique involved). *Nitrates*: Both the GISSI-3 and the ISIS-4 trials have failed to demonstrate a mortality benefit for nitrate therapy in asymptomatic patients (an infrequent occurrence in STEMI patients presenting to the ER). After long term use, tolerance may develop, reducing nitrate effectiveness. Several mechanisms have been proposed. Clinically, the problem is dealt with by avoiding continuous use of nitrates; discontinuous use makes it possible to recover sensitivity to these agents. Patients with endothelial dysfunction are more prone to develop nitrate tolerance; thus, nitrates

Table 2.39 EKG differential diagnosis of MI

Condition	Similarity to MI	Difference from MI
Pseudo-anterior wall MI (changes in V_1–V_3[a])		
LV aneurysm	ST elevations	"Frozen" changes, do not have the usual MI dynamic
LVH	Poor R progression	S (V_1)+R (V_5 or V_6, whichever is larger) ≥35 mm; R (aVL) ≥11 mm
LBBB	QS or poor R progression	QRS ≥120 ms; QS or rS in V_1; monophasic R in L I, V6
Pulmonary emphysema and cor pulmonale	Loss of R waves[b]	Right axis deviation; microvoltage
Left anterior fascicular block	Occasionally, q waves	Left axis deviation; q waves are small
Type B WPW	Negative QRS[a]	Presence of the delta wave
Pneumothorax	Loss of R waves	Microvoltage, clinical context
Brugada syndrome	ST elevations	"Coved" (Type I) or "saddle back" (Types II, III) pattern ST elevation
Pseudo-lateral wall MI (changes in L I, aVF, V5–V6)		
HOCM	Deep Q waves	Associated LVH
Pseudo- posterior wall MI (changes in V_1–V_2)		
Type A WPW	Tall R waves	Presence of the delta wave
RVH	Tall R waves	Associated incomplete RBBB, RV "strain"
Diffuse ST–T changes		
Acute pericarditis	ST elevations	Lack of mirror image changes, morphology of ST elevations[c]
CNS disease	Diffuse ST–T wave changes	Often, associated bradycardia; clinical context
Early repolarization[d]	ST elevations	The "J wave," a slurring or notching preceding the ST segment
Hyperkalemia	Peaked T waves (mimic hyper-acute phase of MI); in more severe cases, widened QRS	Reduction of the size of the P waves
Myocardial fibrosis	Q waves	Clinical context

[a]With WPW, the changes are often restricted to V_1
[b]May associate inferior Q waves
[c]Chap. 7
[d]Changes may also be localized in anterior or inferior leads; there is some concern that this latter location may be associated to life-threatening arrhythmia

appear least effective in the patients who need them most. Nitrates can cause severe headaches, hypotension, and occasional paradoxical bradycardia. *Morphine* is not to be viewed merely as a "pain-killer," as it also helps control sympathetic activation (and is thus effective in reducing the size and complication incidence of STEMI); additionally, it helps improve hemodynamic conditions in patients with pulmonary edema. In the pre-reperfusion era, *β-blockers* were shown to significantly reduce STEMI mortality; in light of the sound rationale behind their use, the Class I indication is maintained in the current thrombolytic era. Smaller studies have suggested a higher efficacy with IV administration, but the large-scale COMIT CCS-2 trial has found no reduction in mortality, as reduced incidence of VF and of early reinfarction was offset by a higher

Fig. 2.4 The evolution phases of acute MI vs. those of acute pericarditis (explanations in the text)

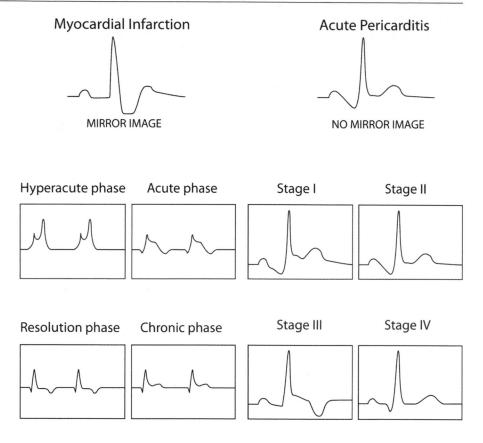

prevalence of cardiogenic shock. Therefore, while early IV β-blockade may be considered (Class IIb indication) in case of excessive adrenergic discharge (tachycardia, HTN), the preferred approach is oral therapy, started as soon as the patient has recovered from the acute phase of STEMI. The dosages are similar to the ones used in HTN. Some popular regimens include: *Atenolol (Tenormin)* 100 mg q.d. or 50 mg b.i.d., continued indefinitely (of note, the available data only refer to the first 6–9 days post-MI; the extension of this treatment is empirical). If a choice has been made to administer Atenolol in the early post-MI phase, this is given (in the absence of HF or hypotension) as a slow IV dose of 5 mg over 5 min, with another 5 mg 10 min after uneventful completion of the first dose; oral Atenolol is subsequently started; *Metoprolol (Lopressor)*: start at PO 50 mg q.i.d. for 48 h then switch to 100 mg b.i.d.; continue indefinitely. If administered early post-MI, three sequential IV doses of 5 mg at 2-min intervals are used, with oral therapy started at 15 min after the eventless administration of the IV therapy. The oral dosage may be reduced if the IV administration was not well tolerated and in the elderly. In the event of HF (whether MI-related or not), indefinite β-blocker therapy is mandatory, in the absence of contraindications. Preliminary data seem to demonstrate the feasibility of *Ivabradine* treatment as an alternative to Metoprolol in STEMI patients.

β-Blockade and HF: A Double Standard

β-Blockers are an integral part of *chronic* HF treatment; however, in *acute* HF (such as with acute MI), these agents are contraindicated.

ACEI, started within 24 h of STEMI onset in the absence of contraindications, produce a small but significant decrease in mortality. ACE-inhibitors appear to possess an antiatherogenic effect, irrespectively of LV function and of the presence of HTN. Such an effect has not been proven for ARB drugs. It is not clear whether these agents benefit all STEMI patients (Class IIa recommendation), or if they should be reserved for high-risk patients (Class I recommendation). High-risk patients have LVEF <40% or clinical HF; the benefit is smallest in patients with small inferior MI. Some popular regimens include: *Captopril*: PO initial dose of 6.25 mg, followed by 12.5 mg t.i.d., and increased to 25, then 50 mg t.i.d.; *Ramipril*: PO initial dose 2.5 mg q.d. for 1 week, then 5 mg q.d. for the next 3 weeks, then increase as tolerated to 10 mg q.d. (or 5 mg b.i.d.); *Lisinopril* 5 mg q.d., increase to 10 mg q.d.; *Trandolapril*, test dose of 0.5 mg, target dose 4 mg q.d.; *Quinapril*: PO 5 mg q.d. or b.i.d., titrated at weekly intervals to 20–40 mg daily in two divided doses. In HF, the target dose is 20 mg b.i.d. These doses may be increased as discussed in Chap. 4, in patients with overt HF. The duration of post-MI ACEI treatment is a matter of debate. While these agents should be continued indefinitely in patients with LV dysfunction or with overt HF, chronic use is not justified in asymptomatic patients with intact LV function. Patients unable to tolerate an ACEI should be treated with an *ARB agent*. The agent of choice is Valsartan 160 mg q.d., started at low doses (20 mg) and uptitrated slowly. Losartan 50 mg q.d. failed to replicate the protection offered by Captopril 50 mg t.i.d. In patients with LV dysfunction (EF <40%) and diabetes or HF *aldosterone antagonists* are used on top of ACEI or ARB agents, under close monitoring of the serum potassium levels. The main agents include *Spironolactone* 25–50 mg q.d. and *Eplerenone*, also dosed at 25–50 mg q.d. Eplerenone has been proven (EPHESUS trial) to reduce mortality as compared to placebo in post-MI patients, and represents an alternative in patients with LVEF <40% and creatinine <2.5 mg/dL in men (2.0 mg/dL in women). As hyperkalemia is common, potassium levels should be monitored, and the drug should not be started at potassium levels >5 mEq/L. Eplerenone has a much lower incidence of gynecomastia than Spironolactone.

Contraindicated or nonindicated therapies, suggested along the decades but proven ineffective or even deleterious include: *CCB*, which, as as a class, are associated with a (nonsignificant) trend towards adverse clinical outcomes; Diltiazem and Verapamil are contraindicated in STEMI patients with associated systolic LV dysfunction and CHF. Immediate-release Nifedipine is contraindicated, as it causes reflex sympathetic activation, tachycardia, and hypotension. *Prophylactic antiarrhythmic therapy*: while prophylactic Lidocaine may decrease the incidence of

malignant ventricular arrhythmia, there is no decrease in mortality, as the incidence of asystole increases; therefore, prophylactic Lidocaine in MI patients is contraindicated; *Prophylactic IV magnesium supplements* were found, in some smaller, open-labeled trials, to reduce MI mortality; however, the ISIS-4 trial and the specially-designed, optimally-dosed MAGIC trial have disproven this hypothesis; *glucose–insulin–potassium (GIK) therapy* was postulated to improve myocardial energy production and ventricular function and to decrease the incidence of serious ventricular arrhythmias in MI patients. Unfortunately, the CREATE-ECLA study has disproven this hypothesis as well; *COX-2 inhibitors* were suggested to complement the action of Aspirin and to overcome resistance to the latter, as Aspirin is only effective on the COX-1 receptors. However, COX-2 inhibitors were actually proven to increase mortality in CAD patients, as they reduce production of prostacyclin, a vasodilatory agent; enhance atherogenesis and thrombogenesis; and cause HTN (In fact, NSAIDs are contraindicated in CAD, as they, too, may increase mortality. However, Naproxen and possibly Diclofenac appear relatively safe.); *HRT*: it was hoped that an *estrogen/progestin* combination would replicate the protective action of natural estrogens, but this was found ineffective in secondary prevention, and actually deleterious (increased risk of CAD and of breast cancer), if used in primary prevention. *Torcetrapib* was developed to raise HDL, but was abandoned due to increased mortality; *Antioxidant therapy,* especially as vitamins E, C and A (β-carotene) have not been proven effective and are not recommended. Nevertheless, due to their intuitive appeal and their over-the-counter availability, they are frequently self-administrated in the population.

Special therapeutic considerations: *RV MI* is usually associated to inferior MI, but occasionally presents in isolation, causing hypotension in a patient with clear lung fields and enhanced jugular veins. Patients with RV MI are especially preload-sensitive, and IV saline infusions (initially, given rapidly) are the mainstay of therapy, while the use of vasodilators (including nitrates, opiates, ACEI, ARB) must be minimized. This is in stark contrast to the aggressive vasodilator and diuretic therapy used in LV MI-related shock. Additional frequent features include *AF* (which must be rapidly converted to NSR, as the atrial kick is especially important in these preload-sensitive patients) and *AV block*, which requires dual AV pacing, to restore physiologic AV activation sequence and optimize CO. Primary PCI is especially effective; the second-choice alternative, IV thrombolysis, may have suboptimal results. *MI in diabetics*: The mortality of STEMI is double than in non-diabetics, due to an often atypical presentation, with HF onset or exacerbation, rather than anginal symptoms; more diffuse and more severe coronary atherosclerosis; and frequent glucose imbalances in the acute stage. Glycemic control is of paramount importance in these patients (as, indeed, in any MI patient), but the optimal treatment for acute hyperglycemia is unclear (notably, the DIGAMI-2 trial has failed to show any advantage for Insulin, administered in isolation or in the first 24 h of presentation, as opposed to conventional therapy alone). In critically ill patients, insulin therapy should be used to decrease glucose levels to a range of 140–180 mg/dL (7.8–10.0 mmol/L), under frequent monitoring, to avoid hypoglycemia. The previous target levels of 90–140 mg/dL (5–7.8 mmol/L) were only attainable at the cost of a significant increase in poorly-tolerated hypoglycemia episodes, and are no longer recommended. However, tight *chronic* glycemic control does bring about a reduction in the incidence of macrovascular complications, and the recommendation to aim at a HbA1C level <7% has not changed.

MI in patients with renal failure is associated to increased mortality, partly due to underuse of invasive strategy, for fear of renal failure exacerbation under contrast material; on the other hand, if this complication does occur, the mortality is also increased.

MI Treatment : Acute Reperfusion Therapy
General remarks: Reperfusion restores blood flow to ischemic tissues, and is achieved by IV thrombolysis (STEMI only), or by primary PCI. In MI, CABG serves for rescue after failed PCI (due to time constraints and tissue friability after MI). Acute reperfusion improves survival by reducing MI size, myocardial remodeling, and arrhythmic potential. The absolute benefit from acute reperfusion is highest with new LBBB, anterior MI, and large at-risk myocardial areas, and lowest with inferior STEMI (except for the subgroup with associated RV MI or anterior ST-segment depression). However, benefit may be obtained regardless of MI location, patient age, and clinical presentation. Whatever the approach, the main concern is for speediness. The main cause for underuse of acute

reperfusion therapy in MI patients remains the delay between symptom onset and presentation to the medical caregiver. In this respect, the education of the public regarding the warning symptoms of a possible "heart attack" cannot be overstressed. The greatest benefit occurs within the first 2 h (when MI can actually be aborted or significantly limited in size); conversely, most of the damage is accomplished by 12 h, and only select patients are candidates for acute reperfusion therapy after this point. After presentation, prompt diagnosis and treatment are just as important. While the target "door-to-needle" and "door-to-balloon" times are of 30 and 90 min, respectively, shorter delays can often be attained, further improving prognosis. These demanding time frames partly compensate for the between symptom onset and presentation.

The absolute benefit from acute reperfusion therapy is highest in patients with new LBBB, anterior MI, and a large at-risk myocardial area (highest number of ECG leads affected, greatest total ST deviation) and lowest with inferior STEMI (except for the subgroup with associated RV MI or anterior ST-segment depression). However, benefit may be obtained regardless of MI location, patient age, and clinical presentation.

Fibrinolytics: Pharmacological reperfusion is indi-

Thrombolysis is indicated despite the absence of the ST elevations

- In postero-basal STEMI, manifesting with ST depressions in V_1–V_3 (posterior leads and echo are helpful for diagnosis)
- In the very early phase of STEMI, with giant hyperacute T waves preceding ST elevation
- In acute LBBB (in a suggestive setting)

---

cated in patients presenting within 12 h of chest pain and ST elevation or LBBB onset.

Occasionally, STEMI is asymptomatic or associates atypical discomfort; if, by chance, the diagnosis is established in a timely manner, reperfusion therapy is recommended as usual. Coronary occlusion is a dynamic process, involving multiple phases of artery occlusion (occasionally, complete) and spontaneous thrombolysis; thus, some patients actually suffer a series of *successive infarcts*, obscuring the definition of

Table 2.40 Contraindications to IV fibrinolytic therapy

Condition	Absolute contraindications	Relative contraindications
CNS conditions	Any past stroke of hemorrhagic or unknown origin; ischemic stroke in the past 6 months; brain neoplasms	TIA within the past 6 months
Trauma	Major trauma, surgery, or head injury within the past 3 weeks	Traumatic resuscitation
High risk of hemorrhage[a]	Bleeding disorders (predisposition to bleeding) or active bleeding	Oral anticoagulant therapy; advanced liver disease; non-compressible vascular punctures
GI disorders	GI bleeding within the past month	Active peptic ulcer
Other	Aortic dissection	IE; refractory HTN; pregnancy or within 1 week postpartum

[a]Not including menses

the 12-h window of opportunity for reperfusion therapy. If there is evidence of such successive episodes (e.g., sudden significant chest pain worsening), the most recent episode should be taken into account. IV fibrinolytics restore coronary TIMI II or III flow at 90 min in 50–85% of patients with STEMI. However, the pooling of TIMI flow II and III cases has been criticized, due to the significant differences in prognosis between the two populations. Pooled data indicate that TIMI III flow is achieved in only 50–60% of cases, as contrasted with a >90% rate for primary PCI.

The choice of the specific thrombolytic agent depends, besides availability and cost issues, on several factors. SK, by far the cheapest and the most available in developing countries, is *dispreferred* in patients presenting >4–6 h after symptom onset (more fibrin-specific agents, such as alteplase (tPA) or tenecteplase (TNK-tPA) are indicated); in allergic patients (SK is allergenic); and when, in the absence of the PCI option, an initial failed attempt at thrombolysis is followed by a second attempt. The contraindications to pharmacological thrombolysis are reviewed in Table 2.40.

The available IV thrombolytic agents include: SK; tPA; r-PA; and TNK-tPA. All of these agents bind to plasminogen, which is the precursor of the natural fibrinolytic, plasmin. The most important characteristics of these agents are reviewed in Table 2.41.

Hemorrhage, the main complication of thrombolysis and of antithrombotic therapy, is discussed in Sect. 2.2.

Glycoprotein IIb/IIIa inhibitors have been empirically found to occasionally achieve reperfusion by themselves, i.e., without being associated with either IV fibrinolytics or primary PCI. However, restoration of TIMI III flow by these agents alone was not seen in a sufficient number of patients to warrant relying on this approach in acute MI. *Combination therapy with IV thrombolytics and GP IIb/IIIa inhibitors* uses half a dose of a fibrinolytic agent (r-PA or TNK-tPA) associated to Abciximab (to overcome the initial platelet activation induced by thrombolysis). This combination regimen was assessed in the GUSTO-V and ASSENT-III trials; while 1- and 12-month mortality was not reduced as compared to full-dose thrombolytic alone, the rate of non-fatal reinfarction was significantly reduced. Unfortunately, as ICH was found to be twice as frequent in the combination therapy group, this approach is reserved for high-risk STEMI patients (large anterior MI), <75 years of age, and not at high risk for bleeding.

Interventional reperfusion in MI: *Primary PCI* has the same theoretical indications as fibrinolytic therapy, and is especially important in patients with large MI, shock, RV MI, or when fibrinolytic therapy is contraindicated or has failed. In patients with large MI, the main benefit consists in lower rates of nonfatal recurrent MI. Importantly however, PCI is not limited to these groups, and is in fact suitable for ≥90% of patients with acute MI. If expertly performed within 90 min of presentation, primary PCI generally has better results (as to overall prognosis and TIMI-3 flow in the infarct-related artery) than IV fibrinolytics. TIMI 3 flow is obtained in 70–90% of patients receiving primary PCI, with a 15% reocclusion rate after simple balloon angioplasty (5% if a coronary stent is used). In the real world, however, the logistic burden limits the general

Table 2.41 The commonly used fibrinolytics

	Dosage (all IV)	T1/2 (min[a])	Activated plasminogen	Complications (besides bleeding[b])	Heparin treatment[c]	Comments
Streptokinase	1.5mil.u. in 100 mL dextrose 5 or 0.9% saline, over 30–60 min.	20	Systemic	Allergy[d], hypotension, fever	Optional[e], for 24–48 h	Re-treatment with SK is most hazardous between 5 days and 4 years of initial use
Alteplase (tPA)	15 mg bolus, then 0.75 mg/kg over 30 min, and then 0.5 mg/kg over 60 min.; total dose ≤100 mg.	4	Clot-bound	May cause hypotension, nausea, vomiting	mandatory, for 24–48 h	
Reteplase (r-tPA)	2 boluses of 10 mg each, at a 30-min interval.	15	Clot-bound	May cause hypotension	mandatory, for 24–48 h	
Tenecteplase (TNK-tPA)	One 30 mg bolus for a patient <60 kg; increase bolus by 5 mg for every 10 kg over 60 kg; maximum dose 50 mg (≥90 kg)	60–90	Clot-bound	May cause hypotension	mandatory, for 24–48 h	

[a] This is relevant in case of hemorrhagic complications, when reversal of fibrinolysis is contemplated; for alteplase, for instance, by the time FFP is obtained, most of the fibrinolytic activity may have spontaneously abated

[b] Generally, the risk of intra-cranial hemorrhage is lowest with SK; with the other agents, risk is greatest in patients aged >65 and weighing <70 kg

[c] IV bolus of 60 U/kg, maximum 4,000 U, followed by a continuous infusion of 12 U/kg for 24–28 h, not to exceed 1,000 U/h. aPTT is monitored (target 1.5–2.0 times control) at 3, 6, 12, 24 h in the first day, and with similar frequency if a second day of treatment is necessary. With SK, if Heparin is used, it is started 3–4 h after infusion completion 1,000 units/h, after PTT measurement

[d] Bronchospasm, angioedema, rash, urticaria, up to anaphylaxis

[e] SK produces fibrin and fibrinogen degradation products, themselves anticoagulants, possibly obviating the need for Heparin; on the other hand, SK induces extensive plasmin-mediated thrombin activity, an argument in favor of ancillary antithrombotic therapy. No difference was found between the patients with and without adjunct *subcutaneous* Heparin therapy in the GUSTO-I trial

Table 2.42 Time Constraints in Primary PCI

90 min of presentation	12 h of symptom onset[b]	18 h of symptom onset	20 h of symptom onset
Primary PCI better than IV fibrinolytics	Ideal time frame for primary PCI in STEMI	Acceptable time frame for primary PCI in cardiogenic shock[a]	Acceptable time frame for primary[b] PCI in patients with Killip III HF, hemodynamic or electrical instability, or persistent ischemic symptoms

[a]Provided shock onset was ≤36 h from STEMI onset

[b]*Any* PCI aiming at acute revascularization is "primary." Within the first 12 h, this means PCI was chosen over IV fibrinolysis; beyond 12 h, PCI is chosen over CABG or over no reperfusion therapy whatsoever

applicability of primary PCI. Primary PCI is almost universally carried out with stent deployment, to reduce the incidence of late restenosis. However, stenting does not significantly affect the mortality (3.0%) or reinfarction (2%) rates. PCI complications include problems with the arterial access site; technical complications of angioplasty; pulmonary congestion due to volume overload; CIN; excess bleeding due to antithrombotic medications; and early reocclusion or late restenosis. Of note, primary PCI can be performed up to 24 h of symptom onset in patients with severe HF (but no cardiogenic shock), hemodynamic or electrical instability, or persistent ischemic symptoms. The culprit lesion is often eccentric and has irregular, "shaggy," ulcerated borders, and may demonstrate haziness associated with intracoronary thrombus. Vasoconstriction may increase the apparent severity of the stenosis, and is countered by intracoronary administration of Nitroglycerin. In patients with either widespread or angiographically unapparent coronary atherosclerosis, identification of the culprit lesion requires correlation with the EKG and echo findings. Angiographically non-significant (<50%) culprit plaques should not be intervened upon, as "plaque sealing" with a stent does not improve outcomes. (Of note, however, the concept of "plaque sealing" may still prove valid, by using a specially designed stent, which is flexible and self-expanding, rather than balloon expandable. This device exerts a mild "push" on the vessel wall, to prevent plaque rupture.) Most PCI procedures in the current era involve the use of stents. DES cause an increased incidence of acute or subacute thrombosis; the exact clinical impact is heatedly debated. If the patient is scheduled to undergo surgery which will require interruption of dual antiplatelet therapy, a bare-metal stent (BMS) is preferable. By and large, most patients are amenable to PCI, the rest being referred for surgery. PCI and surgery are not mutually exclusive, as either may offer "rescue" from failure of the other procedure. A staged approach may also be considered, involving first PCI of the culprit lesion, and later full revascularization by elective CABG (at >12 months after PCI, as CABG requires discontinuation of antiplatelet therapy). The somewhat complex time constraints regarding primary PCI are summarized in Table 2.42.

"Facilitated PCI" (PCI following different combinations of fibrinolytics, and/or GP IIb/IIIa inhibitors, generally in reduced dosages, meant to "clear the field" for PCI) was assessed by the FINESSE and the ASSENT IV trials. No advantage was found for this approach, while the risk of peri-procedure adverse events might actually increase. However, this approach may have a role in STEMI patients facing delays in proceeding to the cath lab.

Occasionally, STEMI presents with angiographically normal coronary arteries, as may do patients with NSTEMI or UA. These cases are discussed in Table 2.43.

Angioplasty in Acute STEMI: Beyond Primary PCI

Primary PCI is, by and large, superior to IV thrombolysis, but the two modalities are not mutually exclusive. Thus, PCI can be used after failed thrombolysis (rescue PCI) or after successful thrombolysis, to provide definitive treatment of the culprit plaque. *Rescue angioplasty* is an important option after failed thrombolysis. The REACT trial demonstrated an up to 50% reduction in the composite end-point of death, reinfarction, stroke, and severe HF at 6 months, in patients

Table 2.43 ACS with angiographically normal coronary arteries

Entity	Mechanism	Clinical manifestations	Therapy
Coronary spasm (Prinzmetal's angina)	Spasm at the site of plaque, or in an apparently normal segment, due to ED[a]	Transient ST segment elevations, occasionally syncope, mainly at night, in younger, heavy-smoking patients	Risk factor management, CCB
Intramural plaque with thrombosis	Pseudonormal coronaries; diffuse atherosclerosis, with positive remodeling (vessel expansion)	General ACS presentation	As for any CAD, but revascularization is not an option
Coronary embolism	Normal coronaries, embolus formed at a distance, (e.g., AF)	General ACS presentation	Therapy of the underlying disorder
Syndrome X	ED,[a] increased sensitivity to pain and to sympathetic stimulation	Typical chest pain, on exercise or at rest; positive stress test (ST depressions); excellent prognosis	Nitrates, β-blockers, or CCB
Apical ballooning syndrome[b]	Not clear; high circulating levels of catecholamines may cause microvascular spasm	Apical and mid-ventricular akinesis (Mimicking anterior MI), mainly in post-menopausal women after severe emotional stress. Occasional HF. Usually fully reversible	Supportive; treatment of HF (Occasionally, inotropic agents or IABP are necessary)

[a]Endothelial dysfunction

[b]Alternative names include: Takotsubo syndrome (Japanese for turtle trap, alluding to the shape of the heart during the attack); broken-heart-syndrome (severe emotional stress, usually the loss of a loved one); and stress CMP

undergoing rescue PCI after failed IV thrombolysis. However, even rescue PCI may fail to restore epicardial blood flow in up to 10% of patients, with a variable number of additional patients undergoing reocclusion. The decision in favor of rescue PCI (as opposed to conservative therapy or to CABG) is based on the importance of the myocardium at jeopardy, as judged by the Killip class; the ischemic symptoms; electrical instability; and the results of post-MI risk stratification (There is a Class IIb recommendation for rescue PCI in all patients after failed thrombolysis. If a policy of routine PCI after IV thrombolysis is implemented regardless of the initial success rates, the notion of "rescue PCI" becomes redundant). In occasional patients a relatively small area of jeopardized myocardium may cause electrical instability (with potentially lethal ventricular arrhythmia), justifying rescue PCI. *PCI after successful thrombolysis* has been assessed in the acute setting (within 24 h) and in the late setting. The CARESS-in AMI study, carried out in *high-risk* STEMI patients initially treated with IV thrombolysis (primary PCI unavailable), and then immediately transported to another hospital for elective PCI (regardless of the initial success of IV thrombolysis) has demonstrated improved outcomes in the intervention group. Whether this policy can be extended to *all*

post-thrombolysis patients (regardless of MI size and clinical status) is unclear. The TRANSFER-AMI study has confirmed the advantages of the "pharmacoinvasive" strategy as compared with standard treatment, without excess bleeding: post-thrombolysis patients transferred for PCI within 6 h of fibrinolysis fared better than patients treated conservatively (with PCI used for rescue only). *PCI late after IV thrombolysis* has been extensively studied, in light of the *late open artery hypothesis*, proposing that coronary patency may improve prognosis despite lack of myocardial salvage (in older trials, LV dilatation and arrhythmia were more frequent and the overall prognosis was poorer, in patients with a persistently occluded infarct-related artery). Several prospective trials have reached diverging conclusions in this respect, possibly due to the different study populations. Thus, the Occluded Artery Trial (OAT) trial, carried out in *asymptomatic* patients with an occluded epicardial coronary artery, but without three-vessel or left main CAD and with no demonstrable residual ischemia, found no benefit for routine PCI. However, the BRAVE-2 trial, evaluating *symptomatic* elderly patients early after MI, did find both mortality and quality-of-life benefit for PCI at >12 h. These findings suggest that the "late artery hypothesis" is just another way of stating the obvious, i.e., that patients with residual ischemia fare worse than those without it, and consequently may benefit from intervention. These findings must be extrapolated cautiously to patients with severe LV dysfunction, as 98% of patients in the BRAVE-2 trial were in NYHA Classes I or II. These patients may present symptoms of HF, rather than of ischemia, or can be asymptomatic; hibernation may play an important role.

Surgical reperfusion is an impractical *primary* option in STEMI. If available in patients with a *coronary anatomy unsuited for PCI,* presenting within 12 h of STEMI onset, emergency CABG is an option, especially in presence of hemodynamic or electrical instability, or of severe HF. Left main stenosis ≥50% and/or triple-vessel disease have classically been considered "unsuitable for PCI," an example of conventional wisdom challenged by contemporary PCI techniques. Primary CABG is also indicated in *mechanical complications of MI* (post-MI VSD or MR). By and large, however, the main use of CABG in MI that of a *rescue procedure* after failed PCI (persistent or recurrent pain or hemodynamic instability). The best results are obtained with arterial revascularization, using LIMA, RIMA, or both. CABG is a major surgical procedure, with a 3–4% overall mortality (higher in the elderly, in diabetics, in patients with decreased LV function, renal failure, COPD, or left main artery disease). The main complications include periprocedural MI, stroke, bleeding, distal embolism, and a systemic pro-inflammatory response.

Acute Reperfusion Strategies: A Comparison

Primary PCI preferred to IV Thrombolysis

- In patients without cardiogenic shock, STEMI prognosis is better with primary PCI than with IV fibrinolytics, only if performed (1) *expertly* (i.e., the operator performs ≥75 cases yearly, and the catheterization laboratory performs ≥36 cases yearly); (2) *promptly* (door-to-balloon time <90 min[#]); (3) *safely*: i.e., the risk of PCI is smaller than that of thrombolysis (risk of intracranial bleeding under thrombolysis >4%, as assessed clinically).
- In patients with cardiogenic shock, if performed within 18 h of shock onset and shock has developed ≤36 h after STEMI and the patient age is <75 years[§].

- When symptom onset was >3 h, and not over the admissible maximum delay for the specific type of clinical presentation (i.e., "later" presentation, but still within the window of opportunity).
- When the diagnosis of STEMI is not certain (if the patient suffers from NSTEMI, the indicated therapy is PCI).

While in select centers primary PCI is the default option for all eligible patients, the highest benefit (justifying transport to a hospital with primary PCI capabilities) is seen with larger MI, and when IV thrombolysis is contraindicated.

[#]In itself, primary PCI is *effective* in this group within 12 h of symptom onset, just like IV thrombolytics. PCI is *more effective* than IV thrombolysis if logistics allow artery opening within 90 min of presentation; otherwise the better vascular patency rates are offset by the greater amount of myocardial necrosis. Of note, the ideal door-to-needle time, in case of IV thrombolysis, is *shorter*, i.e., 30 min; however, due to the much simpler logistics, this is often easier to achieve than the more "lenient" 90-min window for primary PCI. If the preparations for primary PCI would take more than 1 h beyond the point when thrombolysis can be administered ("door-to-balloon" – "door-to-needle" = 90−30 = 60 min), then IV thrombolysis is preferred.
[§]In the absence of these characteristics, the decision of IV fibrinolysis vs. no revascularization therapy is individually based. A useful milestone is a ≥4% risk of ICH, as a reason to withhold IV thrombolysis.

The intraaortic counterpulsation balloon pump (IABP) is a device used to decrease myocardial O_2 demand and increase CO. The balloon is introduced by catheter into the descending aorta, after the take-off of the left subclavian artery. The device is inflated in diastole (increasing blood flow to the coronary arteries) and deflated in systole (reducing afterload and increasing forward blood flow). The inflation/deflation are computer-controlled, under EKG or intracardiac pressure gating. IABP is used in patients with *intractable angina*, as a bridge to revascularization or transplant; *after angioplasty,* to support recovery of the ischemic segments; *after CABG,* for gradual weaning from cardiopulmonary bypass; *in case of myocardial rupture after MI* (acute MR, VSD, free wall rupture), as a bridge to surgery; *cardiogenic shock,* as a bridge to heart transplant; *in preoperative patients with unstable angina with a ≥70% LMCA stenosis and LVEF <35%.* Aortic dissection, AI, and severe aortoiliac atherosclerosis are *absolute contraindications*, while aortic aneurysm or aortic/aortofemoral grafts represent relative contraindications. The main complications include lower limb ischemia and compartment syndrome; renal artery occlusion and renal failure; cerebral embolism during insertion or removal; infection, aortic or iliac dissection or perforation (occasionally, with mediastinal hemorrhage); and thrombocytopenia. Due to these complications, the use of IABP must be restricted to a few days at most.

Assessment of Reperfusion in MI

At first glance, this topic is only relevant in patients undergoing IV thrombolysis, as coronary patency is readily assessed with primary PCI. However, "reperfusion" refers to restoration of *microvascular* circulation; while optimal tissue perfusion requires epicardial TIMI grade III flow, the latter does not guarantee that myocardial perfusion is optimal (or indeed present). The "no-reflow" phenomenon is explained by two strongly interrelated events: *microvascular damage,* (mainly due to distal embolization of atherothrombotic debris) and *reperfusion injury,* due to active mediator release from the microemboli. These mediators cause tissue edema and microvascular spasm, free radical formation, cytokine activation (the first step of an intense inflammatory reaction), calcium overload, and apoptosis.

At the time of primary PCI, reperfusion is assessed in patients with postprocedure TIMI III flow, by the myocardial blush score. Myocardial blush assessment is only possible at the time of coronary angiography. It was hoped that contrast echo would allow bedside evaluation of myocardial perfusion, but this promise it yet unfulfilled. On the other hand, other perfusion-detecting methods (nuclear scan, perfusion MRI) are logistically impractical in acute MI patients. Therefore, evaluation of reperfusion is based on remission of pain and on a greater than or equal to ≥50% reduction in the initial ST elevations 60–90 min after initiation of therapy. Unfortunately, the clinical parameters have low predictive value for the *cause* of lack of reperfusion (failed epicardial reperfusion/subacute thrombosis after PCI vs. no-reflow phenomenon). If the findings persist after IV thrombolysis, or if they recur after an initially successful primary PCI procedure, rescue, respectively "redo" PCI is an option. *Reperfusion arrhythmias* are bursts of ventricular ectopy associated to epicardial vessel recanalization, and as such have long been regarded as a favorable prognostic factor. On the other hand, reperfusion arrhythmias are also a sign of reperfusion injury. These rhythms appear within 6 h after start of thrombolysis and include, most typically, accelerated idioventricular rhythm (AIVR), but also frequent PVCs >8/h, nonsustained VT, sinus bradycardia and possibly high-degree AVB. Reperfusion arrhythmia has a high specificity, but a low sensitivity for the diagnosis of arterial recanalization.

Antithrombotic Therapy

Antithrombotic therapy (a) facilitates and maintains co-ronary reperfusion, (b) limits the consequences of myocardial ischemia, enhances myocardial healing, and (c) reduces the likelihood of recurrent events. Strategies to counter arterial thrombosis include: *measures addressing the atherosclerotic plaque* (primary prevention, i.e., preventing plaque formation or progression; secondary prevention, i.e., preventing recurrent thrombosis on a plaque formerly involved in STEMI occurrence) and *measures addressing the coronary thrombus,* i.e., preventing platelet activation and aggregation; if a platelet clot does form, stopping it from activating the coagulation cascade, either by decreasing the hepatic synthesis of coagulation factors or by preventing the activation of these factors (mainly thrombin); and, if thrombin has not been adequately counteracted, i.e., if a fibrin clot has formed, dismantling the clot. These aims are reached using antiplatelet agents, vitamin K inhibitors, thrombin inhibitors, fibrinolytics, and PCI (primary PCI combines clot lysis and plaque therapy). Of these approaches, antiplatelet and antithrombin therapy are universally used, whether revascularization is undertaken or not. Ideally, percutaneous revascularization should be routine, as primary PCI, or, at the very least, within the first day of STEMI symptoms. In patients with large MI, early PCI is indicated regardless of IV thrombolysis results. *Measures addressing the atherosclerotic plaque* include antihyperlipemic therapy (Sect. 2.1) and PCI, whether primary or early after STEMI. *Measures addressing the coronary thrombus* include antiplatelet therapy; antithrombin therapy;

and fibrinolytic therapy, reviewed above. VKA (oral anticoagulants) are reviewed in Chap. 6. Their role in the management of CAD in general, and of ACS in particular, is relatively modest (they serve as an alternative to Clopidogrel in intolerant patients, and for treatment of intraventricular thrombus, most often formed in a LV aneurysm, itself a consequence of acute MI).

Antiplatelet Therapy

The main antiplatelet agents are reviewed in Sect. 2.2. Antiplatelet therapy in STEMI patients is reviewed in Table 2.44.

Aspirin: Aspirin, started as early as possible, is effective in MI patients, whether they did or did not receive

Table 2.44 Antiplatelet agents in STEMI patients

	No reperfusion therapy	Thrombolysis	PCI[a]
NSAID[b]			
Aspirin	PO[c] 150–325 mg q.d., continue indefinitely	PO[c] 150–325 mg q.d., continue indefinitely	PO 150–325 mg q.d., continue indefinitely
Thienopyridines			
Clopidogrel	PO 75 mg q.d., continue for up to 1 year[d]	PO loading 300 mg[e]; continue for up to 1 year[d]	PO loading dose of 600 mg, then 75 mg q.d., for ≥1 mo. with bare metal stents, ≥12 months (or indefinitely) with DES
Prasugrel	No data to date[f]	No data to date[f]	PO 60 mg loading dose, then 10 mg q.d., for 6–15 months[g]
Ticlopidine	N/A[h]	250 mg b.i.d. for up to 1 year[i]	250 mg b.i.d. for up to 1 year[i]
IIb/IIIa inhibitors			
Abciximab	–	–	IV bolus 0.25 mg/kg, then infusion of 0.125 μg/kg/min over 12 h, not to exceed 10 μg/min
Eptifibatide	–	–	180 μg/kg over 1–2 min at diagnosis, then infusion of 2 μg/kg/min, until PCI, not to exceed 72 h
Tirofiban	–	–	IV infusion 0.4 μg/kg/min, for 30 min, then 0.1 μg/kg/min for ≥12 h, not to exceed 24 h after angioplasty

[a]Primary, rescue, or routine PCI after IV thrombolysis
[b]Other NSAID drugs, including COX-2 inhibitors are contraindicated in ACS; NSAIDS (with the exception of COX-2 inhibitors) may be given for post-MI pericarditis, but the onset of this condition is generally well outside the acute phase of MI
[c]In patients with severe nausea or vomiting, Aspirin can be given IV, in doses of 250–500 mg; older guidelines also suggest Aspirin suppositories of 300 mg; non–enteric-coated formulations are recommended; In patients already on Aspirin, the acute dose may in principle be omitted, but in practice it is frequently administered nonetheless
[d]The risk/benefit ratio must be carefully assessed. The recommendation is based mainly on extrapolation of the data regarding non-STEMI ACS (the CURE trial); A daily dose of 150 mg of Clopidogrel in the week following PCI might improve outcomes, while not increasing bleeding rates
[e]No loading dose in the elderly, except if routine PCI is planned regardless of IV fibrinolytic therapy results (consider lower loading doses); Many advocate a loading dose of 600 mg, even if the patient is already on Clopidogrel (Clopidogrel "reload")
[f]The pivotal study regarding Prasugrel, TRITON-TIMI 38, was carried out in patients with moderate-to-high-risk ACS scheduled for PCI; a 60 mg loading dose was followed by administration of 10 mg q.d., for 6–15 months
[g]This regimen was used in the TRITON TIMI-28 trial, but was not incorporated in the 2008 ESC Guidelines
[h]By extrapolation of data regarding Clopidogrel, 250 mg q 12 h for a total duration similar to that with Clopidogrel appears reasonable. Of note, the current European Guidelines for the treatment of STEMI (2008) do not mention Ticlopidine at all; the recommended alternative in Clopidogrel-intolerant patients is Warfarin
[i]No longer included in the 2009 ESC guidelines

fibrinolytic therapy. It confers as high a benefit as SK, and the combination shows additive benefit. Immediate Aspirin administration is mandatory in all MI patients, with the sole exception of those truly allergic (and not simply intolerant) to the drug. The dose is of 300–325 mg (four chewable tablets of 81 mg, for rapid absorbtion; or one nonchewable tablet of 325 mg). IV Aspirin 250–500 mg, or one suppository (300 mg) are used in case of nausea and vomiting. Technically, the standing recommendation in case of Aspirin allergy is to "replace" this drug with Clopidogrel. Practically, however, as there is a Class I indication for Clopidogrel administration at presentation *in addition* to Aspirin, this amounts to simply omitting Aspirin in these patients. Aspirin 75–162 mg q.d. is continued indefinitely. *Thienopyridines*: Since the landmark CLARITY-TIMI 28 and COMIT/CCS-2 trials, *Clopidogrel* (Plavix) administration at presentation of all STEMI patients (irrespective of subsequent therapeutic strategies) has become routine. Clopidogrel decreases the incidence of hard endpoints such as all-cause mortality, cardiovascular death, reinfarction, or revascularization, without an increased risk of bleeding. A loading dose of 300 mg (600 mg before primary PCI) is followed by 75 mg q.d.; the optimal duration of combined therapy is unknown. If CABG is planned, a 5–7 day waiting period after initial Clopidogrel loading is recommended, if clinically acceptable. Older guidelines notwithstanding, Clopidogrel should be continued for at least 12 months after stent implantation, and possibly indefinitely in DES stents. Therefore, a high risk of bleeding is a relative contraindication to DES implantation. *Prasugrel* (Effient), the latest thienopyridine developed to date, has been shown by the TRITON-TIMI 38 trial to be superior to Clopidogrel in moderate-to-high risk ACS patients, a conclusion also valid in the STEMI subgroup of the patient cohort. Prasugrel significantly reduced the risk for the combined endpoint of cardiovascular death, non-fatal heart attack or non-fatal stroke at both 30 days and 15 months. In the STEMI subgroup, there was no excess bleeding with Prasugrel, unlike the main cohort, where Prasugrel decreased cardiovascular mortality, but increased mortality due to major bleeding, with no difference in mortality between the Clopidogrel and Prasugrel groups. The multiple side effects of *Ticlopidine,* the first clinically available thienopyridine, have lead to its almost universal replacement by Clopidogrel. Ticlopidine can cause neutropenia (1%) and thrombotic thrombocytopenic purpura (TTP; 3%), which mandate CBC follow-up q 2 weeks

for the first 3 months of use. Additionally, up to 20% of patients experience nausea, diarrhea, and rash, mandating therapy discontinuation. There are no direct data as to the optimal duration of therapy after DES use, but it is reasonable to follow the guidelines for Clopidogrel. *IIb/IIIa antagonists*: *Abciximab* (ReoPro) can be used (a) *in combination with half-dose reteplase or TNK-tPA* for prevention of reinfarction and other complications of STEMI in patients <75 years with an anterior MI, and no increased risk for bleeding. If an early invasive strategy is planned (transportation to a PCI-capable facility), this strategy is no longer recommended (see "facilitated PCI," above); (b) *in patients undergoing primary PCI,* Abciximab (IV bolus of 0.25 mg/kg, followed by an infusion of 0.125 µg/kg/min over 12 h), started immediately after diagnosis, reduces by 50% the incidence of death, MI, or urgent total revascularization at 30 days. *Eptifibatide* (Integrilin) is effective in unstable angina and NSTEMI; in STEMI, it is used by extrapolation, and also based on a smaller-scale trial, EVA-AMI, which found it non-inferior to Abciximab. As Eptifibatidide is several-fold cheaper than Abciximab, the issue is of great importance. The recommended doses are of 180 µg/kg over 1–2 min at diagnosis, followed by continuous IV infusion of 2 µg/kg/min, until hospital discharge, initiation of coronary revascularization, or the completion of a 72-h course, whichever occurs first. *Tirofiban* (Aggrastat) is administered as an IV infusion of 0.4 µg/kg/min, for 30 min, followed by a continuous infusion, at 0.1 µg/kg/min. The ON-TIME 2 study showed that Tirofiban significantly improved ST-segment resolution at 1 h after primary PCI. The drug is continued for ≥12 h, but not more than 24 h after angioplasty.

Antithrombin Therapy in MI Thrombin inhibition can be achieved indirectly (by AT III activation), or indirectly (by direct binding to thrombin and inactivation of its active site). The main antithrombin agents are reviewed in Sect. 2.2, and their use in STEMI patients is presented in Table 2.45. *Heparin* is recommended in all MI patients, with the possible exception of those treated with SK. In STEMI patients not undergoing fibrinolysis, Heparin is believed to confer a mortality benefit, based on a metaanalysis of pre-reperfusion era studies. While there is no indication for or against Heparin use in the current guidelines, this agent is routinely used, but only if Fondaparinux is not available (Table 2.43).

VKA have a relatively modest place in the treatment of CAD. They are to be continued, in addition to

Table 2.45 Antithrombin therapy in STEMI patients[a]

	No reperf. Tx	Thrombolysis			Primary PCI
Indirect thrombin inhibitors					
UFH	Alternative to Fondaparinux; adjust by weight	IV bolus 60 U/kg, ≤4,000 U, followed by IV 12 U/kg, ≤1,000 U/h for 24–48 h[b]; target aPTT 50–50 s, monitored at 3, 6, 12, 24 h			Loading dose IV 100 U/kg[c], then infusion, for the duration of the procedure only, at an ACT[d] of 250–350 s[e]
Low-molecular weight heparin (LMWH)					
Fondaparinux	As for thrombolysis; it is the preferred agent in this setting	IV bolus 2.5 mg the following day, start S.C. 2.5 mg q.d. ≤8 days			No; OASIS-6 trial: higher rate of catheter thrombosis and coronary complications (abrupt closure, thrombosis, no reflow, dissection, or perforation) with Fondaparinux[f]
Enoxaparin[g]	As for thrombolysis	RFT	Age		Insufficient data; a suggested strategy involves one S.C. dose of 1 mg/kg, supplemented by an IV dose 0.3–0.5 mg/kg, ideally under anti-factor Xa monitoring (target: 0.5–1.5 U/mL; risk of bleeding increases at >1.U/mL)
			≤75	>75	
		Creat. <2.5 g/L (♂), <2 g/L (♀)	IV bolus 30 mg; 15 min. later, start S.C. 1 mg/kg q 12 h ≤8 days[h]	No IV bolus; first S.C. dose 0.75 mg/kg[i]	
		CRCL <30	S.C. doses repeated at 24 h		
Direct thrombin inhibitors					
Argatroban[j]	In HIT or HIT-prone patients; not approved for general STEMI patients	In HIT or HIT-prone patients; not approved for general STEMI patients			In HIT or HIT-prone patients only
Bivalirudin	Insufficient data	HERO-2 study: Bivalirudin does not improve mortality, but may decrease reinfarction, and increases ≤moderate bleeding as compared to UFH			Loading dose IV 0.75 mg/kg, then infusion, usually for the duration of the procedure only, at 1.75 mg/kg/h (based on the HORIZONS trial[k])
Lepirudin	HIT or HIT-prone patients only	HIT or HIT-prone patients only			HIT or HIT-prone patients only
Dabigatran	Under study (RE-DEEM trial)				

[a]Comments about non-indicated regimens are in italics

[b]Optional after SK; recent data suggests post-thrombolysis anticoagulation should be maintained for ≥48 h, and preferably throughout the entire hospitalization, in which case a non-UFH agent (Enoxaparin, Bivalirudin, or Fondaparinux) is indicated beyond the first 24 h

[c]If a IIb/IIIa agent is being used, the loading dose is decreased to 60 mg/kg

[d]Activated clotting time, measured with the HemoTec device; (300–350 s with the Hemochron device)

[e]UFH loading dose reduced to 50–70 U/kg, target ACT 200 s (measured with either the HemoTec or Hemochron device) if a IIb/IIIa agent is being used

[f]This has led the ESC, but not the ACC/AHA to withhold recommendation in patients undergoing PCI. However, the same study has shown the efficacy of Fondaparinux for non-primary PCI, e.g., rescue PCI or routine transportation to a PCI-capable center after initial IV thrombolytic therapy

[g]The EXTRACT-TIMI-25, comparing Enoxaparin to UFH in STEMI patients eligible for IV fibrinolysis, found a higher efficacy, but also a higher rate of major bleeding, in the Enoxaparin group

[h]The first two doses should not exceed 100 mg in total

[i]The first two doses should not exceed 76 mg in total

[j]Argatroban falsely increases INR

[k]The HORIZONS trial has shown a lower rate of major bleeding and adverse events at 30 days with Bivalirudin compared with UFH + a GP IIb/IIIa blocker in STEMI patients undergoing primary PCI

antiplatelet therapy, in patients in with another indication for their use. VKA are indicated in case of LV thrombus (target INR 2–3), on a long-time basis, as the cause of LV thrombosis is most frequently LV aneurysm, a chronic condition. In high-risk patients allergic in whom Clopidogrel is not available (or there is resistance to it as well), Warfarin is added, with a target INR of 2–2.5. The same target is used for Aspirin-resistant patients, in whom Clopidogrel is unavailable or ineffective.

V - Novel Therapies in MI

Beside the quest for newer and safer percutaneous devices and antithrombotic agents, a few novel directions are being explored. Thus, anti-inflammatory compounds are being tested in patients with ACS, under the hypothesis that their addition to a standard optimal regimen will improve clinical outcomes. A fluid bioresorbable material injected percutaneously into the infarcted myocardium may limit MI expansion and improve LV function, by replacing destroyed extracellular matrix, and leading to formation of a smaller and thicker scar.

Post-STEMI Risk Stratification

Post-STEMI risk stratification (all the considerations below also apply to ACS as a whole): Successful ACS therapy implies not only resolution of the acute episode, but also avoidance of recurrent ischemia in the culprit artery and avoidance of late complications (HF and/or arrhythmia). The risk for these events is in the center of attention even as the patient is being treated for the acute disease, and splits the ACS population in several risk strata, hence the term, risk stratification (Table 2.46). Due to its profound influence on therapy, risk assessment is actually carried out, formally and informally, from the time of the patient's presentation. In this respect, it ought to be discussed immediately following the "Diagnosis" section; however, for the sake of fluency, it is discussed in the current section.

Risk stratification is accomplished formally or informally, by using clinical, EKG, and imaging data (obtained at rest or under stress). These individual assessments are used as such, or grouped in more complex, multifactorial risk scores. Some indicators are specific for a group of entities (e.g., enzyme elevation in all MI patients), while others refer to a single entity (e.g., ST segment elevation in STEMI patients only). Assessment methods and scores will be reviewed next. The practical implication of a positive result of risk stratification is that angiography should be carried out, if not already performed; that an ICD device should be implanted as discussed in Chap. 4; and that appropriate medical therapy should be adopted for ventricular dysfunction or HF. Importantly, risk stratification preserves its importance even in affluent countries, where PCI is readily available. Indeed, routine PCI has not been proven to improve prognosis in ACS all-comers. The OAT trial has found no advantage to routine PCI in asymptomatic post-MI patients without three-vessel or left main CAD and with no demonstrable residual ischemia. Similarly, the ICTUS trial has found no advantage to routine invasive therapy in all NSTEMI patients.

Clinical assessment is based on the presence (or absence) of the following elements: Killip class at

Table 2.46 Risk stratification after ACS: aims and means

What risk is being assessed	Method of assessment	Therapeutic implications (acute phase)	Therapeutic implications (long-term)
Of myocardial necrosis, should the culprit artery reocclude	Stress imaging to detect myocardium at jeopardy[a]	Primary, rescue, or post-fibrinolysis PCI[b] improve prognosis as compared to IV thrombolysis (where applicable) or to conservative therapy only	Early PCI decreases late cardiovascular morbidity and mortality
Of late cardiovascular morbidity and mortality	Echo, to detect LV dysfunction; EKG,[c] to detect the risk of arrhythmia	None	Early PCI decreases late cardiovascular morbidity and mortality

[a]The larger the area at risk, the higher the risk, and the stronger the indication for PCI
[b]If routine primary or post-fibrinolysis PCI is undertaken, this aspect of risk stratification is implicitly accomplished
[c]Including Holter, SAECG, and other newer modalities outlined in Sect. 2.2

presentation; clinical signs of reperfusion; recurrent ischemia; arrhythmia beyond the first 24 h; and mechanical complications of MI.

EKG assessment includes: *a resting tracing,* indicating the type and extent of ischemia. The greater the number of involved leads, the larger the ischemic myocardial area, and consequently, the higher the risk. With STEMI, the number of involved EKG leads and the sum elevation of ST segments allow calculation of different severity scores. While the practical utility of scores is questionable, a larger number of involved EKG leads remains correlated to more severe MI. EKG data from the early thrombolytic era have suggested a prognostically important MI classification as large (extensive anterior MI, culprit artery: proximal LAD; extensive posterior MI, culprit artery: proximal dominant or RCA proximal dominant LCx), small (mainly inferior MI, culprit artery: distal RCA or distal LCx), or intermediate-size (all other MI). An additional EKG negative prognostic factor is the presence of Q waves. The resting tracing is also prognostically useful in regard to the risk of late lethal ventricular arrhythmia. Ventricular arrhythmia >24–48 h is an indicator of high risk for SCD. In the past, this was an indication for *EP study* (considered positive if sustained monomorphic VT is inducible). Current guidelines recommend ICD implantation in post-MI patients with decreased EF (see Chap. 4), occasionally making EPS redundant in this setting (assuming ICD devices are readily available). *Additional EKG techniques* to evaluate the late risk of SCD include: SAECG, T wave alternans, HR variability and turbulence, QT dispersion, and baroreceptor sensitivity. The place of these methods in clinical practice remains to be defined. *An EKG stress test* (submaximal or pharmacological test at 4–5 days; symptom-limited test at 2 weeks; or pharmacological test at 4–6 weeks) is integral part of risk stratification.

Echo is occasionally used for MI diagnosis; otherwise, the first echo examination is carried out within 24–48 h of the acute event, to evaluate LV function and identify a possible LV thrombus. An LVEF EF <40% justifies an invasive approach, as it is a strong predictor of cardiovascular morbidity and mortality (late ventricular arrhythmia, HF). A follow-up echo is carried out at some point >2 weeks from the acute event; in the absence of recurrent acute ischemia or of hibernation, systolic LV dysfunction generally reflects myocardial necrosis. An *echo stress test* can be used for risk stratification, in place of an EKG stress test.

Biomarker-based risk assessment: The area under the curve of *CK or its isoform CK-MB* levels plotted against time is proportional to MI size. However, this method is cumbersome, as serial CK levels need to be measured; a surrogate assessment is that of peak CK, which correlates fairly well with MI size. However, there are several problems with this measurement as well: (a) CK increases normalize shortly after the acute phase of MI, and frequent blood sampling is necessary to avoid missing the true peak value; (b) CK elevations are strongly influenced by the reperfusion status. Thus, a high (but short-lived) CK peak may simply correspond to good reperfusion, with "in bulk" spillage of biomarker; conversely, low (but protracted) elevations may reflect non-reperfusion. In practice, it is often difficult to correlate the pattern of CK increase to one or another of these possible causes. *Troponin* can also be used to assess MI size. Only early troponin release is influenced by the reperfusion status; troponin values at 72 h are not substantially influenced. One study has found that toponin T levels >2.98 μg/L predicted a LVEF <40% at 3 months with a sensitivity and specificity in excess of 80%. *Novel biomarkers for MI,* currently under development, aim at very early detection of myocardial necrosis, some as early as a few minutes after the beginning of the ischemic injury.

There are several risk scores, integrating the available clinical, enzymatic, and imaging information (Table 2.47). All scores are used for STEMI and NSTEMI patients alike. For NSTEMI, the most favored risk score is GRACE, using an online calculator to classify the risk as low, intermediate, or high. This classification is established at admission (risk of in-hospital death) and reassessed at discharge (risk of death at 6 months postdischarge).

Even patients without a high-risk score require urgent therapy

ACS requires immediate treatment. Emergency PCI may be required despite the absence of a formally calculated high risk score. High-risk prognostic factors not included in the scores above include: ventricular arrhythmia (other than cardiac arrest, which is included in the GRACE score), hemodynamic instability, LV dysfunction (LVEF <40% or HF); refractory or recurrent ischemia; previous CAD and/or interventions.

Table 2.47 Risk scores in ACS

The score	Common elements	Additional elements	What it predicts	Comments
GRACE	Age, BP,[a] creatinine levels, ST deviation, and elevated cardiac biomarkers	Killip class, the presence of cardiac arrest at admission, HR	Death in hospital and at 6 months	Uses computerized calculator[b]
TIMI	Age, BP,[a] creatinine levels, ST deviation, and elevated cardiac biomarkers	Other risk factors beside systolic BP and creatinine; known CAD (stenosis ≥50%); Aspirin use in the past week; severity of angina (≥2 episodes within 24 hrs = severe)	Death at 14 days	Easily calculated, thus very popular; based on a point sytem[c]
FRISC	Age, BP,[a] creatinine levels, ST deviation, and elevated cardiac biomarkers	Male sex, previous MI, diabetes, markers of inflammation; invasive	Will early invasive strategy decrease death at 1 year?	Easily calculated, based on a point sytem[d]
PURSUIT	Age, BP,[a] creatinine levels, ST deviation, and elevated cardiac biomarkers	HR, HF	Death at 30 days	Difficult to calculate

[a]Systolic BP only, with the GRACE score
[b]http://www.outcomes.org/grace; a PDA- downloadable version allows bedside use
[c]Maximum score – 7 points; ≤2 is low risk, ≥4 points is high risk of death or MI
[d]Maximum score – 6 points; a score of 0–2 corresponds to a low risk, ≥4 points corresponds to a very increased risk of death or MI
With scores ≥2, an early invasive strategy reduces mortality; the higher the score, the greater the gain of the early invasive therapy

> **Even patients without a high-risk score may have a severe prognosis**
>
> Importantly, the risk scores above refer to the *outcome of NSTE-ACS*; however, *the outcome of the hospitalization* also critically depends on the complications of therapy, mainly bleeding or CIN.

Management of Uncomplicated STEMI Beyond the Acute Stage

All patients should be confined to bed for the first 12–24 h, for initial stabilization. In the absence of complications, self-care, including the use of a bedside commode, is allowed by the end of the first day, and ambulation is allowed by the second day, with a total hospitalization of a few days; in complicated cases, clinical judgment is necessary. In case of recurrent ischemia (whether clinical or by EKG) after initial symptom relief, repeat revascularization therapy is indicated. In patients initially treated with IV fibrinolytics, angiography and, according to the results, PCI or CABG are strongly indicated, whether at the original medical facility, or by transportation to another facility. If this option is unavailable, repeat IV thrombolysis should be given (if SK was initially used, strong consideration should be given to a thrombus-specific agent; if this is unavailable,

repeat SK is only acceptable within the first 5 days after initial administration, in patients in whom the first dose was well tolerated). In patients initially treated with PCI or CABG, repeat coronarography and repeat angioplasty or redo CABG are indicated.

Table 2.48 reviews the main issues related to the social reinsertion of a post-MI patient.

Secondary prevention after MI. Risk factor control: Primary prevention principles are carried forth for secondary prevention as well, but with more drastic targets. *Smoking cessation* (including passive smoking) must be advocated at every single meeting with the patient; if necessary, Bupropion or Nicotine replacement therapy is indicated. *Physical activity* is recommended as moderate-intensity (as defined by a preliminary exercise stress test) aerobic exercise five times a week; in high-risk patients, exercise is performed in dedicated facilities, capable of medical supervision and treatment, if necessary. Rehabilitation programs often also function as informal support groups. *Diabetes* should be treated and monitored (target HbA1C <6.5%). ACEI or ARB drugs are especially indicated, as they benefit both CAD and renal function; additionally, HTN is frequent in diabetics. *Weight reduction* is indicated in patients with BMI >30 kg/m^2 and in men with a waist circumference >102 cm (88 cm in women). A high intake of vegetables, fruit, and fish (especially "oily fish," rich in ω-3 fatty acids), with a

Table 2.48 Work and leisure after discharge in the NSTE-ACS patient

LVEF (%)		Inducible ischemia	Work[a]		Leisure and sexual activity
			Office	Manual	
>40	*and*	No	May resume normal work, 8 h a day, after discharge	At 50% of maximum capacity achieved in a stress test, 4 h a day, for 1 month, increase by 2 h daily every month	Mild effort (<3 METs): sex, slow walking, desk activities; moderate effort (3–6 METs): calisthenics, slow bicycling. Intense effort: >6 METs; personalize recommendations according to stress test results
30–40	*or*	Mild	As above	Only static manual work allowed	
<30	*or*	Significant, but no symptoms at a stress ≤5 METs[b]	As above; otherwise, work contraindicated	Work contraindicated, regardless of degree of stress eliciting inducible ischemia	

[a]There are no guidelines regarding the duration of sick leave after NSTE-ACS
[c]On a Bruce stress test, this corresponds to very mild physical exertion. For orientation, Bruce protocol starts at 4.7 METs (Stage I), and increases demands by 2–3 METs per stage

low intake of saturated fats and of salt are indicated. Recent data show that even a small reduction in daily salt intake would have a huge public-health impact.

Alcohol consumption (especially red wine) is not discouraged; however, due to concerns about possible abuse, the guidelines do not actually recommend it. Moderate consumption may decrease cardiac mortality due to atherosclerosis, while abstainers and heavy drinkers are at higher risk (J curve). The beneficial effects are attributable to flavonoids present in red wine and purple grape juice and several fruits and vegetables. The mechanisms include antiplatelet actions, increased HDL levels, an antioxidant effect, reduced endothelin-1 production, and increased endothelial NO production. *BP control* is indicated, with target values <130/80 mmHg. If (as is often the case) this is not achieved with β-blockers alone, the second drug of choice is an ACEI or an ARB, which are indicated in any event, in post-MI patients. *Lipid management* is indicated in all patients. Despite past concern that immediate post-MI values may not accurately reflect chronic lipid levels, it appears that, by the end of the fourth day, the levels stabilize sufficiently to establish a therapeutic strategy, allowing patient discharge with this cornerstone issue already addressed. The survival benefit of early, aggressive statin therapy (started within 1–4 days of admission, with rapid uptitration to attain target) is partly due to mechanisms such as plaque stabilization and anti-inflammatory activity. Statins reduce hsCRP levels, but the meaning of this decrease (direct antiinflammatory effect of statins vs. plaque stabilization, with secondary hsCRP decrease) is not clear. The target LDL is <100 mg/dL (<2.5 mmol/L) or, in high-risk patients, <80 or even <70 mg/dL (2, respectively 1.8 mmol/L). LDL lowering to <70 mg/dL

was shown by the prospective PROVE-IT study to offer an additional benefit. The target TG level is <150 mg/dL (1.7 mmol/L), and the desirable HDL level (not considered a "target," as there is no specific therapy for low HDL) is >40 mg/L (1.0 mmol/L). HDL decrease often covaries with TG increase; mild abnormalities are treated by emphasizing life style changes, while more severe ones are addressed by newer-generation statins. In statin-intolerant patients, fibrates and ω-3 unsaturated fatty acid supplements are indicated. The value of Ezetimibe as a routine addition to statins (i.e., even if the latter do achieve the LDL targets) is being explored by the IMPROVE-IT study. The impact of HDL increase using a combination of niacin and Simvastatin is being tested in the AIM-HIGH study, while another study (HPS2-THRIVE) is testing niacin in association with a prostaglandin inhibitor, to prevent the main adverse effect of niacin, i.e., flushing.

Medical therapy includes *antithrombotic therapy* (Aspirin, Clopidogrel, or – in patients intolerant to both – Warfarin to a target INR of 2–3); *β-blockers* in all patients, *ACEI or ARB* in all patients, or, at the very least, in those with LVEF <40%; *statins and/or fibrates* as discussed above (practically, a majority of post-STEMI patients require them); and *influenza immunization,* indicated in all patients.

Device therapy includes biventricular pacing and ICD therapy in suitable candidates; these are reviewed under "STEMI complications."

STEMI management: beyond medicine: STEMI mandates optimal patient-caregiver communication. Depression, poor self-image, etc., are common after STEMI, and must be addressed, to achieve optimal long-term results and compliance. A typical example is sexual dysfunction in males receiving β-blockers and diuretics, often ascribed by the patient to the supposedly crippling effects of the "heart attack." In other patients, the omission to perform a late postdischarge echo (a few weeks after the acute event) may result in unrealistic assessment of the myocardial necrosis extent. The patient must understand that part of the damage identified by an early echo may have been salvaged by reperfusion therapy – a fact confirmed by the late echo. A few sentences may clarify this issue and dispel unnecessary worry or the misperception of a discordance between the diagnoses established "by the different doctors." The patient must also be made aware that atherosclerosis is a chronic disease, and that the acute ischemic event has brought not so much a *new disease*, as *new awareness* regarding a long-standing condition. Health-issue awareness must be presented as an important gain in the otherwise negative experience of disease, and this gain must now be used as leverage to obtain optimal compliance to therapy. Conversely, patients overly concerned regarding their disease must be reassured. Except for terminal cases, some truthful but artfully phrased positive insight can almost always be given to the patient. Thus, in the presence of intact or only mildly affected ventricular function, it is fully justified to tell the patient that, far from being crippled by their heart attack, they are in fact (after successful revascularization and with optimal therapy in place), "safer" than they have been in many years (yet, at the same time, they are at increased risk for a subsequent MI, especially in the first year). Conversely, in the patient with extensive myocardial necrosis, the crucial distinction between LV dysfunction and HF must be explained: many patients live (near-) normal lives despite a severely decreased LVEF. Having the patient function as a "goodwill medical ambassador" and promoting primary prevention measures among their siblings or children is also important. Finally, like any chronic disease, atherosclerosis and its complications affect not only the patient, but also his/her significant others. This, too, must be put to use; the spouse's input is often invaluable in ensuring compliance with life style changes and medical therapy on the long run, when compliance tends to decrease.

Complications of STEMI

The complications of STEMI reflect the impact of necrosis on the myocardial function, including: a *negative inotropic effect*, both direct (decreased myocardial function due to ischemia) and indirect (e.g., MI-related RV dysfunction causing suboptimal LV filling and contraction); *myocardial rupture* (decreased resistance of the necrosed tissue); *arrhythmia*, due to altered myocardial excitability and conduction; and *pericardial complications* (pericarditis, tamponade). *Iatrogenic* complications include bleeding, complications of PCI, etc. *Hypotension* may result from cardiogenic shock in extensive MI; suboptimal LV filling due to RV MI; the Bezold–Jarisch effect, in inferior MI; arrhythmia; tamponade; or hypovolemia due to bleeding or excessive diuresis.

Arrhythmia: *Supraventricular tachyarrhythmia* mainly includes paroxysmal AF, which may precipitate HF, by depriving the preload-dependent ischemic LV of the atrial kick. AF is especially common in the elderly and in those with extensive LV dysfunction or RV MI. STEMI-associated AF is associated to higher rates of mortality and stroke. However, many episodes are brief and do not require therapy. In case of rapid AF, which increases O_2 consumption MI size, HR is controlled with an IV β-blocker, a non-dihydropyridine CCB, or Amiodarone, while electrical cardioversion is the procedure of choice in case of hemodynamic compromise. AF therapy includes anticoagulation, often already in place for MI-related indications. *Supraventricular bradyarrhythmia* is mainly seen in inferior MI, due to excessive vagal activation (there is preferential distribution of the vagal nerve in the inferior wall); this is termed *the Bezold–Jarisch reflex*. Occasionally, bradycardia results from opioid therapy or from β-blockade. *Peri-MI AV block* is reviewed in Table 2.49.

Table 2.49 STEMI-associated heart block

MI location	Mechanism	Manifestations	Prognostic significance	Therapy
Inferior	Bezold–Jarisch reflex or AV node artery ischemia	HR >40 bpm, narrow escape rhythm	Benign	IV Atropine, occasionally transvenous pacing
Anterior	extensive myocardial damage	HR <40 bpm, wide-QRS escape rhythm	Severe	Transvenous pacing[a] (atropine not effective)

[a]Even, prophylactically, in cases of MI-associated BBB, with a high probability of later evolution to complete AV block

The significance and impact of *ventricular arrhythmia* (Table 2.50) strongly depend on the time of occurrence in the post-MI evolution (Table 2.48) and on the setting of occurrence (in- vs. out-of-hospital)

The risk for SCD is highest in the first month(s) after MI. SCD is discussed in Chap. 6. In the hospitalized STEMI patient, asymptomatic PVCs (even of the "R-on-T" variety) and hemodynamically stable, non-sustained VT do not require therapy, as their value as predictors of impending VF is poor, and prophylactic Lidocaine is associated to an increased risk of asystole. The only antiarrhythmic therapy indicated in post-MI patients is β-blockade. Hemodynamically unstable ventricular arrhythmia and sustained VT are treated as usual (Chap. 6). Occasionally, the arrhythmia is refractory to therapy. Assuming electrolyte derangements or drug (e.g., digitalis) toxicity are absent, ongoing ischemia should be ruled out by emergency angiography. Transvenous overdrive pacing is often useful for refractory ventricular arrhythmia.

Ventricular dysfunction may be due to irreversible or reversible myocardial damage; to arrhythmia; or to mechanical complications of MI. It manifests by the usual clinical complaints and physical findings, and its severity is quantified by the Killip score. The treatment is the same as that for any HF, as discussed in Chap. 4.

In addition to the usual measures, prompt revascularization and/or rupture repair are recommended, especially in case of advanced ventricular dysfunction. The most severe form of HF, cardiogenic shock, may occasionally be due to RV dysfunction, rather than to extensive LV damage. In these patients, volemic support and prompt revascularization are crucial.

Mechanical complications of MI are most frequent within the first 24 h or at 3–5 days and involve myocardial rupture. These frequently fatal events are reviewed in Table 2.51. A case of ruptured papillary muscle is shown in Fig. 2.5.

STEMI in Special Populations

The elderly: Age >75 doubles mortality, due to the characteristics of both ACS as such, and of ACS therapy. Thus, ACS is underdiagnosed in the elderly, as the symptoms are often non-specific. Invasive strategy is often withheld, despite its proven benefit in the elderly; on the other hand, the elderly are also at increased risk for bleeding. Unfortunately, as clinical trials usually enroll healthier-than-average subpopulations, the validity of result extrapolation to the general population is unclear. *Female gender*:

Table 2.50 MI-related ventricular arrhythmia

Time of occurrence	Direct consequences	Long-term prognostic signification	Remarks
Out of hospital			
As the first manifestation of MI	SCD	Fatal/severe	Patients found in VT have the least severe prognosis, followed by those found in VF; asystole is almost universally fatal
In hospital			
At the time of IV thrombolysis	Possible bleeding complications, if CPR is required[a]	None	Reperfusion vs. malignant ventricular arrhythmia
During primary PCI	Minimized by prompt treatment[a]	None	As above
Early (≤48 h after MI onset)	Minimized by prompt treatment[b]	None	Frequency decreased by thrombolytics and β-blockers
Either in hospital or out of hospital			
Late (>48 h)		Severe	In the absence of recurrent acute ischemia, this is an indication for ICD implantation[c]

[a]Reperfusion arrhythmia is generally benign. However, patients with successful reperfusion and *absent* reperfusion arrhythmias have a better prognosis
[b]As for reperfusion arrhythmia
[c]See Chap. 4

Table 2.51 Mechanical complications of MI

Manifestation	IVS rupture	LV free wall rupture	Papillary muscle rupture or dysfunction
Incidence	Up to 3% without, 0.3% with reperfusion therapy	Up to 6%; PCI, but not IV thrombolysis, might reduce its incidence	About 1%; incidence reduced by thrombolytic therapy
Manifestations	Chest pain, pulmonary edema, shock; loud new pansystolic murmur, precordial thrill; S_3; RV failure	Tamponade, presenting as SCD (EMD) in 75% of cases; in 25%, a sealing clot provides opportunity for intervention. Subacute cases may mimic reinfarction, (recurrent ST elevation).	Acute MR[a]; chest pain, pulmonary edema, shock; occasionally soft murmur, no thrill; RV failure
Echo	VSD flow; RV overload	Tamponade; pericardial sealing clot; occasionally, visualization of the site of rupture	Ruptured papillary muscle, with a flail leaflet; severe MR, eccentric jet
Right heart cathterization	Oxygen step-up from RA to RV; large V waves on RA pressure tracing	Non-specific findings	Large V waves, no O_2 step-up, severely elevated PCWP
Treatment[b]	Surgery (problematic, due to friable necrotic tissue) or percutaneous closure; Nitroprusside may decrease the shunt volume, but in occasional patients it may cause pulmonary vasodilatation in excess of the systemic one and actually increases the shunt[c]	Immediate surgery	Surgery, after initial stabilization (MV replacement, occasionally repair). Nitroprusside improves hemodynamics by decreasing the regurgitant volume.
Prognosis[d]	Mortality 20–50%	Untreated, 100% mortality (50%, in presence of a sealing clot)	Mortality 20–40%

[a]Acute MR (Chap. 5) is usually due to papillary muscle dysfunction, rather than rupture. The posteromedial papillary muscle is more frequently affected than the anterolateral one
[c]For the treatment of pulmonary edema and of cardiogenic shock, see Chap. 4
[c]Used as a bridge to intervention.
[d]Mortality is significantly increased in presence of cardiogenic shock

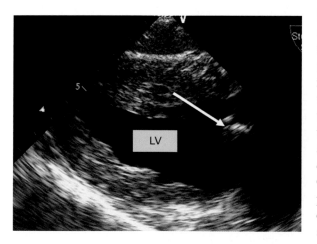

Fig. 2.5 Ruptured papillary muscle in a patient with acute inferior wall MI. Color Doppler demonstrated severe MR

Different studies have found a protective, deleterious, or absent impact of female gender on ACS outcome; therefore, the current guidelines do not recommend gender-based treatment distinction. Of note, European registries show significantly lower aggressive interventional and antithrombotic treatment rates in women, as compared to men. *Diabetes mellitus*: Up to two-third of ACS patients have glucose regulation abnormalities, and one-third have clinically apparent diabetes. These abnormalities increase the risk for CAD and aggravate prognosis; the risk is highest in patients with clinically apparent diabetes. Glycemic control is important in both the chronic and the acute setting, yet tight control increases the risk of hypoglycemia and significantly affects ACS prognosis. Diabetics benefit from early aggressive interventional and antithrombotic therapy. The risk of CIN is higher in diabetics; contrast material may cause renal failure and lactic acidosis in Metformin-treated diabetics. Metformin must be stopped 24 h before angiography, or at least on the same day, to be resumed after 48 h of uneventful recovery. *Anemia* (of any cause) portends a worse prognosis in ACS patients. However, blood transfusions must be used only if absolutely necessary (generally, with Hb levels <8g/L), as (somewhat counterintuitively) they may increase mortality, especially in NSTE-ACS patients. *Chronic kidney disease (CKD)* is associated with a higher prevalence and severity of ACS, due to coexisting diabetes, HTN, hyperhomocysteinemia, as well as to the prothrombotic state and general inflammation prevalent in CKD patients. The risk is higher in severe renal failure, but the correlation is not linear, with the highest risk seen with CrCl decreases <60 mL/min/1.73 m^2 BSA (normal ≥90). In other words, any patient with more than mild renal dysfunction is at increased risk. Patients with CKD are underrepresented in clinical trials (CKD usually

represents an exclusion criterion). CKD also influences ACS treatment, as renally excreted drugs must be either adjusted in dosage, or altogether avoided. An especially important population is that of hemodialysis patients, with a vastly increased risk of cardiovascular morbidity and mortality, due to several mechanisms, pertaining to the dialysis mechanism as such, in addition to the inherent risk represented by the underlying renal failure. Hemodialysis patients are more prone to develop myocardial ischemia, hibernation, and stunning; HF; arrhythmia and SCD; LV hypertrophy; microvascular damage, dependent and independent of the frequently associated severe atherosclerosis; increased peripheral artery stiffness; defective BP control; and myocardial injury, expressed as cardiac troponin elevation. The deleterious effects of hemodialysis are countered by different technical interventions, which are beyond the scope of this text.

The restrictions in the type and dosage of pharmacological therapy in CKD patients are outlined in Table 2.52.

Table 2.52 Dose adjustments and contraindications in ACS patients with CKD

Medication	Dose adjustment
General medication[a]	
Statins	Caution at CrCl <30 mL/min
ACEI	Dose reduction at CrCl <30 mL/min
ARB	Dose reduction at CrCl <30 mL/min
β-blockers	Metoprolol: halve/quarter the dose at CrCl <30, respectively, <15 mL/min
Nitrates	No (poor correlation between nitrate blood levels and clinical action)
Antithrombotic medication	
NSAIDs	
Aspirin	No, but Aspirin (especially in analgesic dosages, i.e., much higher than cardiological dosages) may decrease renal function
Thienopyridines	
Clopidogrel	No[b]
Prasugrel	Insufficient data[c]
Ticlopidine	Probably not; insufficient data[c]
IIb/IIIa inhibitors	
Abciximab	No
Eptifibatide	At CrCl <50 mL/min, keep bolus unchanged, reduce infusion to 1 μg/kg/min; contraindicated at CrCl <30 mL/min
Tirofiban	Reduce dosage to 1 μg/kg/min at CrCl <60 mL/min

(continued)

Table 2.52 (continued)

Medication	Dose adjustment
Indirect thrombin inhibitors	
UFH	
LMWH	*Enoxaparin, Fondaparinux, Dalteparin, Tinzaparin:* reduce dosage at CrCl <60 mL/min, consider withholding at CrCl <30 mL/min[d]
Direct thrombin inhibitors	
Argatroban	No
Bivalirudin	At CrCl <30 mL/min, keep bolus unchanged, reduce infusion to 1 µg/kg/min
Lepirudin	At CrCl <60 mL/min or serum creatinine >1.5 mg/dL, adjust dosage
Dabigatran	At CrCl <60 mL/min or serum creatinine >1.5 mg/dL, adjust dosage; contraindicated at CrCl <30 mL/min
VKA	
Warfarin, Acenocoumarol	No, but exercise caution in severe CKD, as this may affect coagulation by other mechanisms

[a]Data extrapolated from specific agents
[b]Clopidogrel metabolite level appears to be in fact *lower* in patients with more severe renal function, but this finding does not seem clinically relevant
[c]Concerns have been raised about the use in patients with CKD
[d]Due to an abundance of caution, Fondaparinux is contraindicated at CrCl <30 mL/min, but it might in fact be safer in this setting than Enoxaparin, which, in CKD patients, is contraindicated in certain countries only

Preexisting CKD carries a high risk of contrast-induced nephropathy (CIN), occurring up to 3 days after angiography. The main risk factors include diabetes, old age, dehydration, and the use of high-osmolality (as opposed to low-osmolality, nonionic) agents, especially in large amounts. Proper hydration and minimizing the number of angiographic injections are crucial. Some studies (but not others) have found *N*-acetylcysteine effective in preventing CIN. A typical regimen involves two daily oral doses of 600 mg, on the day of angiography and one day before.

2.3.2.3 Non-ST-Elevation MI and Unstable Angina (NSTEMI/UA)

Unsurprisingly, the discussion of UA/NSTEMI is very similar to that of STEMI. There are some differences, however, as reviewed in Sect. 2.3.2.2. Similarly, the therapy of NSTEMI/UA generally follows the same lines as that of STEMI; beside the issue of IV thrombolytic therapy (indicated in STEMI only), there are a few additional differences, as reviewed in Table 2.53. Some of these differences may simply reflect the design of the existing trials, while others may genuinely mirror the differences between STEMI and NSTEMI-ACS.

NSTEMI vs. UA: These two entities represent a continuum, differentiated by the presence or absence of biomarker level elevation (in part dependent on the available measuring technology), and by the prognosis, which is worse with NSTEMI. *Clinically,* NSTEMI/UA presents with at least two of the following three criteria: *resting angina* (can also occur with minimal exertion, and usually lasts >10 min); *new-onset angina* (onset within the prior 4–6 weeks); and crescendo angina (more severe, prolonged, or frequent than previously). *The Braunwald classification* was proposed in order to better quantify the severity and prognosis of NSTEMI/UA. The classification is based on the severity of UA (rated between I and III) and the clinical setting of its appearance (the presence or absence of extracardiac conditions or of recent MI), marked as A, B, or C. Thus, each individual case is designated by a numeral and a letter. Good as a descriptive tool, this classification boils down to the conclusion that patients with resting angina <48 h in duration are at increased risk, especially if they are troponin-positive. *The EKG* presents with ST depressions ≥0.5 mm; the more severe the depression, the worse the prognosis; prompt intervention is mandatory with depressions ≥2 mm. ST depressions in V_1–V_3 may be the mirror image of a posterior MI; the posterior EKG leads (V7–V9) clarify this issue (The LCx and the distal RCA

Table 2.53 STEMI and NSTEMI/UA: a comparison

	STEMI	NSTEMI/UA
Pathogenesis	Fully occlusive thrombus	Less than fully occlusive thrombus
Incidence		Higher than that of STEMI
Patient profile		Older; higher co-morbidity (diabetes, renal failure) than STEMI patients
Time course	Minutes to hours	Up to a few days
Clinical manifestations		Similar to STEMI
Imaging studies		Similar to STEMI
EKG	ST elevations	No ST elevations[a]
Biomarkers	Elevated	Elevated
Therapy	See Table 2.54	See Table 2.54
Rehabilitation		Similar to STEMI
Complications		Similar to STEMI
Prognosis		Mortality lower in-hospital, higher at 6 months and 4 years than with STEMI

[a]ST elevations may be seen in Prinzmetal's angina

Table 2.54 NSTEMI vs. STEMI therapy[a]

Agent	STEMI	NSTEMI	NSTEMI-remarks
β-blockers	√	√	Might decrease progression to STEMI; however, the current guidelines call for β-blockers only in NSTE-ACS patients with LV dysfunction; optional, in all patients, but there is no evidence of long-term benefit
Nitrates	√	√	
ACEI	√	√	In NSTE-ACS patients with LV dysfunction (EF <40%), or with other indications for ACEI; optional, in all patients, but there is no evidence of long-term benefit. Only Ramipril and Perindopril have been proven effective
ARB	√	√	In patients with intolerance to ACEI
Aldosterone antagonists	√	√	
CCB	C/I	Non-dihydropyridine agents (Diltiazem) may be considered if symptomatic despite β-blockers and nitrates; agents of choice in vasospastic angina.	In patients symptomatic despite polytherapy, PCI should be strongly considered
Newer agents, useful in stable angina[b]			
Ivabradine	Insufficient data[c]	May be used (off-label) in patients with a C/I to β-blockers	
Trimetazidine	Insufficient data	Insufficient data	Trimetazidine might decrease the MI size in PCI-treated NSTEMI-ACS patients

(*continued*)

antiplatelet therapy in patients after ACS, especially if they underwent stent implantation, is strongly discouraged, but may be mandatory, especially with surgical procedures where even light bleeding may be life-threatening, such as CNS surgery. Emergency surgery is performed as indicated; however, if a few days' delay is admissible, LMWH can be used empirically, while awaiting the washout of antiplatelet drugs. *NSTEMI/UA: Interventional therapy* – Several metaanalyses have concluded that a routine invasive strategy in all NSTE-ACS patients improves long-term prognosis, but at the cost of an increased early mortality. However, when investigated prospectively (the ICTUS trial), there was no advantage to routine invasive therapy in all ACS patients. All low-risk patients require early risk stratification, and, in the absence of significant inducible ischemia, can be managed conservatively. Conversely, up to two-third of NSTE-ACS patients with moderate or severe clinical manifestations (severe arrhythmia, hemodynamic instability, refractory or recurrent ischemia, dynamic ST segment changes, or HF) have multivessel disease, requiring invasive therapy, usually avoiding left ventriculography; IABP is also frequently used. The optimal timing of non-emergent PCI in NSTE-ACS patients is unclear, as some of the studies have not found early intervention beneficial (For instance, the ICTUS trial found an increased incidence of MI in patients intervened upon within the first 48 h). However, it is not recommended to delay intervention beyond 72 h from presentation.

Prinzmetal's (variant/vasospastic) angina is a distinct entity, akin to UA. It manifests as anginal pain, mainly at night or in the early morning, typically with ST elevations (but occasionally, with ST depressions or even with a normal EKG); nitrates and CCB relieve pain within a few minutes. Most patients have severe atherosclerosis. The etiology appears to be multifactorial, involving endothelial dysfunction; smooth muscle hyperreactivity; autonomic system hyperactivation; and excess endothelin. There is some overlap with syndrome X, as the latter occasionally involves vasospasm as well. Typically, vasospasm occurs at rest, with no symptoms present on exertion. Factors leading to vasospasm include, among others, cocaine abuse, smoking, electrolyte disturbances, cold stimulation, autoimmune disease, hyperventilation, and insulin resistance. The diagnosis involves demonstration of the typical EKG changes, occasionally by Holter monitoring or by loop recorder implantation. Focal or diffuse coronary spasm, demonstrated angiographically

(lumen reduction >75% under intracoronary acetylcholine or Ergonovine as compared to maximum diameter under Nitroglycerin) confirms the diagnosis. Prognosis depends on the extent of atherosclerosis. The treatment is based on CCB and nitrates, in the usual doses.

2.3.3 Stable Angina Pectoris

The pathogenesis of stable angina differs from that of ACS in that the coronary flow is decreased not by a thrombus, but by a gradual decrease of the lumen, caused by increasing atherosclerotic plaque dimensions. A comparison between stable angina and ACS is reviewed in Table 2.55.

The severity of stable angina is quantified by the degree in which it impairs everyday life. This is evaluated by different scores, important for establishing therapy and for assessing its efficacy. *The Canadian Cardiovascular Society score* is the most widely used. Class IV corresponds to resting angina, in principle a type of unstable angina. In some extreme cases, however, a severe anginal score can be otherwise "stable," insofar the severity or frequency of the attacks is unchanged. The *Duke Activity Status Index* is a questionnaire applying a number of points for the ability to perform certain tasks (from self-care to competitive sports); the final score is incorporated in a formula, yielding an estimate of peak O_2 consumption, an important prognostic predictor. VO_2 max is approximately 3.5 L/min (45 mL/kg/min) and

Table 2.55 O_2 supply and demand in stable angina and ACS: a comparison

	Stable angina	ACS
Supply	May be decreased by changes of coronary vascular tone or of platelet activation	Is decreased by coronary thrombosis and distal micro-embolization
Demand	May be increased by physical or emotional stress	Is not necessarily increased; however, ACS may be triggered in a patient previously suffering from stable angina by plaque destabilization caused, among others, by increased sympathetic discharge

2.0 L/min (38 mL/kg/min) in the average young untrained male and female, respectively. The 19-item *Seattle Angina Questionnaire* explores physical limitation, angina stability, angina frequency, treatment satisfaction, and disease perception. This questionnaire is sensitive to both small and important changes in anginal status. Of note, stable angina may be mimicked by DCM, HOCM, or AS, esophageal, pulmonary, or thoracic disease.

Workup for stable angina follows the general rules reviewed in Sect. 2.2. Non-invasive assessment plays an important role. The EKG manifestations are similar to those of ACS. The various diagnostic tests are reviewed in Table 2.56. *Coronarography* is indicated *for diagnosis* in patients with severe angina or severe ventricular arrhythmia; with nonsevere manifestations and non-diagnostic non-invasive test results; and in survivors of cardiac arrest; and *for follow-up* in patients with known coronary disease (recurrent angina after PCI or CABG) or in asymptomatic patients after complex intervention on a large coronary artery (long lesion, multiple stents, suboptimal stent deployment, etc.)

Prognosis: Stable angina has an annual mortality of 0.9–1.4%, with a 0.5–2.6% incidence of non-fatal MI. The risk of cardiovascular mortality is considered high, intermediate, or low, if it is >2, 1–2, or <1%, respectively. The prognosis varies widely, according to the degree of LV dysfunction (LVEF <40%); the severity and distribution of CAD (three-vessel disease, LMCA artery or proximal LAD involvement have the worst prognosis); the presence of risk factors or of full-blown atherosclerosis; and the angina score, calculated based on 16 variables (age, gender, risk factors, existing atherosclerosis, as well as additional clinical and EKG parameters).

Table 2.56 Tests used in the diagnosis of stable angina

Test	Sensitivity	Specificity
Exercise EKG	68	77
Exercise echo	80–85	84–86
Exercise nuclear scan	85–90	70–75
Vasodilator stress myocardial perfusion	83–94	64–90
Dobutamine stress echo	40–100	62–100
Vasodilator stress echo	56–92	97–100

Stable angina – treatment: As with the other ischemic syndromes, the treatment of stable angina can be pharmacological or interventional. Risk factor management follows the usual principles. The main *pharmacological agents* are reviewed in Sect. 2.2. These include most of the agents already discussed regarding ACS, as well as some agents dedicated to the therapy of stable angina. *Aspirin* 81–325 mg PO q.d. (replace with *Clopidogrel* 75 mg q.d. in case of intolerance) is indicated in all patients, in the usual dosages, as are *β-blockers* (Metoprolol 50–200 mg PO b.i.d., Atenolol 50–200 mg PO q.d.). If the latter are not sufficient to prevent the anginal attacks, they are supplemented with CCB. *Amlodipine* 5–10 mg PO q.d. has been shown to reduce progression to unstable angina, the need for revascularization, and the degree of carotid atherosclerosis measured by ultrasound; whether this can be extrapolated to the other CCB is not clear. Popular agents include *Diltiazem* (120–480 mg PO q.d. for the slow-release preparation; 120–360 mg PO divided t.i.d./q.i.d. with the immediate-release preparation); *Verapamil* (120–240 mg PO q.d./b.i.d. for the slow-release preparation; 80–120 mg PO divided t.i.d./q.i.d. with the immediate-release preparation). *Nitrates* may be used either on a daily basis, or reserved for the anginal attacks. *Nitroglycerin* (0.3–0.6 mg SL PRN; 0.4 mg metered-dose spray, PRN; 0.1–0.8 mg/h patch TD q.d.); *Isosorbide dinitrate*: 2.5–10 mg SL PRN; 80–120 mg PO q.d. slow release, 10–30 mg PO b.i.d./t.i.d., immediate-release. Occasionally, angina can be anticipated by the patient, and nitrates may be taken preventively. *ACEI* were shown to reduce rates of death, MI, stroke, and need for revascularization in patients with CAD or diabetes mellitus and at least one other cardiovascular risk factor, irrespective of the presence of HTN or HF. An example is Ramipril, 2.5–5 mg PO q.d., not to exceed 20 mg/d; *Other agents* include *Ranolazine* 500 mg PO b.i.d. initially; if necessary, may increase to 1,000 mg PO b.i.d.; *Nicorandil*, starting at 10 mg b.i.d. (5 mg b.i.d., in patients particularly susceptible to headache), titrated upward, usually to 10–20 mg b.i.d., and up to 30 mg b.i.d.; *Ivabradine* 5 mg b.i.d., increased to 7.5 mg b.i.d. In the elderly, the starting dose is 2.5 mg b.i.d.; *Trimetazidine* 20 mg t.i.d. *Enhanced external counterpulsation* (EECP) is a therapeutic option in stable angina, capitalizing on the same principle as IABP. Briefly, balloons wrapped around the lower limbs are inflated at the beginning of diastole, and deflated before atrial systole, under EKG gating. Subjective and objective (perfusion scan) improvement in stable angina patients has been demonstrated.

Investigational approaches in stable angina involve injection of vascular growth factor (e.g., VEGF), or gene therapy, to determine overexpression of these factors. *Spinal cord stimulation* has been recently proven effective in patients with refractory angina pectoris due to end-stage CAD.

The decision regarding *pharmacological vs. interventional therapy* in stable angina has been addressed by the COURAGE trial, which has not found any reduction in the incidence of death or MI in stable angina patients initially treated with PCI, as compared to those treated with optimal medical therapy alone. Thus, initial conservative therapy appears appropriate in all patients with stable angina, as well as in asymptomatic CAD patients. On the other hand, there was substantial symptomatic improvement in PCI-treated patients, and a substantial rate of cross-over to PCI from the group initially managed by conservative therapy alone, making the interventional community interpret the study as actually encouraging an early interventional approach. Importantly, Class IV angina patients were not included in the study, neither were patients with refractory CHF, EF <30%, or LMCA artery stenosis >50%, and the results cannot be extrapolated to these populations. In patients in whom medical management alone is not sufficient, an additional decision refers to the type of revascularization therapy to be implemented: PCI vs. CABG. Older data suggest that CABG is the procedure of choice with LM stenosis >50%; LM disease equivalent (combined proximal LAD and proximal LCx stenosis); proximal 3VD (>70%); significant 2VD if one of the involved vessels is the proximal LAD; for significant CAD with impaired LV function; in diabetics; and after severe arrhythmia. However, the tremendous progress in PCI techniques allows to solve many of the above-mentioned problems by PCI. Unsurprisingly, the "CABG-vs.-PCI" debate is just as lively as the "conservative-vs.-interventional" debate, as shown by the SYNTAX trial, comparing the safety and efficacy of CABG vs. PCI with TAXUS DES in patients with 3VD or LMCA disease, who were eligible for either procedure. PCI was found inferior for the primary composite end point of major adverse cardiac or cerebrovascular events (MACCE); however, when the actual results are examined, it turns out that the differences are actually small (numerous CABG procedures needed, to avoid just one repeat PCI), with a fourfold increase in the number of strokes in the CABG group. This has prompted the interventional community to interpret SYNTAX as proof of the appropriateness of PCI in this population. This debate illustrates the necessity of individual decision tailoring. Despite widespread use, there is no evidence that adding a GP IIb/IIIa inhibitor to an optimal dual antiplatelet regimen is of benefit in low-risk patients with uncomplicated lesions.

Syndrome X is a particular instance of stable angina, where typical chest pain, usually in a female patient, is associated to a positive stress test; this prompts coronary angiography, which, however, fails to demonstrate significant atherosclerosis. Occasionally, angiography demonstrates vasospasm (on intracoronary acetylcholine administration). The pathogenesis of this syndrome is unclear, a classic explanation being that of microvascular dysfunction ("microvascular angina"), possibly associated to epicardial coronary endothelial dysfunction. Many patients are hypertensive and suffer from LVH with relative ischemia, as well as perivascular fibrosis with structural changes of both the myocardium and the coronaries. The prognosis is very good, with the possible exception of patients with angiographically demonstrated coronary vasospasm. The treatment follows the general lines of stable angina therapy. Therapy is usually started with slow-release CCB s; if the angiogram reveals epicardial coronary disease, nitrates are added. Aminophylline 400 mg/day, divided t.i.d. or q.i.d.; and Imipramine 50 mg/d may be tried if other measures fail.

Bilbliography

Guidelines

1. Fourth joint task force of the European Society of Cardiology and other societies on cardiovascular disease prevention in clinical practice (constituted by representatives of nine societies and by invited experts). European Guidelines on Cardiovascular Disease Prevention in Clinical Practice. *Eur J Cardiovasc Prev Rehabil.* 2007; 14(suppl 2):E1–40.
2. The task force on the management of ST-segment elevation acute myocardial infarction of the European Society of Cardiology: Management of acute myocardial infarction in patients presenting with persistent ST-Segment elevation. *Eur Heart J.* 2008;29:2909–45.
3. The task force for the diagnosis and treatment of non-ST-segment elevation acute coronary syndromes of the European Society of Cardiology: Guidelines for the diagnosis and

treatment of non-ST-segment elevation acute coronary syndromes. *Eur Heart J.* 2007;28:1598–60.

4. Antman EM, Hand M, Armstrong PW, et al. 2007 Focused update of the ACC/AHA 2004 guidelines for the management of patients with ST-elevation myocardial infarction: a report of the American College of Cardiology/American Heart Association task force on practice guidelines (writing group to review new evidence and update the ACC/AHA 2004: Guidelines for the management of patients with ST-elevation myocardial infarction). *Circulation.* 2008;117:296-329.

5. Fraker TD Jr, Fihn SD; writing on behalf of the 2002 chronic stable angina writing committee. 2007 Chronic angina focused update of the ACC/AHA 2002 guidelines for the management of patients with chronic stable angina: a report of the American College of Cardiology/American Heart Association task force on practice guidelines writing group to develop the focused update of the 2002 guidelines for the management of patients with chronic stable angina. *Circulation.* 2007;116:2762–72.

6. Anderson JL, Adams CD, Antman EM, et al. ACC/AHA 2007 guidelines for the management of patients with unstable angina/non-ST-elevation myocardial infarction: executive summary: a report of the American College of Cardiology/American Heart Association task force on practice guidelines (writing committee to revise the 2002 guidelines for the management of patients with unstable angina/non–ST-elevation myocardial infarction). *Circulation.* 2007;116:803-77.

7. Smith SC, Allen J, Blair SN, et al. AHA/ACC guidelines for secondary prevention for patients with coronary and other atherosclerotic vascular disease: 2006 update. *Circulation.* 2006;113:2363-72.

8. The task force on the management of stable angina pectoris of The European Society of Cardiology guidelines on the management of stable angina pectoris. *Eur Heart J.* 2006;27(11):1341–81; doi:10.1093/eurheartj/ehl002.

Suggested Reading

9. Falk E, Shah PK, Fuster V. Coronary plaque disruption. *Circulation.* 1995;92:657-71.

10. Sabatine MS, Cannon CP, Gibson CM, et al. For the CLARITY–TIMI 28 Investigators. Addition of clopidogrel to aspirin and fibrinolytic therapy for myocardial infarction with ST-segment elevation. *N Engl J Med.* 2005;352:1179-89.

11. Chen ZM, Jiang LX, Chen YP, et al. Addition of clopidogrel to aspirin in 45, 852 patients with acute myocardial infarction: randomized placebo-controlled trial. *Lancet.* 2005;366:1607-21.

12. Assessment of the safety and efficacy of a new treatment strategy with percutaneous coronary intervention (ASSENT-4 PCI) investigators. Primary versus tenecteplase-facilitated percutaneous coronary intervention in patients with ST-segment elevation acute myocardial infarction (ASSENT-4 PCI): randomised trial. *Lancet.* 2006; 367:569–78.

13. Hochman JS, Lamas GA, Buller CE, et al. For the Occluded Artery Trial Investigators. coronary intervention for persistent occlusion after myocardial infarction. *N Engl J Med.* 2006;355:2395-407.

14. Antman EM, Morrow DA, McCabe CH; for the ExTRACT-TIMI 25 Investigators. Enoxaparin versus unfractionated heparin with fibrinolysis for ST-elevation myocardial infarction. *N Engl J Med.* 2006;354:1477–88.

15. Kober L, Torp-Pedersen C, Carlsen JE, et al. A clinical trial of the angiotensin-converting-enzyme inhibitor trandolapril in patients with left ventricular dysfunction after myocardial infarction. Trandolapril cardiac evaluation (TRACE) study group. *N Engl J Med.* 1995;333(25):1670–76.

16. Dagenais GR, Yusuf S, Bourassa MG, et al. Effects of ramipril on coronary events in high-risk persons: results of the heart outcomes prevention evaluation study. *Circulation.* 2001;104(5):522-6.

17. Boden WE, O'Rourke RA, Teo KK, Hartigan PM, et al; COURAGE Trial Research Group. Optimal medical therapy with or without PCI for stable coronary disease. *N Engl J Med.* 2007;356(15):1503–16.

18. Bhatt DL, Fox KA, Hacke W, et al. CHARISMA Investigators. Clopidogrel and aspirin versus aspirin alone for the prevention of atherothrombotic events. *N Engl J Med.* 2006;354:1706–17.

19. Serruys PW, Morice MC, Kappetein AP, Colombo A, et al.; SYNTAX Investigators. Percutaneous coronary intervention versus coronary-artery bypass grafting for severe coronary artery disease. *N Engl J Med.* 2009;360(10):961–72.

20. Wallentin L, Becker RC, Budaj A, et al. Ticagrelor versus clopidogrel in patients with acute coronary syndromes. *N Engl J Med.* 2009;361:1045-57.

21. Bavry AA, Kumbhani DJ, Rassi AN, et al. Benefit of early invasive therapy in acute coronary syndromes: a meta-analysis of contemporary randomized clinical trials. *J Am Coll Cardiol.* 2006;48(7):1319-25.

22. Campbell CL, Smyth S, Montalescot G, Steinhubl SR. Aspirin dose for the prevention of cardiovascular disease: a systematic review. *JAMA.* 2007;297(18):2018-24.

23. Oestreich JH, Smyth SS, Campbell CL. Platelet function analysis: at the edge of meaning. *Thromb Haemost.* 2009; 101(2):217-9.

24. Bugiardini R, Bairey Merz CN. Angina with "normal" coronary arteries: a changing philosophy. *JAMA.* 2005;293(4):477–84.

25. Stone GW, Grines CL, Cox DA, et al. Comparison of angioplasty with stenting, with or without abciximab, in acute myocardial infarction. *N Engl J Med.* 2002;346:957-66.

26. Antman EM, Morrow DA, McCabe CH, et al. Enoxaparin versus unfractionated heparin with fibrinolysis for ST-elevation myocardial infarction. *N Engl J Med.* 2006;354:1477-88.

27. Yusuf S, Mehta SR, Chrolavicius S, et al. Effects of fondaparinux on mortality and reinfarction in patients with acute ST-segment elevation myocardial infarction: the OASIS-6 randomized trial. *JAMA.* 2006;295:1519-30.

28. Wiviott SD, Braunwald E, McCabe CH, et al. Prasugrel vs clopigogrel in patients with acute coronary syndromes. *N Engl J Med.* 2007;357:2001-15.

Disorders of Blood Pressure

3

Contents

3.1 Normal and Abnormal Blood Pressure (BP)

BP is defined as the tension in the blood vessel wall, resulting from blood flow through the lumen. Normal BP, one of the main parameters of cardiovascular function, reflects the ability of blood to reach the vascular bed of the organs; abnormal BP may cause serious complications. BP regards arteries, veins, and lymphatics alike, and abnormalities may consist either in excessive increase (HTN) or decrease (hypotension). In current usage, the term "HTN" refers to *arterial* BP. BP depends on

- *CO,* in turn conditioned by LV contractility and size; HR;and AV and MV function.
- *Blood volume,* determined by the balance between *fluid intake* and (a) *elimination* through urine, feces, sweat, and insensible perspiration; (b) *distribution of body water* between the intracellular, intravascular, and extravascular spaces (conjunctive tissue, pleural, pericardial space, etc.); and (c) *distribution of blood* between the arterial and the venous bed.
- *Blood viscosity* (dependent on blood cell number and protein levels).
- *SVR,* dependent on the integrity of the aorta and great vessels (e.g., aortic coarctation may cause HTN in the upper limb), arterial wall elasticity (decreased elasticity increases passive vascular resistance to flow), and active vasoconstriction in the medium-sized arteries.

G.A. Adelmann, *Cardiology Essentials in Clinical Practice,*
DOI: 10.1007/978-1-84996-305-3_3, © Springer-Verlag London Limited 2011

The role of baroreceptors in BP regulation

An important role in BP and HR regulation is played by pressure receptors ("baroreceptors"), nerve endings in the different "key areas" of the circulatory system. Baroreceptors are sensitive to local BP changes, sensed as changes in the degree of arterial wall stretch. These changes activate or deactivate the receptors and are transmitted to the CNS, where compensatory measures are initiated. There exist

- *High-pressure baroreceptors* in the aortic arch and the internal carotid arteries. The afferent limb includes terminations of the glossopharyngeal nerve (cranial nerve IX), with the vagus nerve (X) serving as an efferent limb. High BP causes arterial stretch and increased receptor stimulation, while at lower BP, the receptor activation decreases or stops. The receptors respond only to acute (very rapid) BP changes, and in cases of chronic HTN, they are reset ("recalibrated") to perceive high BP levels as "normal." Other stretch-sensitive receptors include the C receptors in the LV wall, activated by LV contractions that are disproportionately strong in relation to the relatively underfilled LV cavity (the Bezold–Jarisch reflex).
- *Low-pressure baroreceptors,* present in the veins and in the atria; they regulate blood volume, by increasing water retention in the presence of decreased BP. Their action is mediated by the RAAS system and by ADH secretion, leading to water retention. These receptors respond more slowly, to long-term changes in BP.

The role of chemoreceptors in BP regulation

Chemoreceptors sense changes in the chemical composition of blood, namely, in pH, pCO_2, and $SatO_2$. These receptors are both central (in the brain) and peripheral (in the carotids and aortic arch). Not all receptors sense all three compounds. The role of chemoreceptors is especially important in severe settings (e.g., shock), when the levels of the triggering compounds become abnormal.

For historical reasons, the measuring unit for BP is the "millimeter of mercury column" (mmHg), the pressure exerted by a 1-mm-tall mercury column. BP is expressed by the systolic and the diastolic pressure. *Systolic pressure* is the result of active transmission of energy by the heart to arterial blood, while *diastolic pressure* results from part of the systolic energy being stored in the walls of the elastic arteries, which passively transmit it back to the blood in diastole. This ensures organ perfusion pressure throughout the cardiac cycle.

BP: a vital parameter

Alongside HR, body temperature, $SatO_2$, and respiratory function, BP is a "vital sign," i.e., a crucial parameter of a patient's "vital inventory." BP can be problematic when excessively high (>140 systolic and/or >90 mmHg diastolic) or excessively low (<80 mmHg systolic and/or <60 mmHg diastolic). While excessively low BP values can straightforwardly be termed "hypotension", increased BP levels require further discussion. BP varies naturally from moment to moment and often increases even "beyond normal" under stress; the term, "HTN" refers to *recurrent or constant* BP increase in the absence of a physiological explanation. Thus, an *isolated* high BP reading should not prompt the diagnosis of HTN, but requires follow-up to rule out HTN. The differences between the terminology and some important characteristics of hypotension and HTN are reviewed in Table 3.1.

Table 3.1 A brief comparison between HTN and hypotension

	HTN	Hypotension
Name	Used only if recurrent values >140/90[a] mmHg	Used even for isolated episodes
Etiology	Most often, primary	Most often, secondary
Clinical manifestations	Mainly a chronic disease	Mainly an acute disease

[a]In children and adolescents, HTN is defined as BP >the 95th percentile for the child's age

A patient can be defined as hypertensive based on either systolic or diastolic BP, and in this respect, the two are equally important. As regards the prognostic signification of BP increase, in patients younger than 50, diastolic increases are more important as a risk factor for CAD, and after 50 years of age, systolic BP increases are a more important risk factor. Hypotension causes organ hypoperfusion and dysfunction (e.g., syncope, ischemic damage, dysfunction, etc.), while HTN is a major risk factor for atherosclerosis, causing CAD, CVA, kidney dysfunction, retinal lesions, aortic aneurysm dissection, etc.

BP in the peripheral vessels vs. the aorta

Most organs have an autoregulation system, maintaining constant local flow despite variations of aortic BP. Local blood flow is regulated (decreased with HTN, increased with hypotension) by means of vasodilatation or vasoconstriction, achieved by local mechanisms, independent of the autonomous nervous system (hence *auto*-regulation). For instance, in the coronary bed, the main concern is that of underperfusion, and autoregulation is achieved by the balance between ATP (a high-energy compound) and adenosine (resulting from degradation of the former); a high adenosine concentration signifies energy depletion and has a vasodilatory action, ensuring availability of O_2 and nutrients for energy store replenishment (rephosphorylation of adenosine to ATP). In extreme situations (BP decrease below certain limits), autoregulation is no longer operative, and other emergency mechanisms are used: increased O_2 extraction from Hb, and, as a last resort, anaerobic metabolism. Similarly, excessive BP increases may not be counteracted by local mechanisms and may cause serious organ damage (e.g., stroke).

3.2 Mechanisms of HTN

3.2.1 Primary HTN

In 85–90% of adults and adolescents, the causes of HTN are unknown (primary HTN). Secondary HTN (mainly caused by renal disease) is most frequent in children. Workup for underlying conditions is only rarely indicated, but, as our knowledge about the mechanisms of HTN increases, this situation might change in the future. Although the *underlying* causes of most cases of HTN are yet unknown, some of the key operative mechanisms (water and salt overload, vasoconstriction, vessel wall stiffening) are well characterized, and, paradoxically, our ability *to treat* primary HTN vastly surpasses the ability *to understand* all the aspects of its genesis. The clinical settings in which some of the mechanisms of HTN are most strongly expressed can be reversible or irreversible. Correction of these situations improves BP values, but the exact operational mechanisms are not always clear. Causes of isolated BP increase, such as physical or emotional stress, excessive caffeine consumption, etc., are not included, but if they become chronic, they can cause a hypertensive burden, no different from that of "true" HTN. The main mechanisms of HTN are reviewed below.

3.2.1.1 Advanced Age

Most hypertensives are elderly, and conversely, the majority of people older than 70–80 are hypertensive (mainly due to arterial and arteriolar stiffening by collagen deposition in the vessel walls). Several mechanisms are operative in this age group:

- *Decreased vessel wall elasticity* (also a cause of pseudo-HTN)
- A high prevalence of *atherosclerosis*
- *Declining renal function* (most individuals lose up to 50% of their functioning nephrons between ages 40 and 70)
- *Increased sodium sensitivity* (i.e., a greater BP increase for the same amount of excess sodium)

3.2.1.2 Excessive Vasoconstriction

Excessive vasoconstriction, is mainly due to increased adrenalin secretion, which can occur in several settings, including

- *Sleep apnea,* either obstructive (by far the most frequent) or central (Chap. 11). Even after statistical adjustment for potential confounders (obesity, diabe-

(continued)

- BP values depend on the conditions under which they are measured, with office readings being systematically higher than values recorded by self-monitoring (a "miniature" version of the white-coat effect).

"Normal" BP values are reviewed in Table 3.3.

Table 3.3 Normal BP values

The setting	Presence of high-risk comorbidities (mmHg)	
	No	Yes[a]
Office	<140/90	<130/80[b]
Self-monitoring	<135/85	<130/80
Holter	<130/80	<130/80

[a]Diabetes, renal dysfunction, S/P MI, S/P CVA
[b]Current trends question the appropriateness of BP lowering <140/90

These apparently small differences are actually very important, not necessarily in obtaining a "pristine" BP picture (almost unattainable, given the natural variability of BP) but rather in establishing a reasonable *target* for BP treatment.

Of note, pre-HTN is not only a risk factor for HTN (mandating close follow-up) but is, in itself, associated with an increased risk of adverse events, mainly CAD. For values >115/75 mmHg, the risk of CAD doubles for every 20/10 mmHg increase; at a BP of 140/90, the risk is double that of patients with BP 120/80 mmHg. As reports regarding the high risk of pre-HTN accumulate, the definition of "normal" BP may change in the future (as, indeed, has already happened in the past). However, tempering these findings, recent research has suggested that BP reductions <140/90 mmHg may in fact not reduce mortality or morbidity, and that values <120 mmHg systolic and <70 mmHg diastolic may in fact be deleterious. This is, in fact, a revival of the time-honored "U"-curve effect of BP lowering.

There is some disagreement between European and US guidelines regarding the different degrees of HTN severity; additionally, many physicians are still familiar with the designations, mild/moderate/severe HTN. All these classifications are presented in Table 3.4.

The greater "fragmentation" adopted by the ESC results from the observation that most of the excess risk attributable to pre-HTN is actually due to "high normal" values; pooling together different BP values is thus misleading. Additionally, the term, "pre-HTN," carries a negative connotation generating excess office visits and financial burden (a state of affairs, however, possibly preferable to the generally very low degree of BP control in the population). Similarly, the degree of risk increase at BP >160/100 mmHg is differentiated according to the actual value of BP. The classical qualifiers, "mild" and "moderate," for what is in fact a highly lethal disease might encourage patients to disregard the importance of therapy; they have been abandoned in favor of the more "neutral" designations, "grade" or "stage."

The importance of BP classifications according to stages (Table 3.4) is useful for calculating the total cardiovascular risk and for guiding therapy.

Table 3.4 Classification of HTN

BP values			ESC classification	AHA classification	Older Terminology
Systolic		Diastolic			
<120	and	<80	Optimal	Normal	
120–129	and/or	80–84	Normal	Pre-HTN	
130–139	and/or	85–89	High normal		
140–159	and/or	90–99	Grade I HTN	HTN stage I	Mild HTN
160–179	and/or	100–109	Grade II HTN	HTN stage II	Moderate HTN
≥180	and/or	≥110	Grade III HTN		Severe HTN
≥140	and	<90	Isol. syst. HTN	N/A	

3.3.3 HTN: Clinical Considerations

HTN is probably the most frequently encountered medical problem, with a worldwide prevalence of approximately one billion, and tens of millions of fatalities annually (MI, CVA, etc.). Unfortunately, HTN is most frequently asymptomatic, causing irreparable damage to the target organs by the time it is diagnosed; when it does cause symptoms of its own, these are nonspecific (typically, occipital headache). Complications are often the first manifestation of HTN, underscoring the enormous importance of proper screening.

3.3.3.1 Workup for HTN

Workup for secondary HTN

The vast majority of HTN cases are primary, and routine workup for underlying diseases would create huge and useless medical expenses. Moreover, it is relatively improbable to miss secondary HTN, as it tends to aggregate in certain populations and/or associate other signs of underlying disease. The suspicion of secondary HTN is highest in cases not manageable by standard therapy. The indications for workup are reviewed in Table 3.5.

Table 3.5 Suggested indications for workup for secondary HTN

Suspected condition	Presentation	Necessary workup	Treatment
Renal HTN			
Renovascular HTN	Sudden-onset severe HTN (normal BP values documented in the past) or if preexistent, well-controlled HTN suddenly becomes unresponsive to therapy; renal artery murmur	Plasma renin activity, renal Duplex, Captopril test[a]	See Chap. 11
Palpable kidneys	PKD	Imaging, genetic testing	Symptomatic therapy, dialysis, transplant
Glomerulonephritis	Associated RFT derangement, edema	Blood and urine tests, renal biopsy	Steroids, Cyclosporine, ACEI, according to type and presentation
Endocrine HTN			
Pheochromocytoma	"Flash" HTN crisis[b]	Catecholamines determination in plasma and urine	Surgery[c]
Hyperthyroidism, hyperparathyroidism	Signs of thyroid or parathyroid disease	TSH, FT4, PTH, plasma calcium levels; thyroid and parathyroid imaging	Medical/surgical treatment
Cushing's syndrome	Features of Cushing's syndrome	Dexamethasone suppression test; 24-h urinary Cortisol measurement; suprarenal or pituitary gland imaging	Surgical; if possible, wean from steroid therapy
Congenital conditions			
Aortic coarctation	Children, especially if HTN is present in upper limbs only	TEE, CT, MRI	Chap. 10
Neurofibromatosis	Neurofibromas, freckles, café-au-lait spots	Clinical diagnosis	Symptomatic; resect tumors, if compressive
Substance abuse			
Cocaine, Ecstasy, metamphetamine use	Patients with other symptoms of intoxication	Tox. screen	Abstinence; treat. of HTN crisis (see below)

[a]See Chap. 11
[b]Rarely, hypotensive episodes
[c]Preceded by pharmacological α-blockade (Phenoxybenzamine) or combined α- and β-blockade (Labetalol); pure β-blockade is contraindicated, as it leaves all the adrenergic receptors at the disposal of catecholamines and may cause HTN crisis

3.3.3.2 Complications

The main importance of HTN resides in the possible disease- or treatment-associated complications. HTN complications can affect practically any organ, but "target organs" (heart, brain, kidneys) are especially vulnerable.

Mechanisms of hypertensive damage to the blood vessels, myocardium, and peripheral organs

A few decades into the era of effective antihypertensive therapy, these mechanisms are still imperfectly understood. An important role is played by inflammatory mediators and reactive O_2 species (H_2O_2, O_2^-), affecting cellular growth, hypertrophy, remodeling, fibrosis, apoptosis (programmed cell death), and vascular tone. In turn, these events cause

- Damage to the endothelium and to the vascular smooth muscle, affecting vascular tone, decreasing organ perfusion, and increasing SVR.
- Damage to the organ parenchyma, including, among many others, myocardial fibrosis.
- Rarefaction and fibrosis of the microcirculation and of the intercellular matrix, contributing to organ hypooxygenation and damage.
- Lipid oxidation, a key atherogenetic event, increasing vessel wall rigidity and perpetuating HTN ("HTN begets HTN").

HTN and the heart: HTN is the leading cause of HF, by several mechanisms:

- *CAD,* for which HTN is the main reversible risk factor; importantly, HTN is associated to CAD not only causally, but by covariation as well: both HTN and CAD are an expression of atherosclerosis.
- *LVH,* causing diastolic (and, in the later stages, combined systolic and diastolic) dysfunction, as well as relative ischemia in the hypertrophic muscle, as angiogenesis cannot keep pace with advanced muscle hypertrophy.
- Myocardial fibrosis.

HTN-related cerebral damage manifests as stroke, either ischemic or hemorrhagic, or as hypertensive encephalopathy. HTN is the leading cause of stroke. The responsible mechanisms include *damage to the cerebral vessels,* rendering them brittle and susceptible both to bleeding and to thrombosis; *damage to the carotid endothelium* and to the myocardium, causing thrombosis and cerebral embolism; *cerebral overperfusion,* due to failure of the autoregulatory mechanisms, resulting in cerebral edema and hypertensive encephalopathy, a major emergency manifesting with neurological signs, both cognitive and motor; *disruption of the blood–brain barrier* in conditions such as eclampsia, allowing access of toxic compounds to the brain parenchyma.

HTN and the kidneys: a dual relationship

The relationship between the kidneys and HTN includes

- *Renal disease caused by HTN* (hypertensive nephropathy, also termed nephrosclerosis), with deposition of an amorphous ("hyaline") material in the renal arterioles. This causes intrarenal stenosis and ischemia, contributing to HTN and, in the late stages causes, renal tubule atrophy, glomerular atrophy and sclerosis, renal fibrosis, and renal failure. HTN is the leading cause of end-stage renal disease.
- *Renal disease causing HTN:* renovascular HTN, a type of secondary HTN.

Hypertensive ocular damage includes *hypertensive retinopathy,* resulting from retinal atherosclerosis and ischemia, causing retinal microinfarcts and hemorrhage. This occurs mainly in middle-aged or older patients and generally does not affect visual function; and *papilledema,* i.e., edema of the head of the optic nerve, probably as an expression of cerebral edema; this is seen with HTN crisis (extreme BP increases, in the range of 250/150 mmHg), and represents a major medical emergency (risk of cardiovascular complications).

Ocular HTN is not related to HTN

Ocular HTN refers to increased pressure of the fluid filling the anterior ocular chamber and is *not* related to HTN. It is commonly seen in patients with glaucoma.

Funduscopy (ophthalmoscopy) in the diagnosis of HTN

This essential component of the ophthalmological examination consists in observation of the retina for pathological changes of the arteries and veins. For decades, funduscopy was integral part of the workup of HTN patients, for direct assessment of hypertensive retinal damage and for indirect assessment of the risk for target-organ damage. However, the importance of this practice is unclear, as there is poor correlation between retinal changes and target-organ damage, and as there is no specific treatment for hypertensive retinopathy. Moreover, there is relatively poor interobserver agreement regarding funduscopic findings.

The use of funduscopy in hypertensives is currently reserved for diagnosis of papilledema, a hallmark of malignant HTN. However, as funduscopy is often considered part and parcel of the standard physical examination, many "all-comer hypertensives" actually still undergo this examination. The absence of hypertensive retinal changes must, however, not lure the physician into a false sense of security; rather, the general principles of HTN diagnosis and treatment must be applied.

Hypertensive damage to the peripheral arteries: HTN is the main risk factor for PVD. As with CAD, the relationship is both causal (vascular damage caused by HTN favors atherosclerosis) and one of covariation (atherosclerosis, the main cause of PVD, is also a risk factor for HTN).

3.4 HTN Emergencies

The main *cause* of HTN emergencies is suboptimally treated chronic HTN; with the increase in medical awareness in developed countries, the incidence of malignant HTN has decreased. Additional causes include secondary HTN; perioperative HTN; preeclampsia and eclampsia; and HTN caused by recreational drugs (Amphetamines, LSD, Cocaine, Ecstasy). The *pathogenesis* of organ damage in malignant HTN involves breakdown of BP autoregulation, with excessive vessel wall permeability, focal hemorrhages, and edema. The vessel wall changes (myointimal proliferation, etc.) are of an intensity proportionate to the duration and severity of increased BP. *Complications*: Malignant HTN is an extremely severe condition, with a 50% of 1-year mortality in untreated patients. HTN emergencies generally include one or several of the following organ complications: *cardiac complications*: pulmonary edema, ACS; *aortic dissection; cerebral complications*: hypertensive encephalopathy, subarachnoid hemorrhage, CVA; and *renal complications*: hypertensive nephropathy (acute renal failure, with hematuria and proteinuria). The different manifestations listed above are discussed in the relevant chapters. The manifestations of *hypertensive encephalopathy* are *neurological* (severe headache, disturbed mental

HTN-related emergent clinical situations

Spectrum[a]	Entity	BP value (mmHg)	Acute organ damage	Papilledema
Hypertensive urgency[b]	Hypertensive urgency	>180/120	No	No
Hypertensive emergency[c]	Malignant HTN	Diastolic BP usually >140	Yes[d]	Yes
	Accelerated HTN[e]	Diastolic BP usually >140	Yes	No

[a]The term, "hypertensive crisis," is occasionally used to cover both urgencies and emergencies
[b]This term is used especially in the US
[c]In pregnant women, BP >170 (systolic) or >110 (diastolic) is considered an emergency
[d]Chronic organ damage and evolving organ damage due to suboptimally treated HTN are not considered HTN emergencies; on the other hand, most cases of malignant HTN originate from suboptimally treated "run of the mill" HTN, with corresponding chronic organ damage
[e]Note that the treatment of HTN emergencies is immediate and aggressive regardless of the presence or absence of papilledema

status, and visual impairment); *renal* (acute renal failure, occasionally irreversible and requiring chronic dialysis or renal transplant); and *hematological* (hemoloytic anemia; disseminated intravascular coagulation, with multiple tissue infarction and hemorrhage due to consumption of coagulation factors).

3.5 HTN Diagnosis

The medical workup in hypertensive patients aims at assessing the presence and severity of (a) *associated risk factors,* since the impact of HTN – and the

necessity for aggressive treatment – is defined based not only on BP values, but also on global cardiovascular risk; (b) *complications;* and (c) *underlying conditions* (secondary HTN), in select populations (Table 3.6).

3.6 The Treatment of HTN

The *treatment of HTN* is mainly aimed at preventing cardiovascular and renal complications. As the risk of complications depends on comorbidity, the target BP is more stringent (i.e., lower) if the total cardiovascular risk is increased. There are four classes of added risk

Table 3.6 Recommended workup in the HTN patient

	Routine tests	More advanced tests[a]
The cause of HTN		
	None	Tests for renovascular HTN (Ch. 11); aortic coarctation; endocrine disease, etc
The severity of HTN		
	Routine BP measurement in the office	BP self-monitoring, BP Holter
Associated risk factors for CAD		
Metabolic syndrome	Fasting plasma glucose, HDL, TG	N/A
Other metabolic derangements	LDL, Na, K, uric acid[b]	Glucose tolerance test[c] (if fasting glucose >5.6 mmol/L = 100 mg/dL)
Increased arterial stiffness	Not routinely assessed	Pulse wave velocity measurement[d]
Complications of HTN		
Renal involvement	Creatinine, estimated CrCl[e,f]; urinalysis, microalbuminuria dipstick test[g], microscopic exam[h]	Quantitative proteinuria (if dipstick test positive)[i]
Cardiovascular involvement	EKG	Echo, carotid ultrasound,[j] ankle-brachial BP index[k]
Cerebral involvement	Routine neurological exam	CNS imaging

[a]In complicated HTN, more complex diagnostic methods (myocardial or renal nuclear scan, angiography, brain imaging, etc.) may be used

[b]Increased uric acid levels are often associated with cardiovascular disease; it is unclear whether uric acid is a cause or a marker of atherosclerosis, or (since uric acid can act as an antioxidant) a protective mechanism against it

[c]An impaired glucose tolerance test carries a risk of progression to diabetes and development of cardiovascular disease

[d]Aortic PWV quantifies arterial stiffness and, in hypertensives, it is a marker of CV risk independently of BP; not surprisingly, it is increased particularly in the elderly. PWV assessment is based on simultaneous pulse wave measurement at two different positions and determination of the pulse transit time between these points, separated by a known (or assessed) distance

[e]Using the Cockcroft–Gault formula, $GFR = (140\text{-age}) \times (\text{weight in kg}) \times (0.85 \text{ if female})/(72 \times Cr)$

[f]The MDRD formula is a more accurate indicator of GFR in patients with chronic CKD: $GFR \text{ (mg/dL)} = 186.3 \times SerumCr^{-1.154} \times age^{-0.203} \times 1.212 \text{ (if patient is black)} \times 0.742 \text{ (if female)}$; these calculations can be carried out using an online "calculator"

[g]In patients with CKD, proteinuria increases sixfold the incidence of MI, most likely, via proteinuria-associated lipid abnormalities

[h]Hyaline casts

[i]There is a quantitative relationship between proteinuria reduction on one hand and decrease in LDL and TG on the other

[j]Carotid intimal-media thickness (IMT, the echographically measured layer between the intima-lumen and the media-adventitia borders) >1.3 mm is associated to a high probability of coronary atherosclerosis and its sequellae

[k]See Chap. 11

Table 3.7 Mandatory and optional drug treatment in HTN patients

BP	Drug treatment		
	None	Optional	Mandatory
Optimal or normal	Always[a]	N/A	N/A
High–normal	If no criteria for "optional" or "mandatory"	If ≥3 risk factors[b], metabolic syndrome, or subclinical organ damage	Established CV or renal disease or diabetes
HTN grade I	Lifestyle-change-only regimen acceptable (a) for a few months, if 1–2 risk factors[b] or (b) for a few weeks, if ≥3 risk factors, metabolic syndrome, or subclinical organ damage; if BP fails to normalize, drug treatment is mandatory	If lifestyle changes unlikely to be implemented, may immediately start therapy	Established CV or renal disease or diabetes
HTN grade II	Lifestyle-change-only regimen acceptable for a few weeks, if ≤1–2 risk factors; if BP fails to normalize, drug treatment is mandatory	If lifestyle changes unlikely to be implemented, may immediately start therapy	Established CV or renal disease or diabetes, or ≥3 risk factors
HTN grade III	Never	Never	Always

[a]Note that, in presence of associated CAD or HTN, the patient is often treated with diuretics, β-blockers, CCB, nitrates, and/or α-blockers, which decrease BP in addition to their primary effect. In fact, in these patients, one of the important goals is avoiding *hypo*tension (BP<90/60 mmHg), while still optimally managing the primary condition

[b]Excluding diabetes, which mandates drug therapy

(low, moderate, high, very high), i.e., of risk posed by associated non-HTN conditions, in addition to the baseline HTN risk. Established CV disease always represents a very high associated risk; the other risk classes, however, are defined using a "sliding-scale" definition, i.e., the risk class depends not only on the cluster of associated conditions, but also on the baseline BP. In other words, less of an associated burden is necessary to qualify as "severe," if the patient has more advanced (higher-grade) HTN. For instance, the presence of 1–2 associated risk factors represents a low added risk for high-normal BP, a moderate added risk for HTN grades I and II, and very severe added risk for grade III HTN. These considerations influence practically the aggressiveness of BP treatment. Table 3.7 translates these concepts into real-life guidelines for the practitioner. It is assumed that in *any* case, lifestyle changes have been thoroughly discussed with the patient.

Importantly, just as the presence of additional risk factors has a significant bearing on the treatment of HTN, the presence of HTN influences the therapy of coexisting conditions. Thus, low-dose Aspirin is generally indicated in hypertensive patients >50 years of age and in those with moderate or severe creatinine increases, regardless of the presence of underlying heart disease. (However, recent work questions the value of Aspirin for cardiovascular event prevention in patients with asymptomatic atherosclerosis.) Similarly, in diabetics, HTN mandates strict glycemic control, with fasting glucose levels <6 mmol/L (108 mg/dL) and glycated Hb <6.5%. In addition, the combination between HTN and diabetes also mandates cholesterol control to values <175 mg/dL (4.5 mmol/L) for total cholesterol, and <100 mg/dL (2.5 mmol/L) for LDL cholesterol.

3.6.1 Nonpharmacologic Therapy

Lifestyle changes, the staple of primary and secondary prevention of HTN, include *smoking cessation; weight reduction* (and stabilization); *reduction of excessive alcohol intake* (≤2 drinks a day); *physical exercise* (strongest effects with endurance exercise; both systolic and diastolic BP decrease by approximately 5–7 mmHg after an exercise session or following exercise training); *reduction of salt intake:* the extent of BP reduction is proportional with HTN grade, with age, and, if applicable, with the degree of excess body weight. It may take >1 month for BP to decrease after reducing sodium intake. Increased salt intake in overweight patients may increase cardiovascular risk, even in the absence of HTN; *increased fruit and vegetable intake; and decreased saturated and total fat intake.* The DASH diet (Dietary Approaches to Stop HTN) encourages consumption of nuts, whole grains, fish, poultry, fruit, and vegetables and limits intake of red meats, sweets, and sugar.

Lifestyle-changes benefits in HTN

The mechanisms of action of lifestyle changes are incompletely understood and may include

- *Prevention of atherosclerosis* (smoking cessation, weight loss, dietary interventions, e.g., the Mediterranean diet, the DASH diet)
- *Decreased sympathetic activity* (smoking cessation, physical exercise, weight loss, avoidance of alcohol abuse)
- *Avoidance of blood volume overexpansion* (reduced salt consumption)
- *Improved insulin sensitivity* (weight loss, physical exercise, avoidance of alcohol abuse)
- *Other:* RAAS axis inhibition, modulation of transmembrane ionic flux in the vascular myocytes, influence on cortisol secretion, etc.

Recommendations for physical exercise in hypertensive patients regard *frequency:* on most, and preferably on all, days of the week; *intensity:* moderate, i.e., at 40–60% of VO_2 max, assessed by a cardiorespiratory exercise test (Chap. 4) or approximated as the level of exercise increasing HR to 50–70% of maximal HR (220-age); *duration:* 30 min of continuous or cumulated physical activity per day; *type:* primarily endurance physical activity supplemented by resistance exercise. Endurance activity is aerobic activity, i.e., repetitive, rhythmical, relatively low-intensity exercise involving large muscle groups. Typical activities include cycling, walking, running, hiking, swimming, playing tennis, etc.

3.6.2 Pharmacological Therapy

Pharmacological therapy is reviewed in the following section. All antihypertensives can cause hypotension, with excessive fatigue, dizziness, syncope, etc.; these manifestations will not be reiterated for the individual classes of drugs. The mentioned dosages are the maximal dosages for monotherapy. As the current trend is to use ≥2 agents from the beginning, even for moderate HTN, these theoretical dosages are rarely used (Table 3.8).

Table 3.8 Antihypertensive drugs and their mechanisms of action

General mechanism	Specific mechanism	Class of drugs
Decrease in CO (by decreasing LV contractility and HR)		
Adrenergic activity modulation	Cardiac β-receptor *blockade*	β-blockers
	Brain (central) $α_2$-receptor *stimulation*	Clonidine
	Brain (central) $α_2$-receptor *stimulation*	Methyldopa[a]
	Catecholamine depletion from peripheral sympathetic nerve endings	Reserpine[b]
	Nonselective sympathetic (and parasympathetic) blockade	Trimetaphan
Interference with calcium ion activity	Calcium channel blockade	CCB
Decrease in SVR		
By direct action on the vessel wall	Inhibition of Ca influx, which stimulates muscular cell contraction	CCB
	Desensitization of vessel wall myocytes to calcium	Thiazide diuretics, chronic use (other mech. possible)
	Donors of NO, a vasodilator	Nitrates, Nitroprusside
	Incompletely understood; may inhibit intracellular Ca release and function as an NO donor	Hydralazine
	Increases membrane permeability to K ions, which inhibits Ca influx.	Diazoxide
	Incompletely understood; may function as an NO donor	Minoxidil
	Activation of Dopamine vascular receptors	Dopamine, Fenoldopam

Table 3.8 (continued)

General mechanism	Specific mechanism	Class of drugs
By interference with the action of direct vasoconstrictor agents	Inhibition of angiotensin generation	ACEI
	Inhibition of angiotensin action on the vessel wall	ARB
	Inhibition of renin action on the vessel wall	Aliskiren
By interference with α-adrenergic stimulation	Peripheral α-receptor blockade	α-blocking agents
	Catecholamine depletion from peripheral sympathetic nerve endings	Reserpine[b]
	Stimulating central (brain) α_2 receptors	Clonidine[c]
	Stimulating central (brain) α_2 receptors; decreasing peripheral sympathetic activity	Methyldopa[a]
Decrease in blood volume (diuretics)		
Stimulation of glomerular filtration	Increase of primary urine volume, by attracting an "obligatory" volume of water	Osmotic diuretics[c]
Inhibition of tubular reabsorption	In the *proximal tubule* (inhibition of bicarbonate reabsorption)	Acetazolamide[c]; Dopamine; Fenoldopam
	In the *descending portion of Henle's loop*	Osmotic diuretics
	In *Henle's loop*	Loop diuretics
	In *the proximal portion of the distal tubule*	Thiazides and thiazide-like diuretics
	In the *terminal portion of the distal tubule*	Osmotic diuretics, K⁺-sparing diuretics
	In *the collecting tubule*	Osmotic diuretics

[a]Once the mainstay of antihypertensive therapy, it has been largely superseded by newer drugs and is only used nowadays for treatment of pregnancy-induced HTN (it is relatively safe for the fetus)

[b]Reserpine is rarely used today but is still available in some countries, mainly as a combination pill also including a diuretic and/or a vasodilator such as Hydralazine; it is a second-line drug, due to its many adverse effects

[c]Presented here for completeness, they are not (or for Clonidine, no longer) used in cardiology. The main use of osmotic diuretics is for treatment of cerebral edema; of Acetazolamide, for treatment of glaucoma and seizures; and of Clonidine, for relief of withdrawal symptoms after long-term use of narcotics, alcohol, and nicotine (as cigarettes); for migraine headaches; for hot flashes associated with menopause; and for ADD

[d]Diazoxide acts as a CCB; it is, however, classified separately

3.6.2.1 Adrenergic Blocking Agents

Table 3.9 reviews the different types of adrenergic receptors, their blockers, and the corresponding recommended dosages. Noncardiological therapeutic uses are not reviewed. The dosages refer to HTN treatment only and may vary widely from country to country and obviously, from patient to patient; they are presented for illustration purposes only. *α-blockers: Selective α_1-blockers* are generally well tolerated, the main adverse effect being the "first dose phenomenon," i.e., sudden and severe orthostatic hypotension, when the drug is first taken or is resumed after a long interruption. (These drugs are up-titrated carefully and administered at bedtime, to avoid having the peak action occur at the time of orthostatic position.) The mechanism is unclear, but the phenomenon occurs mostly in volume-depleted patients (mainly under diuretic therapy), as well as in patients treated with β-blockers. It is most often seen with Prazosin and is less frequent with newer α_1-blockers. *Nonselective α-blockers* (Phentolamine) have no cardiological application.

3.6.2.2 β-Blockers: β_1 Receptor Blockade

This mainly causes hypotension and AVB (both of which can cause dizziness, weakness, or syncope); exacerbation of HF; and CNS effects (hallucinations, insomnia, nightmares, depression, etc.), especially with lipophilic agents, able to cross the blood–brain barrier (Metoprolol, Propranolol, Sotalol, Oxprenolol); *β_2 receptor blockade* (caused by nonselective β-blockers alongside β_1 blockade) causes bronchospasm, inhibition

Table 3.9 Adrenergic receptors and blockers

The receptor	Receptor mainly in	Function relevant to the cardiovascular system	Blockers used in cardiology (recommended doses, mg/day)
α_1	Vascular smooth muscle[a]	Vasoconstriction	*α_1-Blockers:* Prazosin (start at 1 b.i.d., uptitrate[7] slowly to 10 b.i.d., rarely up to 20 b.i.d.); Terazosin (start at 1 q.d., uptitrate slowly to 10 q.d., rarely up to 20 q.d.); Doxazosin (start at 1 q.d., uptitrate slowly to 16 q.d.); Trimazosin; Alfuzosin (10 q.d., extended-release)[b]
			β-blockers with α_1-blocking activity: Carvedilol[c]- (start at 6.25 b.i.d., double dose[d] every 7–14 days, up to 25 b.i.d.); Celiprolol (200 q.d., may increase to 400 q.d.)-; Labetalol -Tablets 100 b.i.d., may increase every 3 days, up to 400 b.i.d.; in HTN emergencies, up to 1,200–2,400 mg/day orally; *or,* IV initial dose: 20 mg over 2 min; follow with 20–80 mg q.10–15 min until BP controlled, *and* maintenance dose: 2 mg/min continuous IV infusion; titrate up to 5–20 mg/min, not to exceed 300 mg/24 h
α_2	Pancreas, vascular smooth muscle	Inhibition of insulin secretion; stimulation of glucagon secretion; vasoconstriction	See below, "nonselective α-adrenergic blockers"
$\alpha_{1 \text{ and } 2}$ (nonselect. α-blockers)	All of the above	All of the above	Phentolamine[e] (IM/IV 5 mg)
β_1[f]	Heart; kidneys	Positive chrono- and inotropic action (myocardial automaticity and contractility); stimulate renin secretion	Acebuto[g,h]- (200–600 b.i.d.), Ateno- (50–100 q.d.), Betaxo[i]- (start at 5 q.d., uptitrate slowly to 20 q.d., rarely up to 40 q.d.), Bisopro- (start at 2.5–5 q.d., uptitrate slowly to 20 q.d.), Esmo- (IV use in HTN crisis: 500 µg/kg/min for 1 min, followed by a 4-min maintenance infusion of 50 µg/kg/min; if needed, may repeat as above and follow with a maintenance infusion at 100 µg/kg/min), Metopro- (100–450 q.d., if extended-release tablets, or same amount in two daily doses, if nonslow release tablets); Nebivolol[c] (start at 5 q.d., uptitrate slowly up to 20 q.d.)
β_2	Vascular smooth muscle; kidney	Vasodilation, stimulation of renin secretion	See nonselective β-blockers
β_3	Fatty cells	Fatty acid mobilization (lipolysis); uncertain clin. importance	See nonselective β-blockers
β_{1-3} (nonselective β-blockers)	All of the above	All of the above	Alpreno-, Carteo[i]- (2.5–10 q.d.), Mepindo-, Nado-, (40–80 q.d., rarely up to 320 q.d.), Oxpreno[g,i]- (start at 20 t.i.d., uptitrate slowly to 40–120 t.i.d., then switch to slow-release, same dosage; not to exceed 480 mg daily), Penbuto- (20 q.d.), Pindo[g,h] – (start at 5 b.i.d., uptitrate slowly up to 30 b.i.d.), Proprano[h]-, Sota-, Timolol

[a]Also present on the myocardial cells; activation may cause a positive inotropic effect, of unclear clinical relevance (receptor blockade does not cause LV dysfunction)

[b]The agent, Tamsulosin, is for urologic use only

[c]These agents also possess antioxidant actvity, theoretically potentiating the favorable cardiovascular effect

[d]Maximum dose; lower doses are often sufficient

[e]Used in pheochromocytoma- or sympathomimetic-related HTN crises

[f]Agents of choice in patients with PVD, asthma, or diabetes that may be exacerbated by β_2-blockade

[g]These agents also possess intrinsic sympathomimetic actvity, with a theoretically decreased incidence of excessive hypotension and bradycardia

[h]These agents also possess central β-blocking activity, responsible for the CNS effects

[i]Also used as ophthalmic solution, in glaucoma patients

of peripheral vasodilation, hyperglycemia, increased TG, and decreased HDL levels. The effect on glucose metabolism has received a great deal of attention, as β-blockers (especially in association with Thiazides) may favor the appearance of diabetes; therefore, they are contraindicated in patients with the metabolic syndrome or impaired glucose tolerance test. Other adverse effects include nausea, diarrhea; endocrine manifestations (decreased renin secretion, with hypoaldosteronism and hyperkalemia); and blunting of the sympathetically mediated warning symptoms of hypoglycemia (tremor, perspiration, agitation, etc.). The importance of this latter mechanism may have been overestimated in the past. Carvedilol may also cause peripheral edema. Beta-blockers may cause hypertensive crisis in patients using Cocaine, Amphetamine, or other sympathomimetic agents, as β-blockade diverts all of the adrenergic effect to the α-receptors, with significant vasoconstriction. The treatment includes vasodilators (Nitroglycerine, Phentolamine) and diuretics. Finally, β-blockers may cause erectile dysfunction, exacerbation of Raynaud's syndrome, and vision disturbances.

> ## Cardiological uses of β-blockers
>
> β-blockers are among the most important cardiological medications. Their indications include CAD (angina pectoris, post-MI patients); atrial and ventricular arrhythmia; HF; HOCM; and HTN.

3.6.2.3 RAAS Blockers

The RAAS axis is an enzymatic cascade, where each agent stimulates the secretion/activation of the next agent. Sympathetic stimulation and renal underperfusion stimulate renin secretion, which enzymatically cleaves hepatic angiotensinogen into angiotensin I, further cleaved into angiotensin II by the pulmonary "angiotensin conversion enzyme" (ACE). RAAS axis activation causes water retention and vasoconstriction, with increased renal perfusion (local effect) and increased BP (systemic effect). The cascade continues with formation of angiotensins III (the actual stimulant of aldosterone secretion) and IV (a weaker vasoconstrictor). For simplification, these compounds are usually not mentioned.

> ## Positive and negative feedback in biological systems
>
> The RAAS illustrates the two main types of feedback operating in a biological system:
>
> - *Negative (regulatory) feedback:* RAAS activation causes increased renal perfusion, i.e., resolution of the cause for increased renin secretion (the effect inhibits the original cause).
> - *Positive feedback,* a self-maintenance mechanism: RAAS activates the sympathetic nervous system, via angiotensin II (the effect stimulates further expression of its own cause, as sympathetic activation stimulates renin secretion).

Pharmacological inhibition of water retention and vasoconstriction can be achieved by specific action on components of the RAAS system, or by countering their net effects. The medications in question are: ACEI; ARB (angiotensin II receptor blocker); aldosterone agonists; direct renin antagonists (Aliskiren); β-blockers; diuretics, and vasodilators. An additional negative effect of aldosterone, inhibited by ACEI therapy, is ventricular remodeling. This covers a spectrum of changes affecting the shape, size, and function of the LV, as a result of myocardial injury and of the adaptatsion to it. LV dysfunction results in renal hypoperfusion, activation of the RAAS system, and secretion of angiotensin II. In the case of HTN, remodeling mainly consists of myocardial hypertrophy, followed, in late stages, by cardiac dilatation. Inhibition or reversal of remodeling by medication is termed "reverse remodeling."

ACE Inhibitors (ACEI)

ACEI have the following beneficial effects:

- *Antihypertensive effects,* by *arteriolar dilatation* (decreasing SVR) and *increased venous capacity.* This, in turn, decreases BP by decreasing the circulating blood volume, absolutely (natriuresis) and relatively (by storing blood in the venous bed); this results in decreased LV filling and contractility.
- *Cardioprotective effects, by vasodilation,* which decrease SVR, thus increasing CO. By this mechanism, ACEI are effective both in normotensive

patients with LV dysfunction and in hypertensives; and *by inhibition of cardiac remodeling,* an important contributor to HF.

- *Nephroprotective effects,* possibly by lowering of the intraglomerular pressure.

The antihypertensive effect of the different ACEI agents is similar, but the action duration of Captopril is much shorter than with other agents, often leading to its replacement later-generation ACEI agents. The main adverse effects of ACEI include

- *Hyperkalemia,* by indirect inhibition of aldosterone action (aldosterone causes sodium and water reabsorption and potassium excretion).
- *Renal failure,* especially in patients with bilateral RAS. This may be due to inhibition of angiotensin-related vasoconstriction of the efferent renal arterioles, thus: the renal glomerulus, responsible for urine filtration, is situated between the afferent and efferent renal arterioles (upstream, respectively downstream from the glomerulus). When renal perfusion pressure decreases, the driving pressure for urine filtration and the amount of primary urine decrease as well. As a compensatory mechanism, the efferent arterioles contract (under the effect of angiotensin II), increasing intraglomerular pressure and improving filtration. Inhibition of this mechanism by efferent arteriolar vasodilation is the classical explanation for ACEI-related renal failure, a partly unconvincing explanation, since ACEI equally dilate the afferent arterioles, *increasing* glomerular perfusion. The risk of renal failure is increased by diuretics, which further decrease glomerular perfusion by reducing blood volume, as well as by NSAIDs, which inhibit secretion of vasodilatatory prostaglandins.
- *Other effects: cutaneous rash* (rarely); *taste disturbances* (especially with Captopril); *cough; neutropenia,* by medullary depression, with possible serious infections; *hepatic damage* (hepatocellular or cholestatic), generally reversible; *severe allergic reactions,* up to anaphyactic shock, especially in renal failure patients in whom a certain type of dialysis membrane is being used; *angioedema* (severe edema of the face and tongue, with possible asphyxia); *nausea and vomiting; fetal malformations*: ACEI are contraindicated in pregnancy. ACEI are eliminated through the human milk, but the quantities are minute, and therefore, nursing is allowed.

ACEI and ARB – both less and more effective than theoretically expected:

- *ACEI:* (1) *less effective:* incompletely inhibit the RAAS axis, as Angiotensin II can also be produced by ACE-independent mechanisms (chymase also cleaves AII from Angiotensin I); (2) *more effective:* ACEI inhibit degradation of bradykinin (a vasodilator). In addition to its beneficial effect, however, bradykinin may cause cough (a frequent adverse effect) and angioedema. These adverse effects are dealt with by switching from ACEI to ARB.
- *ARB:* (1) *less effective:* ARB have no influence on bradykinin; (2) ARBs completely inhibit the RAAS axis.

Dual ACEI and ARB blockade, to increase bradykinin levels while completely inhibiting the RAAS axis, is recommended in HF treatment but is generally not used in HTN in the absence of HF.

ACEI are administrated orally, unless otherwise specified. Submaximal doses are often sufficient. For all agents, doses must be decreased in case of renal failure. The main agents include *Captopril:* 25–50 mg b.i.d. or t.i.d, titrate up to 150 mg t.i.d.; *Benazepril:* start at 10 mg q.d., titrate up to 40 mg q.d. (rarely, 80 mg q.d.); may divide into two doses; *Enalapril:* PO: start at 2.5–5 mg q.d.; usual daily maintenance dose: 10–40 mg; may divide into two doses; IV (Enalaprilat): 1.25 mg over 5 min, q. 6 h, up to 5 mg q. 6 h; *Fosinopril:* start at 10 mg q.d., titrate up to 40 mg q.d. (rarely, 80 mg q.d.); may divide into two doses; *Lisinopril:* start at 10 mg q.d., titrate up to 40 mg q.d. (rarely, 80 mg q.d.); may divide into two doses; *Moexipril:* start at 7.5 mg q.d., titrate up to 30 mg q.d.; may divide into two doses; *Perindopril:* start at 4 mg q.d., titrate up to 16 mg q.d. (usual dose, 4–8 mg/day); max 8 mg/day in the elderly (>65); *Quinapril:* start at 10–20 mg q.d., titrate up to 80 mg q.d.; may divide into two doses; *Ramipril:* start at 2.5 mg q.d., titrate up to 20 mg q.d.; may divide into two doses; *Trandolapril:* start at 1 mg q.d. (2 mg in black patients), titrate up to 8 mg q.d.; may divide into two doses.

Angiotensin II Receptor Blockers

There are two types of receptors for angiotensin II, AT_1 and AT_2. AT_1 receptor inhibition decreases BP by vasodilatation and reduced secretion of vasopressin and aldosterone. The degree of selectivity for the AT_1 receptors, an indicator of agent potency, is lowest for Losartan, and highest for Valsartan. ARB drugs are generally well tolerated, the most frequent adverse effects being hypotension and hyperkalemia. Infrequent adverse effects include first-dose orthostatic hypotension, rash, GI manifestations (diarrhea, dyspepsia, abnormal LFT), muscle cramps, back pain, nasal congestion, cough, pharyngitis, as well as angioedema, insomnia, anemia, and renal impairment. The low frequency of cough with ARB drugs makes them ideal as replacement drugs for ACEI. According to recent studies, ARB drugs might increase the frequency of MI. The available ARB agents include *Losartan:* start at 25 mg q.d., titrate up to 100 mg q.d.; may divide into two doses; *Irbesartan:* start at 150 mg q.d., titrate up to 300 mg q.d.; *Olmesartan:* start at 20 mg q.d., titrate up to 40 mg q.d.; *Candesartan:* start at 16 mg q.d., titrate up to 32 mg q.d.; may divide into two doses; *Valsartan:* start at 80 mg q.d., titrate up to 320 mg q.d.; *Telmisartan:* start at 20 mg q.d., titrate up to 80 mg q.d.; *Eprosartan:* start at 600 mg q.d., titrate up to 800 mg q.d.; may divide into two doses.

Renin Inhibitors

Aliskiren is the first commercially available direct renin secretion inhibitor; it binds to the catalytic portion of renin, responsible for conversion of angiotensinogen to AT I. Adverse effects are infrequent and include hyperkalemia, hypotension, GI symptoms (mainly diarrhea), rash, elevated uric acid (with gout and/or renal stones), and angioedema. The recommended dosage is 150 mg q.d. (may increase to 300 mg). It is synergistic with diuretics and with ARB (valsartan); no data are available regarding the association with ACEI or β-blockers.

Aldosterone Inhibitors

Aldosterone Inhibitors are used as antihypertensives and as protective agents in HF of any cause, and, for Eplerenone, in post-MI HF. Occasionally, HTN is due to disproportionately high aldosterone activity; in this group, these usually auxiliary drugs may normalize BP by themselves.

The mechanism of action of aldosterone blockers

Beside their weak diuretic and their K^+-sparing actions (indicating these agents as adjuncts to Thiazides and loop diuretics), aldosterone blockers also counteract the myocardial fibrosis and endothelial dysfunction promoted by aldosterone. These actions are especially important in patients with HF.

The available aldosterone inhibitors include *Spironolactone* (25–50 mg b.i.d.) and *Eplerenone* (start at 50 mg q.d., increase up to 50 mg b.i.d.) *The adverse effects of Spironolactone* include hyperkalemia; feminizing effects on male patients (gynecomastia, testicular atrophy, erectile dysfunction); menstrual irregularities; neurological abnormalities (ataxia, drowsiness); rash; renal failure; a possible oncogenic and immunosuppressant effect; and possible inhibition of antidepressive drugs. Spironolactone use is also statistically associated to an increased risk of GI bleeding, but a causal relationship has not been proven. *The adverse effects of Eplerenone* include hyperkalemia, hypotension, dizziness, altered renal function, and increased creatinine concentration.

3.6.2.4 Calcium Channel Blockers (CCB)

Calcium ions are indispensable for muscular contraction. This is relevant to BP both in regard to cardiac contractility (and thus, CO) and in regard to SVR. CCB depress both these functions, by acting on the transmembrane channels that allow ingress of calcium into the cell. The consequent vasodilatation and decreased CO result in decreased BP. Chemically, CCB may be divided into three main classes.

Dihydropyridines

Dihydropyridines are identifiable by the suffix – *pine*. They are potent vasodilators and, besides occasional bradycardia, have relatively little direct effect on the heart;

vasodilatation may trigger reflex tachycardia, precipitating angina pectoris in CAD patients. The tachycardic effect is reduced with the newer, once-daily agents (Amlodipine is marketed both as an antihypertensive and for treatment of chronic angina) and with sustained-release Nifedipine. Other adverse effects include dizziness, headache, flushing, lower limb edema, tachycardia, bradycardia, constipation, and gingival hypertrophy. The contraindications include hypotension and known allergy to the drug. Short-acting Nifedipine is contraindicated in angina pectoris. The main available *dihydropyridines* include *Amlodipine:* Start at 5 mg q.d. (2.5 in the elderly), increase up to 10 mg q.d.; *Azelnidipine:* 8.0 mg q.d.; *Barnidipine:* 10–20 mg q.d.; *Benidipine:* 2–4 mg q.d.; *Efonidipine:* start at 20–40 mg q.d., may increase up to 60 mg q.d.; *Felodipine:* start at 2.5–5 mg q.d., increase slowly up to 10 mg q.d.; *Isradipine:* start at 2.5 mg b.i.d., titrate up to 5 mg b.i.d., rarely up to 10 mg b.i.d.; *Lacidipine:* 4 mg q.d.; *Lercanidipine:* start at 10 mg q.d., increase up to 20 mg q.d.; *Manidipine:* 10–20 q.d.; *Nicardipine:* start at 20 mg t.i.d., increase up to 40 mg t.i.d.; *Nifedipine:* (1) regular tablets: start at 10 mg t.i.d., increase up to 20 mg t.i.d.; (2) extended-release tablets: start at 30 or 60 mg q.d., increase up to 90–120 mg/day q.d., (the maximum dose varies among the available compounds); *Nilvadipine:* start at 4 mg q.d., increase up to 16 mg q.d. (8 mg q.d. in patients with cirrhosis or also taking with Cimetidine); *Nisoldipine:* start at 17 mg q.d., increase up to 34 mg q.d.; *Nitrendipine* (also occasionally spelled "Nitredipine"): start at 20 mg q.d., (10 mg q.d. in the elderly and in patients with liver disease), increase up to 40 mg q.d. *Additional dihydropyridine CCB agents* include *Cilnidipine, Cronidipine, Darodipine, Aranidipine, Dexniguldipine, Elnadipine, Elgodipine, Flordipine, Furnidipine, Iganidipine, Lacidipine, Lemildipine, Mesuldipine, Niguldipine, Niludipine, Olradipine, Oxodipine, Palonidipine, Pranidipine, Sagandipine, Sornidipine, Teludipine, Tiamdipine, Trombodipine, Watanidipine.* Finally, *Nimodipine* is a CCB with a strong specificity for the brain vessels and is used to improve neurological outcomes after subarachnoid hemorrhage. The somewhat surprising use of a vasodilator in the treatment of a hemorrhagic condition is explained by the relief of the postictal vasospasm that generates an ischemic component aggravating the prognosis. An IV CCB agent has also become available: *Clevidipine:* start infusion at 1–2 mg/h; double the dose at 90 s intervals initially, then slower and with lesser increments, up to 4–6 mg/h usually, rarely up to 16–32 mg/h, but not more than 21 mg/h on average, over the 24 h period. The data for administration upon 72 h at any dose are scarce.

Phenylalkylamines

Phenylalkylamines are relatively cardioselective. They depress CO, automatism, and conduction; relieve coronary spasm, with a minimal vasodilator effect; and are used as antihypertensives for HR control in chronic AF, for conversion of atrial flutter and paroxysmal SVT, and for angina treatment. The main available *Phenylalkylamine* is *Verapamil,* dosed PO (1) with nonsustained release tablets, at 40–160 mg t.i.d.; (2) with sustained-release tablets, the doses vary between 100–180 (starting dose) and 400–540 mg q.d. (maximum dose), depending on the preparation. The contraindications include sick sinus syndrome or > first-degree AVB except with functioning pacemaker; BP <90 mmHg systolic; severe LV dysfunction; cardiogenic shock and severe chronic HF, unless secondary to SVT known to be amenable to Verapamil; patients with atrial flutter or AF and an accessory tract (risk of life-threatening ventricular arrhythmia, by AV node blockade and 1:1 transmission of the rapid atrial rhythm to the ventricles); and VT (risk of severe hypotension). *The adverse effects* most frequently include constipation, elevated LFT, nausea, upper respiratory symptoms, flushing, headache and dizziness, fatigue, edema, AVB, bradycardia, hypotension (supine or postural), and paresthesia. A number of more infrequent adverse effects are also occasionally noted. *Gallopamil* is a newer phenylalkylamine agent, and the experience with it is as yet relatively scant.

Benzothiazepines

Benzothiazepines have properties intermediary between those of dihydropyridines and phenylalkylamines. The negative chronotropic effect prevents reflex tachycardia in response to the induced vasodilation. They are used as antihypertensives and for the treatment of angina pectoris.

The main available *Benzothiazepine* is *Diltiazem.* The dosage of the latter is started at 180–240 mg q.d., which may be increased to 360, and rarely, to 480 mg q.d. The most common effects include edema, headache, dizziness, asthenia, first degree AVB, bradycardia, flushing, nausea, and rash. The contraindications are similar to those of Verapamil.

The cardiological uses of CCB

CCB are used as antihypertensives; as antianginotics; for HR control in patients with AF, and, less frequently, in chronic atrial flutter, as well as for conversion of atrial flutter or paroxysmal tachycardia to NSR; and in patients with HOCM.

3.6.2.5 Diuretics

Urine is formed in the functional module of the kidney, the nephron, consisting of the renal corpuscule and the renal tubules. Each kidney has between 800,000 and one million nephrons. The renal corpuscle consists of Bowman's capsule (a double-walled funnel), which harbors the renal glomerulus, a capillary knot with the afferent arteriole upstream, and the efferent arteriole downstream. This anatomic structure distinguishes the glomerulus from other capillary networks, which are situated between a proximal arterial and a distal venous territory, and not between two arterial territories. The structure of the renal glomerulus allows regulation of the glomerular perfusion pressure (the driving force behind primary urine filtration), by balancing the degree of vasoconstriction in the afferent and the efferent arteriole. Urine is formed by the interplay of three main mechanisms: (1) glomerular filtration, i.e., formation of the primary urine (a "preliminary selection" of the candidates for elimination: water, electrolytes, drugs, etc.); (2) reabsorption of the greater part of the initially eliminated substances; (3) excretion into the renal tubules of substances from the efferent arteriole capillaries, which end up being eliminated despite the fact that they were not part of the primary urine. The sites of action of the various classes of diuretics are outlined in Table 3.10.

Osmotic diuretics and carbonic anhydrase inhibitors (Acetazolamide) are not used in cardiology. Dopamine is used as a diuretic in patients with severe HF and is discussed in Chap. 4. Of the K$^+$-saving diuretics, the Aldosterone antagonists (Spironolactone and Eplerenone) were discussed together with the inhibitors of the RAAS; the nonaldosterone-related K-saving diuretics, as well the other classes of diuretics will be reviewed below. The

Table 3.10 Classes of diuretics and their site of action

Nephron segment	Site	Type of diuretic
Renal corpuscle	Glomerulus	Osmotic
Proximal tubule	Proximal contorted tubule	Dopamine, osmotic, carbonic anhydrase inhibitors
Henle's loop	Descending limb of Henle's loop	Osmotic
	Ascending limb of Henle's loop	Loop diuretics
Distal tubule	Proximal part	Thiazides
	Distal part	K-sparing
Collecting tubule	Collecting tubule	K-sparing

adverse effects of diuretics are reviewed in Table 3.11; this list is only partial, and individual agents may possess additional adverse effects.

The "triple whammy" effect

This refers to acute (or acute-on-chronic) renal failure precipitated by the combination of *loop diuretics* (decreased glomerular filtration pressure by contraction of the circulating blood volume), *ACEI* (decreased glomerular filtration pressure by counteracting efferent arteriole vasoconstriction); and *NSAIDs* (counteracting prostaglandin-dependent renal vasodilation).

Loop Diuretics

Loop diuretics are potent diuretics used in HF, renal failure, and treatment of edema (cirrhosis, nephrotic syndrome, cerebral edema). While loop diuretics can be used in chronic uncomplicated HTN, the Thiazides are the diuretics of choice in this setting. Loop diuretics are also called "high-ceiling" diuretics, with an almost linear dose-effect relationship (both in regard to therapeutic action and to adverse effects), as opposed to the relatively rapidly reached plateau of Thiazides ("low-ceiling diuretics"). Loop diuretics are contraindicated in anuria, in case of known allergy, and in hypovolemic patients. They are used mainly in the

Table 3.11 Main adverse effects of diuretics

Class of adverse effect	Specific manifestation	Responsible diuretic
Hypovolemia		
	Dehydration, syncope, renal failure, muscle cramps	All classes (mostly Thiazides[a] and loop diuretics)
Electrolyte imbalance		
Hypokalemia	Muscle weakness, arrhythmia	Thiazides, loop diuretics, Acetazolamide
Hyperkalemia	Similar to the manifestations of hypokalemia	Potassium-sparing diuretics
Hyponatremia	CNS symptoms, coma	All classes (mostly Thiazides and loop diuretics)
Hypernatremia	May be seen in dehydration, if water is lost in excess of sodium	Thiazides, loop diuretics (K-sparing diuretics stimulate natriuresis)
Hypercalcemia[b]	CNS symptoms (fatigue, depression, confusion), GI (nausea, vomiting, constipation, pancreatitis), anorexia, polyuria, tissue calcification	Thiazides
Plasma pH derangements		
Metabolic alkalosis	Arrhythmia, CNS symptoms	Thiazides, loop diuretics
Metabolic acidosis	Kussmaul breathing, muscle weakness, seizures, lethargy, coma	Acetazolamide, K-sparing diuretics
Other metabolic derangements		
Hyperuricemia	Gout	Thiazides, loop diuretics
Dyslipidemia	Increased LDL, TG, and total cholesterol-to-HDL ratio	Thiazides in high dosage, loop diuretics
Altered glucose metabolism	Impaired glucose tolerance, diabetes mellitus	
Increased homocysteine levels	Homocysteine is atherogenic; the causal relationship between Thiazides and increased homocysteine levels is unclear, but folic acid supplements are recommended	Thiazides
Folic acid loss	Possible anemia, CNS manifestations	Triamterene
Other adverse effects		
Ototoxicity	Usually tinnitus and vertigo, but deafness possible	Loop diuretics
Hepatic toxicity	LFT derangements; hepatic coma in patients with ascites	Loop diuretics
Impotence		Thiazides

[a]Paradoxically, in patients with diabetes insipidus, Thiazides *decrease* the urinary volume
[b]This effect is actually therapeutic in idiopathic hypercalciuria, where Thiazides are used to prevent excess urinary loss of calcium and nephrolithiasis

treatment of chronic HTN; in HTN emergencies, they have only an auxiliary role, as the effect onset is slow. Loop diuretics are, however, key in the treatment of hypertensive pulmonary edema. They may counteract the fluid retention stimulated by vasodilators; for these indications, they are used in low doses. The main available loop diuretics include *Furosemide:* PO: usual dosage at 40 mg b.i.d. If response is not satisfactory, add other antihypertensive agents; IV 20 mg, may increase as needed; *Torsemide:* PO: usual dose 5 mg q.d.; may increase up to 20 mg; IV 5–20 mg q.d.; *Bumetanide:* 0.5–2 mg q.d., may increase up to 10 mg, in 2–3 doses; IV or IM, 0.5–1 mg q.d. (IV should be given over 1–2 min). May repeat at 2–3 h intervals, not exceeding 10 mg/24 h; *Ethacrynic acid:* PO 50–200 mg q.d.; IV 50 mg (0.5–1 mg/kg) q.d.

Thiazides

Thiazides (including the chemically unrelated Chlortalidone and Metolazone, exhibiting similar clinical effects) are mainly used as antihypertensives; with HF and edema of different etiologies, loop diuretics are generally preferred. Thiazides are contraindicated in anuria and, for the "true" Thiazides, in patients allergic to Sulfa drugs. In addition, Chlorothiazide may exacerbate lupus, and Metolazone is contraindicated in hepatic coma or precoma. The following thiazide or thiazide-like agents are in common use: *Chlorthalidone:* start at 25 mg q.d., may increase up to 100 mg q.d.; *Chlorothiazide:* start at 500 mg q.d., may increase up to 1,000 mg b.i.d.; *Hydrochlorothiazide:* start at 25 mg q.d., may increase up to 100 mg q.d.; Hydrochlorothiazide is the most commonly employed blood-pressure-lowering drug in the US but might in fact have a very low efficacy. *Indapamide:* start at 1.25 mg q.d., may increase up to 5 mg q.d.; *Metolazone:* the dosage depends on the specific preparation being used: it is 0.5–1 mg q.d. for Mykrox, and 2.5–20 mg q.d. for Zaroxolyn.

K-Sparing Diuretics

K-sparing diuretics are generally used as an adjunct to loop diuretics or to Thiazides. They may cause hyperkalemia and are contraindicated in renal failure. Triamterene is also contraindicated in severe liver disease. The main agents are *Amiloride:* start at 5 mg q.d., may carefully increase up to 20 mg q.d.; *Triamterene:* PO 100 mg b.i.d. after meals (max, 300 mg/day); *Spironolactone:* 25–50 mg b.i.d.; and *Eplerenone:* start at 50 mg q.d., increase up to 50 mg b.i.d.

Other Antihypertensives

Antihypertensives Used in HTN Emergencies

Hydralazine: (1) PO, start at 10 mg q.i.d., increase every 3–5 days as needed, up to 125 mg q.i.d.; (2) IV/IM (rarely used) 20–40 mg, repeated as needed.

Hydralazine produces reflex tachycardia and should not be given without β-blockers in patients with possible CAD or aortic dissection. It can also cause a lupus-like syndrome; *Diazoxide* is administered IV, in doses of 1–3 mg/kg (up to a maximum of 150 mg) or 50–100 mg total q. 5–15 min until an adequate reduction in BP is achieved. It can also be administered by constant IV infusion (7.5–30 mg/min, in various dosing schedules). The drug should be used only for short periods and is best combined with a loop diuretic. Diazoxide may cause hyperglycemia; *Minoxidil:* PO, start at 5 mg q.d., increase up to 100 mg q.d. The usual dosage is 10–40 mg daily, in 1 or 2 administrations. A β-blocker (e.g., Propranolol 80–160 mg) is necessary *before* starting Minoxidil therapy, to prevent compensatory tachycardia caused by intense vasodilatation; *Fenoldopam* is a peripheral Dopamine receptor agonist, causing vasodilatation mainly in the renal, mesenteric, and coronary arteries. It also acts on the renal Dopamine receptors, promoting sodium excretion. Fenoldopam is administered IV, starting at 0.1–0.3 µg/kg/min (maximum 0.4 µg/kg/min). There are no known specific contraindications; *Trimethaphan* is a nonselective sympathetic and parasympathetic ganglion blocking agent, nowadays largely replaced by Nitroprusside, but still occasionally used in the treatment of aortic dissection. It is administered with an IV infusion pump (0.5–5 mg/min). The action is apparent at 1–5 min and lasts for 10 min; *IV nitrates:* the most frequently used agent is Nitroglycerin, primarily a venous vasodilator, with a weaker action on the arteries. Nitrates are weaker antihypertensives than Nitroprusside, and are generally reserved for HTN associated to ischemia. The usual dose is 5–100 µg/min. The adverse effects are discussed in Chap. 2; *Nitroprusside* is a direct arteriolar and venous dilator, with a very rapid action onset (seconds). In combination with a β-blocker, it is standard therapy in aortic dissection. Sodium Nitroprusside is one of the most widely used medications for the treatment of HTN crisis. It is administered by IV infusion pump; the dosage is 0.25–8 µg/kg/min. Nitroprusside may cause thiocyanate toxicity, presenting with malaise, headache, abdominal pain, and neurological signs (altered mental status, seizures). The antidote is sodium thiosulfate, 12.5 g IV stat.

Older, largely abandoned agents used in chronic HTN: Clonidine: PO, start at 0.1 mg b.i.d., increase up to 0.3 mg b.i.d.; the theoretical maximal dose is 2.4 mg/day, but this dose was rarely (if ever) used, even in the heyday of this agent. Lower doses are recommended in renal patients. Clonidine can cause oversedation, lightheadedness, dry mouth, dizziness, constipation, or hypotension (supine or orthostatic) and, in association with β-blockers or CCB, excessive bradycardia. Dangerous rebound HTN may be seen on abrupt discontinuation; *Methyldopa:* (1) PO, start at 250 mg b.i.d. or t.i.d., increase up to 3,000 mg daily, in 2–4 doses; (2) IV 250–500 mg q.i.d., increase up to 1 g q.i.d. Methyldopa has numerous adverse effects: hematological (anemia, thrombo- and leukopenia); cardiovascular (angina, bradycardia, pericarditis, orthostatic hypotension); GI (abnormal LFT, hepatitis, pancreatitis); neurologic and muscular (sedation, headaches, dizziness, nightmares, decreased libido, psychosis, depression, parkinsonism, Bell's palsy, paresthesia, myalgia); endocrinological (hyperprolactinaemia and amenorrhoea, gynecomastia), a lupus-like syndrome, ejaculatory failure, impotence, decreased libido, etc.

Novel approaches in the therapy of refractory HTN include an implantable device that activates the carotid sinus baroreceptors; catheter-based renal sympathetic denervation; development of a vaccine against angiotensin II, designed to lower BP (found ineffective in a stage 2 trial, this approach might still be revived in the future); and an antagonist of both endothelin and angiotensin, currently under study.

3.6.3 Strategies of Antihypertensive Therapy

3.6.3.1 Chronic HTN

Any of the major drug classes (Thiazides, CCB, ACEI, ARB, β-blockers) is appropriate for starting antihypertensive therapy and may normalize BP, with an occasionally better response of diastolic BP than of systolic BP. Unfortunately, proper control of systolic BP may at times require antihypertensive dosages that decrease diastolic BP excessively. Monotherapy is occasionally sufficient in patients with mild HTN and a low total cardiovascular risk; however, in most patients, combined therapy is necessary. It is less important which classes of drugs are used, as long as the combinations are logical (Table 3.12), and one keeps in mind the presence of other factors, such as comorbidity, ethnicity (black patients react better to diuretics than to

ACEI), or financial constraints (generics are substantially cheaper). The possibility of drug interaction or adverse reactions is, as always, very important. Single daily dosage with long-acting agents or with combination "2-in-1" pills is often preferable, as it favors patient compliance. Some of the most common antihypertensive combinations are outlined in Table 3.12. These combinations have a greater efficacy than the sum total of the effectiveness of each drug (synergy). This allows minimizing the adverse effects, both by favorable drug interactions (e.g., associating a diuretic to a vasodilator to counteract fluid retention) and by using smaller doses from each agent. HTN treatment in children is similar to that in adults.

HTN patients often suffer from coexisting conditions, such as HF or CAD, treated with the same drugs as those used against HTN itself. For instance, all the antihypertensives, with the exception of CCB, are also used in the treatment of HF and in the post-MI patient. In these patients, the choice may "already have been made," in regard to the antihypertensive therapy. Additionally,

- In diabetics and in patients with chronic renal failure (in the absence of bilateral RAS), ACEI and ARB are indicated for prevention of onset/progression of renal damage.
- ACEI, in association with diuretics, are effective in the secondary prevention of CVA (even in the absence of HTN).
- Spironolactone prolongs survival in HF patients; Eplerenone prolongs survival in patients with MI-related HF.
- In pregnant women, (1) nonemergent therapy includes Methyldopa, CCB, Labetalol, and (less frequently) other β-blockers; (2) emergent therapy includes intravenous Nitroglycerin, Nitroprusside or Labetalol, and oral Methyldopa.

Occasionally, BP remains >140/90 mmHg, despite treatment with antihypertensive drugs from three different classes, including a diuretic. This is termed *resistant HTN;* excluding white-coat HTN and pseudo-HTN, it is generally caused by poor compliance (medication, lifestyle changes); unsuspected or untreated underlying conditions (obstructive sleep apnea, secondary HTN); administration or abuse of agents such as NSAIDs, steroids, contraceptive pills, excessive amounts of decongestant drops, Cocaine, alcohol, etc. The treatment is based on identification and correction of these underlying disorders.

Table 3.12 Common antihypertensive combinations[a]

Agents		1 Thiazides	2 ACEI	3 ARB	4 CCB	5 β-blockers
A	Thiazides	–	√	√	√	See E1
B	ACEI	√	–	See C2	√[b]	See E2
C	ARB	√	Used in HF; uncommon association in HTN	–	√[b]	As for ACEI
D	CCB	√; The Thiazides counteract fluid retention, resulting from vasodilation-related RAAS activation	√	√	–	√; β-blockers counteract vasodilation-related tachycardia; the β-blocker/nondihydropyridine association is C/I (excessive negative inotropic and chronotropic effect)
E	β-blockers	May precipitate diabetes in patients with impaired GCT or metabolic syndrome; discounseled association	β-blockers might counteract the increased renin levels caused by ACE blockade	As for ACEI	See D5	–

[a]α-blocking agents may be associated with any other class of antihypertensives; they are adjunct agents only. Reserpine, Clonidine, Hydralazine, and Methyldopa are rarely used nowadays, except in pregnancy (Methyldopa, CCB, Labetalol, and, less frequently, other β-blockers)

[b]The ACCOMPLISH trial has found the combination Benazepril/Amlodipine more effective than that Benazepril/Hydrochlorothiazide. These findings run contrary to the formerly popular STITCH algorithm, advocating CCB addition only if an ACEI/diuretic combination has failed

Unfortunately, despite this wealth of available agents, the statistics regarding BP control in the population are dismal. Up to 1/3 of hypertensives are never diagnosed, more than 1/3 of those diagnosed are not treated at all, and 2/3 of those who do receive treatment have suboptimal BP control. Proper physician-patient interaction is of the essence, all the more so as HTN is often asymptomatic, and the patient may find it difficult to understand the reason for lifetime therapy. Proper follow-up is also important. The frequency of follow-up depends on the severity of HTN; for instance, in compliant patients with grade I HTN, who can reliably self-monitor BP at home, it is indicated every 6 months or even at longer intervals.

3.6.3.2 HTN Emergencies

The goal of therapy in hypertensive crises is to prevent/reverse organ damage by effective and fast BP reduction. BP must be reduced within a few hours to around 160/100 mmHg; the initial reduction must generally not be >25% from the initial value; precipitous BP lowering may precipitate organ ischemia. (Autoregulation is reset by the high BP values, and normal or near-normal values may be insufficient to ensure organ perfusion.) Therapy is guided by the degree of organ damage, rather than by absolute BP values, as even remarkably high BP values may present without target organ dysfunction. These *"hypertensive urgencies"* generally do not require parenteral therapy, as opposed to *HTN emergencies,* where the latter is often necessary. After successful BP control, the transition to chronic oral therapy should be gradual, in parallel with weaning off the IV medication. In HTN emergencies due to substance abuse and in patients with (pre)eclampsia undergoing C-section, chronic therapy is generally not necessary. The available agents are reviewed below; the dosages are discussed in the previous section.

Parenteral agents used in HTN emergencies:

- *Nitroprusside:* this is the agent of choice, due to its rapid and easily controllable action; it may trigger reflex tachycardia that mandates associating or replacing it with a β-blocker, in patients with myocardial ischemia or aortic dissection. However, Nitroprusside alone is often administered in patients with critical coronary ischemia, as well as after complex coronary angioplasty. Occasionally, Nitroprusside causes tolerance.

- *Intravenous nitrates:* weaker antihypertensives than Nitroprusside; they are the agents of choice in HTN associating coronary ischemia. IV nitrates cause tolerance, which mandates increasing the doses.
- *β-blockers: Labetalol* is the most potent antihypertensive β-blocker and is the preferred agent for patients with aortic dissection. *Esmolol:* less potent than Labetalol, used when gradual β-blockade is necessary, to avoid adverse events.
- *CCB: Nicardipine* is the most potent antihypertensive CCB; association with a β-blocker is recommended, due to the significant compensatory tachycardia.
- *Other agents: Fenoldopam* has a favorable pharmacological profile, especially in regard to the lack of tolerance or rebound HTN after discontinuation. *Enalaprilat:* while the onset of action is relatively rapid (15 min), the peak action may be delayed up to 6 h; therefore, this agent is used as an auxiliary to other antihypertensives. *Diazoxide:* can cause hyperglycemia and fluid retention; combination with a diuretic is recommended; *Hydralazine:* association with a β-blocker is recommended to avoid compensatory tachycardia; *Loop Diuretics:* auxiliary agents, facilitating the response to vasodilators, which may stimulate fluid retention.

Oral agents used in HTN emergencies:

- *Clonidine:* 0.2 mg orally initially, followed by 0.1 mg every hour to a total of 0.8 mg; it requires several hours to lower BP and is therefore rarely used.
- *Captopril:* 12.5–25 mg PO lowers BP in 15–30 min; the response is variable and may be excessive.
- *Nifedipine:* a fast and effective therapeutic modality for HTN emergencies, Nifedipine capsules have fallen in disfavor due to their unpredictable action, with occasional abrupt BP decrease and compensatory tachycardia, possibly leading to MI and CVA.

3.7　Arterial Hypotension

3.7.1　General Considerations

Arterial hypotension (BP <90 mmHg systolic and/or <60 mmHg diastolic) is a complex phenomenon, where the physiological impact (rather than a set "normal" value) is the main issue. This impact is conditioned by factors such as

- *Individual variability:* the spectrum of "normal BP" is wide (90–140 mmHg systolic and 60–90 mmHg diastolic), and different individuals function optimally at different BP values within this span. This is somewhat at variance with the situation of HTN, which is defined more rigidly as BP >140/90 mmHg (or, in select populations, >130/80 mmHg).
- *The clinical timeframe* (abrupt onset is more symptomatic, as cerebral autoregulation does not have the necessary time to counteract the BP decrease, and syncope may ensue).
- *The absolute value* of BP decrease (a drop >20 mmHg, e.g., from 130 to 110 mmHg systolic) can cause severe symptoms and even syncope.

Classification: Hypotension can be classified as *chronic* or *acute,* in turn *nonlife-threatening* (mild BP decreases, in the absence of syncope), *potentially life-threatening* (syncope), or *definitely life-threatening* (shock, cardiac arrest). Cardiac arrest is discussed in Chap. 6, and cardiogenic shock, in Chap. 4; noncardiogenic shock is also characterized by organ ischemia. *Mechanisms:* As opposed to HTN (most often "primary"), hypotension is generally secondary to identifiable conditions, affecting the mechanisms responsible for BP maintenance. Multiple mechanisms often coexist (Table 3.13) and include *decreased blood volume,* e.g., hemorrhage or dehydration (excessive sensible and insensible perspiration, diarrhea, extensive burns, diuretic use, renal incapacity to concentrate urine, etc.); *decreased CO,* due to myocardial dysfunction, bradycardia (including cardioinhibitory syncope), severe AS, HOCM, or other

Table 3.13 Mechanisms of hypotension and syncope

General mechanism[a]	Specific mechanism	Conditions[b]
Decreased CO		
Excessive bradycardia[c]	Sinus bradycardia, AVB, asystole	Toxic, ischemic, traumatic, or inflammatory disease; neurally mediated (cardioinhibitory syncope); idiopathic; CNS causes
Decreased LVEF	Decreased LV contractility	Extensive MI; DCM
	Decreased LV filling	Excessive tachycardia; PAH+exercise; RCM; PT
	Decreased LV emptying	AS or HOCM[d] + exercise
	Decreased RV emptying	RVOT obstruction,[e] PE[f]
	Combined mechanisms	Ventricular tachyarrthyhmia
Decreased circulating blood volume		
Absolute hypovolemia	Dehydration	Decreased water intake or excessive water losses (diuretics, unbalanced diabetes, Addison's disease[g])
	Hemorrhage	Internal/external
	Plasma loss	Severe burns
Relative (distributive) hypovolemia	Fluid storage in the third space	Edema, ascites
	Blood pooling in the lower limb veins	Orthostatic hypotension[h,i]
Decreased peripheral resistance		
	Vasodilation	Septic shock; anaphylactic shock; neurally mediated (vasodepressor mechanisms)[j]; CNS causes

[a]These mechanisms are often combined
[b]Any of these conditions can also be iatrogenic
[c]In extreme cases, cardioinhibitory syncope
[d]Arrhythmic mechanism also possible
[e]The mechanism actually involves a vasodepressor reflex
[f]The mechanism of syncope in PE is incompletely understood
[g]Hypothyroidism and myxedema can also cause hypotension, by complex mechanisms.
[h]Favored by dehydration
[i]In fact, orthostatic hypotension may also be regarded as "excessive *relative* vasodilation," insofar the lower limb and mesenteric veins do not contract appropriately on standing upright
[j]In extreme cases, vasodepressive syncope

diseases such as PT, tension pneumothorax, PE, severe forms of endocrine diseases, or iatrogenic causes; *excessive vasodilation,* resulting from (a) *disease states:* severe pain, shock, acidosis (often coexisting with shock), dysautonomia (significant decrease in sympathetic vasoconstriction, idiopathic, iatrogenic, or resulting from diabetes); (b) *physiologic states:* pregnancy, postprandially, orthostatism, etc. *Compensatory mechanisms* mainly include stimulation of *thirst,* to increase water intake; *increased water retention,* by renal and endocrine mechanisms (stimulation of ADH secretion); and *sympathetic activation,* to increase CO and SVR. *Symptoms:* Hypotension may run an acute course (syncope) or a subacute one (shock). The symptoms of hypotension are related to decreased organ perfusion, mainly affecting the brain and kidneys. The cerebral symptoms of hypotension include fatigue, sweating, pallor, headache, tremulousness, exercise intolerance (frequently, after exercise), nausea, palpitations, etc. The extreme type of hypotension-related symptoms is syncope (rapidly reversible loss of consciousness and of postural tone), discussed in the next section.

3.7.2 Syncope

Syncope ("blackout," "fainting") is defined as a sudden and spontaneously reversible loss of consciousness and postural tone. Occasionally, the patient reports dizziness, lightheadedness, blurred vision, cold and clammy skin, etc., without actual loss of consciousness and postural tone. These symptoms are termed "presyncope," and may be self-limiting or evolve into full-blown syncope, which may occasionally be avoided by squatting, sitting, or lying down. There are several important mechanisms of syncope.

3.7.2.1 Classification

Syncope by neurological mechanisms: Loss of consciousness by neurological mechanism can be caused *by organic brain disease* (seizure, TIA; postictal state; psychogenic pseudo-syncope; not considered "true" syncope) or by *peripheral receptor stimulation*, transmitted to the CNS, and hence to the vagal innervation of the vessels (causing vasodilation) and/or of the heart (causing bradycardia). Peripheral vagal terminations include *the "C fibers"* in the inferior and posterior LV wall, stimulated during cardiac stretch or forceful systolic contraction; *peripheral parasympathetic fibers* in the walls of cavitary organs such as blood vessels, urinary bladder, etc.; and *the sensory fibers in the carotid sinus.* Vagal activation (occasionally associated with an absolute decrease in sympathetic tone) causes "neurally mediated" (vasovagal) syncope, including several entities: *cardioinhibitory syncope* (syncope caused by pure bradycardia); *vasodepressor syncope* (pure vasodilation); or syncope by *combined mechanisms.* These are reviewed in Table 3.14, together with a discussion of the corresponding terminology.

Table 3.14 Syncope involving a neurological mechanism, excluding CNS disease

Condition	Mechanism	Settings of appearance	Terminology-remarks
Neurally mediated syncope	Vagal activation, with or without sympathetic withdrawal	1–3, below	Partly a misnomer, since syncope due to CNS disease is also "neurally mediated"; the synonym, "vasovagal syncope" is partly a misnomer, since "cardiac" syncope can also involve vagal activation (e.g., inferior MI, RVOT obstruction); also called "common faint"
Neurocardiogenic syncope	Triggered by stimulation of the C fibers	Emotional strain, pain, sustained upright posture	"Neurocardiogenic syncope" is partly a misnomer, as *all* the conditions discussed in this table reflect "neural" (i.e., vagal) stimulation of the heart and/or vessels
Situational syncope	Vagally mediated vasodilation + bradycardia, caused by C fiber activation, as a result of decreased venous return to the heart (Valsalva maneuver), causing the myocardium to contract on a relatively empty cavity	Micturition, defecation, cough, trumpet playing	Partly a misnomer, since orthostatic syncope and the much less frequent carotid syncope also occur in well-reproducible "situations"
Carotid sinus syncope	Cardioinhbitory (70%), vasodepressor (10%), or combined mechanism (20%)	Shaving, swimming, turning the head, wearing a tight tie, etc.	
Orthostatic syncope	The extreme form of orthostatic hypotension	Briskly standing up	Partly a misnomer, since sustained upright posture can also cause syncope, by activation of C fibers; viewed as an inadequate neurovegetative response to orthostatism, it relies on neurovegetative involvement as well
Postprandial syncope	Lack of adequate mesenteric vein contraction after meals	After meals, especially when standing up	See "orthostatic syncope"

Cardiac syncope occurs as a result of organic heart disease (as opposed to neurally mediated syncope, which may cause bradycardia in the absence of organic heart disease). This apparently straightforward definition is problematic, since here too, the actual mechanism occasionally consists in vagal activation (syncope of RVOT obstruction or of inferior MI). Cardiac syncope involves decreased CO, caused by mechanical and/or arrhythmic causes.

- *Mechanical causes:* CMP (DCM, HCM, RCM, idiopathic, or secondary); *myocardial ischemia or infarction; PT; AS;* obstructive *atrial myxoma; vegetation*, etc. For some of these diseases, syncope is a prognostic and therapeutic indicator; for instance, syncope is an indication for surgery in patients with severe AS, and an indication for ICD in HOCM patients.
- *Arrhythmic causes:* Some important causes of tachyarrythmia resulting in syncope include *HOCM*, where the characteristic myocardial disarray (a substrate for severe arrhythmia) plays a more important role in syncope generation than does LVOT obstruction; *ARVD; long QT syndrome* and iatrogenic QT segment prolongation, possibly leading to torsades des pointes; *Brugada syndrome; myocardial infarction or CMP; iatrogenic arrhythmia* that may be caused by diuretics (via potassium depletion) or by AAD; *atrial tachyarrhythmia transmitted over an aberrant pathway; pacemaker dysfunction.*

Idiopathic syncope probably also involves one or more of the mechanisms in Table 3.14, but, by definition, the exact sequence of events leading to syncope is unclear. In older studies, up to 50% of cases of syncope were termed idiopathic, although this percentage may have changed with the advent of newer diagnostic modalities.

3.7.2.2 Syncope: Diagnosis

The aims are to establish the presence, etiology, and possible complications of syncope. The *presence* of syncope is established by anamnesis or eyewitness account, Data regarding the duration, frequency, and situations favoring the appearance of syncope are obtained. Of special concern is the presence or absence of premonitory signs, both for teaching the patient to adopt emergency measures (sitting down or squatting, pulling up to the kerb if driving, etc.) and for establishing a tentative causal diagnosis. A few diagnostic clues include the following:

- Sudden syncope suggests carotid hypersensitivity or AVB.
- Syncope arising in certain "typical" settings (unpleasant smells, blood drawing, etc.) is probably situational.
- A primary seizure disorder is suggested by a loss of consciousness *starting* with seizures and/or by post-attack confusion lasting >5 min and by an aura, such as bright lights or a distinctive smell (different from the warning signs of true syncope, heralded by nausea, vomiting, abdominal pain, sweating, etc.). Associated neurologic signs (vertigo, diplopia, etc.) suggest a TIA; and recurrent syncope with multiform-associated manifestations suggests psychiatric pseudo-syncope.
- Syncope while supine, under exertion, or in the presence of known heart disease probably has a cardiac etiology.

The diagnostic modalities are the usual ones, supplemented by carotid massage and tilt test. Every effort (neurological examination, echo) must be made to diagnose syncope with structural disease of the heart/brain, as it has a much poorer prognosis. However, patient individualization is essential as the yield of advanced testing in all-comers (no cardiac murmurs or carotid bruits, normal EKG) is quite low.

EKG techniques useful in the etiologic diagnosis of syncope include *Resting EKG,* achieving a tentative diagnosis in about 5% of patients; typical EKG findings include sinus bradycardia <40 bpm, AVB Mobitz types II or III, alternating LBBB/RBBB, wide (>0.12 s) QRS complexes, rapid ventricular or atrial arrhythmia, prolonged QT, signs of the Brugada, WPW syndromes, etc. *Resting EKG under provocation maneuvers,* nonpharmacological (carotid massage, Valsalva) or pharmacological (rapid IV injection of ATP 20 mg during EKG monitoring normally causes asystole <6 s, or AVB lasting <10s: these durations are exceeded in a subgroup of patients with otherwise unexplained syncope, generally with a benign prognosis.) A special provocation maneuver is the carotid sinus massage.

Holter testing is indicated if the initial EKG is normal. The ideal duration for testing is ≥48 h. Findings such as AVB >first degree, sinus pauses >2 s, and sustained or nonsustained VT warrant further investigation and treatment. However, the correlation between Holter findings and a syncopal spell is very low: only in about 4% of cases does (pre)syncope occur at the same time as a Holter-detected arrhythmic event. This is partly due to the very high incidence of subclinical arrthythmia even in healthy individuals. A syncopal event in the absence of EKG changes rules out an underlying arrhythmic mechanism. *Loop monitoring* is a very helpful alternative to Holter. The device can be activated by the patient at the time of syncope prodrome (if there is one) or immediately upon recovering consciousness, in which case the device will permanently record the past 5–15 min of EKG tracing, stored on a running basis, and updated continuously. A new generation of implantable loop recorders is available, with a severalfold higher diagnostic yield than that of combined EP, tilt testing, and patient-activated loop recording. *Signal-averaged EKG (SAECG,* Chap. 6): In the syncope patient, this method allows to nonivasively predict the population in whom EP testing will be positive (only about 5% of patients with normal SAECG have inducible arrhythmia on EPS). The shortcomings are that (a) unlike EP testing, for which it proposes to serve as a "gate-keeper," it does not diagnose sinus- or AV-node-related pathology; (b) in patients with low LVEF (with or without syncope), an ICD is indicated in any event (Chap. 4). Therefore, SAECG is best reserved for patients with patients with unexplained syncope and no structural heart disease. *Electrophysiological (EP) testing* is mainly indicated in the syncope patient with structural heart disease and may reveal sinus bradycardia and a sinus node recovery time >3 s; infrahisian block; bifascicular block associating a baseline His-ventricle conduction delay ≥100 ms or II-d or III-d degree His-Purkinje block under incremental atrial pacing or pharmacological stimulation (IV Ajmaline, Procainamide, or Disopyramide); sustained monomorphic VT; or supraventricular tachyarrhythmia with hypotension. As with Holter monitoring, there is often poor correlation between induced arrhythmia and syncope, and thus, EPS only rarely represents definite "proof" of the etiology of syncope. However, the prognosis in patients with inducible VT is substantially worse, a fact especially relevant in patients with syncope and LVEF decrease not <40%. *Exercise stress testing* is recommended in patients undergoing syncope on exertion or immediately thereafter and is considered positive if it elicits syncope and/or second or third degree AVB.

Other diagnostic tests in the patient with syncope: Carotid sinus massage is performed in the supine and the orthostatic positions, on both sides in turn, for ≥5 but ≤10 s, under EKG and BP monitoring. It is considered positive if it elicits asystole ≥3 s or a BP drop ≥50 mmHg. Carotid massage should be avoided in patients with a history of stroke or with carotid bruits. Auscultation is mandatory in all patients, as the carotid sinus, a dilated portion of the carotid artery, may harbor thrombi that can migrate and cause CVA. In the elderly, carotid sinus hypersensitivity may be present even in the absence of disease. *The tilt test* consists in BP and HR measurement with the patient strapped to a table inclined at 60–70°, for 20–45 min, with or without pharmacological stimulation (Isoproterenol), according to different protocols. In patients with neurally mediated syncope, the upright position may cause hypotension and/or bradycardia (i.e., a vasodepressor or a cardioinhibitory response). While the mechanism is incompletely understood, activation of the Bezold–Jarisch reflex is suspected (see "orthostatic hypotension"). Isoproterenol, a nonselective β-agonist, induces baroreceptor stimulation, increasing the susceptibility to vasodilatation, bradycardia, and syncope. It is administered in incremental doses of 1–3 μg/min, to increase HR 20–25% over baseline. Pharmacological stimulation may also be achieved with Nitroglycerin, as one sublingual spray dose of 400 μg, administered in the upright position. The test is considered positive if it induces syncope. There is a divergence of opinion regarding the significance of presyncope induction. Some authorities include, as a positive response, an absolute drop in systolic BP to 80 mmHg or of HR to <40 bpm, or a relative drop in BP >60% or of HR by >30 bpm, as compared to baseline. This occurs in about half of the patients in the absence of Isoproterenol, and in about 2/3 in its presence; the number of positive cases increases with an increased tilting angle and test duration. The sensitivity of the test for diagnosing a vasovagal mechanism of syncope is about 70%, while the reported specificity varies widely among centers (35–92%). The types of positive response to the tilt test are outlined in Table 3.15. All elements considered, the tilt test is indicated in patients with recurrent, otherwise unexplained syncope, in the absence of structural heart disease, or in the presence of a negative EPS. The tilt test is also useful for differentiating syncope with jerking movements from epilepsy, as well as for evaluating patients with recurrent falls, recurrent presyncope, or dizziness. A positive test rules out the necessity of tests for more severe causes of syncope, mainly ventricular tachyarrhythmias. *Echocardiography* is important for (a) *etiologic diagnosis* in patients with atrial myxoma, AS, HOCM, or CAD (tentative diagnosis, based on regional LV dysfunction);

Table 3.15 Types of response to tilt testing

Type	Reponse[a]	HR	BP	Comments
1	Mixed	Falls to <40 bpm for <10 s or not at all; asystole absent, or lasts <3 s	Falls[b]	BP falls before HR
2A	Cardioinhibition without asystole	Falls to <40 bpm for >10 s; asystole absent, or lasts <3 s	Falls	BP falls before HR
2B	Cardioinhibition with asystole	Asystole >3 s	Falls	BP falls before HR or at the same time
3	Vasodepressor	Falls <10% or not at all	Falls	

[a]There are two exceptions to these main types of response on tilting: chronotropic incompetence (<10% HR increase on tilting) or POTS (>HR 130 bpm), both also considered positive responses[b]A BP fall to <90 mmHg associates signs of impending syncope, and one to <60 mmHg, full-blown syncope

(b) *establishing an ICD indication,* in patients with syncope and decreased LVEF. *Cardiac catheeterization* is recommended in patients with a suspected ischemic cause of syncope. *Neurological or psychiatric consult* is indicated as needed.

3.7.2.3 Syncope: Treatment

The treatment of syncope includes therapy of the acute episode and prevention of recurrences. By definition, syncope is self-limiting, and especially if it occurs while sitting, lying down, or squatting, it may require no further immediate treatment. If the patient falls to the ground, it is customary to delay standing up by a few minutes. Venous return to the heart can be increased by raising the patient's legs, for instance by placing them on a tilted chair. The rare patient with severe cranial or spinal trauma must be moved with caution. Workup for complications of trauma may be required. *Prevention of syncope recurrence* is achieved according to the underlying mechanism. *Prevention of cardiogenic syncope* is discussed in Chaps. 4 and 6. *Prevention of stroke* is discussed in Chap. 11. *Prevention of neurally mediated syncope* is discussed below. As carotid-mediated syncope does not have premonitory symptoms, avoidance of the culprit situations and cardiac pacing sum up the management principles; the available measures for vasovagal syncope are reviewed below.

Nonpharmacological Therapy

Nonpharmacological therapy is crucial in syncope patients. Dietary measures, patient-generated maneuvers, or cardiac pacing may be required. *Dietary measures* involve a liberal fluid and salt intake, if not otherwise contraindicated. Adopting *a squatting position* during "graying out" spells helps avoid true syncope. Squatting is easier than sitting or lying down; it increases SVR (correcting hypotension), and if syncope does occur, the patient falls from a minimal height. With situational syncope, the *offending situation must be avoided* (prescribe stool softeners to lessen straining and involuntary Valsalva during bowel movements; males with micturition syncope should urinate while sitting, etc.). Brisk orthostatism should be avoided in case of orthostatic hypotension (it is recommended to first sit on the border of the bed, with the legs hanging down, for about 1 min, before standing up); patients with postprandial syncope should eat multiple small meals and avoid brisk orthostatism after meals, etc. An additional helpful and simple maneuver is *"isometric leg and arm counterpressure,"* i.e., leg crossing or hand grip/arm tensing, increasing BP by sympathetic stimulation, and preventing vasovagal syncope. Some centers offer *"tilt training"* programs, to desensitize the mechanoreceptors, but patient compliance to this arduous and physically unpleasant program is generally modest. *Head-up tilt sleeping* is also an option. Finally, *elastic stockings or support hose* may be useful in patients with orthostatic hypotension. *DDD pacing* is indicated for cardioinhibitory or mixed carotid syncope, as well as for vasovagal syncope. Guidelines only prescribe pacing for recurrent and/or physically injuring vasovagal syncope, but the real issue revolves around resource availability.

Pharmacological Therapy

See Table 3.16.

Table 3.16 Pharmacological therapy of syncope

Drugs[a]	Rationale	Efficacy proven in clinical trials	
		Vasovagal	Orthost.
Stimulants of fluid retention			
Fludrocortisone[b]	Volume expansion, to prevent hypotension	No	Yes
Erythropoietin[c]		Possibly	Also corrects the anemia often associated to dysautonomia (due to decreased bone marrow sympathetic innervation)
α-Adrenomimetics			
Midodrine[d]	Increase SVR and venous return to the heart	Somewhat effective	Yes
Etilefrine		No	No
Pyridostigmine[e]		Possibly	Yes
β-blockers			
Metoprolol[g]	Inhibition of the Bezold–Jarisch reflex, by decreasing inotropism; additional central mechanisms	No	No
Other medications			
Antidepressants : SSRI or SNRI Paroxetine	Cerebral uptake of serotonin causes vasodilation	Variable results	Variable results
Amphetamines (Amphetamine, Dextroamphetamine; Methylphenidate)	Indirect sympathomimetic action	Variable results	Variable results
Clonidine	Central α-adrenergic stimulation	Variable results	Variable results
Octeotride[a]	Mesenteric vasoconstrictor	Variable results	Variable results

[a]Suggested dose SC 0.5–1 μg/kg t.i.d
[b]PO, 0.05–0.2 mg/day. The main adverse effects include potassium loss (possible arrhythmia); Na+ retention (possible HTN and HF exacerbation); C/I in systemic fungal infections
[c]IV/SC, 50 U/kg initially once or twice weekly, subsequently as needed
[d]PO up to 10 mg t.i.d.; adverse effects include HTN (should be administered ≥3–4 h before bedtime, to avoid nighttime HTN), urinary retention, scalp pruritus, chills, and "goose bumps"
[e]Pyridostigmine, 60 mg q.d.; adverse effects: nausea, vomiting, diarrhea, abdominal pain, bronchial hypersecretion, muscle fasciculation or cramps, muscle weakness, perspiration, myosis. Has a complex influence on the CNS, resulting in BP increase in the orthostatic position only, an advantage over Mydodrine, which causes BP increase regardless of the patient's position
[f]Mentioned here for completeness; clinical trials do not support their efficacy

3.7.2.4 Specific Types of Syncope

Orthostatic Hypotension and Syncope

Normally, blood pooling in the lower limb veins on standing up is prevented by (1) *the skeletal muscle pump* (venous compression by the contracting muscles, with "milking" of blood towards the heart, against gravitation); (2) *neurovascular adjustment,* consisting in constriction of peripheral arteries (increasing SVR and shunting away blood from the venous bed) and veins (increasing venous return to the heart). This is triggered by pressure receptor (baroreceptor) activation in the carotid sinus, aortic arch, and, possibly, the proximal coronary arteries; (3) *neurohumoral adjustment,* consisting in RAAS axis activation and increased adrenalin release. This mechanism is operational on a more chronic basis than the first two. Adaptive mechanism dysfunction may lead to pooling of up to 700 mL of blood in the lower limb veins, decreasing cardiac filling by 25% and causing cerebral hypoperfusion and syncope. Orthostatic hypotension is defined as a decrease in systolic BP by >20 mmHg and/or a decrease of diastolic BP >10 mmHg, occurring when briskly standing up from the sitting or lying position. (Hypotension/syncope can also occur after prolonged orthostatism, by activation of the Bezold–Jarisch reflex, but the designation, "orthostatic hypotension," is usually reserved for the cases occurring after briskly standing up.) The diagnosis is confirmed by measuring BP, first with the patient supine, and subsequently, after 2 min of orthostatism. These patients often present compensatory tachycardia (an increase in HR >20 bpm).

Orthostatic hypotension and syncope are favored by *old age,* as in the elderly, suboptimal cerebral autoregulation makes cerebral blood flow strongly dependent on systemic BP. In these patients, orthostatic hypotension or syncope is but the "tip of the iceberg" of a more widespread impairment of the neurovegetative function: *dehydration* (BP decrease by circulating volume contraction); *prolonged bed rest,* which deconditions both the muscles and the baroreceptors in the great vessels; *pregnancy,* which decreases both SVR and venous return (IVC compression by the pregnant uterus). During the first 24 weeks of pregnancy, systolic BP drops by 5–10 mmHg, and diastolic pressure by up to 10–15 mmHg; and *iatrogenic factors.*

> *Drugs causing orthostatic hypotension and syncope* include virtually all the *antihypertensives;* α-blockers and Clonidine are especially notable, but ACEI, ARB, diuretics, and β-blockers, used much more commonly, are usually the ones involved; nitrates, administered mainly in CAD patients; *antidepressants* (mainly tricyclics, MAOI, Nefazodone), *drugs for Parkinson's* disease; *Sildenafil* (Viagra), particularly in combination with nitrates; *narcotics;* and *alcohol.*

A number of conditions are typically associated with orthostatic hypotension and/or syncope. These include

- *Dysautonomic syndromes,* i.e., vegetative system dysfunction. *Primary forms* include *pure autonomic failure* (the Bradbury–Eggleston syndrome); *multisystem athrophy* (the Shy–Drager syndrome); this also associates muscle tremor, problems with coordination and speech, sphincter incontinence, and a typical dissociation between very high supine and very low orthostatic BP values. There is no known treatment, and the condition is usually fatal within 10 years of diagnosis. *Secondary causes* of dysautonomia include amyloidosis, spinal syphilis, multiple sclerosis, diabetes (affecting the sympathetic vascular terminations), etc.

- *Parkinson's disease,* causing a dysautonomia-like syndrome.
- *Varicose veins,* large reservoirs of blood pooling, uninfluenced by the muscular pump or by vasoconstriction.
- *POTS* ("postural othostatic tachycardia syndrome"), characterized by a HR increase >30 bpm from the supine to upright position or a HR >120 bpm within 10 min of head-up tilt. Orthostatic hypotension is often associated.

There are no specific *diagnostic tests* for orthostatic hypotension or syncope, except for comparison of upright and sitting BP. Syncope workup, however, includes a battery of tests, as discussed above. Literally speaking, *the treatment* of orthostatic hypotension consists in its prevention, by avoiding brisk orthostatism and by gradually weaning the patient off the suspected responsible medication (if possible). The *prognosis* of orthostatic hypotension or syncope per se is generally benign and depends on the underlying condition and on any associated trauma. In CAD patients, in the absence of an iatrogenic mechanism, orthostatic hypotension generally indicates advanced atherosclerosis, with increased morbidity and mortality.

Postprandial Hypotension and Syncope

Postprandial hypotension with syncope almost exclusively affects older patients and has generally the same risk factors as orthostatic hypotension. It generally appears 30–75 min after a substantial meal. Prevention modalities are discussed above.

Carotid Syncope

Carotid syncope is infrequent (1% of cases of syncope). Just like the other types of neurally mediated syncope, carotid syncope can be purely cardioinhibitory (70%), purely vasodepressor (10%), or mixed (20%). Carotid syncope is generally abrupt, i.e., has no warning symptoms. The typical settings (Table 3.14), in a patient in whom other causes for syncope have been ruled out, are sufficient to establish the diagnosis. If necessary, confirmation is obtained by carotid sinus massage, as discussed above.

3.8 Abnormalities in Venous and Lymphatic Pressure

Abnormally high or low pressures can also be encountered in the venous and lymphatic systems. These are generally not the object of cardiovascular medicine.

- *HTN in peripheral venous territories* includes portal HTN, cavernous sinus thrombosis, DVT, the SVC syndrome etc., all discussed in Chap. 11. Central systemic HTN is mainly seen in RV failure (often itself a result of LV failure) and causes increased CVP.
- *Pulmonary venous HTN* is generally secondary to LV failure (Chap. 4) but can also be encountered in some congenital syndromes (Chap. 10). It is measured as increased PCWP.
- *Systemic venous hypotension* is seen in dehydration or shock and may prevent administration of IV medications. In emergencies, a central vein (the internal jugular or the subclavian) can be cannulated, or drugs can be administrated intraosseously. The CVP is decreased.
- *Lymphatic HTN* is seen in disorders of the lymphatic system, while hypotension can occur in disruption of the large lymphatic vessels (Chap. 11), typically manifesting as chylothorax. Lymphatic pressures are generally not measured clinically.

Bibliography

Guidelines

The Task Force for the Management of Arterial Hypertension of the European Society of Hypertension (ESH) and of the European Society of Cardiology (ESC). 2007 Guidelines for the management of arterial hypertension *Eur Heart J.* 2007;28:1462-1536.

Suggested Reading

Jamerson K, Weber MA, Bakris GL, et al.; for the ACCOMPLISH Trial Investigators. Benazepril plus amlodipine or hydrochlorothiazide for hypertension in high-risk patients. *N Engl J Med.* 2008;359:2417-2428.

Aggarwal M, Khan IA. Hypertensive crisis: hypertensive emergencies and urgencies. *Cardiol Clin.* 2006;24(1):135-146.

Feldstein C. Management of hypertensive crises. *Am J Ther.* 2007;14(2):135-139.

Chobanian AV, Bakris GL, Black HR, et al. Seventh report of the Joint National Committee on Prevention, Detection, Evaluation, and Treatment of High Blood Pressure. *Hypertension.* 2003;42:1206-1252.

Antihypertensive and Lipid-Lowering Treatment to Prevent Heart Attack Collaborative Research Group. Diuretic versus alpha-blocker as first-step antihypertensive therapy: Final results from the Antihypertensive and Lipid-Lowering Treatment to Prevent Heart Attack Trial (ALLHAT). *Hypertension.* 2003;43:239-246.

The ALLHAT Officers and Coordinators for the ALLHAT Collaborative Research Group. Major outcomes in high-risk hypertensive patients randomized to angiotensin-converting enzyme inhibitor or calcium channel blocker vs. diuretic: The Antihypertensive and Lipid Lowering Treatment to Prevent Heart Attack Trial (ALLHAT). *JAMA.* 2002;288: 2981-2997.

Julius S, Kjeldsen SE, Weber M, et al.; VALUE trial group. Outcomes in hypertensive patients at high cardiovascular risk treated with regimens based on or amlodipine: the VALUE randomised trial. *Lancet.* 2004;363:2022-2031.

Staessen JA, Gasowski J, Wang JG, et al. Risks of untreated and treated isolated systolic hypertension in the elderly: meta-analysis of outcome trials. *Lancet.* 2000;355:865-872.

Psaty BM, Lumley T, Furberg CD, et al. Health outcomes associated with variousantihypertensive therapies used as first-line agents: a network meta-analysis. *JAMA.* 2003;289: 2534-2544.

Yusuf S, Sleight P, Pogue J, Bosch J, Davies R, Dagenais G. Effects of an angiotensinconverting enzyme inhibitor, ramipril, on death from cardiovascular causes, myocardial-infarction, and stroke in high-risk patients. The Heart Outcomes Prevention Evaluation Study Investigators. *N Engl J Med.* 2000;342:145-153.

Contents

4.1 The Syndrome of Heart Failure

4.1.1 Ventricular Function: General Remarks

4.1.1.1 Normal Ventricular Function requires

- *Structural integrity* (myocytes, conjunctive tissue, endocardium, coronary endothelium, pericardium, cardiac nerves). Of note, disturbed integrity occasionally consists not in lack, but in *excess* of tissue. For instance, increased LV mass is a strong independent risk factor for subsequent HF.
- *Optimal interaction between the heart cardiac matrix and the myocytes:* derangement of this interaction is an important contributor to myocardial dysfunction and HF.
- *Optimal interaction between the heart and the peripheral organs:* this involves, among others, normal SVR and PVR *(i.e., afterload);* optimal activation of the RAAS axis; and normal metabolic function of the tissues.
- *Optimal filling of the heart (i.e., preload):* this depends on *extracardiac factors,* mainly optimal blood volume (dehydration causes decreased filling, i.e., decreased preload, while overhydration abnormally increases preload); *cardiac factors,* mainly normal myocardial compliance and the absence of valvular regurgitation (which causes diastolic filling with additional, abnormal volumes of blood). For instance, AI increases LV preload, as LV fills in diastole not only from the LA, but also from the aorta. A normal preload is crucial to normal ventricular function, because (1) in order to properly eject blood, the ventricles have to fill adequately; (2) there is a strong

relationship between optimal contraction and diastolic myocyte stretch: within certain limits, the more a myocyte is stretched, the better it contracts (the Frank–Startling mechanism); the spectrum of optimal myocyte stretch, however, is quite narrow, and excessive decreases or increases in preload may cause suboptimal myocyte contraction.

- *A gradual onset of hemodynamic changes,* allowing the heart to adapt correspondingly.

Cardiac performance is evaluated by several parameters, reviewed in Table 4.1.

Cardiac performance assessment: what indicator to use?

In all patients, LVEF is the main indicator of LV function and is routinely assessed by echo or by nuclear scan. In the critically ill patient, CO is also measured, generally invasively, by means of a Swan–Ganz catheter. For research purposes, other methods (echo, MRI, CT) are also used.

Cardiac output can be calculated invasively or noninvasively, as reviewed in Table 4.2. For a discussion of the interplay between LVEF, CO, and HF, see below, under "LV dysfunction and HF."

4.1.1.2 Ventricular Dysfunction

Several mechanisms may interfere with normal cardiac function, causing disturbances in the parameters mentioned above.

- *Structural lesions* of the myocytes and cardiac connective tissue may affect contraction (systole) and relaxation (diastole). VHD and abnormal communications between the heart chambers and/or great vessels or direct AV communication (without interposition of the capillary bed) may cause abnormal loading conditions (increased pre or afterload).
- *Suboptimal interaction between the atria and the ventricles:* NSR is the ideal rhythm for optimal ventricular function, since, in combination with the slight impulse delay in the AV node, it allows sequential contraction of the atria and the ventricles and full benefit from the atrial kick. The atrial systole pumps a relatively small volume of blood into the ventricles,

and contributes to ventricular filling and optimal activation of the Frank–Starling mechanism. Absence of the "atrial kick" decreases LVEF by a few percentages; usually not very important, this can be crucial in HF patients. Unfortunately, maintaining NSR is not always easy, and indeed not always profitable: for instance, in chronic AF, maintenance of NSR has the same clinical outcome as simple maintenance of adequate HR (approximately 80/min); this is mainly due to the side effects of AAD.

- *Suboptimal interaction with the peripheral organs* mainly results from exaggerated metabolic requirements; increased SVR or PVR; or fluid overload, by excessive RAAS axis activation.
- *Abnormal filling conditions* cause myocardial dysfunction by suboptimal activation of the Frank–Starling mechanism (suboptimal LV contraction due to an excessively *decreased* preload) or by excessive myocardial stretch (excessively *increased* preload).

Ventricular Dysfunction: Adaptive Mechanisms

The disturbances reviewed above activate cardiac and noncardiac adaptive mechanisms, as outlined in Table 4.3.

LV Dysfunction and HF

HF and LV dysfunction: interrelated, but distinct

The dysfunctional ventricles display abnormal systolic and/or diastolic function by failure of the adaptive mechanisms. LV dysfunction is often asymptomatic; conversely, HF is a clinical entity, diagnosed based on symptoms and signs. The interplay between HF and ventricular dysfunction is highly complex.

The incremental value of HF symptoms over objective quantitation of cardiac function:

LVEF, CO, and diastolic function parameters are not sufficient for defining a normally functioning heart (i.e., no LV dysfunction) and full adequacy of the heart in providing O_2 to the peripheral organs (i.e., no HF). Thus,

- *A normal LVEF* is compatible with LV dysfunction in several situations, such as diastolic dysfunction, or in patients with severe MR and a "normal" LVEF, which in fact must count as inordinately low, as in severe MR and a truly preserved LV function, the LVEF exceeds the upper limits of normal.
- *A normal CO*, on the other hand, is compatible with decreased LVEF, compensated for by tachycardia and/or LV dilatation.
- Furthermore, even *the combination of a normal LVED and a normal CO* is still compatible with significant heart disease (diastolic dysfunction).
- Finally, *the combination of a normal LVEF, a normal CO, and normal diastolic function* does guarantee the absence of heart disease (as best assessed with the available technology), but is still compatible with high-output HF.

Patients who had clinical symptoms and signs of HF in the past but are now asymptomatic, while technically not in HF, suffer from "compensated HF," a reminder that the "healthy status" comes at the cost of being medicated, and that, under suboptimal treatment, HF could recur. "Congestive HF" is a synonym for HF, inherited from an era when only advanced cases of HF were diagnosed, the hallmark being fluid accumulation (congestion). Since HF does not necessarily imply congestion (e.g., compensated HF or high-output HF), and congestion can occur without HF, this designation is obsolete; yet, the acronym "CHF," easy to pronounce and age-honored, is still frequently used. (The acronym has also been "recycled" to signify "chronic HF"). Not all decrease of blood flow to the organs is termed HF. Thus, *ischemia* (decreased organ perfusion) may result from either HF or from local mechanisms, such as vessel thrombosis or embolism, while *cardiac arrest* is a general term causing the cessation (not merely the decrease) of perfusion to all the organs, resulting from the incapacity of the heart to contract at all.

Table 4.1 Quantitative indicators of cardiac function

Parameter	Definition	Measuring units	Normal[a]	Measuring techniques	Remarks[b]
Parameters evaluating systolic function					
LVEF/RVEF	Percentage of end-diastolic volume ejected into aorta in systole	%	>55% (LV); >45% (RV)	Echo, nuclear scan, MRI, CT, ventriculography	Assessment by echo = semiquantitative, nuclear = quantitative; at cardiac catheterization; or by MRI or CT
Stroke volume (SV)	The volume of blood ejected into the aorta by each beat	ml	At rest: 70	Swan–Ganz catheter	
CO (LV = RV)	The volume of blood ejected into the aorta each min.	ml/min	at rest: 4–8	Swan–Ganz catheter,[d] echo, MRI, other	Gold standard = Swan–Ganz; 2D echo laborious, error-fraught; MRI, CT very accurate, but less commonly used
Cardiac Index (CI)	CO divided by estimated BSA	l/min × m²	2.6–4.2	Calculated	Better individualization of CO for very small /large patients; estimated average BSA = 1.73 m². In normal subjects, the CO of the LV and RV is equal
Parameters evaluating diastolic function					
E/A waves	Transmitral flow velocity	E = m/s; E/A = ratio	E < 2 m/s; E/A > 1	Echo	Conventional Doppler or tissue Doppler
E deceleration time	Peak-to-zero E wave duration	ms	<140	Echo	Increased in early diastolic dysfunction ("impaired relaxation pattern"); decreased in late stages ("pseudonormalization")

(*continued*)

Table 4.1 (continued)

Parameter	Definition	Measuring units	Normal[a]	Measuring techniques	Remarks[b]
IVRT[e]	Isovolumic relaxation time	ms	80–110	Echo	As above
Parameters evaluating systolic and diastolic function					
PCWP	Pressure in the small PA branches	mmHg	<10	Swan–Ganz catheter	Approximates LA pressure , which in turn approximates LVEDP, an indicator of LV function
CVP	Pressure in the SVC	cm H$_2$O[f]	<10	Swan–Ganz catheter or CVP	Approximates RA pressure = RVEDP. May be secondary to RV or, indirectly, to LV dysfunction (the latter associates with high PCWP)
LVEDP	Intracavitary pressure at end-diastole	mmHg	10–13	Left ventriculography or Swan–Ganz (for RV)	Noninvasive assessment (2D echo) laborious, error-fraught

[a]Measured values differ according to measuring technique
[b]Techniques not mentioned in Chap. 1 are discussed under "HF treatment"
[c]Systolic dysfunction always associates with diastolic dysfunction; however, some indices are particular for systolic or diastolic dysfunction, while others are common
[d]Swan–Ganz catheterization also assesses SVR and PVR, indicating the cause and the adaptive mechanisms in face of decreased CO; normal SVR = 900–1,200 dyn·s/cm^5 (90–120 mpa·s/m^3); normal PVR = 100–200 dyn·s/cm^5 (10–20 mPa·s/m^3)
[e]Isovolumic relaxation time, assessed on Doppler as the lag between the end of systolic aortic flow and the beginning of the mitral diastolic E wave
[f]This measuring unit reflects the measuring technique by CVP

Table 4.2 Measuring CO

Method	Principle	Remarks
Invasive		
Fick's principle	CO = VO$_2$/(Ca−Cv), where VO$_2$ is the O$_2$ consumption per minute; Cv, the O$_2$ content in the PA; and Ca, the O$_2$ content in a peripheral artery	Invasive methods are gradually being replaced with noninvasive approaches. Changes in vascular function, the position of the catheter tip, or damping of the pressure waveform signal affect accuracy of PP measurements
Thermodilution	Injection of 10 ml of cold glucose at a known temperature into the PA and measuring the temperature 6–10 cm downstream	
Invasive pulse pressure measurement	Inserting a manometer into the radial or femoral artery; analysis of the PP waveform provides a measure of the CO	
Noninvasive		
Echocardiogram	CO = AV flow TVI × LVOT transsectional area, calculated based on 2D LVOT diameter measurement	LVOT measurement can be difficult, and any error is squared in area calculation.
PP methods	Proprietary devices, or Q (ml/min) = 2 × PP × HR	See above, for shortcomings
Impedance cardiography (ICG)	The higher the intrathoracic fluid volume, the higher the transthoracic impedance. Impedance variations are used to calculate CO	Suboptimal reliability and reproducibility
Electrical cardiometry	A variant of ICG	Under evaluation
MRI	Velocity-encoded MRI measures CO by multiplying the average aortic velocity or PA by the cross-sectional area of the vessel	Not applicable where most needed, i.e., in the ICU setting

Table 4.3 Adaptive mechanisms in HF/ventricular dysfunction

Mechanism	Rationale	Disadvantage	Remarks
Cardiac mechanisms			
Increased ventricular contraction	To increase CO	N/A	In time, the ventricles "burn out"
LVH/RVH	Increases systolic function and decreases myocyte tension caused by the high LVEDP	Diastolic dysfunction; relative ischemia[a]	Counteracts increased afterload
Cardiac dilatation	LVEF is expressed from a larger end-diastolic volume, and translates into a higher CO	Diastolic dysfunction; relative ischemia[b]; LV sphericization[c]	Counteracts increased preload; also present in late stages of increased afterload
Frank–Starling mechanism	Increased preload increases myocyte stretch and optimizes contraction	N/A	Suboptimal myocyte stretch causes suboptimal activation of the mechanism
Tachycardia	Compensates stroke volume decrease by increasing the number of systoles/min	Increases O_2 demands; chronic tachycardia may cause DCM	Mostly in high-output, acute, or chronic severe HF
Extracardiac mechanisms			
Vasoconstriction	Helps maintain BP	Increases afterload	
CO redistribution	Blood is diverted from skin, kidneys, and skeletal muscle to the brain and heart	Dysfunction of deprived organs; RAAS activation	Mostly in acute or chronic severe HF
Increased tissue O_2 extraction capacity	Increases O_2 delivery/ml perfused blood	N/A	Causes cyanosis
Limited daily exertion	Decreased metabolic demands	Muscle deconditioning	May mask true severity of HF

[a]Development of new blood vessels cannot keep pace with myocardial hypertrophy
[b]Cardiac dilatation increases myocyte stretch and O_2 demands
[c]The normal shape of the LV is elliptic, which optimizes myocyte contraction; for the same degree of preserved myocyte function, a spherical heart contracts less than an elliptical one

4.1.2 Heart Failure

4.1.2.1 Prevalence and Classification

HF affects approximately 2% of the population and is the main cause of hospital admission in patients >65. The prognosis depends on the type of HF (HFPEF has a lower mortality than HF patients with impaired EF); the NYHA class (severe prognosis for NYHA class ≥3); therapy (ACEI, β-blockers, and CRT prolong survival); and comorbidity. On an average, out of 100 patients with HF of any degree, approximately 10 will die every year, most of them from the advanced-HF group (mortality up to 50% per year). The different classifications of HF overlap, as they describe the same phenomenon from different perspectives:

- *Cause:* HF of cardiac/noncardiac cause
- *CO:* high/normal/low output HF

- *LVEF:* HF with decreased vs. preserved EF
- *The affected part of the cardiac cycle:* systolic or diastolic HF
- *Symptoms:* forward failure (i.e., decreased organ perfusion) vs. backward failure (i.e., blood pooling in lungs and veins)
- *The affected ventricle:* left vs. right HF
- *Time course:* acute vs. chronic HF

Table 4.4 shows the correspondence between these classifications. EF is preserved in diastolic failure, and decreased in combined systolic HF and HFPEF (systolic failure associated with diastolic failure). The table also includes a classification based on "type of CMP," i.e., the type of physiological and structural derangement in the heart muscle function leading to HF. These clinical entities will be discussed in Sect. 4.2.

The parameters relevant to the different types of HF are schematically presented in Table 4.5.

Table 4.4 The classifications of HF

Parameter	Isolated failure		Combined failure
	Forward	Backward	
CO	Increased	Normal[a]	Decreased
LVEF	Increased	Normal[a] or decreased	Decreased
Cardiac cause	No	Yes	Yes
CMP type	N/A	HCM or RCM	DCM
Part of cardiac cycle	N/A	Diastole	Systole and diastole
Time course	Acute or chronic		
Affected ventricle	Severe isolated right or left failure rare, due to ventricular interdependence		

[a]See the discussion below, referring to the correspondence between CO and LVEF

Table 4.5 Cardiac and extracardiac functional parameters in HF of different types

HF	↑ output	HFPEF	↓ EF HF
CO (ml)=	↑	N	N[a]/↓
LVEF (%) ×	N/↑	N	↓
Metabolic needs (mlO$_2$/min[c])	↑	N/↓[d]	N/↓[d]
Forward failure	Y	No	Yes
Backward failure	No	Yes	Yes
SVR	↓	N/↑	↑
PVR	No	↑	↑
LV relaxation	No	↓	↓
EDV (ml)	N/↓	N/↓[b]	N/↑
HR (bpm)	↑	N	N/↑

[a]Normal CO may be maintained in face of a decreased LVEF
[b]Severe LVH may cause a decrease in ventricular volume
[c]Metabolic requirements are expressed as mlO$_2$/min = SatO$_2 \times$ Hematocrit $\times$ CO
[d]Decreased activity and, in severe cases, diversion of blood flow to the heart and brain may decrease metabolic requirements

In the following section, we shall review HF with increased CO (which often associates. increased EF as well); with normal EF (HFPEF); and with decreased EF. While this classification is also valid for the RV, we shall concentrate on the manifestations relative to the LV, which are clinically the most relevant. The RV is dealt with separately, with the focus on low-EF RV failure. For both LV and RV HF, a distinction will be made between "forward/backward failure" manifestations.

In parallel with the discussion outlined above, we shall also focus on the acute vs. chronic presentation of HF. This distinction is valid for all classes of HF (regardless of EF or CO), but is most relevant for low-EF HF, and will be discussed as a separate section for both LV and RV low-EF HF.

We shall conclude with a discussion of ventricular interdependence, in order to place the LV/RV failure dichotomy in the proper perspective.

High-Output HF

High-output HF occurs when the metabolic requirements demand an excessively high CO, which cannot be provided despite cardiac and extracardiac adaptive mechanisms. This is a rather infrequent occurrence, vastly surpassed in frequency by HF with normal or decreased LVEF. High-output HF manifests as forward failure, generally chronic, but occasionally presenting acutely (e.g., acute traumatic AV aneurysm). The CO is increased, and LVEF is high or normal. This condition typically affects the LV. As with low-output HF, decreased organ perfusion (in this case, a relative decrease) triggers tachycardia, further increasing CO. In the later stages, these mechanisms are no longer sufficient, and the LV dilates. In time, even this mechanism is overwhelmed and CO decreases. High-output HF may be due to

- *Hyperthyroidism (thyrotoxicosis),* the most frequent situation; excess thyroid hormone increases metabolism and thus O$_2$ and nutrient demand.
- *AV malformation* (abnormal communication between arteries and veins, shunting the normal connecting capillary bed); arterial and venous blood admixture decreases SatO$_2$ and causes a compensatory increase in cardiac contractility and HR.
- *Pregnancy,* in women with previously asymptomatic or compensated HF; onset of high-output HF is due to the presence of the fetus, with its own metabolic demands, and to decreased BP, due to the connection of the mother's vascular system to the low-resistance placenta.
- *Fever, anemia, etc.,* in patients with previously asymptomatic/compensated HF; fever increases metabolic demands, while anemia decreases the O$_2$-carrying capacity of the blood, causing decreased O$_2$ delivery

despite normal cardiac contraction. Anemia is linked to a poor prognosis in HF patients, but it is not clear whether it is a pathophysiologic mechanism or simply a risk marker of HF, or whether anemia correction improves HF prognosis. The latter issue is currently being examined in large-scale trials.

HF with Preserved LVEF (HFPEF)

Classically regarded as a purely passive process, based on gradient-driven LA-to-LV blood "suction," diastole is in fact a complex, energy-dependent, and difficult to quantitate phenomenon. Abnormal diastolic relaxation allows cardiac filling only under increased LVEDP conditions, at the cost of increased energy expenditure. This situation is termed *diastolic LV dysfunction* while asymptomatic; HFPEF consists of symptoms of HF in presence of LVEF >50%, determined within 3 days of symptom onset. HFPEF manifests as backward failure (causing pulmonary and peripheral organ congestion). The CO and LVEF are normal. HFPEF can be acute (it is the first effect of acute ischemia on ventricular function) or chronic, and may affect either ventricle. Approximately 30% of patients presenting with shortness of breath and pulmonary or peripheral edema have disturbed diastolic function but normal LVEF, a fact explaining the terminological shift from "diastolic HF" to "HFPEF" (to better underscore that HF is not a synonym for decreased ventricular contraction) Virtually any type of myocardial injury can cause HFPEF, and thus a complete list of the underlying conditions necessarily includes the causes of systolic HF. For clarity, we shall refer to isolated diastolic dysfunction/failure, while keeping in mind that, in the later stages (and in the absence of treatment), most cases associate with a systolic component. The main scenarios, then, include

- *Quantitative alterations of the myocardium,* which becomes either thinner (in some cases of dilated cardiomyopathy (DCM)) or hypertrophic. Hypertrophy can be *secondary* to increased SVR (especially with HTN or AS) or *primary* (idiopathic HCM).
- *Qualitative alterations of the myocardium,* including infiltrative diseases, where chemical compounds or cells become seated between the myocytes, with or without LV wall thickening. When the latter occurs, it is not "true" LVH, so this condition is not listed as HCM. Although there exist signs of diastolic dysfunction by

echo, MRI, etc., the diagnosis remains essentially clinical: in a patient with dyspnea and edema, yet without evidence of systolic LV dysfunction or pulmonary disease, HFPEF is always suspected, all the more so in the presence of LVH, myocardial scarring, etc.

HFPEF can coexist with decreased-EF HF or be isolated. While most cases of systolic dysfunction associate with a component of diastolic dysfunction, some cases of normal or increased LV contraction may coexist with diastolic dysfunction or HFPEF (e.g., HCM).

HF with Decreased LVEF

Low-EF HF manifests as acute or chronic, combined forward and backward failure, affecting either ventricle. The CO and LVEF are both decreased. HTN and CAD are the most frequent causes (Table 4.6).

HF: Clinical Manifestations

The symptoms and signs of LV failure are those of *"forward"* and *"backward" failure.*

Forward failure is typically seen with acute HF and manifests as pallor, cyanosis (due to increased peripheral O_2 extraction), and organ dysfunction (renal, hepatic, etc.; see Chap. 11). The extreme form of forward failure is cardiogenic shock (typically associating pulmonary edema, a sign of backward failure). The most frequent *symptom of* "backward failure" is dyspnea due to pulmonary overload. Depending on HF severity, dyspnea can occur only during exertion or even at rest (allowing clinical classification of HF by severity, as discussed below). The supine position counteracts gravity-driven blood accumulation in the legs and exacerbates pulmonary congestion and dyspnea. This redistribution of the circulating blood volume causes patients to sleep with their head elevated on more pillows than usual *(orthopnea)*, or to sleep in a chair. Redistribution does increase renal perfusion and diuresis at night *(nocturia)*. Acute episodes of HF decompensation are termed *paroxysmal nocturnal dyspnea (PND)*. The extreme form of backward LV failure is pulmonary edema.

The physical examination reveals pulmonary crackles on auscultation, similar to the sound of gas bubbles in soda water, and mainly heard in inspiration. Crackles are heard in both acute and chronic HF. According to the severity of congestion, the crackles can be limited

Table 4.7 The diagnosis of HF

| | LVEF | | |
	Increased[a]	Normal	Decreased
Failure type	Forward	Backward	Forward + backward
Mechanism			
LV	Decreased[b] organ perfusion; (liver, kidney, etc)	Pulmonary congestion	Decreased perfusion,[c] pulmonary congestion
RV	Decreased[b] amount of blood to lungs	Systemic vein congestion	Systemic vein congestion
Symptoms[d]			
LV	Nonspecific	Dyspnea of different degrees	Combined
RV	Nonspecific	Right subcostal pain, bloating, edema	Combined
Signs			
LV	Renal, hepatic failure, etc; pallor or cyanosis	Lung crackles, pleural effusion	Combined
RV	Nonspecific	Liver enlarged; peripheral edema; ascites	Combined
Labs[e]			
LV	Echo: hyperdynamic LV[f]; EKG: tachycardia	Echo: normokinetic LV; diastolic dysfunction; LVH ± AS; Swan–Ganz: increased PCWP; increased BNP[g]	LV hypo/a/dyskinesia ± dilatation; the rest, as above
RV	Hyperdynamic RV	Echo: enlarged, nonpulsatile IVC; RV dilatation, TR	RV hypokinetic, the rest as above

[a]HF of noncardiac causes

[b]*Relatively* decreased

[c]*Absolutely* decreased

[d]Only the symptoms and signs of cardiac dysfunction are mentioned in the table; additionally, the symptoms and signs of the underlying cardiac or noncardiac condition are present (angina, hyperthyrodism, etc.)

[e]Only the findings expressing the ventricular dysfunction are mentioned; cardiac and noncardiac findings pertaining to the underlying condition (coronary angiography demonstrating stenosis, noninvasive testing for ischemia, lab tests for hyperthyroidism, etc.) are also routinely performed

[f]In the late stages, the LVEF and the CO decrease

[g]Or B-type natriuretic peptide (NT-proBNP)

Table 4.8 The NYHA classification of HF severity

Class	Severity	Intensity of activity necessary for symptom onset	Degree of impairment in everyday life
I	Mild	Higher than usual	Nil
II	Mild to moderate	Usual	Mild
III	Moderate	Modest	Moderate
IV	Severe	Minimal or nil (at rest)	Severe

Table 4.9 The ACC/AHA classification of HF severity

Stage	Heart disease	Symptom intensity
I	Absent, but risk factors present	Nil
II	Present, but asymptomatic	Nil
III	Present	Present
IV	Advanced	Severe

An additional classification refers to MI-related acute HF (the Killip score, Chap. 2). However, the Killip score is geared at assessing *the prognosis of acute MI,* not that of HF per se.

HF: Workup

Since HF is a clinical syndrome, workup is not instrumental in its diagnosis as such, but is crucial for assessing the severity of the underlying LV dysfunction as well as its etiology. The main tests carried out in the patient with HF include:

A. Non-invasive or minimally invasive methods of assessment of LV dysfunction

HF workup: echocardiography

B mode echo is the standard tool for detecting *the anatomical basis of LV dysfunction* (cardiac dilatation, LV aneurysm, etc.) and *the type and severity of LV dysfunction as such.* Systolic dysfunction locally or globally decreases LV contraction. The distinction between regional and global systolic dysfunction helps prioritize the workup differently, since the most frequent cause of regional LV dysfunction is CAD, whereas global dysfunction is more often caused by CMP. However, there are notable exceptions both ways, as CMP can manifest in a patchy pattern, and ischemic CMP can manifest as global dysfunction. The relationship between the degree of LVEF decrease and the severity of HF is complex due to the highly effective adaptive mechanisms. These require time to develop, so it is not unusual to see patients with chronic severe LVEF decreases in NYHA classes I–II, or conversely, patients with pulmonary edema despite only moderate, acute-onset dysfunction (e.g., acute MI).

The main echo method for LVEF assessment is Simpson's method, where LV volumes are obtained by measuring LV surface at end-systole and end-diastole (under the occasionally wrong assumption of a regular LV shape); LVEF (%) = (EDV-ESV)/EDV × 100. (The calculation is performed by the echo machine; the underlying principle is the division of the LV into a "stack" of superimposed cylinders, visualized from two orthogonal views, with summation of the different cylinder volumes.) The advent of 3D echo is expected to increase the precision of noninvasive LVEF measurement.

The correspondence between visual semiquantitation and quantitation using Simpson's method is reviewed in Table 4.10.

Diastolic dysfunction as such cannot be diagnosed based on 2D or 3D images, but LVH and systolic dysfunction virtually always associate diastolic dysfunction.

Table 4.10 Echo quantitation and semiquantitation of LVEF

Visual assessment (semiquantitative)	Simpson's method (quantitative) (%)
Normal	60–65
Mild decrease	40–60
Moderate decrease	25–40
Severe decrease	<25

M mode echo has an ancillary role in the assessment of cardiac function.

Doppler echo is the main diagnostic tool for diastolic dysfunction. Transmitral diastolic flow is biphasic, the first wave corresponding to blood suction from the LA (E wave, as for "early"), while the second (A wave, as for "atrial") corresponds to atrial systole. Normally, E is taller than A, but diastolic dysfunction reverses this ratio. Of note, in late cases of diastolic dysfunction, there is "pseudonormalization" of the E/A ratio (Fig. 4.1). Diastolic dysfunction is graded as described in Table 4.11; much more difficult to detect than systolic dysfunction, it is generally substantially underdiagnosed. The most important indicators are Doppler flow through the MV; tissue Doppler signs; and LVH.

Additional methods of LV function evaluation by echo include:

- *Tissue Doppler echo,* mainly based on the assessment of mitral annulus motion in diastole. This motion includes E' and A' waves that can be analyzed similarly to E and A, their counterparts obtained by mitral flow Doppler interrogation. Tissue Doppler mitral annulus velocities may be more accurate in the assessment of diastolic dysfunction than transmitral Doppler, but the technique is time-intensive and not routinely performed. Numerous other tissue Doppler parameters have been proposed, some also integrating information from conventional Doppler (e.g., the ratio between the E waves obtained by both methods).
- *Speckle tracking,* to assess *LV torsion,* is a newer index for LV function assessment.
- *Global circumferential strain (GCS),* measured by Doppler or by speckle tracking, more directly reflects changes in ventricular wall thickening than LVEF, and might prove an even more accurate measure of LV function.
- *Combined echo techniques,* used, for instance, for calculating CO: Doppler LVOT flow and B or M mode LVOT diameter measurements are combined to yield stroke volume, and then multiplied by HR, to obtain CO. With 2D echo, the method is fraught with error due to the assumption that the geometry and flow dynamics observed in a 2D echo section apply to the heart as a whole (3D), which may be false in patients with deformed cardiac anatomy, for example, after MI. The occasional difficulty in precisely measuring the LVOT diameter is also a possible source of error; as the diameter is squared in the calculations, the magnitude of error increases further. Therefore,

Fig. 4.1 Investigating diastole by Doppler echo (from left to right, diastolic dysfunction grade 1, 2, 3/4). The *black arrows* point at the closure of the AV and PV, as signaled by the second heart sound (S$_2$). *IVRT*- isovolumic relaxation time; E_{DECEL}- deceleration time of the E wave; *S, D*- systolic and diastolic components of the pulmonary vein flow. The last set of three superimposed panels indicates blunting, canceling, or reversal of the systolic component, which is normally directed towards the LA and is greater than the diastolic component (see text)

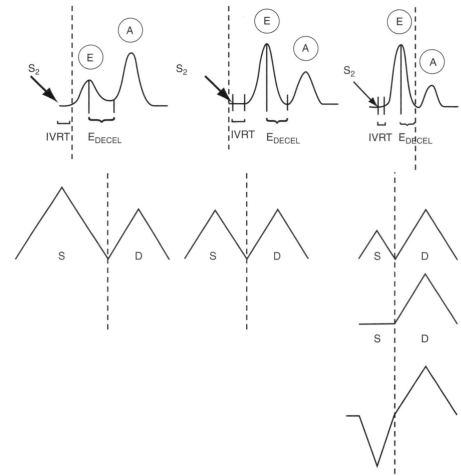

Table 4.11 Grading of diastolic dysfunction

Parameter	Grade			
	1	2	3	4
	Impaired relaxation	Pseudonormal	Restrictive (reversible)	Restrictive (irreversible)
Clinical parameters				
NYHA	I–II	II–III	III–IV	IV
Echo parameters				
Mitral deceleration time (ms)	Increased (>220)	Normal (150–200)	Decreased (<150)	Decreased (<150)
IVRT (ms)	Increased (>100)	Normal (60–100)	Decreased (<60)	Decreased (<60)
Pulmonary vein flow S/D ratio	Normal (>1)	Normal or abnormal (>/<1)	Abnormal (<1)	Abnormal (<1)
Catheterization parameters				
LA pressure	N/↑	↑↑	↑↑↑	↑↑↑

this method is not widely used in clinical practice. 3D echo may change this situation.

HF workup: X-ray techniques

Chest X-ray may show

- *Pulmonary changes,* in turn including (1) thus *fluid overload, with moderately increased PCWP,* vasodilation in the upper lobes and vasoconstriction in the lower lobes, causing "cranial redistribution" of pulmonary vasculature. Normally, the lower lobes are better vascularized, due to gravity; *with moderate-to-severe PCWP increases,* "interstitial" pulmonary edema (edema in the interstitial tissue, but not in the alveoli) and vessel blurring in the upper lobes, presenting as a reticular pattern on the lung fields; *with severe PCWP increases,* blurring of the entire lung field surface (alveolar pulmonary edema). Importantly, the relationship between the degree of PCWP increase and that of X-ray pulmonary congestion is imprecise; patients with full-blown pulmonary edema can present without X-ray pulmonary congestion (despite abruptly increased PCWP, as in acute MI), and conversely, patients recovering from pulmonary edema may still present with pulmonary X-ray changes, which may take up to 24 h to clear. Similarly, patients with asymptomatic chronic HF may present with X-ray congestion; (2) *Kerley B lines,* horizontal lines in the periphery of the lung fields, corresponding to decreased lymphatic drainage in chronic HF patients; and (3) *pleural effusion,* especially on the left side.
- *Cardiac shadow enlargement,* due to either cardiomegaly or pericardial effusion. The diagnosis is based on the following findings: *an increased cardio-thoracic index* (the ratio between the largest diameter of the cardiac shadow and of the thorax, normal <0.5); *the RV/sternum contact line,* observed on the lateral chest X-ray, extends more than normal cranially, an early sign of RV dilatation; *the shape and size of the cardiac shadow:* in later stages, the *LV apex* is pushed by the dilated RV; an enlarged cardiac shadow may correspond to cardiomegaly or to pericardial effusion (Chap. 7).
- *Other findings:* (1) *pulmonary lesions unrelated to HF* that may show the alternative true diagnosis, in case of noncardiac; (2) *assessment after medical procedures: in patients with indwelling devices* (Swan–Ganz catheter, IABP, CVP catheter), chest X-ray helps confirm the correct position of the catheter;

chest X-ray is also routinely performed *to assess the possible complications after thorax puncture* for pleural or pericardial drainage, CVP insertion, etc.

CT can assess systolic parameters much like echo; diastolic assessment is based on demonstrating increased LV mass (this can also be assessed by echo, but the method is laborious and error-fraught; this may change with the advent of 3D echo). In practice, CT is rarely used for the assessment of HF severity, but is useful for assessing its cause, especially in CHD.

Left ventriculography: see "invasive assessment of ventricular dysfunction."

HF workup: *MRI*
Rarely used, provides data similar to those provided by CT.

HF workup: *Nuclear Scan*

Nuclear Scan precisely assesses global and regional systolic function; nuclear LVEF assessment is specifically indicated with Adriamycin treatment. The assessment is based on measuring end-systolic and end-diastolic radioactive count, under EKG gating. Nuclear perfusion scan assesses LV dysfunction reversibility (hibernating areas in CAD related HF) and is a key component of systolic dysfunction workup. With the advent of the Metaiodobenzylguanidine (MIBG) scan to investigate cardiac sympathetic innervation, risk stratification in HF patients might be entering a new era, as the status of the sympathetic cardiac innervation is a good predictor of late arrhythmia and SCD.

HF workup: Other Noninvasive or Minimally Invasive Methods of LV Dysfunction Assessment.

- *Noninvasive SatO₂ measurement (pulse oxymetry),* based on noninvasive analysis of the capillary blood in the nail bed.
- *Chemical blood analysis:* (1) *measuring blood gases: O₂ saturation (Sat O₂,* normal >95%) and *partial pressure of CO₂ (pCO₂,* normal <45 mmHg) measure the effectiveness of pulmonary function, and indirectly, the degree of pulmonary congestion; (2) *diagnosis of ventricular dysfunction,* based on increased levels of BNP, helps monitor the treatment in chronic HF and distinguish cardiac from pulmonary dyspnea; (3) *monitoring of blood drug levels:* digoxin levels require periodical monitoring, especially in case of renal dysfunction (the recommended concentrations are 1–2.6 nmol/l, to ensure efficacy and avoid toxicity); (4) *monitoring for*

possible adverse events of medication: of special concern are BUN (values >20 mg/dl, common in diuretic-treated patients, indicate dehydration), K$^+$ levels (usually decreased with regular diuretics, but occasionally increased with aldosterone antagonists; normal 3.7–5.2 mEq/l), and Na$^+$ levels, often decreased with chronic diuretic use (normal 135–145 mEq/l); (5) *novel markers: copeptin,* a vasopressin-related agent, has been recently suggested as a prognostic predictor in chronic HF; increased *resistin* levels in the circulating blood appear to be directly associated with the incidence of HF in at-risk patients.

HF workup: *EKG*

EKG shows nonspecific changes, all of which may be caused by the organic cardiac lesions or by drug toxicity. *Ventricular and atrial tachyarrhythmia* includes *AT with variable AVB,* especially suggestive of Digitalis toxicity; *AF,* which is occasionally not the complication, but the cause of HF; and the entire spectrum of ventricular arrhythmia, including VF. *AVB* of different degrees may also be seen. EKG may also help diagnose *electrolyte disturbances* (e.g., hypo- and hyperkalemia), often encountered in diuretic-treated patients; in Digoxin-treated patients, a typical EKG pattern, "the Digitalis effect," must not be confused with ischemia. This includes a shortened QT interval and a characteristic down-sloping ST depression ("reverse tick appearance"). The arrhythmia and AVB occasionally caused by Digitalis are technically not a component of the "Digitalis effect."

HF workup: other methods to assess CO:

- *pulse pressure (PP) methods* use the waveform of arterial pressure variation over time to measure CO; unfortunately, these methods are influenced by the properties of the peripheral vessels, and thus do not offer an universally reliable CO assessment;
- *impedance cardiography (ICG)* is based on the variations of impedance (resistance to the electrical current) in the blood-filled aorta, as detected by electrodes on the chest. It is still not sufficiently precise for clinical use; *MRI* accurately measures CO, but is used for research only.

B. Invasive or minimally invasive methods of assessment of LV dysfunction

Invasive pressure monitoring:

- *Arterial:* of a peripheral artery (generally, the radial) by arterial line, to measure BP in severe cases of

HF, in the ICU; or *of the LV and aortic pressure,* in the cath lab (increased LVEDP shows LV dysfunction).
- *Venous,* by Swan–Ganz monitoring: increased PCWP shows LV failure; *an isolated increase in CVP in the presence of normal PCWP shows isolated RV dysfunction.*

Left ventriculography:

- At the conclusion of coronary catheterization, assesses global and regional LV function, the presence of VSD or LV rupture, the presence, severity, and mechanism of MR, etc.

Myocardial biopsy:

- Is used for diagnosis of infiltrative myocardial disease, such as amyloidosis. It is also key for post-transplant follow-up.

4.1.2.4　HF: Treatment

The present discussion focuses on the LV, but similar considerations apply to the RV as well (with the possible exception of Digoxin, which has little effect on the RV). High-output HF therapy mainly addresses the underlying disease (hyperthyroidism, A-V aneurysm, etc.), and is not further discussed.

Several theoretical goals emerge for HF treatment:

- To improve myocardial contractility (inotropic treatment) and diastolic relaxation, or, as an extreme measure, to ensure cardiac function by transplant or artificial devices
- To optimize preload and afterload
- To counteract remodeling (dilatation, hypertrophy, aneurysm, sphericization)
- To counteract excessive sympathetic stimulation

Contractility is improved mainly in acute HF by short-term IV treatment; despite decades-long research (and several unfulfilled promises), the only inotropic agent in chronic HF remains Digitalis. There is still no convincing evidence of a truly effective drug specifically aimed at improving diastolic function. The other points in the list are thus the mainstay of HF treatment. A few important points of strategy:

- *LV dysfunction vs. overt HF:* asymptomatic LV dysfunction also requires treatment.

- *Systolic HF vs. HFPEF:* in principle, both require treatment, but the only effective way to improve diastolic function is therapy of systolic dysfunction.
- *Acute vs. chronic HF:* the treatment differs in several points (discussed below).
- *RV vs. LV failure:* the treatment of isolated RV failure involves a partly different strategy (discussed below). However, as the most frequent cause of RV failure is LV failure, this distinction is often of little relevance.

Tables 4.12–4.16 review the most frequently used therapeutic approaches to HF, both pharmacological and device-based. After this general introduction, the treatment of chronic and acute HF shall be individually discussed. Cardiogenic shock, which can complicate either acute or chronic HF, is reviewed separately. Only the contraindications and adverse effects of agents not previously discussed are reviewed here.

Table 4.12 Treatment strategies in HF

Strategy	Mechanism	Treatment	Acute HF	Chronic HF
Lifestyle changes		Dietary measures, physical exercise		
	Blood volume reduction	Salt and (in severe HF) fluid restriction	Yes	Yes
	Decreasing metabolic requirements	Weight loss, if overweight	N/A	Yes
	Optimize O_2 extraction by the tissues	Physical exercise	N/A	Yes
	Nutritional supplements	Coenzyme Q10	No	Possibly
Medication	Pre- and afterload reduction	Vasodilators		
		ACEI, ARB	No	Yes
		Na nitroprusside	Yes	In severe failure/shock
		Nitrates	Yes	Yes
		Pulmonary vasodilators	No	RV failure due to PAH
	Preload reduction	Diuretics	Yes	Yes
		Furosemide	Yes	Yes
		Metolazone	No	Yes
		Thiazides	No	Yes
		K-sparing diuretics	No	Yes
		Eplerenone	No	Yes
	Stimulating LV contraction	Inotropic agents		
		Digitalis	No	Yes
		IV adrenergic agents	Yes	In severe HF/shock
	Counteract excess sympathetic stimulation	β-blockers	No	Yes
	Improving LV relaxation	Calcium blockers	No	Possibly, in HFPEF
	Replacing electrolyte loss D/T diuretics	Supplements (mainly K, Mg)	Yes	Yes
	Treating HF complications			
	AAD	Amiodarone	Select pat.	Select patients
	Anticoagulation	Warfarin	Post-PCI	If AF or LV thrombus
Ensuring support in terminal patients	End-of-life care	Hospice treatment	No	Yes

Table 4.13 Vasodilators in HF[a]

Class/ representatives	Starting dose[a] (mg)	Target dose[b]	Remarks
Chronic HF			
ACEI			
Captopril	6.25 t.i.d.	50–100 t.i.d.	ACEI, associated with diuretics, are first-line therapy. They can be combined with ARB, for complete RAAS inhibition. Also indicated in asymptomatic LV dysfunction with LVEF <40%
Enalapril	2.5 b.i.d.	10–20 b.i.d.	
Lisinopril	2.5–5 q.d.	20–35 q.d.	
Ramipril	2.5 q.d.	5 q.d.	
Trandolapril	0.5 q.d.	4 q.d.	
ARB			
Candesartan	4–8 q.d.	32 q.d.	ARB associated with diuretics are first-line therapy for HF, if the patient is intolerant to ACEI
Valsartan	40 b.i.d.	160 b.i.d.	
Hydralazine/nitrates (ISDN[c])	37.5/20 t.i.d.	75/40 t.i.d.	Can be administered separately, but the existing data refers to the combination of the two drugs
Aliskiren[d]	150 mg q.d.	300 mg q.d.	Association to ACEI and ARB may produce complete RAAS blockade
Acute HF			
Nitroprusside	0.3 μg/kg/min	5 μg/kg/min	See text
ISDN	1 μg/h	10 μg/h	See text
Nitroglycerine	10–20 μg/min	200 μg/min	See text
Nesiritide	Bolus 2 μg/kg	→Drip 0.015–0.033 μg/kg/min	See text

Table adapted from "ESC Guideline Desk Reference," Wolters Kluwer/LippincottWilliams & Wilkins, 2008
[a]This table does not mention relaxin, a vasodilatory peptide, with a potential role in the therapy of acute HF (at present, of research interest); α_1-blocking agents (generally reserved as adjunct therapy of HTN – Ch. 3); and the vasodilatory effect of dopamine and dobutamine (which decreases afterload, but may limit the ability to use these agents in hypotensive patients)
[b]In milligrams
[c]Isosorbide dinitrate
[d]The only medication in this table not included, at the time of writing, in the ESC guidelines

Some of the therapeutic measures reviewed above are commented on in the following paragraph. The commentary is individualized for acute and for chronic HF.

Treatment of Chronic HF

Medical Therapy

Lifestyle changes: limiting Na intake helps decrease blood osmolality, as salt attracts water into the intravascular space. *In advanced cases,* fluid restriction is added, also to limit the circulating blood volume. Fluid restriction requires individualization, since it may precipitate renal hypoperfusion with ensuing renal failure and RAAS axis stimulation. Indeed, many HF patients have a contracted circulating volume despite excess body fluid (combined effect of diuretics and fluid storage in the "third space"). *Weight reduction* in the obese decreases the metabolic burden on the heart; excess weight also impairs the diaphragm and thorax wall inspiratory excursion, adding restrictive respiratory limitations to an already limited blood oxygenation, as a result of LV dysfunction-driven lung congestion. *Physical exercise* improves the peripheral use of the available blood (endothelial function/vasodilation, blood O_2 extraction, etc.); additionally, physical exercise has a positive psychological impact; it improves self-image and, in dedicated facilities, allows contact with patients experiencing similar problems – an informal but highly efficient support group.

Vasodilators decrease both afterload (by arterial dilatation and SVR decrease), and preload (venous dilatation decreases the venous return to the heart and the CVP).

Table 4.14 Diuretics and dialysis in HF

Chronic HF			
Class/representatives	Starting dose (mg/24 h)	Target dose (mg/24 h)	Remarks
Loop diuretics			
Furosemide	20–40	40–240	First-line therapy, associated with ACEI
Bumetanide	0.5–1.0	1–5	
Torasemide	5–10	10–20	
Thiazides			
Bendroflumethiazide	2.5	2.5–10	Isolated or associated with loop diuretics; contraindicated if eGFR[a] <30 ml/min
Hydrochlorothiazide	25	12.5–100	
Metolazone	2.5	2.5–10	
Indapamide	2.5	2.5–5	
K-sparing diuretics			
Spironolactone	50	100–200	Halve doses when associating these drugs to ACEI/ARB
Eplerenone	50	100–200	
Amiloride	5	40	
Triamterene	50	200	
Acute HF			
Class/representatives	Moderate (daily, mg)	Severe (daily, mg)	Remarks
Loop diuretics			
Furosemide	20–40	40–100 bolus, 5–40 mg/h infusion	PO/IV according to symptoms
Bumetanide	0.5–1.0	1–4	PO/IV
Torasemide	10–20	20–100	PO
Others			
Hydrochlorothiazide	50–100		In acute HF refractory to loop diuretics; the combination is more effective than very high doses of loop diuretics alone
Metolazone[b]	2.5–10		
Spironolactone[c]	25–50		
Acetazolamide	0.5		In cases of alkalosis
Dopamine	See "inotropes"		Produces renal vasodilation
Dobutamine	See "inotropes"		Increases BP, and thus renal perfusion
Ultrafiltration/hemodialysis			In case of renal failure or hyponatremia[d]

Table adapted from "ESC Guideline Desk Reference," Wolters Kluwer/LippincottWilliams & Wilkins, 2008

[a]eGFR estimated glomerular filtration rate, the volume of fluid filtered from the renal (kidney) glomerular capillaries into the Bowman's capsule per unit of time; normal >90 ml/min/1.73 m²; <30 signifies severe renal failure

[b]Effective especially with eGFR <30 ml/min/1.73 m²

[c]Best choice if no renal failure or hyperkalemia

[d]Hyponatremia can result from hemodilution, when there is excessive water retention/Na depletion

Table 4.15 Inotropic agents used in HF

Chronic HF			
Class/representatives	Daily dose (mg)		Remarks
Digitalis			
Digoxin	0.125–0.25		IV administration in HF rarely used today, except if rapid AF causes acute HF
Acute HF			
Class/ representatives	Bolus	Infusion	Remarks
Adrenergic agents			
Dobutamine	No	2–20 µg/kg/min	
Dopamine	No	1–2 to >5 µg/kg/min	See discussion of effects according to dose
Norepinephrine	No	0.2–1.0 µg/kg/min	
Epinephrine	No	0.05–0.5 µg/kg/min	
Phosphodiesterase inhibitors			
Milrinone	25–75 µg/kg, over 10–20 min	0.375–0.75 µg/kg/min	
Enoximone	0.25–0.75 mg/kg	1.25–7.5 µg/kg/min	
ATP-sensitive K channel opening, Ca sensitizing agents			
Levosimendan	12 µg/kg over 10 min	0.05–0.2 µg/kg/min	

Table adapted from "ESC Guideline Desk Reference," Wolters Kluwer/LippincottWilliams & Wilkins, 2008

ACEI counteract RAAS axis activation (Chap. 2), acting as *vasodilators; inhibitors/reversors of LV remodeling* (dilatation, hypertrophy, sphericization): reversal of cardiac remodeling is called *reverse remodeling*. Although this provides theoretical support for ACEI efficacy in HFPEF, HPEF patients derive significantly less benefit than patients with decreased LVEF; *inhibitors of aldosterone secretion,* and thus of Na and water retention, with stimulation of urinary K retention; *preventors of diabetic renal damage,* an important comorbidity in some HF patients.

ACEI are first-line therapy in chronic HF, indicated in patients with systolic and/or diastolic LV dysfunction, whether symptomatic (HF), or not. ACEI are associated with β-blockers and, in HF, with diuretics as well.

Long-term ACEI treatment

- Delays onset of overt HF in patients with asymptomatic LV dysfunction
- Improves symptoms (decreases NYHA class) and reduces hospitalization in HF patients
- Increases long-time survival in HF patients

ARB have, by and large, the same clinical effect as ACEI, and are indicated in case of ACEI intolerance. ARB can also be *added to* ACEI, a second-line strategy in patients with LVEF <40%, symptomatic despite the mandatory ACEI/diuretic/β-blockers combination. This association is justified by properties exclusive to each of the two classes of drugs. Indeed, ACEI increase the levels of bradykinin, a vasodilator (also responsible, however, for the occasional ACEI-associated cough), while ARB completely block the AII activity; this is not true of ACEI, since AII can also be produced by ACE-independent mechanisms (AII cleavage from AI under the action of the chymase system). The interplay of these characteristics is outlined below (Table 4.17).

Aliskiren is the first commercially available direct renin inhibitor (β-blockers indirectly inhibit the sympathetic-activated renin secretion). This action results in vasodilation both directly (renin itself is a potent vasoconstrictor) and indirectly (renin activates the rest of the RAAS). At present, Aliskiren is indicated only for HTN treatment, but there are reports about its efficacy in HF as well. Theoretically, associating it to the ACEI/ARB combination would result in a total inhibition of the RAAS. Aliskiren is indicated in HTN in doses of 150–300 mg, once daily. Whether these doses

Table 4.16 Nonpharmacological strategies in HF

Aim	Mechanism	Modality	Use
Increase the amount of contractile myocardium	Restore decreased coronary flow	Coronary revascularization	Common
	Add contractile cells	Stem cell therapy[a]	Experimental/early clinical
Improve function of the existing myocardium	Decrease afterload	IABP[b]	Common
	Reverse ventricular dyssynergy	CRT	Common
	Improve myocardial, pulmonary, and muscular function[c]	Exercise training program	Common
	Improve contraction coordination by RV electrode stimulation	A set of transvenous endocardial leads	Experimental
	Decrease heart-damaging systemic inflammation	10 ml of the patient's blood exposed ex vivo to oxidative stress, then reinjected IM	Experimental
Decrease O_2 consumption by decreasing myocardial wall tension; reduce MR	Prevent remodeling	The ACORN device	In select centers
	Create a favorable remodeling	The Myosplint device[d] or surgical remodeling[e]	Rarely or not at all
		The Rheos system[f]	Experimental/early clinical
		The Dor procedure (LV aneurysm resection and artificial patching)	Uncommon
Increase blood oxygenation	Oxygenate blood ex vivo and reinfuse	Extracorporeal membrane oxygenator (ECMO)	Rarely
Augment the myocardium's own contractile capacity	Long- and short-term pumps	Miniature LVAD[g]	Experimental/early clinical
	Wrap the heart in the mobilized latissimus dorsi muscle, made to contract by an electric stimulator	Dynamic cardiomyoplasty	Abandoned
Decrease circulating blood volume	Eliminate excess water	Intermittent peripheral ultrafiltration	Experimental
Render the terminal LV dysfunction irrelevant	Replace heart with donor heart	Transplant	Common
	Replace heart with pumping device	LVAD[h]	Common
Ensure support in terminal patients	End-of-life care	Hospice treatment	Common

[a]Currently of research interest only

[b]Also improves coronary perfusion

[c]Exercise training probably only modestly improves morbidity and mortality, but significantly improves quality of life

[d]May actually worsen MR

[e]The Dor procedure consists of LV aneurysm or anterior wall scar exclusion with a purse-string stitch and a Dacron patch; in 90% of patients, CABG is also performed. The recent STITCH trial has found no outcome impact to the Dor procedure. The Batista procedure, consisting of partial myocardial resection and mitral annuloplasty, has been abandoned

[f]The implantable carotid sinus baroreceptor activator, suggested as a therapeutic modality in HTN might produce favorable atrial and ventricular remodeling

[g]One such device is no larger than a man's thumb

[h]Most require systemic anticoagulation or antiplatelet therapy. Some are used over the short term (≤5 days), others are used for longer periods

Table 4.17 The rationale for associating ACEI and ARB

	Bradykinin buildup	Complete AII blockade	Vasodilation
ACEI	Yes	No	Submaximal
ARB	No	Yes	Submaximal
ACEI + ARB	Yes	Yes	Maximal

are optimal in HF as well remains to be clarified.

Nitrates: in combination with hydralazine, nitrates have been shown to be effective in chronic HF. However, they are indicated only if more modern therapeutic agents are ineffective.

Diuretics: by stimulating the renal elimination of water and Na, diuretics decrease cardiac preload. Furosemide also has venodilator activity, which helps relieve preload; in fact, with IV administration, dyspnea is relieved even before diuresis onset. Alongside ACEI, and in combination with them, diuretics are first-line therapy in HF. As opposed to ACEI, diuretics are not indicated in patients with asymptomatic ventricular dysfunction. The most important adverse effects of diuretics (Chap. 2) are *hypokalemia,* or, in case of K-sparing diuretics, *hyperkalemia; dehydration,* with possible worsening of HF due to ventricular underfilling; and *RAAS axis activation* (due to decreased renal perfusion). Due to their high efficacy, *loop diuretics* are the preferred diuretics in HF. In chronic HF, body weight fluctuations generally reflect fluid balance, and must be monitored to adjust diuretic dosage. Loop diuretics can be combined with thiazides for greater efficacy. *Thiazides* can be used in all stages of HF, but in severe HF, they serve as adjuncts to loop diuretics. They are contraindicated in severe renal failure, unless associated with loop diuretics. In this setting, the preferred agent is Metolazone, chemically not a thiazide, but displaying thiazide-like effects. Loop diuretics and thiazides are often associated with medication for electrolyte replacement, administered (1) *as tablets:* K (typically, 600 mg/tablet; dosage, 1–4 tablet/day, or more); Mg (typically, 200–300 mg/tablet, usual dose 1–2 tablet/day); (2) *by encouraging consumption of electrolyte-rich foods.* *Potassium* is mainly found in fresh fruit and vegetables (bananas, water melon, cantaloupe, avocado, potatoes); dried fruit and vegetables (figs, apricots, raisins, beans, lentils); fruit and vegetable juices (carrots, oranges, plums/prunes); yogurt; and fish (especially codfish and tuna); *magnesium* is mainly found in whole-flour baked

goods and cereals, different types of nuts, beans, cornmeal, spinach; *phosphorus* (occasionally also depleted by diuretics), is mainly found in milk, yogurt, fish and lentils, with lesser amounts found in eggs, beef and turkey. *K-sparing diuretics* are indicated *in combination with loop diuretics* (to potentiate their action and avoid K wasting), and *as aldosterone antagonists,* if the combination ACEI/diuretic/β-blocker is not sufficiently effective. In this case, Spironolactone, Eplerenone (in postinfarction HF) or ARB (unless already aboard, in ACEI-intolerant patients) can be used.

Inotropic agents: the only currently available inotropic agent for chronic HF is Digitalis; once the mainstay of HF treatment, Digitalis is much less used today, unless the patient has AF-associated HF (Digitalis used for HR control). Digitalis may be considered in patients with LVEF <40% still symptomatic despite the diuretic/ACEI and/or ARB/β-blocker combination; it may be administered orally or (infrequently today), IV. Digitalis is contraindicated in WPW patients, since it may slow AV conduction and favor conduction over the aberrant pathway, leading to life-threatening ventricular arrhythmia; in idiopathic HCM (increased LV contraction may increase subvalvular obstruction); and with hypokalemia (risk of life-threatening arrhythmia; hypokalemia is indeed frequent in HF patients, due to diuretic use). The adverse effects of Digitalis include GI symptoms (nausea, vomiting, diarrhea, anorexia); cardiac symptoms (AVB of different degrees, atrial and ventricular arrhythmia of variable severity); and other symptoms: (xanthopsia, vision with a peculiar yellow coloring; neurological and psychiatric symptoms, including delirium and convulsions).

β-blockers have a prominent place in HF therapy. Abolishing compensatory tachycardia may precipitate HF decompensation, and β-blockers were considered strictly contraindicated in HF ever since first used, in the 1960s. While this is still true in occasional patients (and in many cases of acute HF), in most *chronic* HF patients, the adaptive adrenergic stimulation is excessive and actually contributes to morbidity and mortality. Consequently, β-blockers have become an essential part of therapy in chronic HF. They are indicated in patients with LVEF <40% and mild, moderate or severe HF symptoms, after reaching optimal therapy with ACEI and diuretics. In other words, any patient with LVEF <40% and chronic HF has to take, at the very least, ACEI (or ARB), diuretics, and β-blockers. The first two classes are introduced simultaneously, and after dosage optimization, β-blockers are added. As β-blockers occasionally do not add symptomatic benefit, compliance problems are not uncommon; patient education is essential in regard to the survival benefit, even in the absence of any symptomatic improvement. β-blockers should be initiated in small doses and up-titrated slowly, every 2–4 weeks, under careful follow-up of worsening HF, hypotension, or bradycardia (HR <50 beats/min. mandates caution or cessation of upti-tration). In patients with post-MI asymptomatic LV dysfunction, long-term β-blocker therapy is indicated regardless of LV systolic dysfunction and symptomatic status. While there are no clear guidelines regarding use in asymptomatic LV dysfunction of other etiology, β-blockers are usually administered in these patients in addition to ACEI. If the patient presents with chronic tachycardia or HTN, the indication is even stronger. The main β-blockers used in HF are presented in Table 4.18. These agents are started in clinically stable patients, with no recent changes in the dosage of other drugs (especially diuretics). β-blockers are contraindicated in patients with decompensated HF (although recent registry data suggests that if the patient hospitalized for acute HF is already on β-blocker therapy, it may not be necessary to discontinue it); with recent changes in dosage of other medications; or with excessive bradycardia, in the absence of a pacemaker. (For relative contraindications, see Chap. 3.)

Ca channel blockers (CCB): often used for the treatment of HTN and/or CAD (the most frequent causes of HF), CCB have an unclear place as primary

Table 4.18 β-blockers in HF

Stable chronic HF		
Representatives	Starting dose	Target dose (mg q.d.)
Bisoprolol	1.25 mg q.d.	10
Carvedilol	3.125 mg b.i.d.	25–50
Metoprolol	12.5–25 mg q.d.	200
Nebivolol	1.25 mg q.d.	10

Table adapted from "ESC Guideline Desk Reference," Wolters Kluwer/Lippincott Williams & Wilkins, 2008

HF therapy, and are not included in the HF treatment guidelines. CCB may help increase CO by peripheral vasodilation and also be effective in HFPEF, but the data are inconclusive. Nondihydropyridine CCB (Verapamil, Diltiazem) have a negative inotropic action, deleterious in case of associated systolic dysfunction.

HF: CAVE NSAIDs

- NSAID inhibit prostaglandin action, which mediates not only inflammation, but also the renal effect of diuretics. In diuretic-compensated HF patients, NSAID use may lead to HF decompensation.
- Other prostaglandin-mediated effects inhibited by NSAID include systemic and renal vasodilation, the former increasing CO and the latter stimulating diuresis; decreased renal perfusion activates the RAAS, a notoriously harmful process in HF.

In the HF patient, β-blockers

- Decrease HR and O_2 requirements; this improves systolic and diastolic function
- Decrease the incidence of arrhythmia
- Are effective antianginal agents (CAD is often present)
- Help manage HTN
- Counteract catecholamine-mediated cardiac remodeling
- Carvedilol also has vasodilatory and antioxidant action (the former, by peripheral vascular α-blockade)

AAD may be cautiously considered in (1) *ventricular arrhythmia:* despite the increased risk of life-threatening arrhythmia in patients with cardiac dilatation and LVEF <35–40%, routine AAD treatment for primary prevention is contraindicated, due to AAD-related arrhythmia. Even ventricular arrhythmia (if nonsustained and asymptomatic) is not an indication for AAD. However, AAD may be considered in patients with decreased LVEF and sustained, symptomatic ventricular arrhythmia. In fact, in these patients, there is an indication for ICD, which however may not be accessible, especially in developing countries. AAD can also be used in ICD-bearing patients, to reduce the number of electrical discharges. For this indication, Amiodarone is the preferred drug. Of note, HF treatment includes β-blockers, with an important antiarrhythmic action of their own. (2) *Atrial arrhythmia,* most frequently AF with rapid ventricular response: digoxin is the drug of choice. If ineffective, Amiodarone can be used.

Anticoagulants: blood flow in dilated hearts is slower than normal, and may even be stagnant in LV aneurysms; therefore, prophylactic anticoagulation in HF patients appears intuitively appropriate. However, this has never been found effective, and in unselected HF populations, adverse events (bleeding) exceed possible benefits (thromboembolism prevention). The indications for anticoagulation in HF include: chronic or recurrent paroxysmal AF; LV thrombus diagnosis by echo; on a case-to-case basis, thromboembolic episodes (especially if recurring) of suspected cardiac etiology. For all of the above, VKA are the drugs of choice. Primary prevention of DVT and thromboembolism in bedridden patients is based on LMWH.

Other agents: the blood levels of *Coenzyme Q10,* a compound essential to life, are decreased in chronic diseases, including HF. However, the value of supplementation is unclear, and Q10 is not included in HF treatment guidelines. It may occasionally be tried, as an adjunct to conventional treatment. The same applies for a number of nutritional supplements suggested as beneficial in HF, but never conclusively proven as such.

Interventional therapy. Revascularization: in chronic HF, revascularization is indicated in the presence of significant myocardial hibernation, identified noninvasively. Surgical risk/benefit ratio must be carefully assessed, since in severe HF, both the potential benefit and the surgical risk are high. *Valvular surgery:* VHD may cause or intensify HF, by different mechanisms.

- *AS* causes increased peripheral resistance (afterload), responsible for LVH (diastolic dysfunction), and, ultimately, for LV dilatation (combined systolic and diastolic dysfunction).
- *AI* causes increased preload (LV fills both normally, from the LA, and abnormally, from the aorta), and causes LV dilatation, with combined systolic and diastolic LV dysfunction.
- *MR* causes increased preload (LV fills both normally, from the pulmonary veins, and abnormally,

with blood regurgitated into the LA in the previous systole), producing LV dilatation (combined systolic and diastolic HF).

The indications for surgery in VHD are reviewed in Chap. 5. While patients with severe HF are at high surgical risk, surgery may represent the only chance of survival.

HF in the setting of severe MR

MR can be the cause or the result of LV dysfunction. In the former setting, LV ensues due to a chronic increase in preload, whereas in the latter, LV dilatation of another cause (e.g., from ischemic or toxic CMP) leads to annulus dilatation, leaflet malcoaptation, and MR. MR increases the severity of the LV dysfunction, with further increase in regurgitant volume – *"MR begets MR."* Compensatory mechanisms allow maintaining a low-normal LVEF despite severe myocardial dysfunction; surgery before the onset of irreversible LV dysfunction is thus essential. The most severe challenge is the management of patients with severe LV dysfunction *and* severe MR (Chap. 5).

LV aneurysmectomy: LV aneurysms are not only a potential source of arrhythmia and embolism, but also decrease stroke volume; additionally, there is increased tension and O_2 demand in the myocardial wall. Aneurysm resection, a logical solution, is, however, a major undertaking, recommended only in large aneurysms causing intractable HF. LV aneurysmectomy is performed at the end of the usual bypass surgery; it can be part of the Dor procedure (see below).

Conventional pacing: the indications for cardiac pacing are reviewed in Chap. 6. In HF patients, DDD systems are preferred, being better tolerated and maintaining the atrial kick. RV-only pacing causes LBBB and ventricular dyssynchrony, potentially aggravating HF.

Cardiac resynchronization therapy (CRT): in many HF patients, the ventricles contract a few milliseconds apart (not simultaneously, as in normal individuals), due to conduction delays through the dilated, often scarred myocardium. This translates as a widened QRS complex (>12 ms), and LVEF lower than that predicted based on myocardial damage alone. CRT is achieved by biventricular pacing, using three leads, one each in the RA, RV, and the coronary sinus. The latter vein drains the blood from the myocardium into the RA and allows inserting a pacing lead in very close proximity to the LV, avoiding the necessity for intraventricular leads that would be difficult to introduce and to maintain in place (due to the turbulent intraventricular flow). The ventricles are paced in perfect synchrony. The CRT device can function as a pacemaker only (CRT-P) or also possess an ICD function (CRT-D, "D" for "defibrillation"). CRT with or without an ICD is indicated in association to optimal medical therapy (including an ACEI, a diuretic, a β blocker, and an aldosterone antagonist, either ARB, Spironolactone, or Eplerenone), in patients with LVEF ≤35%, QRS ≥0.12 s, and

- NYHA Class III or ambulatory Class IV in NSR (Class I indication) or AF (Class IIa indication)
- NYHA Class I or II, undergoing implantation of a permanent pacemaker and/or ICD with anticipated frequent ventricular pacing (Class IIb indication)

CRT was found effective in patients with prolonged QRS and LV systolic dysfunction (LVEF <40%) that is mildly symptomatic or altogether asymptomatic (MADIT-CRT trial). CRT generally increases EF only modestly, but sufficiently to substantially improve symptoms (NYHA class regression) and to prolong survival. CRT-D are the ideal alternative, since ICD is indicated anyway in these patients; they are, however, severalfold more expensive than CRT-P. Up to 30% of properly selected patients do not respond to CRT. The causes may be: the absence of dyssynchrony, despite QRS prolongation; pacing at the site of LV free wall scar; and use of the same pacing electrode positioning in LV dysfunction of different etiologies, where the LV activation sequence

may actually be different. Conversely, some patients with QRS complexes <12 ms may have contraction dyssynchrony, as evidenced by echo. While these patients might also benefit from CRT, there is no consensus to date in regard to non-EKG dyssynchrony definition. The (not yet universally validated) echo parameters of dyssynchrony include:

- *Pulsed-wave Doppler parameters* (a delay between the onset of RV and LV contraction >40 ms is considered increased).
- *M-mode parameters* (a septal-to-posterior-wall motion delay >130 ms is considered increased).
- *Tissue Doppler parameters* (a delay between QRS onset and the onset/peak of basal septum/basal lateral wall contraction >62–65 ms is abnormal).
- *Strain imaging* and *speckle tracking* parameters.

Tagged MRI imaging also measures strain, but MRI is contraindicated in many pacemaker bearers, and the measuring method itself is highly complex.

ICD: as opposed to previously discussed treatments, ICD is not meant to improve LV function or HF symptoms, but to prevent cardiac arrest. LVEF decreases of any nature carry the risk of fatal ventricular arrhythmia, but routine AAD therapy is contraindicated, due to its own arrhythmic potential. The indications for ICD related to LVEF decreases are reviewed in Table 4.19; of note, these represent only a component of the indications for ICD implantation, as discussed in Chap. 6. All patients should be on optimal medical therapy and with a life expectancy >1 year. (The latter criterion is not satisfied in many NYHA class IV patients, in whom the only option is transplant).

LV assist devices (LVAD): at present, LVAD is indicated as a bridge to transplant (while awaiting availability of a donor) and in severe acute myocarditis

Table 4.19 Indications for ICD implantation related to LVEF decrease

LVEF		NYHA		Etiology		Arrhythmia	Indication class
≤35%	and	Class II /III	and	Any[a]			I
≤30%	and	Class I	and	Post-MI[a]			I
≤40%			and	Post-MI[b]	and	NSVT and inducible VF or sustained VT at EPS	I
Normal or near-normal					and	Sustained VT	IIa
≤35%	and	Class I	and	Nonischemic			IIb

[a]If post-MI, should be ≥40 days after the acute event
[b]>48 h after the acute event

(occasional recovery after various periods of LVAD use). These indications are rapidly evolving, as is the degree of device miniaturization.

Cardiac transplant, a last-resort measure in severe HF refractory to optimal treatment, involves using a heart harvested from a donor. Donors are either recently (<6 h) dead patients, or patients with preserved vital functions, but no cerebral function ("brain-dead"). The most severe scenario requiring heart transplant is cardiogenic shock, dependent on inotropic treatment for adequate organ perfusion. In suitable candidates with chronic HF, VO$_2$ max <10–12 ml/kg on cardiopulmonary stress testing is an indication for transplant. (Documentation of VO$_2$ max is required before entering a patient on the transplant waiting list). Non-HF related indications for cardiac transplant include patients with refractory myocardial ischemia on maximal conservative therapy and where revascularization is not, or is no longer possible and patients with severe arrhythmia, refractory to medical therapy, and/or triggering exceedingly frequent ICD discharges. Overall, about 50% suffer from CAD, most of the rest being accounted for by myocarditis and other CMP; only about 1% of candidates suffer from CHD. *The contraindications* for cardiac transplant include: severe noncardiac disease such as kidney, lung, or liver disease, severe diabetes, severe vascular disease, HIV infection, most malignancies, etc., due to the high risk of complications (surgery, chronic immunosuppressive therapy) and to the noncardiac decrease in life expectancy.

Selection and matching of the donor heart

The main donor characteristics making a heart *unusable* for transplant include: age >55; prolonged cardiac arrest, severe hypotension, or prolonged dependence on inotropes; traumatic heart injury; sepsis; malignancy (except for primary, nonmetastatic brain cancer); and positive serology for HIV and hepatitis B or C.

There are three tiers of medical examination of the donor's heart: *general screening; cardiac function assessment,* by EKG, chest X-ray, arterial blood gas report, and, in the US (but not in Europe), for possible severe VHD or CAD. In the presence of risk factors for CAD, as well as in male donors >45 years of age and in females >50, routine cardiac catheterization is carried out. Significant coronary stenosis makes the heart unusable; and *direct examination in the OR,* at the time of cardiac harvesting.

If a donor heart has been found appropriate for transplant, it is matched to a maximum-priority recipient from the waiting list, according to blood group (ABO) compatibility and the size of the patient's body and the donor heart.

The cardiac transplant procedure is performed using cardiopulmonary bypass. Patients with severe PAH (e.g., CHD-related HF) may require combined heart/lung transplant. Most frequently, the patient's own heart is removed *(orthotopic procedure);* actually, the LA roof, containing the pulmonary vein ostia, is kept in place, and the corresponding portion of the donor heart is trimmed at the time of surgery. This portion of tissue is the first one to be sutured in place, followed by suture of the great arteries. The most frequent *complications* are infection or graft rejection in the early posttransplant period, and transplant vasculopathy later on. (Each may occur at any time, but is most frequent in the mentioned periods): *infection* manifests and is treated in the usual fashion. The main pathogens are *CMV* (from the donor or by the reactivation of the recipient's own, formerly quiescent disease; the treatment is with IV Gancyclovir, followed by oral Valgancyclovir or Acyclovir); and *P. carinii,* treated with TMP-SMX. *Rejection* may manifest as HF and ventricular arrhythmia or present insidiously, with dyspnea, excessive fatigue, and nonspecific general symptoms. Some patients are almost asymptomatic, despite their life-threatening condition. Therefore, a high index of suspicion must be maintained, as well as a low threshold for extensive workup, in collaboration with the transplant team. Depending on severity, rejection can be treated with steroids alone or in conjunction with polyclonal or monoclonal anti-lymphocyte antibody therapy and/or IL-2 inhibitors. *Transplant vasculopathy* is nonatherosclerotic concentric intimal hypertrophy that can occur as early as 3 months after transplant. CMV infection and the trauma of repeated blunted rejection episodes are the suspected cause. Due to the diffuse nature of the lesions, revascularization is usually not feasible. Noninvasive testing for ischemia is much less valuable than with atherosclerotic CAD. Compounding these difficulties, the clinical manifestations are also often misleading (fatigue, perspiration, left arm pain, GI symptoms, etc.), since surgical severing of sensory nerves often precludes typical angina. The only resort for severe posttransplant vasculopathy is retransplantation. *Malignancy* is related to chronic immunosuppressive therapy. *HTN* is mainly related to Cyclosporine- or Tacrolimus-induced renal vasoconstriction, with a secondary increase in sodium concentration and plasma volume. The treatment is not different from that of run-of-the-mill HTN. The preferred strategy is a combination of ACEI and CCB.

Posttransplant maintenance therapy includes steroids and immunosuppressors, while *follow-up* focuses on transplant rejection and vasculopathy. Immunosuppressive therapy after cardiac transplant typically includes a calcineurin inhibitor (cyclosporine or tacrolimus), an antiproliferative agent (cyclosporine or mycophenolate Mofetil, MMF), and a corticosteroid. The regimens vary widely, from center to center and even among patients. An additional group of agents are the TOR group (inhibitors of the "target of rapamycin"), including Evrolimus and Sirolimus. Repeated endomyocardial biopsies are required (in the immediate posttransplant period, as frequently as once weekly). Follow-up for vasculopathy is challenging due to the poor performance of noninvasive testing in these patients (certain centers perform annual routine coronary catheterization). Ultimately, problem-free transplant patients are seen once a year. Considering the dismal prognosis of end-stage HF, *the survival rates after cardiac transplant are nothing short of spectacular:* approximately 70% of patients are alive at 5 years (figures slightly better for males). The veteran tranplantee worldwide was operated on three decades ago. Moreover, there are virtually no lifestyle limitations after cardiac transplant, except for the frequent medical visits early on.

The logistics of cardiac transplant

Most countries maintain a list of transplant candidates, due to the severe shortage of donors (Only a few thousand candidates, i.e., a small fraction of the total, undergo transplant each year). Transplant candidates have by definition intractable HF and severe prognosis, yet there are several categories of emergency; the highest is designated as "zero-degree," and refers to cardiogenic shock, dependent on IV inotropes for peripheral perfusion.

Zero-degree candidates are hospitalized, but many of the others aren't; in order to be readily accessible in case a suitable donor emerges (an unpredictable occurrence, since many donors are road accident victims), the candidates have a special beeper, by which they can be summoned to the hospital by a nurse coordinator. This psychologically traumatic strategy will hopefully be altered by the new method of "beating heart" transplantation (see below).

New frontiers in cardiac transplant

- New technology might help prolong the "shelf-life" of excised hearts, by preserving them not on ice (as is the current practice) but at body temperature, connected to a pulsatile pump irrigating them with blood.
- Intensive research pursues the generation of transgenic pigs, free of species-specific membrane antigens (the porcine and the human heart have similar sizes).
- The notion of cardiac transplant is being extended from the "whole-organ" to the "cell transplant" approach: stem cells (from the bone marrow) or myoblasts (undifferentiated muscle cells from the patient's own limbs) are implanted into the myocardium, to differentiate into mature muscular cells and restore the systolic function. This investigational technique has encouraging preliminary results.

Implanted devices for inotropic support are last-resort options, reserved for patients with intractable HF awaiting transplantation, and for severe myocarditis. These devices supplant cardiac function totally ("artificial heart") or partially (LVAD=LV assist device). The difference is a practical one: the artificial heart requires removal of the patient's own heart, while the LVAD does not. Artificial hearts remain in the patient's body for all the rest of their lives; unfortunately, this span is generally not much longer than 1 year. LVAD may be temporary or definitive (months or years). There have been reports of cardiac recovery after months or years of LVAD assistance, especially in myocarditis and myocardial hibernation. LVAD-assisted survival can span several years. LVADs use two cannulas, one in the ventricular apex (LV, RV, or both) and one in the aorta, connected via a pumping device. Flow may be pulsatile (mimicking normal cardiac function) or continuous. The miniature pump, powered by batteries, is implanted subcutaneously (in the abdominal wall).

Devices and procedures for prevention or correction of cardiac remodeling include: (1) *wrapping up the LV* in different materials, either synthetic or native to the body (muscular bundles from the thorax or upper limbs). These function as "harnesses" preventing excessive LV dilatation. One of the best known devices is the "Acorn," a fine mesh of synthetic material wrapped around the heart; (2) *the Dor procedure,* consisting of resection of LV aneurysm and restoring the LV elliptical geometry (in advanced HF, the heart shape is globular, rather than elliptical). It is usually carried out at the conclusion of CABG, in patients with MRI-confirmed large areas of myocardial scarring and LV aneurysm, presenting with intractable angina and/or HF. The Dor procedure is contraindicated in patients with RV dysfunction; PAH; and dysfunction at the base (rather than the apex) of the LV. Despite substantial LVEF increase, the incremental survival benefit over that of CABG alone is modest.

Hospice (end-of-life) care: terminal HF represents a huge physical, psychological, and financial burden not only for the patient, but also for their family. Hospice care ensures a humane and professional multidisciplinary approach to this difficult period.

Chronic HF requires a coherent therapeutic strategy

The underlying diseases are treated as indicated (revascularization, VHD surgery, etc.). The treatment algorithm of HF per se is based on several decision tiers, the different medications or procedures being indicated with various degrees of emphasis. Thus:

- The first-choice drugs are ACEI, diuretics, and β-blockers. The first two classes are started simultaneously, and when the dosage is optimized, β-blockers are started and up-titrated cautiously. If the patient is ACEI-intolerant, ARB may be used. If this treatment results in asymptomatic status, LVEF is assessed again, and an ICD is implanted as indicated.
- If the patient is still symptomatic, an aldosterone antagonist or (unless already on board) an ARB is added. Again, the necessity of ICD is assessed.

- If, at this point, the patient is still symptomatic and has a QRS complex >120 ms, CRT is indicated (very frequently, these patients have an LVEF <35%). If the QRS is not >120 ms or if the patient is still symptomatic, Digoxin, Hydralazine/nitrate, LVAD, or transplant are considered. (Despite the marginal role reserved by guidelines to Digoxin, this is usually administered in earlier stages. Digoxin has a much more prominent place in patients with HF and AF.)
- ACEI and β-blockers are indicated in patients with asymptomatic LV dysfunction (LVEF <40%).

Treatment of Acute HF

In acute HF, the main task is safeguarding the patient's vital functions, by relief of pulmonary congestion; improvement of peripheral perfusion; preservation of systolic BP >90 mmHg; and preservation of $SatO_2$ >90%.

Achieving these goals often requires invasive monitoring (arterial line for BP, Swan–Ganz catheter to monitor PCWP and CO), as well as invasive treatment (angioplasty in CAD-related HF, IABP, mechanical ventilation). As opposed to the case of chronic HF, the medications are typically administered IV. The main drugs include:

- IV fluids, to optimize LV filling pressures; these are crucial in cardiogenic shock, but contraindicated in pulmonary edema in the absence of shock.
- Morphine (3–5 mg boluses, under BP follow-up), to relieve anxiety, dyspnea (vasodilation), tachypnea (by respiratory center depression), and ischemic chest pain; the main adverse effects include respiratory depression ($SatO_2$ monitoring is essential) and nausea/vomiting (antiemetics routinely administered).
- Diuretics, a mainstay of treatment in both acute and chronic HF, must be used cautiously or avoided in RV MI-dependent acute HF. IV loop diuretics are the first choice.
- Vasodilators (nitroglycerine, nitroprusside), under BP monitoring and, for nitroprusside, under monitoring for signs of toxicity as well.
- Inotropic agents, in cardiogenic shock (BP<80 mmHg); dopamine can be used in small doses, for its diuretic

effect. The most frequently used inotropic agents include: *adrenergic agents:* (Table 4.11), activating the α and/or β adrenergic receptors, thus: *dobutamine* stimulates β1 receptors, increasing LV contractility and CO, in a dose-dependent manner: higher doses may cause HTN and arrhythmia; *dopamine* has different clinical actions, according to dosage: for infusion rates <3 μg/kg/min, it causes renal vasodilation, and may stimulate diuresis (activation of "dopaminergic" receptors); between 3 and 5 μg/kg/min, it is mainly inotropic, and at >5 μg/kg/min, it causes vasoconstriction, which may help restore BP and organ perfusion, but also increases afterload. Dopamine is usually administered in low doses, combined with higher doses of dobutamine; *epinephrine and norepinephrine* act on α- and β-adrenergic receptors, causing vasoconstriction and increased CO and BP (vasopressor action). Because of the increased afterload, the use of these agents must be of short duration. Classical situations include CPR and shock; for instance, septic shock involves a component of vasodilation which is countered by vasopressors. *Phosphodiesterase inhibitors:* phosphodiesterase degrades mediators of β1-receptor activation by catecholamines; therefore, inhibiting this enzyme indirectly ensures prolonged/intense catecholamine activity. These agents have a net inotropic and vasodilatory action, helping increase CO. *Levosimendan* increases CO by a double mechanism, inotropic and vasodilatory. The former is based on increasing the sensitivity of the myocytes to calcium (without actually affecting the calcium levels), while the latter is based on opening the ATP-sensitive (KATP) K channels.

- Oxygen is routinely administered to reach $SatO_2$ >95% (in COPD patients, >90%, to avoid respiratory depression). O_2 is administered either noninvasively (with a sealed face mask), or invasively (mechanical ventilation). Noninvasive ventilation often uses positive end-expiratory pressure (PEEP), to prevent airway collapse at the end of expirium and improve blood oxygenation.
- IABP is an aortic balloon introduced through the femoral artery, to reduce cardiac workload and improve coronary perfusion in severe acute HF, as well as in severe ischemia. The balloon inflates in diastole (improving coronary perfusion, which, as opposed to other arteries, occurs mainly in diastole), and deflates in systole (decreasing SVR). The net result is an increase in CO and coronary perfusion.

Beside *severe acute HF,* the balloon is also indicated in *CAD* patients, as discussed in Chap. 2.
- LVAD or cardiac transplant, in refractory cardiogenic shock and pulmonary edema.

Acute HF requires a coherent therapeutic strategy

Generally,

- If systolic BP is >100 mmHg, a vasodilator (associated with morphine, as needed) is administered.
- For BP=90–100 mmHg, vasodilators and/or inotropes are administered.
- For BP <90 mmHg (shock), fluids and inotropes are administered, and an IABP is inserted; vasodilators are contraindicated, and diuretics are used with caution (hypovolemia may hinder ventricular filling and further compromise systolic function).

In all cases of acute HF, C-PAP or mechanical ventilation is used as indicated.

The treatment of isolated RV failure includes correction of the underlying disorders: PAH, PS, RV MI, etc. Acute isolated RV failure, as seen in RV infarction, is mainly treated with fluid infusions (Chap. 2); in case this does not correct the problem, inotropes and Nitroprusside may be used. As with LV MI, early (<6 h) reperfusion is key.

4.2 Cardiomyopathy

As is often the case in medicine, the term, "cardiomyopathy," is exceedingly vague: it might, in principle, refer to limited or clinically irrelevant myocardial disease; to the subtle ion channel pathology leading to lethal arrhythmia, as seen, for instance, with the Brugada syndrome; to localized ischemic myocardial dysfunction, etc. In practice, however, the term is reserved for severe myocardial disease leading to heart failure. By and large, cardiomyopathy is classified by the pattern of myocardial involvement, which can consist of dilatation, hypertrophy, or interstitial infiltration, idiopathic or secondary to the underlying conditions. This clinically useful classification is based on the classical diagnostic technology and terminology, and is therefore subject to serious limitations. For instance, potentially lethal HCM abnormalities can be so subtle as to be undetectable by echocardiography; HCM shows a typical pattern of "restrictive physiology"; late cases of HCM may associate cardiac dilatation; myocardial scarring seen with some cases of RCM is histologically similar to that caused by ischemia, in DCM patients; etc., etc. These limitations notwithstanding, the time-honored entities of dilated, hypertrophic, and restrictive CMP (RCM) remain clinically relevant.

4.2.1 Dilated Cardiomyopathy

4.2.1.1 Definition, Mechanisms

The most frequent type of CMP, it consists of cardiac dilatation (in normal individuals, echo-measured LV short axis dimension = 2–4 cm in systole, 3.5–6 cm in diastole; long axis dimension = 4.6–8.4 cm in systole and 6.3–10.3 cm in diastole), occurring either by direct myocardial damage (of known or unknown causes), or as a compensatory mechanism, to help preserve CO despite decreased LVEF. Whether dilatation is the cause of LV dysfunction or a compensatory mechanism against it, it ultimately decreases CO, since

- The more dilated the heart, the higher the myocyte tension and O_2 consumption, resulting in diffuse sub-endocardial ischemia and further LVEF depression.

- Dilated hearts have an abnormal spherical (rather than ovoidal) shape. This further decreases systolic function, since it compromises the normal spiral "wrap-around" allowing myocytes to produce an EF of 55–60%, while only shortening by 15%.

- Cardiac dilatation causes mitral annulus widening and produces or increases MR, which diverts part of the CO into the LA. Dilation and sphericization are, alongside LVH, the main components of "cardiac remodeling" and are partly reversed by optimal treatment (Fig. 4.2).

Surprisingly, there is no strict definition for the degree of LV dilatation and systolic dysfunction justifying the appellation, "DCM." A good rule of thumb is that DCM involves an LVEF decrease <45%, and often much below this threshold.

4.2.1.2 Classification and Etiology

DCM is classified as primary (idiopathic) or secondary (25%, respectively 75% of cases). Suspected etiologic factors in *primary DCM* include viral infections, autoimmune mechanisms, and toxic agents. About 20–30% of cases are inherited (familial DCM); the rest are due to environmentally driven or random mutation. A particular form of primary DCM is ARVC. The most important causes of *secondary DCM* are: CAD (ischemic CMP);

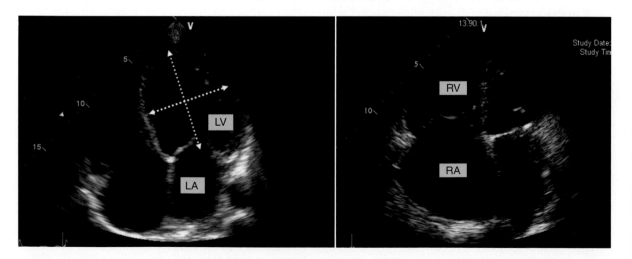

Fig. 4.2 Dilated Cardiomyopathy. *Left panel:* idiopathic DCM. Note the LV dilatation and the almost spherical shape of the LV, a severe form of cardiac remodeling; *Right panel:* secondary DCM: severely dilated right cavities in a patient with chronic severe TR

VHD; inflammation (infectious, especially viral myocarditis; collagen vascular disease and other autoimmune conditions); metabolic and endocrine diseases (hyper- and hypothyroidism, diabetes); the action of physical and chemical agents (radiation, Adriamycin, alcohol, etc.); infiltrative diseases (e.g., sarcoidosis, Fabry's disease); neuromuscular disorders (e.g., Duchenne's muscular dystrophy); peripartum CMP; and chronic tachycardia. Additionally, many cases of HCM present, in their late (final) stages, as DCM.

4.2.1.3 Clinical Picture

DCM typically presents as HF; about a third of all HF cases are due to DCM. Often, the symptoms are mild and the quality of life is preseved, but DCM can cause severe HF, occasionally requiring transplant. In addition to the usual HF signs, DCM can associate with nonspecific chest pain, occasionally difficult to differentiate from angina, especially since CAD is often the underlying cause of DCM. There is a high risk of life-threatening ventricular arrhythmia, and the first manifestation of DCM may be cardiac arrest. Asymptomatic cardiac dilatation also carries the risk of life-threatening arrhythmia. Diagnosis is based on the exclusion of other possible ctiologies. Echo shows global LV hypokinesia, although segmental involvement is possible. Nuclear perfusion scan and coronarography show results in accordance with the ischemic or nonischemic origin of CMP. The myocardial mass is increased, as demonstrated by MRI. In advanced cases, survival rates were classically dismal, but with modern therapy, they have improved substantially. The treatment is nonspecific.

In the following section, the most important causes of DCM will be individually reviewed.

4.2.1.4 Secondary DCM: Underlying Disorders

Ischemic CMP: just as there is no clear definition of the degree of ventricular dilatation and/or LVEF decrease that define DCM, there is no strict definition of the degree of ischemic damage representing "ischemic CMP." As a general rule, if the degree of ischemic LV dysfunction and/or dilatation and/or HF are ≥ moderate, the term appears justified. Ischemic involvement of the myocardium may be macro- and/or microvascular.

If there are significantly large hibernating areas, DCM can be reversible with revascularization.

DCM caused by myocardial inflammation (myocarditis)

1. *Etiology*: The most frequent causes of myocarditis are infective or autoimmune.
   - Infective myocarditis is usually of viral etiology (Coxsackie virus, Influenza virus, HIV, etc.; for an overview of HIV-related cardiac involvement, see Chap. 12). Other infective etiologies include bacterial (generally, after penetrating trauma to the chest or with sepsis) or parasitic myocarditis; the latter is illustrated by Chagas' disease, prevalent in South America, and characterized by a biphasic course, involving: (a) *an acute inflammatory disease,* nonspecific but for the typical eyelid edema on the side where the parasite-carrying bug bit and infested the patient; (b) *a chronic stage,* involving an especially arrhythmia-prone CMP, alongside GI and neurological manifestations.
   - Autoimmune myocarditis is present in cases of systemic inflammatory disease, such as lupus, rheumatoid arthritis, etc. The diagnosis is based on otherwise unexplained diffuse LV systolic dysfunction, in a patient with these diseases; *acute rheumatic fever,* a condition where antibodies directed against Streptococcus group A (generally infecting the throat) also attack the myocardium. Myocarditis occurs only in the first phase of the disease, and is generally self-limiting; it is the second phase (valvular damage and dysfunction, often manifesting decades later) that represents the main problem. *Other causes:* postvaccination, serum sickness, or transplant rejection-related myocarditis

2. The *clinical picture* includes the manifestations of the underlying disease; symptoms and signs reflecting cardiac inflammation (most often, stabbing chest pain, due to involvement of the pericardium – myopericarditis); and HF and/or arrhythmia. Myocarditis is suspected in HF and long-standing unexplained low-grade fever (in post-MI patients, fever is usually self-limiting), and can present either as an overwhelming acute event, or have a slower (subacute) course. Close follow-up is mandatory, since, occasionally, the disease can progress very quickly. Diagnosis is based on the clinical picture, a generally diffuse LV contractile dysfunction by

Table 4.20 Clinical course of myocarditis

Type	Prevalence (%)	Onset	Prognosis
Fulminant	17	Distinct	Complete recovery or death
Acute	65	Indistinct	Usually, incomplete recovery; death not uncommon
Chronic active	11	Indistinct	Usually, incomplete recovery; mild or moderate residual LV dysfunction, occasionally restrictive pattern
Chronic persistent	7	Indistinct	Usually, no LV dysfunction

echo, increased inflammatory markers, and, occasionally, myocardial biopsy. This must be taken from several areas of the RV, due to possible patchy cardiac involvement. Unfortunately, the practical impact of biopsy on management is often limited.

- The clinical course of myocarditis is classified as reviewed in Table 4.20.

3. *The treatment* is generally supportive, but may also involve steroids, and occasionally, LVAD insertion for definitive support, bridging to transplant, or assistance until myocardial recovery. Immunosuppression is not routinely recommended, as several trials have not shown it to be beneficial. Exceptions exist, however; for instance, giant cell myocarditis (diagnosed by biopsy) may benefit from a combination of immunosuppressants and corticosteroids. According to recent research, Interferon beta-1b might be effective in chronic viral CMP.

DCM caused by metabolic and endocrine diseases

- Thyroid disease-related DCM: *hyperthyrodism* can cause both high- and low-output HF. The former is related to increased metabolic demands, and the latter (DCM picture) to chronic tachycardia (occasionally, AF) and HTN. This is seen mainly in elderly patients, with preexisting heart disease. The treatment is that of hyperthyrodism, HF, and HTN; *hypothyroidism* can cause DCM by direct influence of hormone deficiency on the myocytes, as well as by increasing cholesterol levels, a risk factor for CAD. Additionally, hypothyroidism

often causes pericardial effusion, with occasional tamponade.

- Rarer causes of DCM include other endocrine conditions (acromegaly, hypo- or hyperparathyroidism), electrolyte deficiency (zinc, potassium, phosphate, magnesium), or deficiency of vitamins (thiamine – beriberi), aminoacids (carnitine), or protein (starvation).

- Diabetic CMP: the existence of this syndrome has been debated, as diabetes (isolated, or as part of the metabolic syndrome) is a major risk factor for CAD; however, diabetics appear to sustain myocardial damage beyond that expected from associated CAD.

- Abdominal obesity is often part of the metabolic syndrome and is associated with a sedentary lifestyle, both risk factors for CAD. Obesity also affects cardiac function directly, by fatty acid toxicity to the myocytes, and increases cardiac work for perfusion of the highly vascularized fatty tissue.

DCM caused by toxic agents

- Alcohol is one of the most frequent causes of DCM in westernized countries. While moderate consumption increases HDL and decreases BP, excessive consumption may affect the heart *directly,* through myocyte toxicity, with inflammation and fibrosis; and *indirectly,* alcohol causing HTN and vitamin B1 deficiency, both deleterious to the myocardium. The onset of alcoholic CMP does not require prolonged consumption; even a binge is sufficient to cause HF and life-threatening arrhythmia ("the holiday heart syndrome"). Alcoholic CMP may also cause atrial arrhythmia (especially AF or flutter). A high index of suspicion is required, as symptoms tend to be insidious, and the patients often dissimulate them, due to social stigma. The treatment is nonspecific, in addition to vitamin B1 supplements and complete abstinence. The latter may be problematic, but if achieved, even advanced LV dysfunction may improve spectacularly (especially if the history of alcohol abuse is relatively brief).

- Stimulants: cocaine causes coronary spasm, myocardial ischemia, and chronic tachycardia; Amphetamines may cause CMP, acute MI, HF, or arrhythmia.

- Adriamycin (Doxorubicine) is a cytostatic used in breast, bone, stomach, and thyroid cancer, leukemia, etc. Its main toxicity is cardiac, manifesting as dilatation and global systolic dysfunction immediately after treatment or as late as 2–3 years subsequently. (Late onset portends poor prognosis.) Fortunately, LV involvement is generally gradual. Follow-up is performed by nuclear MUGA scan. The following findings require treatment discontinuation: LVEF <45%; >20% LEVF decrease, even if the final value is above 45%; >10% LVEF decrease, if the posttreatment LVEF is <55%. The major determinant of cardiotoxicity is the total administered dose (danger in total doses >400 mg/m^2 of body surface). Cardiotoxicity is generally irreversible. A more recent Adriamycin preparation may be associated to lower cardiotoxicity.

- Other: trastuzumab, a monoclonal antibody used in breast cancer, also causes cardiotoxicity, which is probably reversible. *Rosiglitazone,* an antidiabetic, is linked to an increased incidence of death and of HF. While the recently published RECORD study seems to have exonerated Rosiglitazone, the safety profile of this agent is still not clearly understood. *Pioglitazone,* another thiazolidinedione, has a better cardiovascular safety profile.

DCM caused by infiltrative diseases

- Sarcoidosis is an immunological disease characterized by small inflammatory nodules (granulomas), most often in the lungs and the lymph nodes, but occasionally involving the heart. Cardiac sarcoidosis typically presents as DCM (occasionally, RCM). The signs and symptoms are those of HF, in addition to extracardiac signs of sarcoidosis. *Lab tests: EKG:* possible arrhythmia and conduction disturbances; *chest X-ray:* pulmonary and mediastinal lymph node involvement; *echo:* regional hypokinesia, not following a coronary distribution; occasionally, a typical "speckled" ("snowstorm") myocardial texture; thinning or thickening of the myocardial walls (especially the IVS); RV dilatation (secondary to the sarcoidosis-related PAH; cor pulmonale is the most frequent cardiac complication of sarcoidosis); *nuclear scan* may show perfusion defects not following a coronary distribution; and *myocardial biopsy* shows typical granulomas. Most patients do not require treatment, but if they do, this typically consists of cortisone (Prednisone), with or without associated immunosuppressive agents.
- Hemochromatosis (hyperabsorbtion of iron in the intestine and deposition in the myocardium)

or *hemosiderosis* (transfusional iron overload); *type IV glycogen storage disease,* etc.

DCM caused by physical agents, exposure to high altitudes: see Chap. 12.

DCM caused by neuromuscular disorders: muscular dystrophy (Erb, Duchenne, etc.) is characterized by progressive muscle weakness, severe cases causing death by diaphragm paralysis. A muscle by itself, the myocardium may also be affected (dilated, or occasionally hypertrophic CMP). The diagnosis and treatment are those of HF.

Peripartum CMP is a condition characterized by global LV systolic dysfunction in the last month of pregnancy or in the first 5 months afterward. Its frequency in the US is of 1/1,000–4,000 live births, but may be much higher in other areas of the world. The cause is unknown, but autoimmune and toxic mechanisms (related to pregnancy-specific metabolites) are suspected. Risk factors include previous similar episodes as well as obesity or malnutrition, especially in alcoholics and smokers. It manifests as typical HF, with diffuse LV systolic dysfunction on echo. Many cases are only mild/moderate and self-limiting, but may recur on subsequent pregnancies. The treatment is supportive, and extreme cases may require a transplant.

LV noncompaction is a relatively rare form of CMP, where the LV has an unusual, trabeculated appearance. Other CHD can be associated. This condition progresses over time to DCM.

DCM of high-output states: see Sect. 4.1.

4.2.2 Hypertrophic Cardiomyopathy

Hypertrophic cardiomyopathy is characterized by excessive LV wall thickening, either idiopathic, or due to increased SVR (increased afterload due to HTN or AS). LVH can be symmetrical or preferentially involve a specific wall. The hypertrophic muscle has impaired relaxation (diastolic dysfunction) and is ischemic, since angiogenesis does not keep up with myocyte hypertrophy. *The symptoms and signs* are those of the underlying disease and of HFPEF (in advanced stages, systolic HF is superimposed); asymmetric hypertrophy has specific manifestations (see below). *The treatment* is that of the underlying disease and of HF; in the frequent case of HTN-related HCM, much of the treatment overlaps. Optimal treatment improves symptoms and promotes reverse remodeling of the heart.

4.2.2.1 Idiopathic HCM: Definition, Mechanisms, and Particularities

Idiopathic HCM is genetically determined through inheritance or random mutation.

- As opposed to increased-afterload HCM, it is generally asymmetric, involving mainly the upper IVS. A form mainly involving the LV apex (Yamaguchi's CMP) is relatively frequent (<20% of cases) in, but is not limited to, Japanese people. This form is identified by echo; by EKG (giant negative T waves), and by genetic screening. In addition to HFPEF and arrhythmia, these patients are also at risk of apical MI and aneurysm. Overall, however, the risk is lower than with septal hypertrophy, and this is considered a relatively benign disease.

- It not only represents a change in ventricular thickness, but also disrupts the normal myocyte alignment ("myocardial disarray"), causing abnormal electrical activity and arrhythmia. (HCM is especially known as the main cause of SCD in young athletes). In fact, as opposed to DCM, which involves substantial LV dilatation, some patients with potentially lethal HCM have only modest LVH.

- It may cause flow obstruction from the LV into the aorta, (obstructive idiopathic HCM or HOCM, seen in about 25% of patients), or be nonobstructive. Obstruction can be absent at rest and appear with the Valsalva maneuver (forcibly exhaling against a closed airway) due to a decrease in LV volume. The intraventricular obstruction has earned this disease several acronyms (IHSS=idiopathic hypertrophic subaortic stenosis; HOCM=hypertrophic obstructive CMP).

- It virtually always associates with MV abnormalities, including MR and systolic anterior motion (SAM) of the anterior mitral leaflet, which progresses in midsystole to approximate the IVS, causing obstruction. For many years believed to be due to "suction" of the MV towards the hypertrophic IVS (Venturi phenomenon), SAM is in fact due to abnormal papillary muscle insertion (the papillary muscles tether the mitral leaflets). The septal "bulge" intensifies this phenomenon.

- As with secondary HCM, it is especially affected by the onset of AF, due to loss of the atrial kick. AF is generally a marker of advanced disease.

- As with secondary HCM, the hypertrophic myocardium is relatively ischemic, as angiogenesis cannot keep up with myocyte hypertrophy.

4.2.2.2 The Symptoms of Idiopathic HCM

The symptoms of idiopathic HCM are those of HF, sometimes associating angina-like chest pain and/or light-headedness, syncope, or SCD. There is no linear relationship between symptoms and the magnitude of hypertrophy or of LVOT obstruction; that obstruction does, however, contribute to symptoms, is demonstrated by the favorable effect of septal resection in suitable candidates. In patients with HCM, the onset of AF generally causes clinical deterioration, due to loss of the atrial kick; with rapid HR, diastole is shortened, limiting the time for ventricular filling, a process already disturbed by the impaired ventricular relaxation. Episodes of AF are best treated by electrical cardioversion, and chronic AF benefits from β-blocker or CCB therapy. AV ablation and DDD pacing is an alternative in patients who cannot tolerate loss of the atrial kick.

Risk factors for SCD in idiopathic HCM

- Young age (<30 years) at diagnosis
- Personal or family history of aborted SCD or unexplained syncope
- Sustained AT, VT, or bradyarrhythmia
- IVS thickness >3 cm (normal: 9–11 mm)
- Hypotension on physical exertion
- Specific genetic mutations

The poor prognosis is dramatically changed by ICD implantation. HCM with minimal or no symptoms and nonhigh LVOT gradients has a better prognosis.

4.2.2.3 The Physical Findings in Idiopathic HCM

The physical findings in idiopathic HCM are those of HF, with the addition of a late-systolic murmur caused by the dynamic LVOT obstruction; the murmur intensifies with Valsalva and must not be mistaken for the coexisting systolic murmur of MR, heard over the mitral area and starting with the onset of systole. *Pulsus bisferiens* consists of a "double-impact" pulse wave (normal early- and late-systolic amplitude, mid-systolic decrease).

4.2.2.4 Workup

EKG demonstrates nonspecific LVH; *echo* findings (Fig. 4.3) include septal or apical hypertrophy, SAM, MR, and a late-systolic LVOT flow velocity increase giving the Doppler tracing a particular "dagger" shape,

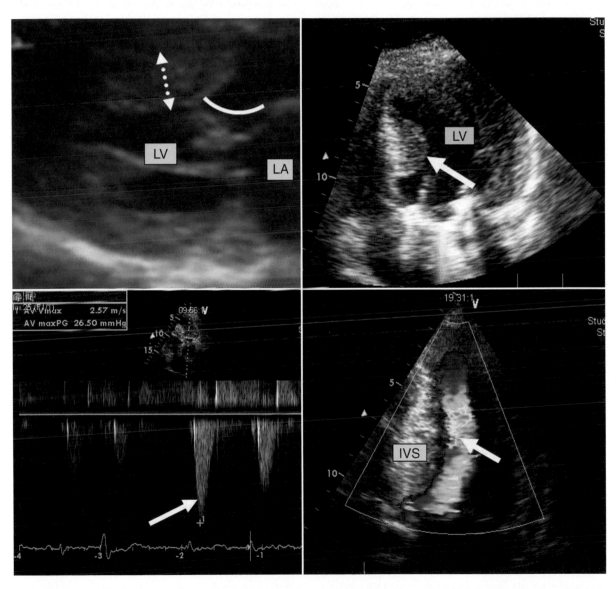

Fig. 4.3 HOCM. *Upper left*: severe IVS hypertrophy and "bending" of the anterior MV leaflet to approximate the IVS (SAM); *upper right*: alcohol septostomy was attempted, but did not succeed to remove the subvalvular stenosis; *lower left*: CW Doppler shows an increased subvalvular gradient, with a characteristic "dagger" shape, as opposed to the rounded shape of transvalvular aortic flow (Ch. 5). Additional confirmation that this is, indeed, subvalvular flow is provided by the small 2D "pilot image" in the *upper portion* of the echo panel. The gradient is higher in one of the beats (the one actually being measured) than in other beats as can be seen from the EKG monitor lead. This beat is the first beat after a VPB; due to the compensatory pause (prolonged diastole), LV filling, contractility, intracavitary flow, and ultimately, intracavitary gradient are increased; *lower right*: mid-LV gradient (brightest color flow, *arrow*, at the midseptal level)

that helps differentiate it from the Doppler tracing reflecting MR. Importantly, many patients with familial HCM have nonhomogenous distribution of the abnormal myocardium, which can be easily missed by conventional echo. This distribution is not seen with secondary LVH, making a strong argument for *cardiac MRI* in patients at risk for HCM. *Cardiac catheterization,* with a catheter in the LV and one in the aorta, shows a disproportionate increase in LVOT pressure (as compared to the aorta) in the beat following a PVC (post-PVC beats have a higher stroke volume, increasing the dynamic obstruction); *genetic testing* is important both for the patient (identifying the risk for SCD) and for their offspring (identifying mutations in the patient's asymptomatic children or parents, to single them out for follow-up).

4.2.2.5 Therapy

Medical Therapy

Patients with absent or mild symptoms do not require treatment. In more severe cases, the drugs of choice are β-blockers, to decrease myocardial contractility and obstruction and counteract ischemia. Alternatively, Verapamil 480 mg/day may be used to depress myocardial contractility and improve relaxation. Disopyramide can be used to decrease SAM, MR, and LVOT obstruction. Association with β-blockers is reccomended, to avoid enhanced AV conduction and high ventricular rates in case of superimposed AF or flutter. Combining β-blockers and CCB is not recommended, due to the risk of bradycardia and pulmonary edema. HF is treated as usual. Caution must be exercised in using diuretics and Digitalis as these agents decrease LV systolic volume and increase obstruction.

Interventional Therapy

Interventional therapy aims at relieving LVOT obstruction, either by removal of a part of the septum, or by permanent pacing, to counteract the functional mechanism of dynamic obstruction. *The surgical approach* consists of LVOT enlargement by septal myotomy/myectomy (the Morrow procedure). A retrospective analysis has found long-term survival to be no different from that of the general population. *MV replacement* can be considered in patients with relatively mild LVH and abnormalities of the mitral apparatus. *Alcohol ablation,*

a percutaneous modality of septal "shrinkage," involves instillation of ethanol into the first and/or second septal perforator coronary arteries, after preliminary definition of the corresponding myocardial territory by myocardial contrast echo. This controlled infarction effectively relieves LVOT obstruction, but may associate with large anterior MI or complete AVB. The procedure is therefore generally reserved to patients who are not candidates for surgical myectomy. *Dual-chamber pacing* has been suggested as an additional option in drug-resistant, surgery-ineligible patients, to create a slight dyssynchrony between the IVS and the LV free wall. Depolarization and contraction involve the RV first, including the septum, which will retract as the anterior mitral leaflet progresses towards it. This decreases the dynamic obstruction. However, the true efficacy of this method is unclear, and it is generally used as a less preferred option. *Cardiac transplant* is the last-resort option for otherwise intractable cases.

4.2.2.6 Secondary HCM

Secondary HCM differs from primary HCM by the generally uniform pattern of LVH, the absence of SAM, and the absence of MR, except for late, "burnt-out" cases, when cardiac dilatation and functional MR ensue. Secondary HCM is generally diagnosed and treated according to the underlying disorder. In hypertensive CMP, myocardial damage starts as LVH and diastolic dysfunction. In later stages, cardiac dilatation ensues. As with primary HCM, the myocardium is relatively ischemic. HTN treatment (especially with ACEI) substantially improves HF symptoms, and may partly reverse LVH and other cardiac remodeling. AS-related HCM is discussed in Chap 5. In the elderly, myocardial hypertrophy may present as a "sigmoid septum," a distinctive bulge of the proximal IVS, which may occasionally cause obstruction or SAM and MR; or as severe concentric LVH, with decreased LV diameter and severe diastolic dysfunction. As even in normal elderly, the mitral E and A wave velocities are usually disturbed (A ≥E), the latter may be difficult to quantify by conventional Doppler.

4.2.2.7 Pseudo-HCM

Fabry's disease, a glycogen storage disease, may manifest as pseudo-HCM, obstructive or not. Specific enzyme replacement is available. *Mutations in the LAMP2 gene* are responsible for a form of CMP mimicking HOCM.

4.2.3 Restrictive CMP

"Restrictive physiology," "restrictive filling," "restrictive CMP"

- *"Restrictive physiology"* refers to LV filling at higher pressures, due to decreased LV compliance. This pattern is intrinsic to diastolic dysfunction, and causes typical changes of the transmitral blood flow (see above).
- *"Restrictive filling"* is (rather confusingly) the name set apart for a specific stage (i.e., the early stage) of the abnormal transmitral blood flow, as assessed by Doppler. Restrictive filling is seen in restrictive physiology, but not all the types/stages of restrictive physiology are designated as "restrictive filling."
- Finally, *"restrictive CMP"* designates severe restrictive physiology occurring in the absence of dilatation or hypertrophy. RCM can be idiopathic or secondary, mainly in patients with amyloidosis or endomyocardial fibrosis.

4.2.3.1 Idiopathic RCM

Idiopathic RCM is diagnosed after secondary RCM has been ruled out. It is the most infrequent type of CMP. Its manifestations and treatment are non-specific.

4.2.3.2 Secondary RCM

- *Cardiac amyloidosis,* a typical example of RCM, is also known as the "stiff heart syndrome." It consists of deposition of amyloid, a protein, between the myocytes, impairing LV diastolic function. This occurs either with multiple myeloma, ("primary amyloidosis"), or, less commonly, in chronic diseases, mainly inflammatory ("secondary amyloidosis"). A form of amyloidosis occasionally seen in the elderly is unrelated to any detectable underlying disease. *The clinical picture* is nonspecific. *Echo*

shows the typical restrictive LV filling pattern, and may occasionally demonstrate a particular "sparkling" texture of the myocardium or endocardium. The *EKG* may show rhythm and conduction disturbances (AF onset is especially deleterious, as it abolishes the atrial kick). Kidney, bone, or abdominal fat *biopsy* confirm amyloidosis as such, while cardiac involvement is diagnosed by myocardial biopsy. *The treatment* is that of HF and of the underlying disease. The prognosis is severe; most patients die within 2 years of diagnosis. Importantly, cardiac transplant is not an option in the most frequent form of amyloidosis (primary) due to widespread amyloid organ damage.

- *Loeffler's endocarditis,* a component of the hypereosinophilic syndrome, typically manifests in middle age, featuring eosinophilia, restrictive physiology, and mural thrombus, alongside nervous system and bone marrow involvement. The therapy is that of HF, supplemented with anticoagulation, corticosteroids, and antineoplastic agents, including tyrosine kinase inhibitors or hydroxyurea. Endocardiectomy may be necessary for advanced fibrosis.
- *Endomyocardial fibrosis,* a rare condition, consists of abnormal endocardial scarring that penetrates the myocardium and causes typical restrictive physiology. The treatment is anti-inflammatory, and in case of failure, surgical (removal of scar tissue).

4.2.4 Primary RV CMP

- *Arrhythmogenic RV CMP (ARVC)* is a cause of life-threatening ventricular arrhythmia, accounting for 15–20% of SCD in the young, especially in males (higher percentages are reported in Italy). ARVC is genetically transmitted, but may skip generations. It usually first manifests in adolescence, as syncope or SCD, most frequently under physical exertion. Additional symptoms include RV, and later on, biventricular failure and occasional PE. The diagnosis is based on workup in patients with syncope or in the asymptomatic offspring of known patients. Currently, there is no available genetic test. *Workup: EKG:* 50% of patients exhibit the "epsilon wave," a small positive deflection at the end of the QRS complex; this wave is usually detected on SAECG. Other EKG findings include: inverted T waves in V1–V3, a nonspecific finding which is actually normal in children; RBBB; and ventricular arrhythmia (VT, VF). *Echo* shows an enlarged and diffusely hypokinetic RV, with a paper-thin free wall, and functional TR (by tricuspid annulus dilatation). Echo can miss the diagnosis of ARVC. *MRI* visualizes the dilated and thinned-out RV (noninvasive procedure of choice). *Right ventriculography* displays diffuse hypokinesia and RV dilatation. *Myocardial biopsy* shows fatty or fibro-fatty RV infiltration, but false positive (nonspecific fatty infiltration) and false negatives (patchy involvement) are frequent. RV biopsy carries the risk of tamponade in patients with severe thinning of the RV wall. *Medical therapy* is based on Sotalol, with Amiodarone as an alternative. *Catheter ablation* is not always successful; moreover, the disease often recurs after ablation; *ICD,* an "obvious" solution, carries the risk of perforation; occasional scarring and infiltration around the ICD lead may cause suboptimal sensing of arrhythmia and decreased shock effectiveness. As there is no specific genetic test, the routine workup in the offspring includes EKG techniques (resting tracing, Holter, SAECG, and stress test), echo, and cardiac MRI.

- *Uhl's anomaly* is a rare form of CMP, usually manifesting in early childhood as RV failure. The RV wall is paper-thin, hence the eponym, "parchment heart disease." This condition is usually refractory to therapy, and may require transplant.

Bibliography

Guidelines

The Task Force For The Diagnosis And Treatment Of Acute And Chronic Heart Failure 2008 Of The European Society Of Cardiology. Developed in collaboration with the heart failure association of the ESC (HFA) and endorsed by the European Society Of Intensive Care Medicine (ESICM). *Eur Heart J.* 2008;29:2388-2442.

Jessup M, Abraham WT, Casey DE, Feldman AM, Francis GS, Ganiats TG, Konstam MA, Mancini DM, Rahko PS, Silver MA, Stevenson LW, Yancy CW, writing on behalf of the 2005 Guideline Update for the Diagnosis and Management of Chronic Heart Failure in the Adult Writing Committee. 2009 Focused update: ACCF/AHA guidelines for the diagnosis and management of heart failure in adults: a report of the American College of Cardiology Foundation/American Heart Association Task Force on Practice Guidelines. *Circulation.* 2009;119:1977-2016.

Suggested Reading

The Beta-Blocker Evaluation of Survival Trial Investigators. A trial of the beta-blocker bucindolol in patients with advanced chronic heart failure. *N Engl J Med.* 2001;344:1659-1667.

The CIBIS-II Investigators. The Cardiac Insufficiency Bisoprolol Study II (CIBIS-II): a randomised trial. *Lancet.* 1999;353(9146):9-13.

Pfeffer M, Swedberg K, Granger C, et al. Effects of candesartan on mortality and morbidity in patients with chronic heart failure: the CHARM-Overall programme. *Lancet.* 2003;362(9386):759-766.

Pitt B, Poole-Wilson PA, Segal R, et al. Effect of losartan compared with captopril on mortality in patients with symptomatic heart failure: randomised trial–the Losartan Heart Failure Survival Study ELITE II. *Lancet.* 2000;355(9215):1582-1587.

The SOLVD Investigators. Effect of enalapril on survival in patients with reduced left ventricular ejection fractions and congestive heart failure. *N Engl J Med.* 1991;325(5):293-302.

Taylor AL, Ziesche S, Yancy C, et al.; African-American Heart Failure Trial Investigators. Combination of isosorbide dinitrate and hydralazine in blacks with heart failure. *N Engl J Med.* 2004;351(20):2049-2057.

Chung ES, Leon AR, Tavazzi L, et al. Results of the predictors of response to CRT (PROSPECT) trial. *Circulation.* 2008; 117:2608-2616.

Moss AJ, Hall WJ, Cannom DS, et al.; for the MADIT-CRT Trial Investigators. Cardiac-resynchronization therapy for the prevention of heart-failure events *N Engl J Med.* 2009; 361:1329-1338.

The MERIT-HF Investigators. Effect of metoprolol CR/XL in chronic heart failure: Metoprolol CR/XL randomised intervention trial in congestive heart failure (MERIT-HF). *Lancet* 1999;353(9169):2001-2007.

Packer M, Coats AJ, Fowler MB, et al. Effect of carvedilol on survival in severe chronic heart failure. *N Engl J Med.* 2001;344(22):1651-1658.

Valvular Heart Disease

5

Contents

5.1 General Remarks

5.1.1 Clinical Diagnosis and Work-Up of VHD

VHD (stenosis, insufficiency, or combined lesions) is a major class of heart disease; if severe and left untreated, it may lead to irreversible myocardial damage and death. VHD may exert its deleterious effect both by a direct decrease of stroke volume (e.g., with critical AS or acute severe MR) and by the ultimately deleterious adaptive cardiac changes it produces (ventricular hypertrophy and dilatation, atrial dilatation, and functional or organic PAH). While preventing symptoms despite severe valvular dysfunction, these changes may lead to irreversible myocardial damage. The different types of VHD may cause systolic and diastolic LV dysfunction and failure; infective endocarditis (IE); PAH; AF or flutter and thromboembolic complications; absolute and relative myocardial ischemia and a tendency to develop larger MI; and the iatrogenic complications related to mechanical valvular prostheses. Most cases of chronic VHD have an insidious evolution, occasionally leading to late diagnosis and increased morbidity and mortality; therefore, careful routine physical examination remains

G.A. Adelmann, *Cardiology Essentials in Clinical Practice*,
DOI: 10.1007/978-1-84996-305-3_5, © Springer-Verlag London Limited 2011

the main screening modality for VHD. The typical *clinical sign* of VHD is a systolic or diastolic heart murmur. Systolic murmurs reflect increased flow velocity through a normal or pathologic connection (cardiac valve, fistula, VSD, etc.) between chambers under different pressures. Thus, high blood flow velocity due to either normal (exercise, pregnancy, etc.) or pathologic states (valve stenosis) may cause a systolic murmur. Most systolic murmurs associate a low probability of underlying disease ("innocent" murmurs, transmitted through the thin chest wall of younger patients); systolic murmurs only require work-up if they have characteristics suggesting increased severity (long, loud murmurs, murmurs associating a thrill, etc.). Conversely, diastolic murmurs are most often pathologic and do require work-up. Continuous murmurs may be innocent (venous hums, mammary souffles) or pathologic (e.g., coronary fistula). The auscultatory characteristics of murmurs include timing in the cardiac cycle, intensity, location, radiation, and quality. Finer characterization distinguishes different murmur configurations (crescendo, decrescendo, crescendo–decrescendo, or plateau). *The timing* of a systolic murmur is important, most innocent murmurs being midsystolic; holo or late-systolic murmurs are often pathologic. Of note, the length of the murmur per se may be related to the severity of the underlying condition (e.g., longer murmur in severe AS) or not connected to it (early systolic murmur in acute MR; early- and midsystolic murmur only, rather than holosystolic murmur, in large VSD). Likewise, *the intensity* of the murmur may be directly related to the severity (i.e., loud systolic murmur in severe chronic MR), unrelated to it (loud systolic murmur in hemodynamically insignificant aortic sclerosis, which may be mistaken for AS), or inversely related (loud systolic murmur in small, i.e., nonsevere VSD) to the severity of the underlying heart disease. Usually, the intensity is graded between grades I and VI (grade I = barely audible; grade ≥ IV = associates a palpatory thrill; grade VI = heard even with the stethoscope not immediately touching the skin). *The radiation* of a mitral systolic murmur is to the left axilla; of an AS murmur, to the left carotid artery; and of a small VSD, to the entire precordium. In contrast, diastolic murmurs tend not to radiate. *The quality* is described as musical (MR murmur due to papillary muscle dysfunction); blowing (other chronic MR); high-pitched and faint (AI); harsh/rasping (AS); rumbling (low-pitch

murmur of MS); or machine-like ("to-and-fro murmur," e.g., with PDA). Occasionally, different interventions are used to alter the intensity of cardiac murmurs, as reviewed in Table 5.1. Additional diagnostic findings in VHD pertain to the heart sounds, as reviewed in Table 5.2.

The work-up of VHD mainly includes *echo*, able to diagnose and quantitate both the valvular dysfunction and its impact on the myocardial and pulmonary vascular function. In addition, echo is the diagnostic method of choice for IE, a major complication of VHD; *Cardiac catheterization* provides information of both imaging and nonimaging nature (visualization of ventricular function and of valvular regurgitation; demonstration of transvalvular pressure tracings). Cardiac catheterization allows calculation of the AV and MV area (relevant in AS, MS), based on Gorlin's equation. This factors in the *CO* (measured with a Swan-Ganz catheter, using Fick's thermodilution principle); the *pressure gradient*, calculated based on the directly-measured LV and aortic pressure (for AS) or PCWP (for MS); *the diastolic filling period* (seconds/beat); the systolic ejection period (seconds/beat); and the *HR* (bpm). Calculating stenotic valve area by Gorlin's formula is influenced by the coexistence of regurgitant lesions, as shown in Table 5.3.

Cardiac catheterization is usually not routinely recommended in VHD, but may be required to clarify disparities between the clinical and the echo manifestations. *Chest X-ray* shows dilatation of the different cardiac chambers, valve calcification, pulmonary congestion, PA, or aortic root dilatation. *Exercise testing* is useful for assessing disparities between the clinical symptoms (severe) and the echo findings (mild); this is commonly the case in combined VHD. The pitfalls of these different methods are discussed in the relevant sections. *Cardiac CT and MRI* have a relatively limited utility, with the exception of VHD associated to CHD and for quantification of pulmonic insufficiency (PI) and of its impact on the RV size and function.

5.1.2 Treatment of VHD: General Principles

According to the patient's condition, the treatment of VHD consists in one or more of the following:

Table 5.1 Clinical maneuvers facilitating the differential diagnosis of cardiac murmurs

	Increase	Mechanism	Decrease	Mechanism
Inspiration	(1) Right-sided murmurs; (2) HOCM, MVP	(1) Increased venous return due to negative thoracic pressure in inspirium; (2) HOCM, MVP: decreased LV volume in inspiration increases intraventricular obstruction and degree of prolapse	Left-sided murmurs (except for HOCM, MVP)	Decreased venous return due to negative thoracic pressure in inspirium
Valsalva	HOCM; MVP	Valsalva decreases preload, increasing dynamic LV obstruction and the degree of valvular prolapse	Most other murmurs	Decreased LV preload → decreased transvalvular flow → decreased murmurs
Exercise	Most murmurs	Increased transvalvular flow		
Positional changes	Standing: HOCM, MVP	Decreased LV volume → increased intraventricular obstruction and valve prolapse	Standing: most other murmurs	Decreased LV volume → decreased flow →decreased murmur
	Squatting or passive leg raising: most murmurs except for those of HOCM, MVP	Increased preload → increased flow → increased valvular murmurs, but decreased intraventricular obstruction and valvular prolapse	Squatting or passive leg raising: HOCM, MVP	See under "increase" (second column)
Pharmacological interventions	Amyl nitrite: AS (in initial hypotensive phase); MS, right-sided lesions	Decreased peripheral resistance → increased systolic flow → increased murmur	MR, VSD, AI	Decreased peripheral resistance → decreased regurgitation → decreased murmur

- Alleviating the symptoms of HF
- Repairing or replacing the diseased valve
- Antithrombotic medication, where indicated (AF, prosthetic heart valve, MS with a previous embolic event; target INR 2.5, range 2–3)
- IE prophylaxis
- Prophylaxis against rheumatic fever

The follow-up of patients with VHD and prosthetic valves is reviewed in Table 5.4.

5.1.3 Rheumatic Fever

The acute phase develops in approximately 3% of untreated patients with group A β-hemolytic Streptococcus infection, such as strep throat or scarlet fever. While the overall incidence in westernized countries has decreased over the past decades, rheumatic fever remains an important cause of morbidity and mortality elsewhere. The disease becomes clinically apparent approximately 20 days after the acute episode and may affect the heart, joints, skin, and brain. The *chronic phase* is apparent decades after the acute phase and mainly affects the cardiac valves and (with the MV and TV) the subvalvular apparatus as well. This involves progressive fibrosis, with leaflet thickening, commissural fusion, and chordal shortening and thickening, causing valve stenosis or insufficiency. The pathogenesis is based on an autoimmune reaction due to the similarity of bacterial and human cellular wall protein components. In the acute phase, the diagnosis is based on *the Jones criteria*, including

Major criteria

- Migratory polyarthritis
- Carditis, manifesting as HF, pericarditis, or a new heart murmur
- Subcutaneous nodules in the wrist, elbow, or knee
- Erythema marginatum, a rash typically clearing in the middle
- Sydenham's chorea, or St. Vitus' dance, consisting in rapid involuntary movements of the face and arms

Minor criteria

- Fever
- Arthralgia
- Elevated ESR and CRP levels

Table 5.2 Other clinical findings in VHD

	S1[a]	S2[b]	Other[c]
AS	–	Soft or absent aortic component of S2 in severe AS	Early aortic systolic ejection sound in bicuspid AV; slow-rising, diminished pulse ("parvus et tardus") in severe AS; ejection click in noncalcified valve
AI	–	–	Increased pulse pressure (several peripheral signs; see text)
MS/TS	Accentuated, due to closure of rigid valves; if the valves are calcified, S1 is soft or inaudible	–	Opening snap, in the absence of severe valvular calcification
MR/TR	Diminished		Midsystolic click, if MVP
Other	Physiologically split in up to 70% of normals; pathological split in RBBB; RV pacing; Ebstein's anomaly; TS (slower RA/RV pressure equalization, hence delayed TV closure)	Fixed splitting in ASD; the split is variable with respiration in MR (faster emptying of LV, hence earlier closure of the AV) and RBBB (delayed RV contraction, thus delayed PV closure); paradoxical split in LBBB (AV closes later than PV, the reverse of normal)	Ejection click in the pulmonic area and at the left sternal border during expiration, with PS

[a]S1 is caused by the sudden block of reverse blood flow due to closure of the AV valves (MV, TV); it is composed of M1 and T1
[b]S2 is caused by the closure of the AV and pulmonary valve at the beginning of ventricular diastole; it is composed of components A2 and P2
[c]S3 is caused by rapid early filling of the ventricles and is benign in the young and in trained athletes, but may reemerge later on as a sign of DCM, when it signifies sudden tensing of the chordae ("S3 gallop"); S4 is sometimes audible in healthy children and trained athletes, or pathologically, in LVH patients in NSR (presystolic or atrial gallop)

Table 5.3 The influence of valvular regurgitation on AV and MV area measurement by the Gorlin formula[a]

	Assessing MV area in MS patients	Assessing AV area in AS patients
AI	Underestimation of valve area, due to shortening of the diastolic filling period[b]	Underestimation of valve area, due to increased LV/aorta gradient[b]
MR	Underestimation of valve area, due to MR-related LA/LV gradient[c] increase	Overestimation of the valve area, since the LV partly decompresses into the LA[d]
TR	Underestimation of CO,[e] and thus of MV area	Underestimation of CO, and thus of AV area

[a]Valve area = CO × diastolic filling period (for MV) or systolic ejection period (for AV) × HR/constant × √ pressure gradient
[b]As the LV fills not only through the MV, but through the AV as well
[c]The LA fills not only from the pulmonary veins (in systole and diastole), but from the LV as well (in systole). The impact of MR is decreased by coexisting LA dilatation
[d]This shortens the systolic ejection period and the net forward flow through the AV
[e]The delay in progression of the cold saline to the PA is misinterpreted as decreased CO

- Leukocytosis
- Heart block
- Elevated or rising ASLO or DNAase titer
- A previous episode of rheumatic fever

Rheumatic fever is diagnosed in the presence of two major criteria, or one major criterion plus two minor criteria.

Primary prevention of rheumatic fever relies on proper diagnosis of streptococcal infection. The "rapid strep test" has a high positive predictive value for streptococcal angina. While a negative test does not allow to confidently rule out the diagnosis, confirmation by culture is required in children only, as both "strep throat" and de novo rheumatic fever are much less frequent in adults. The treatment of streptococcal infection may include: (a) a single IM dose of Benzathine Penicillin G (preferred in low-compliance patients), 600,000 U in children <27 kg (60 lb), 1,200,000 U otherwise; (b) multiple oral doses of Penicillin over 10 days, thus: Penicillin V 250 mg b.i.d. or t.i.d. in children, 500 mg b.i.d. or t.i.d. otherwise; (c) erythromycin (in

Table 5.4 Follow-up of patients with VHD[a,b]

	Mild	Moderate	Severe
AS	*Clinical*: yearly; *Echo*: as required based on clinical findings[b]	As with severe AS	First *clinical and echo* reevaluation at 6 months; subsequent reevaluations at 6–12 months, as dictated by clinical and/or echo progression
AI	*Clinical*: yearly; *Echo*: every 2 years	As with mild AI	*Clinical and echo*: every 6 months, if EF and LV diameter show significant changes; yearly, after stabilization
MS	Every few years	*Clinical, echo*: yearly	*Clinical, echo*: yearly
MR	Every few years	If asymptomatic, *clinical*: yearly; *Echo*: every 2 years	*Clinical*: every 6 years; *Echo*: yearly
Prosthetic heart valves	First assessment immediately after surgery, if carried out under echo supervision; assessment at 6–12 weeks after surgery (if not feasible, at the end of the hospital stay); *clinical* F/U yearly, *echo* F/U as required; yearly echo F/U in patients with biological prosthetic valves after the fifth year		
Other[c]	Patients after PMV followed up just like asymptomatic MS patients		

[a]With any VHD, a sudden change in the clinical status (dyspnea, HF, suspicion of IE, etc.) should prompt immediate clinical and echo assessment

[b]If at any point the indications for surgery are reached, this should be carried out; the follow-up then crosses over to that of postintervention VHD patients

[c]There are no clear-cut guidelines for the frequency of follow-up in patients with tricuspid and PV disease (see the relevant sections)

case of allergy to Penicillin), 20–40 mg/kg/day, 2–4 times a day (upper dose if Erythromycin estolate) for 10 days; of note, the use of Erythromycin is being deemphasized, as resistant Streptococcus species have emerged. (d) Azithromycin over 5 days, 500 mg on the first day and 250 mg q.d. for the next days. Once-daily Amoxicillin 1,500 mg q.d. (or 750 mg if body weight ≤30 kg) is an acceptable alternative to IM Penicillin.

Treatment of acute rheumatic fever includes Aspirin 100 mg/kg/day (for 6–8 weeks, until clinical manifestations and inflammatory markers normalize), and if carditis is present, corticosteroids (Prednisone 2 mg/kg/day PO for 2–4 week), to abate inflammation and prevent valvular complications. If steroids are used, salicylates must be maintained for an additional 2–4 weeks after steroid discontinuation.

Secondary prophylaxis of rheumatic fever is essential, as the tendency of recurrence is very high, and if carditis was a component of the initial picture, it, too, tends to recur. The recommended agents include Benzathine Penicillin G (1,200,000 U IM q.4 weeks, or q.3 weeks in high-risk patients, i.e., those with carditis and those living in economically disadvantaged areas); Penicillin V PO 250 mg b.i.d., or Sulfadiazine, 0.5 mg q.d. for patients weighing ≤27 kg (60 lb), or 1 g q.d. otherwise; or, for individuals allergic to Penicillin, Erythromycin 250 mg b.i.d. The duration of secondary

prevention is controversial, but should be (a) of >10 years since the last episode, and at least until age 40, or even lifelong, in patients with carditis; (b) of >5 years since the last episode, and at least until age 21, whichever is longer, in the absence of carditis.

5.2 Mitral Stenosis (MS)

5.2.1 General Remarks

MS prevents normal diastolic opening of the MV. It is mainly caused by rheumatic fever and affects women twice as often as it does men. Less frequently, MS is caused by congenital valvular malformations (observed mainly in infants and children) or mucopolysaccharidosis or is mimicked by -LA conditions such as myxoma, thrombus, or severe annular calcification.

MS: A Disease not Limited to the Valve Leaflets

MS involves various combinations of leaflet thickening and calcification, commissural and/or chordal fusion, and papillary muscle fibrosis. The chordae and papillary muscles are collectively known as the mitral apparatus.

The normal MV area is 4.0–5.0 cm². Stenosis generally only becomes symptomatic on exercise when the valve area reaches 2.5 cm², and at rest with areas <1.5 cm² (larger patients require higher flow and become symptomatic at relatively larger valve areas). The main pathophysiological impact of MS is an increase in the LA pressure and in the LA/LV diastolic pressure gradient. The LA distends gradually, as an adaptive mechanism aimed at decreasing the LA pressure and the transvalvular gradient. However, this mechanism only partly corrects the increased LA pressure, which propagates retrogradely to the pulmonary veins, resulting in increased pressure and decreased venous compliance, further accentuated by increased endothelin-1 secretion. The increased pressure also involves the pulmonary arterioles, initially by an active vasoconstrictive mechanism, followed by organic changes, including intimal hyperplasia and medial hypertrophy. These changes are collectively known as "the second barrier" in MS (the "first barrier" being the stenosis itself). This barrier allows the patient to remain asymptomatic for decades, but ultimately leads to PAH. Normal LV filling is impeded in case of increased transmitral flow or of shortened diastole; the increased LA and pulmonary venous pressure override the protection offered by the "second barrier," leading to dyspnea, up to pulmonary edema. This explains the initial onset of symptoms under physical stress. However, with further progression of MS (area <1.5 cm²), symptoms ensue at rest as well.

The time course of MS is slow, with a 20–40 year time lag between the initial episode of rheumatic fever and the first manifestations of the disease, and with an additional decade until the symptoms become disabling. In more than half of the patients, the symptoms are not progressive; if they are, however, the prognosis is grim, with a 10-year survival rate ≤15%. Most deaths are due to progressive pulmonary congestion, followed by systemic, or, less frequently, PE or IE. In the Western world, the age of presentation is usually in the fifth or sixth decade.

MS is graded according to the severity of valvular narrowing, the transvalvular gradient, and the PA pressure (Table 5.5). These parameters are generally interrelated, with occasional exceptions (e.g., patients with pulmonary vascular overreactivity and a degree of PAH disproportionate to the severity of the MS).

Table 5.5 Grading the severity of mitral stenosis (MS)

Severity	Valve area (cm²)	Gradient (mmHg)	sPAP (mmHg)
Mild	1.5–4.0	<5	30
Moderate	1.0–1.5	5–10	30–50
Severe	<1.0	>10	>50

5.2.2 MS: Diagnosis

Clinical picture: The classical symptoms of MS (dyspnea, pulmonary edema, fatigue) are caused by pulmonary congestion, initially under exercise-induced or other tachycardia (e.g., AF), and subsequently at rest. Other patients present with embolic events, or infrequently, with hemoptysis (rupture of distended pulmonary capillaries) or with hoarseness/dysphagia secondary to left recurrent laryngeal nerve or esophageal compression by the distended LA or PA. Hoarseness can also occur as a complication of surgery for MS. On auscultation, MS presents as an *accentuated first heart sound* (because of the increased closing force of the noncompliant MV leaflets; when the leaflets are very thickened and calcified, however, S1 decreases in intensity or disappears); an *opening snap* (OS), heard after the aortic component of S2, and due to the sudden tensing of the noncompliant mitral leaflets after completion of the diastolic opening excursion; a *low-pitched middiastolic rumble* (best heard in left lateral decubitus, and accentuated by exercise or amyl nitrate, which increase transmitral flow; the murmur is occasionally accompanied by a thrill); and a *presystolic murmur* (due to the increased flow corresponding to the atrial systole, only present in sinus rhythm). Pulmonary rhales, signs of right HF, a left parasternal heave (RVH due to PAH), and rarely today, a malar flush in patients with advanced disease and severe PAH may also be noted. AF develops in up to 40% of symptomatic MS patients. MS leads to dilatation and electrophysiological alteration of the LA; additionally, rheumatic disease leads to fibrosis of the atrial myocardium, also favoring the onset of AF. Therefore, even successful percutaneous mitral valvuloplasty (PMV) may not prevent AF, the best predictors of which are advanced age and increased LA dimensions.

The Clinical Signs of MS are Neither Specific, Nor Sensitive

The clinical signs above do not necessarily indicate MS (for instance, they may be present with mitral *obstruction* due to LA myxoma). Conversely, the absence of a murmur does not rule out MS and is, in fact, common in patients with severe PAH, low CO, and/or a heavily calcified, immobile MV.

Echo picture: As with all VHD, echo is the main diagnostic technique for MS. The techniques for obtaining the relevant data are reviewed in Table 5.6. Echo also identifies and quantifies coexisting valvular or nonvalvular cardiac pathology and assesses the feasibility of PMV (Wilkins' or Cormier's score – Tables 5.7 and 5.8). Of note, favorable scores are still compatible with noncandidacy for PMV, in case of more than mild MR, LA thrombus, or heavy commissural calcification (the latter, an important prognostic parameter, is not

Table 5.6 Echo assessment of MS

Method	MV area	MV gradient	Other data concerning the MV	Other data regarding the heart and pulmonary circulation
2(3)-D echo	Planimetry from the short axis[a]		*MV morphology*: valvular and subvalvular thickening (valve thickness >5 mm in diastole is abnormal), fusion, and calcification; mitral annular calcification (MAC); *MV function*: "doming" of the anterior leaflet in diastole ("hockey-stick" appearance), immobility of the posterior leaflet, decreased valvular flexibility; "fish-mouth" appearance of the MV in diastole	Coexisting VHD or LA enlargement; LA thrombus and the severity of coexisting MR are assessed by TEE. sPAP[b] (calculated from the TR velocity signal[c] is an indicator of MS severity)
Doppler	The diastolic pressure half-time method[d]	By calculating the TVI of the transmitral CWD signal	Increased E wave velocity, reflecting the increased LA/LV pressure gradient ("torrential" early LV filling)	Severity of associated valvular or nonvalvular cardiac disease
Combined Doppler and 2D assessment	The continuity equation[e]			
M-mode			Flattened descending slope of the early diastolic mitral leaflet motion[f]; leaflet thickening; the posterior leaflet motion is parallel, rather than a mirror image, to that of the anterior leaflet	Coexisting LA enlargement

[a]Problematic if the image quality is poor or in case of severe mitral annulus calcification
[b]Reevaluate every 1–2 years, or every 3 or 5 years in severe, moderate, and mild MS, respectively
[c]Using the modified Bernoulli's equation
[d]The more severe the stenosis, the longer it takes to the LA and LV pressures to equalize, expressed as a flatter CWD transmitral E wave deceleration slope. The time required for a 50% reduction in diastolic transmitral gradient is termed "pressure half-time" (PHT). MV area = 220/PHT (calculated automatically by the echo machine). Factors affecting transmitral gradient equalization (abnormal LA or LV compliance, associated AI or MR) or MV geometry (previous valvotomy) decrease the accuracy of this method. Decreased LV compliance and AI decrease the MV flow, causing underestimation of MS severity; MR increases MV flow → overestimation of MS severity. Beat-to-beat variability in AF requires averaging out of the results over 5–10 beats
[e]Blood flow through the MV = blood flow through the LVOT; as blood flow = sectional area × TVI (time-velocity integral of the blood flow, i.e., the area under the Doppler curve), MVA = LVOT area × LVOT TVI/MV TVI. The LVOT flow is assessed by PWD, and the MV flow, by CWD. The method is mainly affected by coexisting MR (MV flow > LVOT flow → underestimation of MV area) or AI (MV flow < LVOT flow → overestimation of MV area)
[f]Paralleling the prolonged deceleration time of the E wave on CWD

Table 5.7 The Wilkins score in MS

| MS grade | Mobility restriction | Thickening | | Calcification |
		Subvalvular	Leaflet	
1	Mild (only tips of leaflets are restr.)	Just underneath leaflets	<5-mm thickness[a]	Single area
2	Moderate (only tips of leaflets are restricted, but more severely than in grade 1)	≤1/3 of chord length	Thickened at margins <8 mm	Scattered areas on leaflet margins, midportion spared
3	Moderate-to-severe, but valve still moves forward in diastole	>1/3 of chord length; papillary muscles spared	Entire leaflet thickened <8 mm	Scattered areas on leaflet margins, midportion involved
4	Severe (absent or minimal forward valve motion in diastole)[a]	Papillary muscles involved	Entire leaflet thickened >8 mm	Extensive brightness involving most of leaflet tissue

[a]The normal thickness of the MV leaflets is <2 mm

assessed in the Wilkins' score). Finally, echo is useful in guiding PMV itself. Exercise echo may be required in patients with suggestive symptoms, in the presence of nonsevere MS and nonsevere PAH at rest (Fig. 5.1).

Diastolic and Systolic Motion of the MV: Beyond Terminology

In NSR, the normal MV has a biphasic anterior *diastolic* motion, the two phases corresponding to the E and A waves. This motion is assessed as a component of the Wilkins' score. On M-mode echo, only the motion of the anterior MV leaflet is toward the transducer ("anterior" motion), whereas the motion of the posterior leaflet is away from the transducer ("posterior motion"); one of the M-mode signs of MS is the "anterior" motion of this leaflet, i.e., parallel (rather than mirroring) the anterior leaflet, to which the posterior leaflet is tethered. Finally, a particular pattern of *systolic* anterior motion (SAM) is seen in HOCM patients.

Cormier's grading is a simplified version of Wilkins' score and defines three groups of patients, as shown in Table 5.8. The best results are seen in patients from Group 1.

Catheterization allows calculation of the MV area using Gorlin's formula and is useful in patients at risk for CAD and in whom intervention on the MV is indicated, or if there is *a discrepancy* between

Table 5.8 The Cormier score in MS

Finding	Group 1	Group 2	Group 3
Mitral leaflet involvement			
Pliability of the anterior leaflet	Good	Good	Any
Calcification of the MV[a]	No	No	Yes
Subvalvular involvement			
Chordal thickening	No	Yes	Any
Chordal length	≥10 mm	<10 mm	Any

[a]Assessed by fluoroscopy

- The symptomatic status and the noninvasive MS severity assessment
- The noninvasively derived MV area and gradient
- The assessed severity of MS and that of PAH (unexpectedly high PAH, requiring a formal study of the PA pressure and reactivity)

X-ray demonstrates

- LA dilatation (bulging of the posterior cardiac border on lateral chest X-ray; encroachment of the esophagus by a dilated LA, on barium swallow; double contour along the right inferior cardiac border)
- RA dilatation (bulging of the lower arch of the cardiac border on a PA film)
- RV dilatation (increased contact of the lower portion of the cardiac shadow and the sternum, on a lateral chest X-ray; leftward rotation of the heart, with "horizontalization" on the PA chest X-ray)

Fig. 5.1 CW Doppler in a patient with mitral stenosis (MS), to calculate the MV area and the transmitral gradient. Placing the cursor at the tip of the pressure curve automatically displays the deceleration slope and calculates valve area (first cycle). Manually tracing the transvalvular flow curve contour (second cycle) allows automatic calculation of the transvalvular gradient. The patient is in AF, and thus several measurements should be averaged (note the difference in shape between the two complexes being measured)

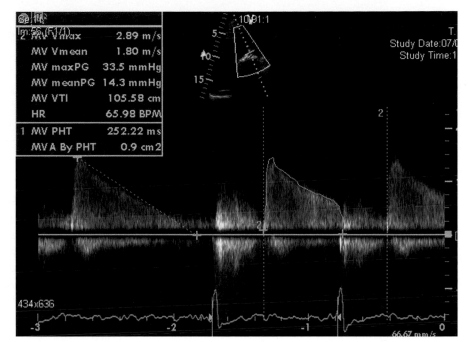

- MV calcification (white speckles on X-ray or fluoroscopy)
- Pulmonary congestion (see Chap. 4)
- Enlargement of the pulmonary trunk (bulging of the left middle cardiac arch on the PA chest X-ray)

The EKG demonstrates LA enlargement (P wave duration >0.12 s, notched P wave in the limb leads), RV enlargement (right axis deviation >90°, tall R waves in V1–V2, deep S-waves in V5–V6), and frequently, AF.

5.2.3 MS Therapy

MS therapy aims to correct the pathophysiological disturbances caused by the VHD, and if necessary, to relieve the stenosis itself. An additional concern is the prevention of complications (IE, thromboembolism) and, if relevant, of rheumatic fever recurrences.

5.2.3.1 Conservative Therapy

No therapy is required in *asymptomatic patients* in NSR, but with nonmild MS, excessive physical exertion must be avoided, to prevent pulmonary congestion resulting from increased transvalvular flow and gradient. Salt restriction is encouraged. In *symptomatic patients*, it must be kept in mind that pharmacological therapy is not a substitute for PMV or surgery in appropriate candidates. Commonly used drugs include diuretics and negative-chronotropic agents (β-blockers, nondihydropyridine CCB). Occasional increased bronchial reactivity is treated with inhaled corticosteroids (sympathomimetic agents may cause tachycardia and worsen symptoms). *AF* onset may cause flash pulmonary edema and death, even in asymptomatic patients, and is best treated by electrical cardioversion, although the chances of obtaining a stable NSR are low in the presence of more than mild LA enlargement. In PMV or valve replacement candidates, cardioversion is best carried out after the procedure, to enhance the chances of durable success. The indications for anticoagulation in AF are discussed in Chap. 6. *Significant PAH* is treated with NO, prostacyclin, or endothelin antagonists, usually after interventional relief of MS. *Anticoagulation* is indicated in patients with MS associated to AF, to a prior embolic event, or to LA thrombus and may also be considered in patients with severe MS and LA dilatation ($\geq$50 mm) or LA "smoke." *IE prophylaxis* is discussed in Sect. 5.13.

5.2.3.2 Interventional Therapy

Interventional therapy for pure MS is indicated in case of severe stenosis (MV area <1.5 cm^2), if the patient displays symptoms or signs of complications or is about to face hemodynamic challenges (major noncardiac surgery, pregnancy). *Absolute indications* include any case of MS that is symptomatic at rest or on mild exertion, but comorbidity (severe PAH or additional VHD) may cause symptoms at lesser degrees of MS severity. The converse is not true, as even severe MS may be clinically silent, especially in sedentary patients. Therefore, true asymptomatic status is defined as the absence of symptoms during exercise test (by the Bruce or modified Bruce protocol, or using Dobutamine); in patients in whom other clinical parameters (old age, comorbidity) dictate a sedentary life style anyway, this point may be moot. PMV, if feasible, is the default option, unless there is another compelling indication for open-heart surgery (e.g., severe CAD); in these patients, surgical valvuloplasty or MV replacement is indicated. *Relative indications* for intervention (valve replacement not indicated, but valvuloplasty may be warranted) generally refer to patients with ongoing or past complications, or at risk of hemodynamic decompensation.

As always, however, the decision to intervene is individually tailored. The common clinical scenarios are presented in Table 5.9.

Percutaneous Mitral Valvuloplasty (PMV)

Feasibility: The feasibility of PMV is assessed by echo and clinically, to evaluate

1. Anatomic suitability:
   - Calculating the *MV score*, based on the degree of MV thickening (normal <2 mm), mobility, and calcification, as well as subvalvular thickening (chordae, papillary muscles). The greater the thickness, the calcification, and the mobility impairment, the lower the chances for successful PMV (effective and uncomplicated, i.e., not leading to severe MR). These elements are individually graded from one (least severe) to four (Table 5.10). A total score <8 implies excellent chances for successful PMV, while a score <10–12 portends a fair chance of success. Although the chances of success for PMV are judged by the global score, certain individual findings carry a special signification unto themselves, as reviewed below.

Table 5.9 MS: indications for percutaneous mitral valvuloplasty (PMV)[a]

	Symptoms at rest/exercise *and/or*	Symptoms at rest/exercise
Past or ongoing complications of MS	any of the following: AF[b]; sPAP >50 mmHg at rest; previous embolism; "smoke" in the LA	
	or	
Risk of hemodynamic decompensation	need for noncardiac major surgery *or* desire for pregnancy	
	or	
Other VHD	nonsevere AV disease[c]	
	and	*and*
Anatomy suitable for PMV[d]	yes	no, as formally assessed, but judged amenable by operator
	and	*and*
Clinical characteristics favorable to PMV	yes	yes[e]

[a]If feasible, PMV may also be considered in patients with moderate PAH at rest (sPAP <50 mmHg), even if asymptomatic
[b]Recurrent or persistent, if of recent onset
[c]PMV may delay the necessity for bivalvular surgery
[d]See text for definition of suitable anatomy
[e]If there is a contraindication for open-heart surgery or in highly experienced centers, where "unfavorable" anatomy is still compatible with good chances of success

- *Severe or bicommissural calcification* is a contraindication for PMV, due to the risk of leaflet tear and severe MR and of calcium embolism (the degree of calcification correlates with reduced valve mobility, factored into the MS score).
- *The presence and degree of commissural fusion*: MS by mechanisms other than commissural fusion is generally not amenable to PMV; on the other hand, the more severe the adherence, the higher the risk of leaflet tear and severe MR after PMV, especially in case of associated heavy commissural calcification.

2. Clinical suitability- absence of:
   - LA thrombus, as the catheter may fragment the clot and cause embolism. Detection of LA thrombus mandates anticoagulation for ≥3 months, at which time the patient's candidacy for PMV is reassessed.
   - More than trace-to-mild MR (risk of severe MR).
   - Severe associated VHD (aortic or tricuspid).
   - An indication for CABG, mandating open-chest surgery.
   - High-risk clinical characteristics, including old age, history of valvuloplasty, or HF NYHA class IV (relative contraindications).

The MV Score: An Indicative Assessment Only

A patient with a favorable MV score may not be a candidate for PMV. Conversely, PMV may be attempted in patients with a score >8 and high risk for surgery; in the worst-case scenario, severe MR may ensue, leading to emergent valve replacement surgery.

PMV Success: A Matter of Experience

The technique of PMV has a very steep learning curve, and good results are only seen in highly experienced, high-volume centers. High operator experience – an essential, difficultly quantifiable element – is the single most important indicator of success.

Technique: PMV is carried out by a transseptal approach, whereby an hourglass-shaped (Inoue) balloon is inserted into the LA from the RA, then threaded through the stenotic MV, and inflated to release the stenosis. The procedure is performed under fluoroscopic guidance and often under echo guidance as well. More recently, a valvotome-based percutaneous technique has been introduced, which, however, is not widely available. Its main advantage is the possibility to reuse the valvotome after sterilization.

Results, complications, and follow-up: PMV has immediate results similar to those of surgical valvotomy, with roughly a doubling of the MV area and a decrease by half of the transmitral gradient. The formal definition for PMV success is a postprocedure valve area >1.5 cm^2 and a decrease in LA pressure to <18 mmHg in the absence of complications. In experienced centers, these results are attained in up to 95% of judiciously selected patients. Postprocedure echo assessment must be deferred for at least 72 h, as early hemodynamic changes make MV area assessment unreliable before this time line. *Complications* of PMV mainly include severe MR and large ASD (small ASDs generally seal off within 6 months of the procedure). In patients with favorable morphology, there is an 80–90% event-free survival rate. Restenosis after PMV occurs with variable frequency; old age, severe MS, severe PAH, advanced NYHA class, AF, and concomitant significant tricuspid regurgitation (TR) are associated with poorer long-term results. In those in whom severe MS does recur, the options include redo PMV or valve replacement. Recurrent symptoms must also prompt a search for alternative causes (e.g., progression of CAD).

Surgical Therapy

Surgical therapy is reserved for MS patients with poor anatomic and clinical suitability for PMV, or in those in whom severe coexistent disease (coronary or valvular) independently mandates open-heart surgery. The indications for intervention are more conservative if valve replacement is necessary, as opposed to percutaneous or surgical valvuloplasty (see above). With this in mind, the available surgical procedures include: (1) *closed valvuloplasty*, by performing cardiotomy in the area of the LA appendage and advancing a valvotome to the MV, with separation of the fused leaflets (initially, this separation was performed manually, by introducing the index finger through the stenotic valve); this is the usual technique of choice in developing countries; (2) *open valvuloplasty*, the current standard method for *surgical* valvuloplasty (but note that the standard method for valvuloplasty as such is percutaneous). Open valvuloplasty allows proper splitting of fused commissures and chordae, as well as proper calcium debridement; the LA appendage is amputated, to minimize long-term risk of embolism; (3) *valve replacement* is indicated in patients who are not candidates for valvuloplasty, or if an experienced center is not available. Whenever possible, the subvalvular apparatus (papillary muscles, chordae) must be preserved, as this helps preserve LV function; artificial chordal reconstruction is possible. In patients with severe rheumatic involvement, preservation of the subvalvular apparatus may not be possible. Postponing surgery until a severe symptomatic status is reached leads to poorer results; however, in patients first diagnosed in advanced stages of the disease, surgery is still indicated.

5.3 Mitral Regurgitation (MR)

MR is defined as the systolic reflux of blood from the LV into the LA. Just like other types of valvular insufficiency, MR can be acute or chronic. As the causes, manifestations, and treatment of acute and chronic MR are different, the two settings will be discussed separately.

5.3.1 Acute MR

The most frequent causes of acute severe MR include rupture of a papillary muscle as a result of acute MI, IE destruction of a mitral leaflet, or complicated balloon PMV. The sudden volume overload of the LA (which has to accommodate the regurgitant volume) and of the LV (which fills in diastole with the "extra" amount of blood previously regurgitated into the LA) give rise to pulmonary congestion, hypotension (despite a somewhat increased LV contractility, as a result of increased preload), and frequently, cardiogenic shock. The physical examination mainly reveals the manifestations of pulmonary edema and cardiogenic shock. Of note, the manifestations of MR as such may be blunted (short systolic murmur), due to rapid equalization of the LA and LV pressures ("fast and dramatic" regurgitation). The nonhypertrophic LV does not produce a hyperdynamic apical impulse. Occasionally, the only physical sign is a third

heart sound. *The treatment* is surgical and must be adapted to the specific underlying disease (leaflet destruction requires insertion of a valvular prosthesis, as does papillary muscle rupture; in some cases, however, the latter is amenable to repair, with native valve preservation and avoidance of long-term anticoagulation). Medical therapy is usually only used for initial stabilization, on the way to emergent surgery. Nitroprusside infusion reduces afterload, the regurgitant fraction, and ultimately, pulmonary congestion, while somewhat improving CO. However, Nitroprusside may accentuate preexisting hypotension. Careful addition of an inotropic agent may be warranted. IABP is commonly used. If the underlying condition is IE, antibiotic treatment is of the essence.

5.3.2 Chronic MR

5.3.2.1 Etiology

Organic MR is usually caused by CAD, the MVP syndrome, rheumatic heart disease (where MR is often associated with MS), IE, or collagen vascular disease. Some diet pills used in the 1990s and early 2000s (the Fenfluramine in the Fen/Phen combination, as well as the parent compound, Dexfenfluramine) have been associated to increased VHD incidence, mostly of the aortic and mitral valves, of mild intensity and at least partly reversible (although severe cases have occurred as well). The risk of PAH is also increased. Histologically, the valve lesions resemble those caused by carcinoid. The treatment is the usual one. *Functional MR* is caused by the impact of LV dysfunction on MV function. It can result from DCM of any etiology (with annular dilatation and leaflet malcoaptation), as well as from tethering of the mitral leaflet to a hypokinetic, ischemic LV segment (most frequently, the posterior LV wall). Occasionally, the same condition may cause both organic and functional MR. For instance, HOCM may involve both hydrodynamic (i.e., functional) and structural (organic) abnormalities of the MV.

5.3.2.2 Pathophysiological Impact

Chronic MR leads to dilatation of the LA (LA dilatation minimizes the LA pressure and the PCWP and

Functional MR and Functional Murmurs: Two Distinct Entities

Importantly, *functional* MR is caused by severe *organic* disease affecting the LV, but sparing the MV; it is usually a sign of significant cardiac disease. In contrast, functional murmurs reflect normally increased flow through the heart valves.

decreases LV afterload) and of the LV. The latter occurs due to the addition of new sarcomeres in series (eccentric hypertrophy), enabling maintenance of forward stroke volume, despite severe MR. Thanks to these compensatory mechanisms, the patient may remain asymptomatic for many years. However, there is gradual onset of myocardial dysfunction, the slightest evidence of which must prompt MV replacement, as in the later stages myocardial changes are irreversible. Of note, even "normal" LVEF (55–60%) is considered a sign of LV dysfunction, as this translates in a decreased forward output, but the greatest risk involves patients with clinically manifest HF. PAH is also an indicator of severe prognosis.

5.3.2.3 Chronic Ischemic MR

Chronic ischemic MR can be either *organic*, by ischemic involvement of a papillary muscle (chronic scarring and shortening; this is in contradistinction to papillary muscle rupture, which causes acute MR), or *functional* (annular dilatation or leaflet tethering to a hypokinetic LV segment). LV dilatation *causing* MR must be distinguished from that *resulting from* long-standing severe MR; while surgery may be indicated even in the latter, the prognosis is much worse. Aside from the clinical history, the two entities can also be distinguished by the echo conformation of the regurgitant jet, which tends to be concentric in primary annular dilatation and eccentric in the setting of MV pathology. If CABG is indicated on grounds of coronary ischemia alone, mitral repair (if feasible) is recommended even for moderate MR. Additionally, coronary revascularization itself may substantially decrease the degree of regurgitation, if the involved myocardial segment is viable.

5.3.2.4 MVP

MVP, the most common nonischemic cause of MR, is described as a >2 mm systolic displacement of the MV into the LA. This displacement must be assessed from the long-axis view (either parasternal or apical), as even the normal MV, with its characteristic saddle shape, may appear as prolapsing, if viewed from other echo windows. MVP is due to excess connective tissue in the mitral leaflets, which appear thickened. The condition is quite frequent, involving 2–3% of the general population, and is more frequent in patients with Marfan's disease. "Classic" MVP involves valve thickening >5 mm ("non-classic prolapse" otherwise). The thickened valves have suboptimal mechanical properties, hence the prolapse. The disease is self-maintaining, in the sense that the greater the prolapse, the higher the tension applied to the chordae, which thin out and offer increasingly weaker mechanical support; occasionally, this process results in chordal rupture and a flail MV (i.e., a totally untethered leaflet, with its point directed to the LA; Fig. 5.2). Flail MV is generally seen with classic prolapse and is a variant of asymmetric MVP (as opposed to

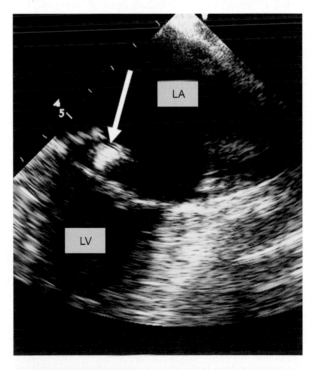

Fig. 5.2 Flail mitral valve (*arrow*); *LA* left atrium; *LV* left ventricle. This was the anatomic substrate of severe mitral regurgitation (MR) identified on color Doppler

"symmetric" MVP, where the two leaflets protrude equally into the LA, but the leaflet tips do meet). Secondary MVP can be seen in patients (especially younger women) with ASD, hyperthyroidism, emphysema, or HCM. While the overall prognosis is dictated by the underlying condition, secondary MVP appears of little significance unto itself and is generally not associated to significant MR.

MVP is asymptomatic in most patients, but it may also cause MR; while this is usually not severe, MVP does remain the most frequent cause of severe nonischemic MR in the Westernized world. Occasional atypical chest pain, palpitations, and anxiety have suggested the existence of an "MVP syndrome"; large populational studies, however, have not found an increased incidence of these manifestations in MVP patients, and this "syndrome" is no longer recognized as a clinical entity. The *physical findings* include a midsystolic click, corresponding to the sudden tensing of the prolapsing leaflets and/or chordae, and, in patients associating MR (the most important complication of MVP), a late-systolic murmur, best heard at the apex. The presence of a murmur portends a more serious prognosis and justifies an echocardiogram. The major predictors of mortality in MVP patients are the severity of MR and of LVEF decrease. *The treatment* involves only reassurance in most patients, β-blockers in patients with palpitations, and surgery in those with severe MR. Surgery is ideally carried out as MV repair in patients who had no time to develop LV dysfunction. If repair is not feasible, MV replacement, with preservation of the mitral apparatus, is the procedure of choice.

5.3.2.5 Chronic MR: Diagnosis

The symptoms (if present) are those of HF. Chest pain may represent underlying ischemia; the mechanism in MVP patients is unclear. The *physical signs* of chronic MR include a typical systolic murmur best heard in the mitral area and irradiated to the left axilla. It has a typical "blowing" quality (as opposed to the harsh/rasping quality of the AS systolic murmur) and is usually holosystolic, but may be late-systolic and be preceded by a click in patients with underlying MVP. The intensity of the murmur does not correlate well with the severity of MR. A third heart sound may be heard in patients with

LV dilatation. Physical signs of left or biventricular dysfunction (pulmonary rhales, peripheral edema) may be found in advanced cases. *Echo*: in most patients, TTE is sufficient, but TEE may be required in case of eccentric jets (visualization from different angles avoids underestimation of MR), as well as in surgical candidates, in whom precise definition of MR mechanisms allows the choice of optimal surgical strategy. Echo allows assessing the severity and mechanism of MR, as well as its impact on the LA and LV structure and function. The methods for MR severity assessment are reviewed in Table 5.10 and illustrated in Fig. 5.3. As a general rule, a central MR jet with a structurally normal mitral apparatus suggests functional MR (annular dilatation). Conversely, an eccentric jet suggests an organic cause, e.g., MVP. Stress echo is useful for the diagnosis of latent LV dysfunction in patients with severe MR and a normal resting LV function.

Cardiac catheterization is generally not required for the diagnosis of MR per se, but may occasionally establish a previously unknown diagnosis of MR, at routine contrast injection into the LV, in a patient with CAD. Provided the injection technique is correct and the hemodynamic status of the patient is the same, catheterization and echo MR severity grading correlate well. In MR patients, Swan-Ganz catheterization may record a tall v wave; as this depends on the compliance (ability to stretch) of the LA, it will be present in all patients with acute MR, but only in some of those with chronic MR. The severity grading of MR by catheterization is reviewed in Table 5.11.

Chest X-ray and EKG may show LA and LV enlargement; the X-ray examination additionally defines the degree of pulmonary congestion.

5.3.2.6 Chronic MR: Therapy

Medical therapy is nonspecific and consists in treatment of HF, if present. However, medical therapy is not a substitute for surgery in suitable candidates. Despite data supporting the use of vasodilators (ACEI or Hydralazine) in asymptomatic MR patients, the current guidelines restrict this therapy to patients with another independent indication for it, such as HTN or HF. These patients may have either organic MR with coexistent HTN or HF, or functional MR, where ACEI, diuretics, and β-blockers are the mainstay of

Table 5.10 Echo assessment of MR severity

Assessment method	Principle	Severe MR	Pitfalls[a]
Semiquantitative	Visual assessment of jet area as trace, mild,[b] moderate, or severe, as compared to LA area	Jet area approximately 1/2 of LA area, and/or reaches bottom of LA	Underestimation of eccentric jets[c]; assessment under different hemodynamic conditions[d]
Quantitative, by color Doppler	Measurement-based comparison of jet area to LA area	Jet area >40% of LA area (mild MR: <20%)	As above
Vena contracta[e]	Measuring jet width immediately after its entrance into the LA	>5 mm	Measuring the vena contracta on a freeze-frame that does not display it at its maximum width
Regurgitant volume (1)	Regurgitant volume = regurgitant valve area[f] × TVI of mitral flow[g]	>60 mL	Incorrect measurements of the radius are squared (and thus amplified), in the formula: area $= \pi r^2$
Regurgitant volume (2)	LVOT blood flow = diastolic MV flow-systolic MR flow	>60 mL	As above
Regurgitant fraction	MR flow/diastolic MV flow	>60%	As above
PISA	MR volume = volume of blood converging in the LV toward the regurgitant orifice; this equation is used to calculate regurgitant orifice area[h]	Effective regurgitant orifice (ERO = regurgitant flow volume/jet velocity) >0.4 cm^2	As above
Additional indicators of severe MR	Torrential early filling of LV, due to increased LA/LV gradient (LA filled from pulmonary veins and from previous systole); increased LA pressure blunts or abolishes pulmonary vein flow	Increased E wave velocity (>1.2 m/s); systolic flow blunting or reversal in the pulmonary veins[i]	LA pressure increases of other etiologies

[a]Any of the described techniques may provide an incorrect assessment, if the echo machine settings are incorrect
[b]Trace or mild MR, seen just behind the mitral leaflets, is considered normal
[c]Visualization from as many angles as possible (if necessary, using TEE) is mandatory. Even with good visualization, however, the jet may have different dimensions from the different angles, and the largest dimension is the one used to assess MR severity
[d]Differences in the loading state (hydration, blood pressure) may lead to real differences in MR severity, and serial testing must be carried out, as far as possible, under similar conditions; BP at the time of the echo must be recorded
[e]At the vena contracta, the blood column is "at its narrowest and fastest"; the vena contracta is situated a few mm above the valve level. The blood flow converges toward the vena contracta and splays distally to it
[f]As blood converges in systole toward the regurgitant orifice, it assumes a hemispheric shape, the radius of which can be calculated and used to approximate the orifice area
[g]TVI, i.e., the area under the CW tracing of the regurgitant flow
[h]Calculated based on the formula, regurgitant orifice area = convergence flow area × convergence flow velocity/MR velocity
[i]The pulmonary blood flow has a systolic and a diastolic wave, both directed toward the LA

therapy. MV surgery, possibly combined with LV reconstruction techniques (Chap. 4), is recommended in these patients only if the conservative strategy fails. *Surgical therapy* may consist of MV repair or replacement. The former is preferable, whenever possible. The eligibility criteria for MV repair are reviewed below. The rule of thumb, in patients with severe organic MR, is that all but the very "healthy" and the very sick patients are to be operated on. The indications for surgery are discussed in Table 5.12. Similarly to AS, MR might benefit in the future from percutaneous intervention.

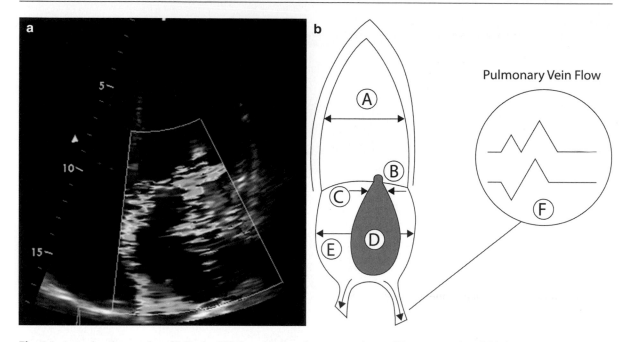

Fig. 5.3 Assessing the severity of MR: *A* – LV dimensions and contractility; *B* – PISA; *C* – vena contracta; *D* – Jet area; *E* – LA size; *F* – pulmonary vein flow (explanations in the text). Note that in this patient there are actually two regurgitant mitral jets. Both featured regurgitant jets are severe, but the very eccentric jet on the left is more difficult to semiquantitate than the more concentric one. The true severity of this jet was not immediately apparent, and required fastidious angulation of the transducer. Meticulous investigation of the jet, often by TEE, is required to define the underlying mechanism and establish the surgical strategy, if warranted. This color study was obtained in the patient with a flail MV presented in Fig. 5.2

Table 5.11 Grading of MR severity by catheterization

Feature	Mild	Moderate	Moderate/severe	Severe
Opacification of the entire LA	No	No	Yes	Yes
Contrast completely clears from LA from beat to beat	Yes	No	No	No
Opacification of LA is less than that of LV	Yes	Yes	No; LA=LV	No; LA=LV
Systolic contrast reflux into pulmonary veins	No	No	No	Yes

Table 5.12 Indications for surgery in patients with severe organic MR

Symptoms		LV involvement (structural and/or functional)		Comorbidity	Feasibility of MV repair	Class of indication
Yes	*or*	LVEF 30–60% *or* LVESD 45–55 mm	*or*	AF *or* sPAP >50 mmHg at rest[a]		I
					Yes[b]	II
		LVEF <30% *or* LVESD >55 mm *and* refractory to medical therapy[a, c]				II

[a]If chronic ischemia is present, CABG at the time of MVR is indicated if feasible

[b]MV repair may be considered (class II indication) even in asymptomatic patients with severe MR and preserved LV function. If this choice is made, this table is redundant

[c]Chances are better if repair is possible and if there is low comorbidity. Otherwise, transplant may be the only solution

> **Eligibility Criteria for MV Repair**
>
> MV repair is generally considered feasible *in the absence* of rheumatic MR with extensive valvular and subvalvular fibrosis; severe prolapse of the anterior leaflet (repair of a prolapsing posterior leaflet is technically easier); or prolapse involving roughly <50% of the leaflet length (there may not exist enough leaflet material for repair).

Percutaneous therapy, recently introduced to clinical practice, is a form of mitral repair (as opposed to percutaneous therapy of AS, which consists in valve replacement). It consists in MV clipping in patients who are surgical candidates due to severe MR and enables restoring systolic coaptation of the mitral leaflets and avoidance or delay of surgery in most patients.

5.4 Aortic Stenosis (AS)

5.4.1 General Remarks

AS consists in narrowing of the LV/aorta connection. This may affect the AV (valvular AS) or the sub- or supravalvular area (SVA). The latter are discussed in Chaps. 4 (HOCM) and 10 (supravalvular stenosis). Valvular AS is caused by valvular calcification (proceeding from the base toward the tip and restricting valve mobility). Most frequently, AS is degenerative, but it can occasionally be of rheumatic (commissural fusion, invariably associated with mitral involvement) or congenital etiology (the latter, mainly seen in young patients). The severity grading of AS is reviewed in Table 5.13.

Table 5.13 Aortic stenosis (AS): severity grading

Severity[a]	Area (cm^2)	Mean gradient (mmHg)	Peak gradient (mmHg)	Jet velocity (m/s)
Mild	>1.5	<25	<36	<3.0
Moderate	1.0–1.5	25–40	30–50	3–4
Severe	<1.0 cm	>40	>50	>4[a]

[a]In the presence of normal CO

> **AV Sclerosis: An Entity Not to be Confused with AS**
>
> In as many as 25% of adults over 65, there is irregular valve thickening, without significant obstruction to LV outflow (peak flow velocity ≤2 m/s), but occasionally producing a systolic murmur, due to the intense vibration of the thickened leaflets in contact with the blood flow. Pathologically, the lesions are similar to those of atherosclerosis. Aortic sclerosis is more frequent in patients with risk factors for CAD, but even after statistical correction, the risk of adverse cardiovascular outcomes in these patients is significantly higher than in the general population.

Pathophysiological changes: The main consequence of AS is concentric LVH, which counters the high intracavitary systolic pressure, maintaining a normal LV afterload (systolic wall stress), and consequently, a normal LVEF, despite the valvular stenosis. Normal LV chamber volume is also maintained. Occasionally, the process of LV hypertrophy may be either too modest (resulting in decreased LVEF early on) or excessive (in elderly patients, especially women); paradoxically, the latter are at high surgical risk, despite an increased LVEF. Concentric hypertrophy allows preservation of the asymptomatic status for many years and is viewed as an adaptive mechanism; this is all the more important, since it is the symptomatic status, rather than the absolute AV area, that represents the indication for surgery (although severe AS is rarely truly asymptomatic). The protection offered by LVH, however, comes at a cost: the hypertrophic myocardium has a reduced coronary blood flow and coronary vasodilator reserve, with various degrees of subendocardial ischemia, contributing to systolic and diastolic LV dysfunction. The hypertrophic muscle is also very vulnerable to ischemic injury, both in terms of absolute risk and of severity (larger MI). An additional consequence of LVH is increased LVEDP, with correspondingly increased dependence on the atrial kick; the onset of AF usually leads to symptomatic deterioration in patients with significant AS. The onset of symptoms in AS patients depends on a combination of factors, including stenosis progression (usually, several decades are required for the onset of severe

AS, but there are wide individual variations), the degree of LVH, and the presence of associated cardiac disease (AF, CAD, VHD). A notable noncardiac complication of severe AS is impaired platelet function and decreased levels of von Willebrand factor, occasionally leading to bleeding. These anomalies are reversible with the relief of stenosis.

5.4.2 AS Diagnosis

The physical signs of AS are especially important, since they are generally present during the asymptomatic stage and allow early diagnosis and optimal follow-up. These signs include: a slow and/or sustained upstroke of the arterial pulse, which may be of low volume (*pulsus parvus et tardus*); *a systolic murmur* heard loudest at the upper right sternal border and irradiating superiorly, to the carotid arteries; in severe AS, the murmur peaks late in systole. The harsh (rather than "blowing") quality and the point of maximum intensity allow to distinguish this murmur from an irradiated MR murmur. The murmur is further distinguished from that of HOCM, as outlined in Table 5.14.

Additional physical findings include: *a thrill*, associated to the AS murmur; *narrowed pulse pressure* (i.e., a reduced difference between the systolic and diastolic BP); *a decreased second heart sound* in severe AS (due to decreased valve pliability); a sustained, *thrusting apex beat*; a *fourth heart sound*, in patients in NSR (atrial contraction, decreased LV compliance); and *a third heart sound*, in case of LV dilation and failure. AS often coexists with some degree of regurgitation (diastolic murmur) and with a particular double-peaked pulse, called *pulsus bisferiens* (also seen with HOCM). *The symptoms* of AS may be absent for decades, while the disease progresses; symptom onset is the milestone to assess candidacy for surgical therapy. The main complaints relate to *HF*, manifesting as dyspnea on exertion, or, in later stages, at rest, and due to systolic or combined systolic and diastolic LV failure. HF may be due to inadequate LV hypertrophy or to LV dysfunction secondary to long-standing AS; *syncope* (rarely, SCD; see below); and *angina* (due to relative ischemia of the hypertrophic myocardium). The average survival after symptom onset is 2–3 years.

> **AS-Related Syncope: A Multifactorial Event**
>
> Possible causes of syncope in the AS patient include: *BP drop due to vasodilatation*, not compensated by an increase in CO (which is precluded by fixed stenosis); in turn, the vasodilatation may be caused either by muscular exertion or by a reflex triggered by the LV filling pressures; *arrhythmia*, due to ischemia of the hypertrophic muscle; and *AV block*, due to involvement of the electrical conduction system in the degenerative process.

Echo: The main echo parameters of AS are similar to those of MS and include *AV area* measurement by direct planimetry or assessment by the continuity equation; of note, the latter uses the LVOT diameter, measured by 2D echo. Any measurement error is squared, when using the formula, area $= \pi r^2$. This error can be avoided by simply calculating the ratio between the peak flow velocity through the AV and through the LVOT, the so-called *dimensionless*

Table 5.14 Distinguishing the murmur of AS from that of HOCM

Maneuver	AS	Mechanism	HOCM	Mechanism
Squatting	Increases	Increased preload, higher LV/aortic gradient	Decreases	Increased LV systolic diameter → decreased dynamic obstruction
Isometric exercise	Decreases	Increases afterload → decreases transvalvular gradient	Increases	Increased CO → increased dynamic obstruction
Orthostatism	Decreases	decreased LV filling → decreased transvalvular flow	Increases	Decreased LV filling → increased dynamic obstruction[a]

[a]The mechanism also involves an increased contractility of the LV

index, a measurement independent of 2D measurements. The dimensionless index is especially useful for the assessment of prosthetic aortic valves, where scintillation from the prosthesis makes LVOT measurement difficult (normal value for prosthetic AVs = 0.3–0.5); Doppler *peak transvalvular gradient*, using Bernoulli's equation: peak gradient = $4v^2$, where v is the transaortic flow velocity, and the LVOT flow velocity is neglected (a misleading assumption in case of increased LVOT flow, e.g., with coexisting significant AI); Doppler *mean transvalvular gradient* (calculated as the time-velocity integral= TVI of the transvalvular flow, i.e., the area under the Doppler flow curve); assessment of the *AV morphology* (leaflet thickening and calcification, various degrees of commissural fusion) *and function* (restricted opening of the AV). With rheumatic AS, there is leaflet fusion at the tips, with "doming" of the leaflets, similar to that seen with bicuspid AV. A particular variant of anatomical anomaly is *aortic bicuspidy*, typically manifesting as the presence of two unequal, rather than of three leaflets (a raphe, often present on the larger leaflet, may be mistaken for a third commissure). This is an extremely frequent form of congenital heart disease, present in 1–2% of the overall population. Bicuspid AV has an oval (football-shaped) opening pattern, rather than the typical opening along three convergent lines ("the Mercedes Benz sign"); in parasternal long-axis view, the valve opening has a "doming" appearance. Aortic coarctation and aneurysmal dilatation of the ascending aorta are often associated. *Unicuspid AV* is a rare entity; often, there is severe stenosis in early childhood and aortic malformations are associated.

Due to the highly unpredictable rate of progression, careful *follow-up* is necessary in patients with nonmild AS (see Table 5.4). Classically, *Dobutamine echo* has played an important role in establishing candidacy for AVR in patients with severe AS. Patients with low contractile reserve were generally deemed inoperable. However, this conventional wisdom has been recently challenged, as even this latter disfavored group was found to do better with surgery (although the risk was very high in patients with a transaortic gradient <20 mmHg). This entire topic will probably be revolutionized by the increasing availability of percutaneous AV implantation.

> **Dobutamine Echo in Severe AS: Two Aims**
>
> - *A diagnostic aim*: *to rule out pseudo-AS*, in patients with low LVEF and suspected severe AS, where the decreased LV function is due to some other cause. In these "low-output, low-gradient" patients, the calculated AV area increases by ≥0.3 cm^2, and the gradient increases little, if at all. Conversely, with true AS, the gradient increases significantly, while the calculated valve area remains constant.
> - *A prognostic aim*: *to assess the LV contractile reserve*, i.e., the ability to increase CO by ≥20 mmHg.

Subaortic stenosis, caused by a subvalvular membrane, manifests like valvular AS and is diagnosed by echo. Its surgical removal is indicated in the presence of symptoms, of a gradient >50 mmHg, and/or of significant associated AI, resulting from damage to the valve leaflets by the turbulent flow in the LVOT.

EKG shows LVH and, occasionally, conduction disturbances due to fibrosis extension to the conduction system (Fig. 5.4).

Chest X-ray is of limited use, as there is no characteristic image of LVH. The main radiographic sign of AS is valvular calcification, especially with degenerative AS; extensive calcification is characteristic of severe disease. *Cardiac catheterization* is reserved for patients with suboptimal TTE images (TEE may be tried first, but aligning the Doppler beam with the blood flow may be problematic.) The main findings on catheterization include an increased systolic gradient between the LV and the aorta, associated AI or MR, LVH (with different degrees of LV dilatation and dysfunction), and, crucially in these generally elderly patients, CAD.

> **AV Gradient: Two Possible Definitions and Two Possible Pitfalls**
>
> The aortic transvalvular gradient can be defined as:
>
> - The maximum gradient that practically occurs between the LV and the aorta; this is measured in real time by Doppler echo.

Fig. 5.4 Severe LVH and "strain pattern" (ST depression and T-wave inversion) in a patient with critical AS

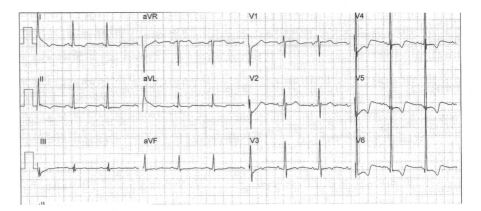

• The difference between the maximum LV pressure and the (nonsimultaneous) maximum aortic pressure; this is measured offline by cardiac catheterization.

As the maximum LV pressure occurs at a time of nonmaximum aortic pressure, the gradient obtained by Doppler is higher than that obtained by catheterization. Additionally, aortic pressure varies along the aortic root and must be measured at its minimal point ("vena contracta"), where the potential energy of the blood column is minimal, and the flow velocity, kinetic energy, and pressure gradient are maximal While CWD echo is set up to detect this maximum gradient, the catheter transducer necessarily measures the pressure at the exact point where the catheter tip is located. Gradual withdrawal of the catheter is necessary to avoid missing the point of the vena contracta, an error that would lead to *gradient underestimation.* Conversely, increased transaortic flow (e.g., with AI, when each systole propels the extra amount of blood regurgitated into the LV in the previous diastole) may lead to Doppler *overestimation* of the gradient.

5.4.3 AS Treatment

Medical therapy mainly consists in the stabilization of patients with HF, angina, or syncope, as a bridge to interventional therapy. *Interventional therapy* has traditionally been synonymous with surgical AV replacement (AVR). The technique of percutaneous AVR

is making rapid progress. The only other nonsurgical interventional approach is aortic balloon valvuloplasty. As opposed to PMV, the latter has a very restricted applicability, namely, in patients with severe AS who are too frail to undergo immediate valve replacement (aortic valvuloplasty as a bridge to surgery) or who require emergent noncardiac major surgery that would be poorly tolerated in the presence of untreated severe AS. The indications for AVR are reviewed in Table 5.15. *The Ross procedure* consists in replacing the stenotic AV with the patient's own PV, while the PV is replaced by a cadaver valve (homograft). This is the procedure of choice in infants and children, as neither graft requires anticoagulation, and both have favorable flow conditions. The isograft grows with the rest of the child's body, and the pulmonary homograft has an overall good survival. However, the use of the Ross procedure in adults is controversial, as the procedure treats a single condition (AS) with *two* valvular prostheses. *Percutaneous AVR* for the treatment of severe AS, mentioned above, uses a biological valve wrapped around a balloon; inflation of the latter relieves the stenosis and deploys the prosthetic valve. This as yet not widely available technique could prove ideal, initially for patients with critical AS too frail to undergo surgery, and hopefully, as an alternative to AVR in general. Another option (potentially useful in patients with significant PVD) is a surgical approach involving minithoracotomy and delivery of the prosthetic valve through a *left ventricular apical puncture* without cardiopulmonary bypass. An older and little-used method (tentatively revived in some centers) is the *aorto-ventricular bypass*, whereby the stenotic AV is rendered irrelevant. The procedure is complex itself, detracting from the potential appeal

Table 5.15 Indications for AV replacement (AVR) in AS[a]

Valve involvement		Symptoms		LV involvement (structural and/or functional)		Comorbidity	Class of indication
Severe stenosis	*and*	at rest or (if relevant) on exercise	*or*	LVEF<50%	*or*	other cardiovascular disease requiring open-heart surgery	I
Severe stenosis	*and*			LVH≥15 mm not due to other causes *or*, on exercise, BP decrease *or* complex ventricular arrhythmia			II
Severe stenosis *and* moderate-to-severe calcification *and* peak velocity rate on Doppler progressing ≥0.3 m/s/year							II
Severe stenosis *and* low gradient (<40 mmHg), whether or not there is LV contractile reserve[b]							II
Moderate stenosis						*and* other cardiovascular disease requiring open-heart surgery	II

[a]As discussed in the text, some of these settings may allow for percutaneous AV implantation, or possibly for a combined or staged surgical/percutaneous approach

[b]Assessed by Dobutamine echo; indication stronger if contractile reserve present. If contractile reserve absent, the surgical risk is high, but surgery may still represent the only available option

of this strategy, especially in the era of catheter-delivered AV prosthesis.

5.5 Aortic Insufficiency (AI)

AI is defined as backward flow from the aorta into the LV, in diastole. AI may be caused by pathological processes involving the valve leaflets or by dilatation of the aortic root, causing malcoaptation of structurally normal aortic leaflets. AI may be chronic or acute, with different causes and manifestations.

5.5.1 Acute AI

Occasionally (in case of IE, aortic dissection, trauma – including balloon valvuloplasty), severe AI develops acutely, with an LV that had no time to adapt, resulting in a steep increase in LVEDP, propagated backwards to the pulmonary circulation. Additionally, there is acute LV dilatation, generating increased wall stress, which is itself a cause of increased oxygen demand and of subendocardial ischemia. Together with the universally present tachycardia, this commonly causes myocardial ischemia, further compromising the LV function (resulting in pulmonary edema and cardiogenic shock) and occasionally causing lethal arrhythmia. These changes are especially severe in patients with significant LVH (e.g., a hypertensive patient now suffering aortic dissection which extends to the aortic root and causes acute AI), as these patients have an already increased LVEDP. The particular hemodynamics prevent full expression of the classical signs seen in chronic AI, occasionally leading to nondetection of acute AI in a severely ill patient. Rapid equilibration of the (increased) LVEDP with the (decreased) aortic pressure diminishes pulse pressure and the period of regurgitation, hence that of the diastolic murmur. This reflects by echo as a short (<300 ms) AI diastolic half-time (i.e., the time by which the LV/aortic gradient is reduced by 50%), and an abnormally rapid LA/LV pressure equalization, causing a shortened (<150 ms) mitral deceleration time and premature closure of the MV (before the end of the EKG diastole).

5.5.2 Chronic AI

Chronic AI may be idiopathic or caused by congenital anomalies (bicuspid valve, Marfan syndrome; less frequently, Ehlers–Danlos syndrome, discrete subaortic stenosis, or VSD with prolapse of an aortic cusp – Chap. 10); calcific or myxomatous degeneration; inflammatory conditions (rheumatic fever, less frequently, infective or noninfective aortitis – Chap. 11); HTN; or by certain anorectic drugs (see "MR"). *Pathophysiology and clinical manifestations*: chronic AI causes LV dilatation, which allows maintaining

- *Normal forward stroke volume* (= total stroke volume − regurgitant volume), by increasing the total stroke volume; LV dilatation makes this possible, since a normal LVEF will translate in a higher absolute blood volume being ejected in each systole

- *Normal LVEDP* (preload), by myocardial fiber rearrangement and addition of new sarcomeres

Cardiac dilatation, however, carries its own complications, as it increases wall stress (afterload) and myocardial oxygen consumption. Ultimately, the preload increases as well, and after a several decades-long asymptomatic stage, the patient becomes symptomatic. The myocardial changes are initially reversible, but become irreversible later on; therefore, as opposed to the case of AS, it is not the onset of symptoms, but that of LV dysfunction that triggers the recommendation for surgery.

Chronic AI: Diagnosis The *symptoms* (when present) mainly include dyspnea and palpitations. The *clinical signs* include *a diastolic murmur* in the aortic area (second intercostal space along the right sternal border), best heard when the patient is seated and leans forward with their breath held in expiration. The murmur has a soft quality. If it irradiates to the right parasternal region, the differential diagnosis includes ascending aortic aneurysm; *a systolic murmur* in the aortic area, due to increased flow (different from the AS murmur by the lack of a harsh quality and of an opening click); *a middiastolic mitral (Austin Flint) murmur* ("rumble"), due to restricted opening of the MV, which is impacted by the aortic regurgitant flow; a third heart sound, due to LV volume overload; *a high pulse pressure*, manifesting as a decreased difference between the systolic and the diastolic BP, and a plethora of peripheral signs (see below); the real usefulness of these signs in the current era is uncertain.

Concentric and Eccentric Ventricular Hypertrophy

The two terms are somewhat confusing, as they may carry a connotation of symmetry with the former and of asymmetry with the latter. In fact, the intended meaning is that, with concentric hypertrophy, the "additional" layers of muscle progress toward the central axis of the heart (sarcomeres added in parallel with the existing ones, resulting in a decreased cardiac volume), whereas with eccentric hypertrophy, the cardiac walls progress away from the axis (sarcomeres added in series, with cardiac dilatation).

Of note, both AI and AS may exhibit the two types of hypertrophy, but eccentric hypertrophy is more specific to AI and concentric hypertrophy, to AS.

Clinical Signs of Increased Pulse Pressure in Chronic Severe AI: A Glossary

- **Watson's water hammer pulse:** bounding peripheral pulses
- **Corrigan's pulse:** rapid upstroke and collapse of the carotid artery pulse
- **de Musset's sign:** head nodding in time with the heart beat
- **Quincke's sign:** pulsation of the nail bed capillaries
- **Duroziez's sign:** a double sound over the femoral artery on distal compression

- **Traube's sign:** "pistol shot" systolic and diastolic murmurs on gradual compression of the femoral artery
- **Becker's sign:** pulsations of the retinal vessels
- **Müller's sign:** pulsations of the uvula
- **Hill's sign:** the systolic popliteal BP is by ≥20 mmHg higher than the brachial systolic BP (as measured by a cuff; this might be an artifact resulting from intense reverberation of the pulse wave in the lax lower limb vessels)

Echo: see Table 5.16. *Catheterization* is rarely necessary for the diagnosis of chronic AI as such, but may be indicated if associated CAD independently requires catheterization. The typical sign is partial opacification of the LV from the aorta in diastole, which can be graded semiquantitatively (with good correlation to the echo grading); an additional finding is rapid equalization of the aortic and LV pressures, measured simultaneously, in severe AI. *EKG signs* are nonspecific and mainly include the manifestations of LVH (tall R waves in L1, aVL, and V5–V6, deep Q waves in V1–V2, left axis deviation ≥−30°, increased QRS duration); occasionally, the T waves in V5–V6, otherwise negative in LVH, are positive ("LV volume overload pattern"). The *chest X-ray* mainly demonstrates tortuosity of the ascending aorta and LV dilatation, in its extreme forms termed "cor bovinum."

Table 5.16 Echo findings in chronic aortic insufficiency (AI)

	Finding	Significance	Mild AI	Severe AI
Color Doppler	Diastolic regurgitant jet from the aorta into the LV	Jet *surface and width* allow semiquantitation of AI as trace, mild, moderate, or severe[a,b]	AI jet width/LVOT width <25%; AI jet surface (at its base)/AV surface <25%	(See mild AI): both parameters >60%
	Diastolic flow reversal in the descending aorta	Indicates severe AI	None	Involves abdominal aorta[c]
Spectral Doppler	CW pressure half-time of the regurgitant flow	The more severe the AI, the faster the aorta/LV pressure equalization	>400–600 ms	<250 ms
	Diastolic flow reversal in the descending aorta	Indicates severe AI	None	Involves abdominal aorta
	Vena contracta (mm)[d]	Normal <0.3		>0.6
Combined Doppler/2D methods	Regurgitant volume	In the absence of MR, AI backflow = aortic outflow − mitral inflow	<30 mL	>60 mL
	Regurgitant fraction	Regurgitant volume/stroke volume	<30%	>60%
	Regurgitant orifice area[e] (cm²)	<0.10	0.11–0.29	>0.30
2D	Pathology of the aortic leaflets and/or root; LV dilatation and hypertrophy	Reveals the mechanism of AI	Variable	Variable

[a]This evaluation correlates well with the angiographic qualitative assessment, as 1+, 2+, 3 or 4+
[b]Jet *length* is an unreliable indicator of AI severity
[c]Moderate AI: in the thoracic descending aorta only
[d]That is, the width of the AI jet at the level of the AV
[e]Calculated using the PISA method or the continuity equation in diastole, using the surface and TVI of the supravalvular area (SVA): regurgitant area = supravalvular area × TVI (supravalvular, by PWD)/TVI (valvular, by CWD). SVA is defined as the surface area of the hemispheric convergence area of the regurgitant flow, in the LV, as it converges toward the regurgitant orifice, on its way to the LA

5.5.3 AI-Therapy

AI has a long asymptomatic phase, which is the ideal time for diagnosis, before the onset of irreversible LV changes. If symptoms appear early on, AI can be corrected before the onset of LV dysfunction. Asymptomatic LV dysfunction generally becomes symptomatic within 2–3 years and may be at least partly irreversible at the time of surgery. Postoperative survival and recovery of LV function mainly depend on the severity of preoperative symptoms or of reduction in exercise tolerance, the severity and duration of LVEF decrease, and the severity and duration of LV dilatation.

5.5.3.1 Medical Therapy

Medical therapy has traditionally consisted of vasodilators, for afterload reduction and decrease of the aortic regurgitant fraction. However, there is no clear proof of their efficacy and their use is debated. The agent of choice is Nifedipine (although ACEI and thiazides, the latter as adjunct therapy, have also been used), but here again, the ideal dosage is not clear. In patients with asymptomatic AI, no reduction or delay in the requirement for AVR has been demonstrated with either Nifedipine 20 mg b.i.d. or Enalapril 20 mg q.d., but these dosages are considered by many as unrealistically low. The ESC guidelines only recommend vasodilator therapy in patients with HF or HTN, as well as in AI patients who become symptomatic during pregnancy, while the ACC/AHA guidelines recommend them (Class I) in all patients with severe AI who are symptomatic and are not candidates for surgery, as well as (Class II) to improve the patient's hemodynamic profile before AVR, or even in asymptomatic patients with LV dilatation and/or

dysfunction. Of note, the latter two indications are explicitly not recognized by the ESC. As AI patients tend to tolerate bradycardia poorly, β-blockers have been traditionally considered contraindicated. Recent retrospective data, however, have challenged this traditional wisdom by finding a favorable effect of β-blockers in this population. This finding requires confirmation from prospective studies.

5.5.3.2 Interventional Therapy

The indications for *AVR* in AI patients are outlined in Table 5.17.

5.6 Tricuspid Stenosis (TS)

The most frequent *etiology* of TS is rheumatic (when TR and some type of MV disease are usually associated), but TS can rarely be caused by congenital abnormalities or by other diseases (carcinoid, Fabry, Whipple). Obstruction to tricuspid flow mimicking TS can be caused by RA masses or IE. In patients in NSR, the clinical manifestations include a giant "a" wave (due to backward propagation of the RA contraction against a stenotic valve), a diminished y descent in the jugular pulse (due to delayed RA emptying), a tricuspid OS, and a middiastolic tricuspid rumble, with presystolic accentuation (again, in patients in NSR). Any associated valve disease presents with the respective signs. The symptoms include hepatic congestion, ascites, and lower limb edema, mimicking RV failure. *Therapy*: TV replacement is indicated for severe TS that remains symptomatic despite medical therapy, or if the patient requires left-sided valve surgery. Biologic prostheses are preferred in the tricuspid position, due to the low-flow conditions, encouraging mechanical valve thrombosis.

Table 5.17 AI: indications for surgery

Degree of regurgitation		Symptoms		Comorbidity
Severe	*and*	NYHA class II-IV *or* angina	*or*	LVEF≤50% *or* diameter >70 mm (end-diastolic) *or* >50 mm (end-systolic[a]) *or* requirement for surgery on coronaries, aorta, or other valves
Any	*and*			Aortic root dilatation >45 mm (Marfan's); 50 mm (bicuspid AV); >55 for all other patients

[a]>25 mm/m^2 BSA

5.7 Tricuspid Regurgitation (TR)

5.7.1 Etiology

TR can be caused by valve leaflet pathology or tricuspid annulus dilatation (functional TR). Leaflet pathology may be caused by rheumatic disease, IE, congenital conditions (Marfan's disease, Ebstein's anomaly, cleft TV), TV prolapse, external trauma, carcinoid disease, or be iatrogenic (repeated myocardial biopsy in cardiac transplantees, valve lesion by catheter or pacemaker, effects of radiation therapy). Tricuspid annular dilatation may occur in any patient with increased RV systolic pressure (MS, LV failure, PS, PAH) or diastolic pressure (RV failure of any cause, RV infarction).

5.7.2 Diagnosis

The symptoms of TR parallel the physical manifestations (e.g., hepatic pulsation) and signs of RV failure or of PAH. *The clinical signs* include *a systolic murmur* along the lower left sternal border, occasionally increasing in inspirium (Carvallo's sign), due to blood suction by the decreased intrathoracic inspiratory pressure; *abnormal systolic waves* in the jugular venous pulse and systolic hepatic pulsation (due to blood reflux toward the great veins in systole, in severe TR); *a middiastolic murmur* in severe regurgitation (relative TS; the diastolic flow is abnormally increased, as it includes the extra volume previously regurgitated into the RA). Coexisting diseases (PAH, LV, or RV failure, other cardiac or noncardiac conditions) have the usual presentation. *The echo signs* of TR include (1) *by Doppler: a systolic regurgitant jet* from the RV to the RA. This is graded semiquantitatively by color imaging as trace, mild, moderate, or severe. Spectral CW tracing allows the assessment of the regurgitant jet velocity; this is used in the Bernoulli equation to calculate the PA pressure as $sPAP = 4v^2$, where v is the maximum regurgitant jet velocity; *increased tricuspid E wave velocity*, due to the increased tricuspid flow in diastole; and *systolic blood flow reversal in the hepatic veins* (with severe TR). Trace or mild TR is frequently seen in healthy subjects and is considered normal; (2) *by 2D assessment*: tricuspid leaflet, LV/RV, PA, or other valve pathology; assessment of tricuspid annulus dilatation, with functional TR. Severe TR displays a jet area >30% of RA area; tricuspid E wave velocity >1 m/s; annular dilatation >4 cm; and/or hepatic vein flow reversal (Fig. 5.5).

TR and PAH: Who Is the Culprit?

sPAP >55 mmHg is likely to provide the explanation for TR (annular dilatation with anatomically normal TV), whereas sPAP <40 mmHg generally does not explain significant TR, which is most likely caused by leaflet pathology.

TR Severity and TR Jet Velocity: Two Distinct Issues

TR severity is assessed by the regurgitant jet area. Even jets with a very small area (mild TR) may have very high velocity (representing severe PAH).

Catheterization in TR patients demonstrates systolic reflux of contrast media from the RA into the RV, allowing semiquantitation of TR. Different degrees of PAH are seen, as well as RV dilatation and tall systolic v waves, corresponding to the backward systolic blood flow. Angiography can lead to either under or overestimation of TR severity (the former due to dehydration, and the latter, to the simple fact of passing a catheter through the TV). *Chest X-ray* demonstrates RV enlargement and the often associated cardiac or pulmonary pathology (MS, chronic lung disease, etc.). The *EKG* is nonspecific and may show signs of RVH in patients with PAH.

5.7.3 TR-Therapy

TR therapy is guided by the severity of TR and of its clinical manifestations and by coexisting cardiac pathology. *Medical therapy* consists in the management of RV failure, PAH, or of rarer causes of TR (e.g., carcinoid);

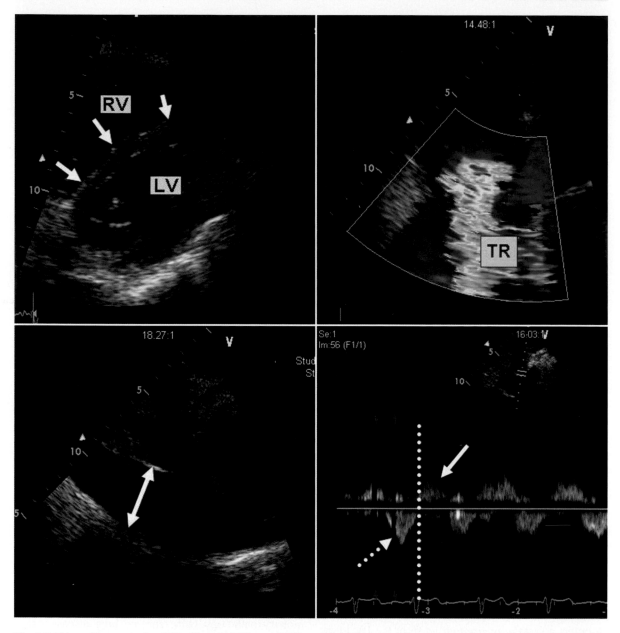

Fig. 5.5 Tricuspid regurgitation (TR). *Upper left*: Flattened IVS (*arrows*) in a patient with severe TR complicated by PAH; *Upper right*: TR flow on color Doppler mode; *Lower left*: severely dilated IVC (*double-headed arrow*) in the same patient, due to severe RV dysfunction; *Lower right*: systolic flow reversal in the hepatic vein (*full arrow*), as opposed to normal diastolic flow toward the RA (*dotted arrow*). The *dotted line* indicates systole onset

Interventional therapy – see Table 5.18. Occasionally, correction of another cardiac problem (e.g., MS or MR) corrects the TV pathology as well. In other patients, however, intervention on the valve itself is often required. If the underlying problem is tricuspid annular dilatation, this can be corrected by annuloplasty; however, if TR is caused by leaflet pathology, TV prosthesis is required. This will usually be a bioprosthesis due to the low-flow velocities through the TV, leading to increased risk of thrombosis. In the absence of surgical correction, severe TR has a poor prognosis, due to the associated RV dysfunction.

Table 5.18 Tricuspid regurgitation (TR): indications for surgery

Regurgitation		Etiology		Symptoms		Comorbidity		Complications
Severe	and	primary	and	yes, despite optimal medical therapy	and no	severe RV dysfunction or severe PAH (defined as sPAP >60 mmHg)		
Severe or moderate	and	primary			and	indication for left-sided valve surgery		
Severe or moderate	and	secondary			and	indication for left-sided valve surgery	and	dilated tricuspid annulus (>40 mm)
Severe					and	indication for left-sided valve surgery	or	progressive RV dilatation and/or dysfunction

5.8 Pulmonic Stenosis

5.8.1 Etiology

Similarly to AS, PS may be valvular, subvalvular, or supravalvular. Subvalvular stenosis is generally seen with severe or long-standing PS, causing infundibular hypertrophy, which regresses after successful balloon valvuloplasty. The vast majority of cases of PS are congenital in origin. Some cases may be caused by carcinoid disease.

5.8.2 Diagnosis

Symptoms are rare even with severe PS; when present, they include dyspnea, fatigue, and the inability to increase CO under exercise or during pregnancy, leading to presyncope or syncope, especially under conditions of dehydration. Additional symptoms include RV failure and functional TR. If there is associated PFO (or if the foramen ovale opens as a result of increased RV and RA pressures), there is cyanosis and an increased risk of paradoxical embolism. Severe cases mostly present in childhood, and most symptomatic cases become so before adolescence. *The clinical findings* include a harsh crescendo–decrescendo systolic murmur at the pulmonic area (second left intercostal space); the murmur irradiates diffusely, may be preceded by a click (if the stenosis is valvular, and the leaflets are pliable), and may be associated to a palpatory thrill. The more severe the stenosis, the louder the murmur, and the longer its total duration and time-to-peak-intensity. S2 is widely split, with a pulmonary component that is soft (due to leaflet rigidity) and delayed (longer time necessary for RV/PA pressure equalization). Occasional patients present with cyanosis. *Echo findings* include data regarding the mean and peak transpulmonic gradient (peak gradient >36 mmHg, corresponding to a jet velocity >3 m/s, represents severe PS) and typically show fusion of the leaflets, giving the valve a dome-like or conical shape. The leaflets may be thickened and dysplastic. Different degrees of RVH, TR, and PAH may be seen. The severity grading of PS is reviewed in Table 5.19.

Chest X-ray may show poststenotic aneurysmal dilatation of the pulmonary trunk and/or the left PA. Most patients with PS have normal pulmonary vasculature, which sets them apart from patients with pulmonary atresia (decreased pulmonary vasculature).

Table 5.19 Severity of PS-grading

Severity	Valve area (cm²)	Peak gradient (mmHg)
Mild	>1	<50
Moderate	0.5–1.0	50–75
Severe	<0.5	>75

5.8.3 PS Management

Echo evaluation is appropriate in case of clinical suspicion of PS. If PS is found to be nonsevere, infrequent follow-up (every 5–10 years) is sufficient; otherwise, catheterization is recommended for the evaluation of candidacy to pulmonary valvuloplasty. Most cases of PS do not require catheterization. Balloon valvotomy is recommended for PS patients with a catheter peak-to-peak gradient >30 mmHg, especially if they are symptomatic; in asymptomatic patients, intervention may be deferred until the catheter gradient becomes >40 mmHg. In patients with PV dysplasia and/or calcification, surgery is usually required.

5.9 Pulmonic Insufficiency (PI)

Trace-to-mild PI is considered normal. Greater degrees of PI are seen with idiopathic PA dilation or with connective tissue disorders. PI can also be iatrogenic, after balloon valvuloplasty for PS, or after surgery for TOF. The *clinical signs* of PI include a diastolic murmur over the PV area; the pulmonic component of S2 is accentuated with PAH, but inaudible in the absence of a pliable PV. With RV dilatation and failure, a third and fourth health sound may be heard. The jugular venous pressure is usually increased, according to the degree of RV dysfunction. While the prognosis is usually good, severe RV dilatation and dysfunction, as well as lethal ventricular arrhythmias (SCD), have been reported. LV dysfunction may result from chronic suboptimal filling. The diagnosis of PI is established semiquantitatively by *color Doppler*; as with AI, the assessment must be based on the width of the regurgitant jet at its base (vena contracta). Occasionally, there is diastolic flow reversal in the PA. *Cardiac MRI* can be useful not only for identification and quantitation of PI, but also for assessment of the RV volume, mass, and function (RVEF). RV dilatation, especially in the presence of QRS prolongation, portends an increased risk of SCD. PV replacement is formally recommended for patients with severe PI and a NYHA class > I, but, as with AI, is advocated also for asymptomatic patients with ventricular dilatation and dysfunction. *The EKG*

demonstrates different degrees of RVH (R wave prominence in V1, right axis deviation).

5.10 Combined VHD

In certain cases (rheumatic disease, CHD), there is multiple valvular involvement. In these cases, one lesion usually predominates and dictates the dominant pathophysiology; however, the nondominant lesion also impacts the clinical picture. The diagnosis of these entities is subject to considerable potential error. As a general rule, significant valvular regurgitation associated to a primarily stenotic lesion leads to underestimation of valve area by the thermodilution method, since the latter only accounts for forward flow. In these cases, the continuity equation (based on Doppler data) is very helpful (Table 5.20). The management of these patients is complex, and solid clinical judgment must be applied to each particular case. If the dominating lesion is AS, even mild symptoms should prompt surgery; if the dominant lesion is AI or MR, surgery may be deferred until the onset of LV dysfunction. In many cases of mixed VHD, exercise testing is necessary for establishing the correct diagnosis.

5.11 Prosthetic Valves

5.11.1 General Remarks

There are two main types of prosthetic valves: mechanical (made of metal, carbon, and fabric) and biological (porcine valves). Mechanical valves are more durable than artificial valves, but are also more thrombogenic, requiring anticoagulant therapy. Recent studies have shown that biological valves implanted in younger patients (in principle, not the ideal recipient population, due to the long life expectancy and the probability of valve degeneration) do have a long survival span (on average, 15 years). The main types of *mechanical valves* include the *ball and cage valves* (Starr–Edwards; the oldest and the most thrombogenic type of valve, discontinued in 2007); *tilting disk valves* (single circular occluder controlled by a metal strut: the Bjork-Shiley valves were the first introduced, the Medtronic-Hall

Table 5.20 Combined valvular lesions[a]

		1 AS	2 AI	3 MS	4 MR	5 TR
A	AS	–	Volume overload of noncompliant LV → pulmonary congestion	See C1	See D1	Nonspecific
B	AI	High-gradient event in nonsevere AS, due to increased transvalvular flow	–	See C2	See D2	Nonspecific
C	MS	AS evaluation is difficult, since MS decreases LV filling; AS murmur predominates; MS produces pulmonary congestion[b]	MS restricts LV filling, blunting the impact of AR on LV volume; thus, even severe AR may fail to exhibit the typical clinical signs and cardiomegaly. MV area measurement by pressure half-time is inaccurate	–	Lack of LV dilatation even with severe MR	The degree of TR dependence on MS may be difficult to estimate[c]
D	MR	[d]AS worsens MR; MR increases LVEF, masking AS-dependent LV dysfunction; MR reduces forward flow, masking the true severity of AS	Both produce LV dilatation	High-gradient event in nonsevere MS, due to increased transvalvular flow		Nonspecific

[a]The combination of "non-severe" lesions may cause hemodynamic compromise and warrant surgery

[b]If AS appears less than severe, PMV may be performed first, to be followed by reassessment of the AV. If symptoms improve, AVR may be delayed; otherwise, bivalvular replacement is indicated

[c]If the TV is rheumatically deformed, it may be safely assumed that TR will not improve after PMV or MV replacement. However, the regression of functional TR (i.e., TR due to annular dilatation) after MV surgery is unpredictable, and tricuspid annuloplasty is advocated, lest a second open-chest surgical procedure become necessary

[d]This combination is usually due to rheumatic fever, but congenital AS combined with MVP-related MR may be seen in young patients; AVR and MV repair is the optimal approach, but AS alone may lead to significant improvement in MR. If MV surgery is indicated due to severe MR, AVR is warranted if aortic gradient is >30 mmHg, as the true AS severity is most likely masked by the MR-dependent reduced forward flow

valves are currently the most frequently used); *bileaflet valves* (two semicircular leaflets rotating about struts attached to the valve housing, ensuring a more physiologic blood flow, with a lower risk of thrombotic complications; the most used are the St. Jude Medical valves); and *tri-leaflet valves*. In turn, biological valves are classified as allografts (cadaver valves), isografts (self-transplantation, as in the Ross procedure), or xenografts (porcine valves).

5.11.2 Prosthetic Valve Choice

The choice of the optimal type of prosthetic valve in a given patient depends on the ability to benefit from the main theoretical advantage, i.e., *avoidance of chronic anticoagulation*. This excludes patients with an independent indication for anticoagulation (e.g., AF or previous stroke), as well as women contemplating pregnancy (there is insufficient evidence in favor of LMWH in this setting, and oral anticoagulants may cause teratogenic complications, especially in the first trimester; low-dose warfarin, i.e., <5 mg/day, may be safe, if the prosthesis is not of a highly thrombogenic type). Conversely, patients with a history of poor compliance to anticoagulation or those with a history of mechanical valve thrombosis are (all other things being equal) ideal beneficiaries. The *relative risk for valve degeneration* (biological valve) vs. *anticoagulation-related bleeding* (mechanical valve) is a key consideration, as are the patient's preferences regarding chronic anticoagulation vs. the prospect of requiring a repeat intervention in the future. Thus, by and large, mechanical prostheses are preferred in patients already on chronic anticoagulation, whatever the

Fig. 5.6 Prosthetic St. Jude valve in the mitral position (diastole, as indicated by the cursor on the simultaneous EKG tracing): *Left* – open valve; *right* – closed valve. Notice the echoes projected by the mechanical valve, projected as whitish shadows. These are separate for each valve in the *left*, and merged into one single echo (*right*)

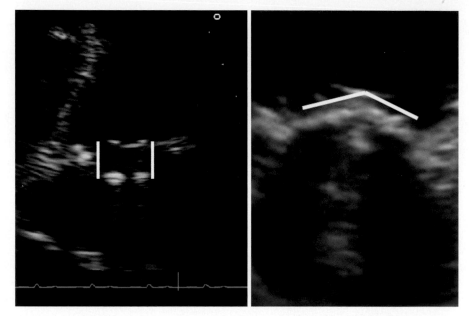

reason; in patients aged <65–70 for whom, in the Western world at least, there is a life expectancy exceeding the average survival time of biological valves; in patients at risk for biological valve degeneration, e.g., those with hypercalcemia due to hyperthyroidism (or possibly associated to CRF); and in patients at high risk for redo surgery (should the need arise to replace a degenerated biological valve). The latter group mainly includes those with poor LV function or with previous open-heart surgery interventions, in whom pleural and pericardial adhesions make future surgical dissection hazardous.

5.11.3 Management of Prosthetic Valves

Follow-up after valve replacement surgery is carried out (1) *clinically*: yearly, and as soon as a new murmur is detected; (2) *by echo*: intraoperatively, if surgery is performed under echo guidance (immediate postprocedural inspection); at 6–12 weeks after surgery, as a baseline assessment after adaptation to the improved hemodynamic conditions; as soon as a new cardiac murmur is detected; and yearly, in patients with a biological prosthesis, after the fifth year since the initial surgery. The most meaningful comparison is that with the patient's baseline transvalvular gradient. The default echo modality is TTE, but TEE should be used

whenever valve dysfunction or IE are suspected, as well as in patients with suboptimal TTE images. Figure 5.6 presents a normally functioning St. Jude bileaflet valve.

Antithrombotic management after valve replacement is indicated lifelong in patients with mechanical prostheses, and for the first 3 months after biological prosthesis insertion (target INR 2.5). The thrombogenicity of mechanical valves is due to platelet and coagulation factor activation, in contact with the foreign materials. The target INR for mechanical valves is established according to (1) *valve-related risk of thrombosis*, as different types of prosthesis carry different risks of thrombosis. Thus, thrombogenicity is *low* for Carbomedics valves in the aortic position, Medtronic-Hall valves, and St Jude Medical valves without Silzone (the latter is a now-discontinued technology of silver coating of the prosthetic valve sewing ring, to decrease the risk of IE; unfortunately, these valves were associated to increased incidence of paravalvular leak, and possibly, of valve thrombosis); *medium*, for Bjork–Shiley and other bileaflet valves; and *high*, for Lillehei–Kaster, Omniscience, and Starr–Edwards valves; (2) *patient-related risks of thrombosis and embolism*: a past history of other valve replacement or of thromboembolism; AF; LA diameter >50 mm; LA spontaneous contrast; MS of any degree; LVEF <35%; or a hypercoagulable state. The target INR is calculated using the following algorithm: start at 2.5, for a low-thrombogenic valve and no patient-related risk factor, and add 0.5 for each superior class of thrombogenicity, as well as for the presence of ≥ 1 patient-related risk factor. For instance, for a highly thrombogenic valve in a patient with AF, the target INR is $2.5 + 0.5 \times 2$ (two thrombogenicity classes above "low") $+ 0.5$ (≥ 1 risk factor) $= 4$. This is the highest recommended target INR. In the example above, the valve-related INR requirements supersede the AF-related ones (target INR for AF $= 2.5$). The antithrombotic agents of choice are oral anticoagulants (see Chap. 6). Antiplatelet drugs can be added in patients with atherosclerotic disease, as well as in those with a past history of embolism. Weekly INR monitoring is recommended in patients requiring coronary PCI and stent deployment, where Clopidogrel addition, mandatory in DES-carrying patients, significantly increases the risk of bleeding.

5.11.4 Management of Complications Related to Prosthetic Valves

Prosthetic valve thrombosis is suspected in case of an embolic event or of recent escalation in HF severity and is confirmed by echo (ideally, by TEE); fluoroscopy may demonstrate decreased valve opening. It is important to distinguish valve thrombosis from fibrin strands (small filamentous structures on both sides of a prosthetic valve) and from pannus (tissue ingrowth due to excessive endothelial proliferation). While fibrin strands are generally benign and require no treatment, pannus occasionally leads to valve obstruction requiring redo valve replacement. Pannus is not amenable to antithrombotic therapy. Therapy depends on the hemodynamic impact of the thrombus (obstructive vs. nonobstructive) and on its embolic potential. Thus: (1) *Surgery* is indicated in all patients with aortic or mitral prosthetic valve thrombosis, unless the thrombi are small (<10 mm) and nonobstructive. Surgery is generally not indicated in patients with prosthetic tricuspid or pulmonary valves (thrombolysis is first-choice therapy in these patients). (2) *Thrombolysis* is indicated in patients with small thrombi (unless the minute dimensions justify a conservative approach), or if surgery is unavailable or high-risk. A typical regimen is the following: 250,000 UI over 30 min followed by an infusion of 100,000 UI/h, for up to 72 h, under repeated echo monitoring for thrombus resolution and tPA (100 mg total dose, administered as a 10 mg bolus followed by a continuous infusion of 5 mg/h). At thrombus resolution, Heparin (50 U/kg/h IV initially, followed by continuous infusion of 15–25 U/kg/h, adjusting dose by 5 U/kg/h q. 4 h, as per aPTT results) and oral anticoagulants are started. Heparin is discontinued when the therapeutic INR is attained. If there is proof that the prethrombosis INR target had been systematically attained, the target is increased (not to exceed INR $= 4$), and antiplatelet agents may be added; (3) *Either surgery or thrombolysis* are indicated in patients with a large mobile thrombus (>5 mm), with previous thromboembolism, or (on a case-by-case basis) in whom initial response to Heparin or oral anticoagulants was unsatisfactory; (4) *Heparin and aspirin* are recommended in all other cases, with subsequent chronic oral anticoagulant treatment in case of success, or crossover to the surgery/thrombolysis group, in case of failure.

Prosthetic valve failure may present either as valve obstruction or as paravalvular regurgitation. Rarely seen with current mechanical valves, it used to be traditionally expected after ≥ 15 years after bioprosthesis implantation. However, biologic prostheses were recently shown to have a significantly longer life span in patients <50. If there is hemodynamic compromise (or, in patients at low risk for surgery, even in the absence of symptoms), surgical correction is required. In asymptomatic patients with a biological valve implanted >10 years previously, prophylactic valve replacement may be considered if another open-heart surgical intervention is indicated.

HF in the patient with prosthetic heart valves may simply reflect progression of preexisting LV dysfunction, but must first and foremost raise the possibility of new-onset prosthesis dysfunction. Echo is urgently required.

Other complications are reviewed in Table 5.21.

5.12 Special Situations in Patients with VHD

5.12.1 Noncardiac Surgery

Noncardiac surgery may cause hemodynamic decompensation or myocardial infarction (Table 5.22) or prosthetic valve thrombosis, as a result of interruption of anticoagulant therapy in patients with valvular prostheses (Table 5.23).

Table 5.21 Other complications of mechanical valve prostheses

Complication	Incidence	Remarks
AF	Up to 50%, in the postoperative stage	Prevented by β-blockers; if extends beyond 24 h, DCC, anticoagulation, and/or AAD are warranted
Conduction disturbances	In 2–3% of patients after AVR; up to 8% after repeat surgery	Calcification, old age, IE, and TV surgery are risk factors
IE	3–6%	Typically, large vegetations. Early IE (<60 days after surgery) is typically caused by *S. epidermidis* and has a very high mortality. Late IE is mainly streptococcal and has lower mortality. TEE is the diagnostic method of choice, therapy is antibiotic and occasionally surgical[a]
Hemolysis	More frequent in caged-ball than in tilting disk or bioprosthetic valves	Small valves, IE, and paraprosthetic leaks are risk factors. Elevated LDL and reticulocyte count frequent. Beta-blockade indicated, prosthesis replacement required
Dehiscence	Variable	Calcification, infection are risk factors. Urgent surgery required
Patient-prosthesis mismatch	Variable	Prostheses with a diameter <21 mm not indicated in large or physically active patients
Pannus formation	In up to 5% of mechanical prostheses/year	More frequent in the aortic than in the mitral position. Often associated to thrombus
Embolic stroke	Variable	Previous stroke a major risk factor. Usual therapy

[a]The indications for surgical therapy in prosthetic valve IE include: persistent bacteremia, tissue invasion (abscess, fistula new or worsening heart block), recurrent embolization, fungal infection, mechanical dysfunction (dehiscence or obstruction), and HF

Table 5.22 VHD and noncardiac surgery: the risk of hemodynamic decompensation

VHD	Low risk	High risk	Recommended action
MR	Preserved LV function	LVEF <30%	Consider valve surgery or avoidance of noncardiac surgery in high-risk patients
AR	Preserved LV function	LVEF <30%	As above
MS	Asymptomatic and/or sPAP <50 mmHg	Symptomatic and/or sPAP >50 mmHg	PMV indicated, if the time and the valve morphology allow it
AS	Asymptomatic and nonvascular surgery	Symptomatic; vascular surgery[a]	In high-risk patients, AVR[b]

[a]Excluding carotid endarterectomy, which is intermediate-risk, alongside intraperitoneal, intrathoracic, head and neck, orthopedic, or prostate surgery. Other types of surgery are considered low-risk for cardiac complications
[b]In the very frail patient, aortic valvuloplasty may be considered; strict perioperative monitoring is essential

Table 5.23 Anticoagulation in patients with mechanical valves undergoing noncardiac surgery

Type of surgery	Emergency surgery	Recommended strategy
Major	Yes	Revert anticoagulation using FFP or prothrombin complex concentrate; start UFH as soon as feasible (or LMWH in therapeutic b.i.d. doses, rather than the q.d. prophylactic doses), resume VKA as usual (consider higher target INR)
Major	No	Electively stop VKA and start UFH (last dose 6 h before surgery) or LMWH[a] (last dose 12–24 h before surgery, according to half-life), then continue as above
Nonmajor[b]	Yes	Consider partial reversal of anticoagulation, to a target INR of 2
Nonmajor	No	Lower VKA dosage to a target INR of 2

[a]If possible, under monitoring of anti-Xa activity (therapeutic range is 0.5–1 IU anti-Xa/mL, between 3 and 4 h after a S.C. injection)
[b]Including dental procedures

5.12.2 *Pregnancy and Delivery*

Severe VHD should be surgically treated before considering pregnancy. This is especially true for severe stenotic lesions, poorly tolerated in pregnancy (which causes increased flow through a fixed obstruction). A baseline echo examination must be performed in any woman with VHD or with a prosthetic valve (to provide recommendations regarding future pregnancies), as well as in pregnant patients with dyspnea or a heart murmur more than trivial in intensity. In patients with severe stenosis, echo should be repeated routinely at 3 and 5 months, and monthly after 5 months. In case of *hemodynamic decompensation*, symptomatic treatment and bed rest are indicated according to the underlying VHD (β-blockers and diuretics for MS, diuretics and possibly vasodilators for AI). These usually suffice to see the patient with regurgitant lesions to term, while in patients with stenotic lesions, balloon valvuloplasty may be required (as definitive treatment for MS, or as a bridge to surgery in AS patients). If valve replacement surgery is necessary and the fetus is viable, preprocedural caesarian section is recommended. Patients with Marfan's disease require treatment with β-blockers for the entire duration of pregnancy, to avoid aortic dissection. An additional concern in women with prosthetic valves is the *teratogenic effect of VKA*, mainly severe CNS and bone abnormalities. In principle, the risk is negligible if the daily requirement of Warfarin is <5 mg, in which case it may be used for the entire duration of the pregnancy, to be replaced by UFH after week 36, in preparation for delivery. In case the required dosage is ≥5 mg daily, or if an abundance of caution is being exercised, Warfarin is replaced by UFH in the first trimester of pregnancy, and beyond week 36. There are no systematic guidelines as to the use of Acenocoumarol in this setting, with some case reports describing uneventful pregnancies, and others, severe fetal toxicity. Theoretically tempting, LMWH prophylaxis has not been conclusively shown to be effective and cannot be recommended. *Caesarian section* is required in women with VHD associated to Marfan's syndrome, unstable stenotic lesions not amenable to balloon valvuloplasty, and in patients with severe LV dysfunction. These findings also justify *early termination of pregnancy*.

5.13 Infective Endocarditis (IE)

See Chap. 8.

Bibliography

Guidelines

Nishimura RA, Carabello BA, Faxon DP, et al. ACC/AHA 2008 Guideline update on valvular heart disease: focused update on infective endocarditis: a report of the American College of Cardiology/American Heart Association Task Force on Practice Guidelines. *Circulation*. 2008; 118:887-896.

Bonow RO, Carabello BA, Chatterjee K, et al. ACC/AHA 2006 guidelines for the management of patients with valvular heart disease: a report of the American College of Cardiology/American Heart Association task force on practice guidelines (writing committee to develop guidelines for the management of patients with valvular heart disease). *Circulation*. 2006;114:e84-e231. doi:10.1161/CIRCULATIONAHA.106.176857.

Suggested Reading

Braunwald E. On the natural history of severe aortic stenosis. *J Am Coll Cardiol*. 1990;15:1018-1020.

Gaasch WH, Sundaram M, Meyer TE. Managing asymptomatic patients with chronic aortic regurgitation. *Chest*. 1997;111(6): 1702-1709.

Zajarias A, Cribier AG. Outcomes and safety of percutaneous aortic valve replacement. *J Am Coll Cardiol*. 2009;53: 1829-1836.

Pereira JJ, Lauer MS, Bashir M. Survival after aortic valve replacement for severe aortic stenosis with low transvalvular gradients and severe left ventricular dysfunction. *J Am Coll Cardiol*. 2002;39(8):1356-1363.

Levine RA, Handschumacher MD, Sanfilippo AJ, et al. Three-dimensional echocardiographic reconstruction of the mitral valve, with implications for the diagnosis of mitral valve prolapse. *Circulation*. 1989;80:589-598.

Han Y, Peters DC, Salton CJ, et al. Cardiovascular magnetic resonance characterization of mitral valve prolapse. *J Am Coll Cardiol Img*. 2008;1:294-303.

Block PC. Percutaneous transcatheter repair for mitral regurgitation. *J Interv Cardiol*. 2006;19(6):547-551

Antunes MJ, Barlow JB. Management of tricuspid valve regurgitation. *Heart*. 2007;93:271-276.

Zoghbi WA, Enriquez-Sarano M, Foster E, et al. Recommendations for evaluation of the severity of native valvular regurgitation with two-dimensional and Doppler echocardiography. *J Am Soc Echocardiogr*. 2003;16(7):777-802.

Zoghbi WA, Chambers JB, Dumesnil JG, et al. Recommendations for evaluation of prosthetic valves with echocardiography and doppler ultrasound: a report From the American Society of Echocardiography's Guidelines and Standards Committee and the Task Force on Prosthetic Valve. *J Am Soc Echocardiogr*. 2009;22(9):975-1014; quiz 1082-1084.

Contents

6.1 Supraventricular Tachyarrhythmia

6.1.1 General Remarks

6.1.1.1 Definition, Prevalence, Importance

Supraventricular tachyarrhythmia (SVT) is a global term for abnormal rhythms generated in one or more of the following structures: the sinus node, the atrial myocardium, the AV node, or the bundle of His, down to its bifurcation. Thus, the designation, "supraventricular" departs from the anatomical landmarks, since the bundle of His is in the upper portion of the IVS; in fact, with one of these rhythms, that is, antidromic AV reentrant tachycardia (AVRT), part of the aberrant circuit is in the ventricular myocardium itself. The acronym "SVT" may stand for supraventricular *tachycardia* or *tachyarrhythmia*. Arbitrarily, the former term generally does not cover atrial flutter (AF) and flutter. During SVT, the HR is usually ≥100 bpm, but can be lower in case of coexisting AV block; the term, "tachycardia," is still justified in these cases, as it applies to the atrial rate. SVT is quite frequent, although the exact incidence remains unclear, partly due to the large number of asymptomatic cases (demonstrated by Holter); however, the incidence of SVT increases with age and with the presence of structural heart disease. SVT may cause symptoms ranging from the sensation of "extra" or of "skipped" heart beats, to palpitations and even syncope. Additionally, in patients with underlying structural heart disease, it may exacerbate angina pectoris, HF, and/or hemodynamic instability. Occasionally, SVT may degenerate into ventricular tachyarrhythmia, with hemodynamic instability or sudden death, a particular concern in patients with professions impacting public safety (e.g., pilots). SVT may be difficult to differentiate from ventricular tachycardia, a condition with a different treatment and a significantly worse prognosis; moreover, the first-line treatments for SVT are generally contraindicated in VT. Additional concerns with SVT include the toxic (including proarrhythmic) effect of chronic AAD treatment and possible bleeding under antithrombotic therapy; the possibility of tachycardia-related CMP, in chronic cases; abolishment of the atrial kick, either due to AV discordance or to absent P waves (AF), precipitating HF in predisposed individuals; the risk of thromboembolism with AF and flutter (leading causes of stroke); and finally, the considerable amount of anxiety SVT generates.

6.1.1.2 Classification

There exist several classification systems for SVT, as discussed below. As the different classification criteria are interrelated, there is substantial overlap.

The mechanism of SVT: There are three possible mechanisms of arrhythmia generation (whether supraventricular or ventricular). These include:

- *Increased automaticity*, that is, the increased ability to reach the threshold for action potential initiation, either in the specialized (sinus node, AV node, His-Purkinje system), or the nonspecialized myocardium (ectopic foci in the atria or ventricles).
- *Triggered activity* is seen when the electrical oscillations in the myocite membrane ("afterdepolarizations" caused by previous electrical impulses) reach levels allowing them to initiate an action potential, and thus an ectopic rhythm. Afterdepolarizations may be of two types: "early," that is, occurring before repolarization of cardiac tissues (mainly causing ventricular arrhythmias) and "delayed," occurring after the depolarization of the surrounding myocardium is complete (causing mainly atrial and digitalis-induced arrhythmias).
- *Reentry* is a mechanism whereby a normal, or, more commonly, an abnormal (premature) impulse is "recycled" over an abnormal circuit, generating an arrhythmia. The two limbs of the circuit may be (1) normal or pathologic conduction pathways (the slow and the fast pathway in the AV node or the normal conduction system on one hand, and an aberrant AV or, infrequently, ventriculo-ventricular pathway, on the other; occasionally, both limbs are aberrant pathways); or (2) acquired, either as distinct physical

entities (e.g., the two halves of the circumference around a myocardial scar), or as functional entities (ischemic myocardial areas conducting at different velocities). If (as often occurs) the two limbs have different conduction velocities and refractory periods, then an impulse blocked down one of the limbs (still in its refractory period) is conducted down the other limb; by the time it has reached the distal extremity, the previously refractory limb has recovered its conductibility, and the electrical impulse now travels up this limb, prematurely depolarizing the myocardium, at a rate dictated by the time necessary for circling the reentry circuit. Reentry circuits may be large (*macroreentry*), as with (a) AVRT, where the circuit involves the atria, the AV node, the His bundle, the ventricular myocardium, and the aberrant pathway; or (b) surgical atriotomy scar reentry circuits (causing reentrant AT, or, in case of even larger circuits within the RA, atypical AF); (c) surgery-independent RA reentrant circuits (typical AF); (d) Mahaim-bundle tachycardias, or small (*microreentry*), as with (a) sinoatrial reentry tachycardia; (b) atrial microreentry tachycardia; (c) some cases of AF; and (d) AV nodal reentrant tachycardia (AVNRT), where the circuit involves the slow and the past pathways within the AV node.

The supraventricular arrhythmias arising by these different mechanisms are reviewed in Table 6.1.

Dependence vs. nondependence of the arrhythmia on the AV node refers to whether the AV node is part of the reentry circuit *generating* the arrhythmia. Most SVTs show AV nodal dependence. Two semantic points are of great importance: (1) With the exception of tachyarrhythmias antegradely conducted through an aberrant pathway, all supraventricular arrhythmias depend on the AV node for *conduction* of the impulses to the ventricles; this does not qualify them as AV node-dependent; (2) AV node dependence must not be mistaken for the entity, AVNRT. AV-node dependence simply requires that the AV node be *part* of the reentry circuit; AVNRT is the particular instance where the *entire* reentry circuit is within the AV node. The distinction between AV node-dependent and -independent arrhythmias is clinically important both for diagnosis and for therapy. Efficacy of AV-inhibitory maneuvers or drugs generally points to an AV node-dependent arrhythmia (although there are some exceptions, outlined below). In patients with AV node-independent

Table 6.1 Supraventricular arrhythmias by responsible mechanism

Site	Automaticity	Triggered activity: delayed afterdep[a]	Reentry
Sinus node	Sinus tachycardia		Sino-atrial reentry tachyc.
Atrial myocardium	AF[b]; automatic AT	AT; digitalis toxicity	AF[b]; atrial flutter[c]
AV node	Junctional escape rhtyhm, nonparox. junctional tachycardia, focal junctional tachycardia	Nonparoxysmal junctional tachycardia	AV nodal reentry tachycardia
Atrial myocardium, accessory pathway, AV node, His bundle, ± ventr. myocardium			AVRT, Mahaim tachycardia

[a]Early afterdepolarizations mainly cause ventricular arrhythmia
[b]The two mechanisms coexist; AF by reentry involves microreentry circuits
[c]Macrorentrant circuit in the RA (for typical AF) or other macroreentrant circuits (e.g., around scar tissue – atypical flutter)

arrhythmias, AV node blockade, while unable to influence arrhythmia *generation*, may still influence its *conduction* to the ventricles. The longer ventricular pauses thus obtained reveal more clearly the atrial electrical activity (often obscured by significant tachycardia), facilitating EKG diagnosis. Of note, an AV-node independent arrhythmia is not necessarily supraventricular; if the QRS complexes are wide, it might be a ventricular tachycardia.

The different possible effects of AV node inhibition in SVT patients

AV node inhibition may

- *Abruptly terminate the arrhythmia* (with AV node-dependent tachycardias, sinoatrial reentry tachycardia, and some forms of AT)
- *Gradually slow down the cardiac (atrial=ventricular) rate*, which subsequently reaccelerates (with sinus tachycardia, some forms of AT, and nonparoxysmal junctional tachycardia)
- *Leave the atrial rhythm unchanged, but slow down the ventricular rate* by inducing a transient AVB (with AF and some forms of AT); often, this allows better examination of the atrial waves, for rhythm diagnosis
- *Leave both the atrial rhythm and the ventricular rate unchanged*, i.e., have no effect at all; this demonstrates AV node-independence, and suggests the possibility of VT

Dependence vs. nondependence on an accessory pathway: This separates AVRT from the other types of SVT, a very important distinction, since rapid conduction of an atrial tachyarrhythmia (in the worst-case scenario, AF) over an aberrant pathway can lead to VF and sudden death. Aberrant pathways are generally identified by EKG, either in NSR (delta wave), or at the time of SVT: if rate-dependent BBB slows down the HR, the bundle branch is part of the reentry circuit (AVRT); otherwise, BBB would simply change the QRS morphology, but not the HR. Occasionally, the only modality to identify an aberrant pathway is EPS.

6.1.1.3 Underlying Conditions

Risk factors for SVT include: female sex, anxiety, fatigue, caffeine, alcohol, cigarettes, and, in patients with an aberrant pathway, a suggestive family history. Though most common in otherwise healthy individuals, SVT can also occur in patients with chronic lung disease (hypoxia typically causes MAT), and, less commonly, in patients with myocardial ischemia or significant MV disease.

6.1.1.4 SVT Diagnosis

Clinical manifestations: The severity of clinical manifestations varies widely: some patients are asymptomatic or complain of palpitations, while others may suffer syncope or SCD. *Asymptomatic* patients are at risk for tachycardia-induced CMP, if SVT is chronic (a characteristic not displayed by all types of SVT). Generally, this CMP takes weeks or months to develop, and is at least partly reversible even in severe cases. *Palpitations* are the most frequent complaint, usually with an abrupt onset and termination (a characteristic of reentrant arrhythmias, the most common mechanism of SVT), and lasting for seconds to hours. Conversely, automatic tachycardias may be nonparoxysmal and have a gradual onset and termination. However, this distinction is not always clinically evident, since stress-induced sympathetic stimulation may cause sinus tachycardia to take over after termination of reentry SVT; as one form of tachycardia supplants another, the transition may be less clearly perceived by the patient. *Chest pain* is occasionally reported; the explanation is unclear, since most patients do not have underlying coronary disease. *The urge to urinate* described by some patients may be related to release of the atrial natriuretic peptide. AV dyssynchrony causes atrial contraction against closed AV valves, with "cannon 'a' waves" and *abnormal pulsations in the neck. Syncope and SCD* are the most severe complications of SVT.

SVT-related syncope: mechanisms

These include:

- Decreased CO, if the SVT is very rapid, or in presence of an aberrant pathway
- Prolonged asystole after termination of the SVT
- A vasovagal reaction to tachycardia

The first two mechanisms can also cause SCD.

EKG manifestations: *The P wave axis* is best assessed in leads II and V1, where it is positive in NSR and in superior atrial rhythms (with an altered morphology), and negative in inferior atrial rhythms, where atrial activation is reversed. *The P-QRS relationship*: The P wave may precede, coincide with or follow the QRS complex, depending on the sequence of atrial vs. ventricular activation: if atrial activation occurs first, P precedes QRS; if it occurs last, P follows QRS; and if they are simultaneous, P and QRS are superimposed. *The position of the P wave relative to the preceding and subsequent R waves* (the R_1P and the PR_2 segments): the tachycardia is of the "long RP" type if R_1P is longer, and of the "short RP" type otherwise. Importantly, during very fast HR, these

differences may be difficult to measure. Despite substantial overlap between the different arrhythmias in regard to the long or short RP feature, a short RP usually corresponds to AVRT or to AVNRT, and a long RP, to AT. Simultaneous activation of the atria and the ventricles (i.e., a very short or zero RP interval) indicates typical slow-fast AVNRT, rather than AVRT; *The PR interval* may be constant or variable (with MAT or with AV dissociation); a shortened PR is typical of the Long-Ganong-Levine (LGL) syndrome. *The QRS complexes*: *QRS morphology* is usually normal (narrow), but the occasional wide-QRS SVT requires differentiation from VT; the underlying mechanisms for QRS widening with SVT are discussed below. Especially with faster tachycardias, the QRS amplitude varies from beat to beat; "*QRS alternans*" has an unclear mechanism, and is virtually never seen with AT; the *ventricular rate* is 150–250 bpm, most commonly <200 bpm. Normally, the atrial and ventricular rates coincide, but the latter may be slower with AV block. A rate of 150 bpm should raise the suspicion of AF with a 2:1 AV block. Relatively slow ventricular rates (<160–170 bpm), in the absence of visible P waves indicate conduction over the slow AV node pathway, and thus AVNRT; *Regularity*: SVT is generally a regular rhythm, with some exceptions, such as the "warm-up" and "cool-off" period of some automatic tachycardias, or the presence of variable AV block; *The mode of onset of the arrhythmia*: (1) Most frequently, reentrant arrhythmias start abruptly ("paroxysmal SVT= PSVT"). The three most frequent types of PSVT are AVRT, AVNRT, and AT. Typically, the initiating event is an APB conducting down one pathway and blocked down the other. Most frequently, these events involve the AV node, with antegrade conduction down the slow pathway (slow-fast AVNRT); this reflects on the EKG as a prolonged PR corresponding to the initiating APB. Atypical (fast-slow) AVNRT may also be initiated by a normal sinus beat; (2) less frequently, the onset is gradual (the "warm-up" phenomenon of automatic SVT); *The mode of termination of the arrhythmia*: tachycardias which terminate by a P wave are most frequently AV-node dependent (i.e., *not* AT). PSVT terminates abruptly, whereas automatic tachycardia may exhibit the "cool-off" phenomenon.

EPS is indicated in patients with poorly tolerated SVT, especially if it is unresponsive to medical therapy and raises the possibility of RF ablation. EPS is a mainstay of management in symptomatic patients with accessory pathways, and is advocated by some even in the absence of symptoms. Similarly, EPS is indicated in patients with AF before RF ablation, which is the procedure of choice for recurrent, poorly tolerated episodes of AF.

Other tests: The various modalities of EKG monitoring (Holter, loop recorder, implantable recorder) are used in patients in whom SVT is suspected, but has not been identified on routine EKG. Echo is routinely used to rule out structural heart disease, and has a particularly important role in the workup of patients with AF. Lab tests, such as CBC to rule out anemia, thyroid function tests to rule out hyperthyroidism, etc., are routinely performed.

6.1.1.5 Therapy of SVT

There are two main aspects to SVT treatment: termination of the acute event and, if indicated, prevention of recurrences.

Antiarrhythmic Drugs

The Vaughn-Williams classification divides AAD into several classes, according to their mechanism of action. This classification has some problematic aspects: thus, it accounts neither for the fact that some AAD act on several phases of the action potential, nor for the cases where a given AAD behaves according to one class, but its metabolites behave according to another class (e.g., procainamide acts by a Class I mechanism, and its metabolite, by a Class III mechanism). Additionally, certain drugs (Digoxin, Adenosine, Magnesium sulfate) are not captured in the classification (unless one accepts the formal solution of a "miscellaneous" Class V). The Vaughn-Williams classification is reviewed in Table 6.2.

The *recommended dosages* of the different AAD are discussed in the relevant sections. The *main adverse effects* of the usual AAD will be briefly listed.

- *β-blockers, CCB*: Chap. 3.
- *Quinidine*: The main symptoms include cinchonism (flush and rash, tinnitus, blurred vision, impaired hearing, confusion, headache, abdominal pain, nausea and vomiting, and diarrhea, dizziness) and thrombocytopenia.
- *Procainamide*: Rash, myalgia, fever, agranulocytosis, drug-induced lupus erythematosus, torsades des pointes.

Table 6.2 The Vaughn-Williams classification

Class	Involved electrolyte channels	Mechanism	Representatives
Ia	Na	Decrease excitability; lengthen the action potential	Quinidine, procainamide, disopyramide
Ib	Na	Decrease excitability; shorten the action potential	Lidocaine, phenytoin, mexiletine
Ic	Na	Decrease excitability; no effect on the action potential	Flecainide, propafenone, moricizine
II		β-blockers	Propranolol, esmolol, metoprolol, atenolol, etc.
III	K	Prolong repolarization, decrease reentry	Amiodarone, sotalol, ibutilide, dofetilide
IV	Ca	CCB	Verapamil, diltiazem

- *Disopyramide*: Acute HF, hypotension, dry mouth, constipation, urinary retention, blurred vision, glaucoma, rash, agranulocytosis.
- *Mexiletine*: Dizziness, pirosis, nausea, nervousness, tremor.
- *Lidocaine*: CNS stimulation (nervousness, tinnitus, tremor, dizziness, blurred vision, seizures), followed by depression (drowsiness, loss of consciousness, apnea). Occasionally, Lidocaine may cause hypotension, arrhythmia, cardiac arrest, or seizures.
- *Flecainide*: Proarrhythmic action in patients with structural heart disease, especially post-MI patients and patients already suffering from ventricular arrhythmia; worsening of HF.
- *Propafenone*: Hypersensitivity reactions, lupus-like syndrome, granulocytopenia, dizziness, gastrointestinal upset, a metallic taste and bronchospasm; worsening of HF.
- *Amiodarone* has a multitude of side effects, including interstitial lung disease (the most severe side effect), occasionally after as little as a week of treatment;

hypo- or hyperthyroidism; asymptomatic corneal microdeposits, vision distorted by a bluish halo, or optical neuropathy; LFT derangement, rarely up to hepatomegaly, hepatitis, or cirrhosis; blue–gray, partly or fully reversible discoloration of the skin; photosensitivity.

- *Sotalol* may cause torsades des pointes and other serious ventricular arrhythmia or bradycardia; dizziness; elevated LFT; and hyperglycemia in diabetics.
- *Dofetilide* may cause torsades des pointes, avoided by hospitalizing the patient for ≥3 days for serial creatinine measurement and telemetry monitoring.
- *Ibutilide* may cause potentially life-threatening ventricular arrhythmia, QT segment prolongation, bradycardia; hypotension (occasionally, postural) or HTN. Hospitalization is recommended.

Acute Therapy of SVT

SVT must be carefully differentiated from other arrhythmias with a similar EKG presentation: *with narrow-complex SVT*, sinus tachycardia (occasionally, very rapid in young subjects) must be ruled out, as the usual SVT treatment would be both redundant and ineffective; and with *wide-complex SVT*, VT must be ruled out, since calcium- and β-blockers, commonly used for SVT, are contraindicated in VT. SVT must also be distinguished from rapid AF (rhythm regularity and the presence of f waves may be difficult to assess with fast HRs), so as to avoid AV nodal blockade in the occasional patient with AF and an aberrant pathway. Like any other guidelines, these recommendations may be superseded by previous experience, in a given patient.

In patients with narrow-complex tachycardia, the treatment depends on the hemodynamic situation. AV node-blocking therapy, either by vagal maneuvers, or pharmacological, is the treatment of choice in the absence of hemodynamic compromise; otherwise, these measures are generally ineffective, and DCC (usually at low energies) is indicated. *Vagal maneuvers* include coughing, Valsalva, or immersing the face in cold water; occasionally, the Trendelenburg position may facilitate the success of vagal maneuvers. Carotid sinus massage can be tried (but carries a risk of stroke in the elderly). *Adenosine* is the drug of choice, but is contraindicated in patients with severe asthma (risk of bronchospasm) or with severe coronary disease ("steal phenomenon," by selective vasodilation in the healthy coronaries).

CCB have a longer duration of action and are preferred in SVT recurring soon after Adenosine therapy (the half-life of Adenosine is of a few seconds only). They are especially effective in the presence of numerous APBs and VPBs, which may trigger subsequent episodes of AVNRT; in this setting, CCB achieve both acute termination of SVT and recurrence prophylaxis. Other therapeutic options include: *β-blockers* (adverse effects are minimized by using the short-acting agent, Esmolol) and *Digoxin*, rarely used today, as it is only modestly effective (the vagal AV node inhibition caused by Digoxin is often superseded by the stress-induced catecholamine stimulation). *If an accessory pathway is known or suspected to exist*, AV-node blocking measures are best avoided, as a narrow-complex SVT is still compatible with the existence of an accessory pathway capable of antegrade conduction. Since the QRS complexes are narrow, this pathway may either be conducting retrogradely or not be involved at all in the current SVT episode; yet, these same pathways are also frequently capable of antegrade conduction, with potential life-threatening ventricular arrhythmia in case of AF or flutter (Adenosine itself may induce AF in up to 15% of cases). While the vast majority of SVT do not involve aberrant pathways, this possibility should be kept in mind, and, especially when treating a first episode, a defibrillator should be available. *The second line of therapy* involves AAD from Classes IA (procainamide), IC (Propafenone, Flecainide), or III (amiodarone, sotalol, ibutilide). Transvenous or transesophageal atrial overdrive pacing is also an option, either acutely, if DCC is contraindicated (e.g., digitalis toxicity), or as chronic antitachycardia pacing, in otherwise treatment-unresponsive patients. An "artificial" tachycardia is created to suppress the reentrant arrhythmia; after discontinuation of overdrive pacing, it is generally the sinus node (rather than the reentrant circuit) that takes over as cardiac pacemaker.

In patients with wide-complex tachycardia, (1) in clear cases of SVT with aberrant conduction, the treatment is as that for narrow-complex tachycardia; (2) in clear cases of SVT with preexcitation (i.e., antidromic SVT), the agents of choice are AAD Class IA (Procainamide, Class IC (Flecainide), or Class III (Ibutilide, Amiodarone). However, in the presence of severe LV dysfunction, the only pharmacological choice remains Amiodarone. In these patients, DCC may be the best option; (3) in unclear cases (ventricular vs. supraventricular arrhythmia), Procainamide, Sotalol, or

Amiodarone should be used (the latter, with depressed LV function), as they are effective against both SVT and VT. Lidocaine can be used, but it will be effective only against VT. Again, DCC is a sound option.

Prevention of recurrences is, in principle, required only for clinically significant AVNRT (recurrent symptomatic cases or hemodynamic compromise); however, RF ablation, effective in most types of SVT, is nowadays popular as definitive therapy, even in milder cases (especially in patients whose profession impacts public safety, e.g., pilots). Alternatively, it may be sufficient to simply teach the patient self-administration of vagal maneuvers or of AAD in case of need (the "pill-in-the-pocket" approach). The most frequently used agents are calcium- and β-blockers, and Digoxin; if these fail, class IC drugs are used; if no other alternative is effective (and RF ablation is refused or unavailable), class III drugs are used.

The various therapeutic options in SVT patients are discussed in Tables 6.3 and 6.4. Table 6. 5 reviews the corresponding recommended drug dosages. Long-term therapy in patients with preexcited tachycardia is discussed in the relevant section. These tables essentially follow the ESC/AHA Guidelines, but the "Classes of recommendation" have been replaced by a scoring system (++ first choice, + useful, − not recommended or contraindicated). The rationale is the following: as the Guidelines are strictly based on the strength of available

Table 6.3 Acute management of hemodynamically stable, regular[a] supraventricular tachyarrhythmia (SVT)

Arrhythmia	DCC[b]	Vagal Man.	Adenosine	CCB	β-blockers	Digoxin	Class IA	Class IB	Class IC	Class III
Narrow-QRS tachycardia										
First-line	++	++	++	++	+	+	−[c]	−	−	+[d]
Second-line	(by definition, second-line therapy is tried if first-line has failed)						++[e]	−	++[f, g]	++[g, h]
Wide-QRS tachycardia										
Clearly SVT with BBB	++	++	++	++	+	+	−	−		+
Clearly SVT with preexcitation										
Reasonably preserved LVEF	++	−	−	−	−	−	++[e]	−	++[f]	++[h]
Depressed LVEF	++	−	−	−	−	−	−	−	−	++
Unknown origin (SVT? VT?)										
Preserved LVEF	++	−	−[i]	−	−	−	++[e]	+[j]	++[f]	++[k]
Depressed LVEF	++	−	−	−	−	−	−	++	−	−

[a]This refers to the atrial rhythm, and, in case no variable AVB is present, to the ventricular rhythm as well

[b]Overdrive pacing is an alternative to DCC, especially in digitalis toxicity, where DCC may precipitate life-threatening ventricular arrhythmia. This is especially an issue with some forms of AT

[c]Procainamide is ++ in focal AT

[d]Amiodarone

[e]Procainamide

[f]Flecainide

[g]In uni- or multifocal AT, combined only with an AV node-blocking agent

[h]Ibutilide, Amiodarone

[i]Adenosine might be safe for the treatment of wide-QRS tachycardia with a reasonably preserved LV function (Class IIB indication)

[j]Lidocaine

[k]Sotalol, Amiodarone

Table 6.4 Chronic management of regular SVT

The arrhythmia	RF abl.[a]	CCB	β-blockers	Digoxin	Class IA	Class IC	Class III
Inappropriate sinus tachycardia	+	+	++	−	−	−	−
Sinoatrial reentry tachycardia	++	++	++	+	−	++	++
Focal AT (FAT)							
Asymptomatic, nonsustained[b]	−	−	−	−	−		−
Asymptomatic, sustained[c] or incessant	++	+[d]	+[d]	−	−	−	−
Symptomatic, recurrent	++	++	++	−	+[e,f]	+[f]	+[f]
Multifocal AT (MAT)							
	++	++	++[g]	−	+	+	+[g]
Nonparoxysmal junctional tachycardia[h,i]							
	[i]	++	++	−	−	[i]	[i]
Focal junctional tachycardia[h]							
	++	+[j]	++	−	−	++	++
AV nodal reentrant tachycardia (AVNRT)							
Minimal symptoms, infrequent episodes[k]	++[l]	++[m]	++[m]	+[n]	−	+[o]	+[o]
Bothersome symptoms and/or hemodynamic compromise[p]	++	++[q]	++[q]	+[n]	−	+[q,r]	+[r]
Hemodynamic compromise during AVRT episodes	++	+	+	+[n]	−	+[r]	+[r]
AV reentrant tachycardia (AVRT)							
Preexcitation (delta wave present)							
Asymptomatic AVRT	+[s]	−	−	−	−	−	−
Symptomatic AVRT, no hemodyn. compromise	++	−	+	−	−	+	+
Symptomatic AVRT, hemodyn. compromise	++	−	+[t]	−	−	+[t]	+[t]
Permanent junctional reentrant tachycardia	++	−	+	−	−	+	+
No preexcitation (delta wave absent)							
Well-tolerated	+	++	++	−	−	+	+
Poorly tolerated (incl. hemodyn. compromise)	++	−	+	−	−	+	+
Atriofascicular type Mahaim tachycardia	++[u]	−	[u]	−	−	[u]	[u]

[a]Permanent antitachycardia overdrive pacing may be an option in some cases of AT
[b]No therapy is required
[c]If rapid and frequently recurrent, then tachycardia-induced CMP may be a concern
[d]Only if RF ablation is unavailable or declined by the patient
[e]Disopyramide
[f]Only associated to AV node-blocking drugs
[g]Contraindicated in the frequent cases of coexisting pulmonary disease
[h]Technically, all the procedures marked ++ carry a Class IIA indication, with no approach designated as Class I; however, in the

Table 6.4 (continued)

conventional system used in these tables, "++" refers to the preferred therapy, not to its efficacy; in this regard, these are "the preferred" therapies, as others simply do not exist. See under the relevant heading, for comments

[i]With this arrhythmia, the accent falls on correction of the underlying disorders. It is in itself a benign arrhythmia, where more drastic measures are generally not indicated; Classes IC or III agents and RF ablation are rarely considered

[j]As second-line therapy

[k]No therapy whatsoever, except for vagal maneuvers; when needed is also ++

[l]In truly infrequent, well-tolerated episodes, the indication mainly depends on the patient's choice of finding a definitive solution to their condition

[m]The "pill-in-the-pocket" strategy is a ++ option

[n]Rarely used today, due to its low efficacy, as its indirect vagal effect is often superseded by the enhanced sympathetic tone

[o]Flecainide, propafenone, or sotalol, used as a second line of therapy, if the ++ agents are ineffective and RF is not available or declined by the patient

[p]If recurrent and symptoms are bothersome to the patient

[q]Caution in HF

[r]For points (b) and (c), these agents are part either of the "first-line" of therapy, i.e., as a first-choice agent (generally not the preferred agents, yet in some patients previous experience may indicate their use), or as a "second-line" therapy, should the ++ agents fail

[s]On a case-by-case basis, especially in patients with a profession affecting public safety (pilots, etc.)

[t]As a second line of therapy, should RF ablation be unavailable or declined by the patient

[u]There is scant data regarding therapy other than RF ablation

Table 6.5 Drug dosage for SVT treatment

Medication	Termination of acute event	Prevention of recurrences
Adenosine	IV 6 mg, rapid bolus over 1–2 s, followed by saline flush; if no response within 1–2 min, may repeat bolus twice, at a dosage of 12 mg each	No (no oral form available)
CCB		
Verapamil	0.075–0.15 mg/kg IV over 2 min (i.e., 5–10 mg in an average adult); may repeat 15–30 min later, as needed	PO, 120–360 mg daily in divided doses; slow release available
Diltiazem	IV 0.25 mg/kg over 2 min (approx. 20 mg on average); may repeat as needed, 0.35 mg/kg IV over 2 min; (maintenance 5–15 mg/h) alternatively, 120–360 mg PO q.d. in divided doses	PO 120–360 mg daily in divided doses; slow release available
Beta-blockers		
Esmolol	500 µg/kg IV over 1 5 min, followed by a maintenance infusion of 60–200 µg/kg/min IV[a]	N/A
Metoprolol	2.5–5 mg IV bolus over 2 min; up to three doses	PO 25–100 mg b.i.d.
Propranolol	0.15 mg/kg IV	PO 80–240 mg daily in divided doses
Cardiac glycosides		
Digoxin	0.5–1 mg IV over 10–15 min, followed by 0.25 mg q2 h; maximum 1.5 mg/day	(1) loading dose PO 0.5 mg daily, for 2 days; (2) maintenance 0.125–0.375 mg daily
Class IA AAD		
Procainamide	Loading dose IV 20 mg/min for 25–30 min, maintenance dose 2–6 mg/min. Can also be administered IM, 50 mg/kg/day in divided doses q3–6 h	PO 50 mg/kg/day, q3 h for regular release, q6–12 h for sustained release (depending on the formulation); rarely used today
Class IC AAD		
Flecainide	PO 200–300 mg; IV 1.5–3.0 mg/kg over 10–20 min	PO 200–300 mg daily, divided doses
Propafenone	PO 600 mg[b]; IV 1.5–2.0 mg/kg over 10–20 min	PO 450–900 mg[b] daily, divided doses

(continued)

Table 6.5 (continued)

Medication	Termination of acute event	Prevention of recurrences
Class III AAD		
Amiodarone	150 mg IV over first 10 min, then 360 mg over next 6 h, then 540 mg over next 18 h	PO 100–400 mg[c]
Sotalol	80 mg PO b.i.d.; increase dose gradually q2–3 day to 240–320 mg/day	PO 160–320 mg daily, in two doses
Ibutilide	IV 1 mg over 10 min, may repeat if necessary 10 min after end of initial infusion.	N/A

[a]An alternative dosing regimen: loading dose IV 250–500 µg/kg/min for 1 min, followed by a 4-min maintenance infusion of 50 µg/kg/min; if no effect within 5 min, repeat loading and maintenance doses (the latter, in 50 µg/kg/min increments). May repeat sequence up to a total of 4–5 cycles; on later cycles, may omit boluses and lower the maintenance dosage/ increase the intervals between infusions

[b]The dosage of the "pill-in-the-pocket" approach can be tailored based on these guidelines

[c]Amiodarone administration involves a PO loading dose of 800 mg daily for 1 week, followed by 600 mg daily for 1 week and 400 mg daily for 4–6 week, before initiating maintenance therapy; if amiodarone was used for AVNRT termination, oral loading may be decreased or avoided

evidence, for some entities, even the best available agents for a given indication may occasionally carry a Class II recommendation (since there may not exist, to date, therapeutic modalities warranting a Class I recommendation). However, by default, these agents are *first-choice* for the clinician, and are consequently marked ++ in the table.

6.1.2 SVT: Clinical Entities

The different clinical entities are reviewed in Fig. 6.1.

6.1.2.1 Supraventricular Arrhythmia Not Involving the AV Node

NSR and Sinus Arrhythmia

The normal cardiac rhythm originates in the specialized myocytes belonging to the sinoatrial node, located in the RA wall, near the entrance of the SVC. The sinoatrial node is vascularized by the RCA in 55% of patients, by the LCx in 35%, and by both, in 10%. Of all the cardiac myocytes, the sinus node has the fastest depolarization rate, and thus assumes the role of physiological pacemaker, its impulses overriding those of subjacent centers. A nonsinus (ectopic) cardiac rhythm may be either a *parasitic* rhythm (if it overrides the NSR) or a *replacement* rhythm (in case of pathologically decreased sinus

node activity or AV block). The spontaneous sinus depolarization rate is at about 100 cycles/min, a rate decreased by the parasympathetic system and increased by the sympathetic system, resulting in a net normal sinus rate of 60–100 bpm. The maximum sinus firing rate is up to 200 bpm in younger subjects, but generally no higher than 150 bpm in older individuals. The electrocardiographic components of NSR are discussed in Chap. 1. Sinus rates <60 bpm are considered bradycardic, and those >100 bpm, tachycardic. Both bradycardia and tachycardia can occur either in normal or in sick subjects.

NSR is fairly regular, but a certain degree of irregularity is not only common, but expected in healthy subjects, as it expresses the sympathetic/parasympathetic balance, in response to the phases of respiration; thermal regulation; day/night variation; centrally generated impulses; or baro-reflex influences. Variations in the sinus node discharge rate can be assessed

- *On a routine basis*: Clinical examination and EKG may reveal "sinus arrhythmia," defined by a cycle-to-cycle difference >0.12 s. Most frequent in children and younger patients, and especially influenced by respiration (*respiratory arrhythmia*), this phenomenon might minimize energy expenditure by avoiding unnecessary heart beats during expiration (when blood oxygenation is minimal).
- *Using special equipment*: (a) Beat-to-beat "HR variability" (HRV) is assessed with a photoplethysmograph that detects the pulse pressure waves.

Fig. 6.1 Supraventricular arrhythmia

I. SUPRAVENTRICULAR ARRHYTHMIA NOT INVOLVING THE AV NODE

1. Rhythms involving the sinus node

- Sinus arrhythmia

- Sinus tachycardia (appropriate)

- Inappropriate sinus tachycardia

- Sinoatrial re-entry tachycardia

2. Rhythms involving the atrial myocardium

- APBs

- Wandering pacemaker

- Focal AT (FAT)

- MultifocalAT (MAT)

- AF

- Atrial flutter

II. SUPRAVENTRICULAR ARRHYTHMIA INVOLVING THE AV NODE

1. Without an aberrant pathway

- Junctional premature beats (JPB)

- Junctional Escape Beats (JEB)

- Junctional Escape Rhythm

- Nonparoxysmal junctional tachycardia

- Focal junctional tachycardia ("automatic" or "ectopic" junctional tachycardia)

- AV nodal reentrant tachycardia (AVNRT)

2. With an aberrant pathway

- AV reentrant tachycardia (AVRT)

- Permanent junctional reentrant tachycardia

- Atriofascicular type Mahaim tachycardia[3]

III. INCREASED AV NODE CONDUCTION OF UNCLEAR SIGNIFICANCE

- LGL syndrome

Decreased HRV is seen in HTN, shock, and after MI, but the clinical value of its assessment is unclear; (b) a related entity is HR turbulence, defined as heart rhythm variability after a ventricular extrasystole. Diminished HR turbulence in a post-MI patient is an independent indicator of poor prognosis. The clinical value of this assessment is yet to be defined.

Appropriate Sinus Tachycardia

Appropriate sinus tachycardia results from sympathetic activation, triggered by stimulation of the peripheral and central chemoreceptors. The former are situated in the common carotid arteries and the aortic arch and sense variations in blood pH, pO_2, and pCO_2; the central chemoreceptors are situated in the medulla oblongata, and are sensitive to pCO_2 variations. A decreased pH and pO_2 and an increased pCO_2 will activate the receptors and trigger sympathetic activation. The settings leading to receptor activation include, among others, cardiac or respiratory failure; venous and arterial blood admixture (in CHD or arterio-venous aneurysm); anemia; O_2 content decrease in the inspired air; and increased metabolic requirements (fever, hyperthyroidism, pregnancy, etc.). In all these settings, sinus tachycardia is a normal adaptive mechanism, and thus is "appropriate."

Inappropriate Sinus Tachycardia

Inappropriate sinus tachycardia is defined as a sinus rate >100 bpm, in the absence of a physiological trigger. This entity is distinct from (1) sinoatrial reentry tachycardia, which, although "inappropriate" and involving the sinus node, involves a reentry circuit through both the sinus node and the atrial myocardium; (2) sick sinus syndrome (SSS)-associated tachycardia, which (despite the name) is nonsinus in origin and appears on the background of sinus bradycardia. Keeping these clarifications in mind, there are two entities manifesting as an inappropriately high sinus discharge rate. These include:

- A syndrome actually termed "*inappropriate sinus tachycardia*," consisting of a permanently increased sinus node discharge rate; this is seen mainly (90%) in otherwise healthy young women, and is diagnosed after ruling out other possible causes of tachycardia (hyperthyroidism, anemia, etc.). In addition to the high resting HR, there is abnormally severe tachycardia on exertion; the onset of tachycardia is gradual ("warm-up" phenomenon). Therapy is driven by the severity of the symptoms and the degree of tachycardia (i.e., risk of tachycardia-related CMP), and consists of β-blockers or nondihydropyridine CCB (Verapamil, Diltiazem). RF "modification" of the sinus node is a last-resort measure. The immediate success rate is approximately 75%, but ulterior recurrences may decrease long-term efficacy to as low as 25%. In most patients, insertion of a permanent pacemaker is necessary, following sinus node modification.
- *The Paroxysmal orthostatic tachycardia syndrome (POTS),* a form of dysautonomia: As opposed to the normal sinus rate increase as an adaptation to orthostatism, POTS-associated tachycardia is excessive (a HR increase >30 bpm on standing up, or an absolute HR >120 bpm within 10 min of head-up tilting).

Sinoatrial Reentry Tachycardia

Sinoatrial reentry tachycardia is a relatively uncommon arrhythmia, based on reentry between the sinus node and the atrial myocardium (and is thus not a "pure" sinus arrhythmia). It presents with sinus-like P wave morphology and an average HR somewhat lower than in other reentrant tachycardias, often leading to confusion with inappropriate sinus tachycardia (as there is no apparent trigger). However, unlike the latter, it has an abrupt onset and termination and can be terminated by vagal maneuvers, verapamil, digoxin, or amiodarone, but usually not by β-blockers. If long-term pharmacological therapy is not desired or fails, RF ablation is an option.

APBs

APBs arise from the atrial myocardium, between a normal sinus beat and the next expected beat. APBs are extremely frequent in both healthy and sick subjects, and they occur in the setting of sympathetic stimulation, smoking, excessive alcohol consumption, myocardial ischemia, fatigue, fever, anxiety, etc. APBs are also seen in patients with pulmonary disease and systemic hypoxia and in those with significant MS or MR. APBs can occur randomly or in a pattern (e.g., every second beat = atrial bigeminy). They have the following characteristics: *EKG features*: *the P waves* have an abnormal morphology, different from that of sinus P waves. Generally, beats arising in the high atrial myocardium are positive in leads II, III, and aVF, and those originating in the low atrial myocardium are negative in the same leads. Occasionally, the premature P waves are buried in the T wave, where they appear as a "hump" or "peak"; *the PR interval* depends on the proximity of the aberrant pacemaker to the AV node, as well as on the degree of prematurity of the extrasystoles. Thus, the PR interval can be normal (if the aberrant focus is not very close to the AV node, and the extrasystole is not excessively early, so that the atrial myocardium and the AV node are not in their refractory period); prolonged, if the APB occurs during the refractory period; or shortened, if the aberrant focus is close to the AV node and is firing outside of the refractory period; *the QRS complex* is usually narrow, but can occasionally be wide, if the APB occurs during the relative refractory period of the ventricular conduction system. Occasionally, the QRS complex is absent, if the APB falls within the absolute refractory period of the ventricular myocardium; *the sinus beat following the APB* occurs after an incomplete compensatory pause, i.e., the interval between the sinus beat before and after the APB is less than two normal sinus cycles; this pattern is due to the fact that the APB propagates not only anterogradely (towards the AV node), but also retrogradely (towards the sinus node, which it depolarizes and resets). *Clinical features*: Clinically, APBs are often asymptomatic (as demonstrated by their almost universal presence on Holter recordings, in the absence of any complaints), but may occasionally be felt as "palpitations," "extra heart beats," or "skipped" beats. If an APB is sufficiently premature to occur before the opening of the TV (i.e., during ventricular systole), the resulting atrial contraction will not be able to propel blood into the ventricles, and will cause retrograde progression of blood from the heart towards the great veins. This causes a "cannon 'a' wave," i.e., a strong, unexpected pulse wave in the internal jugular vein. Occasionally, a critically timed APB can trigger a supraventricular arrhythmia (AT, AF). *Treatment*: Generally, APBs are treated with reassurance only, but if they cause significant palpitations, AAD may be used, most frequently low doses of β-blockers. Lifestyle changes and anxiety management are also recommended.

Wandering Pacemaker

Wandering pacemaker is an atrial arrhythmia consisting of the shifting of the atrial pacemaker from the sinus node to the atrial myocardium, and hence to the AV node and back, as a result of variations in the degree of vagal activation: when the activation is intense, the sinus node becomes bradycardic, allowing subjacent foci to take over the pacemaking activity; when the vagal activation returns to normal, the sinus node resumes its function. Generally, the HR is 45–100 bpm, i.e., not tachycardic. This rhythm is often seen in healthy subjects, as well as in patients with heart disease or COPD. Occasionally, it may be a precursor of the more serious condition, multifocal AT. The EKG characteristics include: *P waves* of ≥3 different morphologies, typically varying from normal positive P waves in leads II, III, and aVF, to isoelectric, and finally to negative waves in these leads, as the pacemaker descends from the sinus node towards the AV node. The QRS complexes are generally narrow. Clinically, the heart rhythm is slightly irregular, and may cause palpitations. This condition generally does not require treatment. Beta-blockers should be avoided, as they would further increase vagal predominance.

Atrial Tachycardia

Atrial tachycardia is an arrhythmia caused by the rapid firing of one or several nonsinus atrial foci (unifocal AT vs. multifocal AT, or MAT). It is generated in the atrial myocardium, by several mechanisms, reviewed in Table 6.6. While AT can occasionally be seen in healthy younger subjects (see "APBs," above), it is more frequent in patients with cardiac disease (e.g., with CAD or after cardiac surgery involving the atria, typically for CHD correction); chronic lung disease, typically, COPD with hypoxia (a cause of MAT); drug toxicity (e.g., digitalis); and electrolyte imbalance. The EKG features include: *P waves* with an abnormal morphology, which can be constant (unifocal AT), or variable (multifocal AT = MAT, displaying ≥3 different P wave morphologies). The atrial rate generally varies between 150 and 200 bpm; the atrial rhythm is generally regular, but automatic tachycardia often exhibits the "warm-up" phenomenon, where the rhythm gradually increases after its initiation, until it stabilizes at a certain level. A similar phenomenon ("cool-down") is noted upon termination of the tachycardia; *the PR segment* is constant with unifocal AT, and variable with MAT; depending on the timing of ectopic beats in regard to the ventricular refractory period and on the proximity of the ectopic focus to the AV node, the PR interval can be normal, shortened, or prolonged; *the QRS complexes* are generally narrow, but can occasionally be wide (AT with aberrant conduction), in which case VT must be ruled out. The ventricular rate may be 150–200 bpm, in case of 1:1 transmission, or lower, in case of AV block. The ventricular rhythm is generally regular, but can be irregular during the warm-up/cool-down phases, and in case of Mobitz type I or variable AV block. Nonspecific *ST-T* changes may be present.

Table 6.6 Atrial tachycardia

(Uni)focal AT			
Mechanism	EKG characteristics	Clinical characteristics	Treatment
Intraatrial reentry	Frequent coexistence of 2:1 AV block; the association of AT and AVB suggests AT by intraatrial reentry	Generally associated to underlying heart disease. May cause AF or flutter; hemodynamic consequences generally modest, due to associated AVB (HR 100–120 bpm)	Variable results of Adenosine and β-blockers for termination; AAD often fail to prevent recurrences; RF ablation is an option
Increased automaticity	The "warm-up" and "cool-down" phenomena	Often seen in younger patients; does not respond to vagal maneuvers; is more likely to be incessant	Propranolol often effective, adenosine and verapamil often ineffective for termination; RF ablation is the therapy of choice for incessant tachycardia
Triggered activity		The least common mechanism; often seen in older patients, typical of digitalis toxicity; is believed to be due to delayed afterdepolarizations	If appropriate, treatment of digitalis toxicity; verapamil and adenosine successful, β-blockers less so, for termination; RF ablation is an option
Multifocal AT (MAT)			
Variable mechanism (automaticity or triggered activity)	≥3 distinct P wave morphologies, at a rate of 100–130 bpm; variable PP, PR, and RR interval length; P waves separated by isoelectric intervals. Rhythm is always irregular (often confused with AF on the EKG)	Most frequent in elderly, critically ill patients, especially with advanced lung disease (mainly COPD); may also be seen in patients with HF; may degenerate to AF	Correction of electrolyte disturbances and of hypoxia; CCB in high doses; RF ablation or DCC not useful; Amiodarone is occasionally useful

Atrial Fibrillation (AF)

Definition, Mechanisms, Prevalence AF is the most frequent type of arrhythmia overall, with a 0.4–1% prevalence in the general population, and as high as 8% in people aged >80. AF is generated by ectopic foci in the LA, especially near the ostia of the pulmonary veins, and is due both to increased automaticity and to multiple reentrant wavelets. The activity of these ectopic foci is modulated by external triggers, such as sympathetic activation, HTN, drugs, etc. The understanding of this focal (as opposed to diffuse intraatrial) mechanism has opened the possibility to use RF ablation for AF treatment. AF is characterized by a chaotic activity of the atria, (1) electrically: multiple wavelets, reflected on the EKG by small-amplitude, ill-defined, irregular deflections ("f waves"), that replace the normal sinus P waves; the atrial rate is very fast, 400–700 bpm; (2) mechanically: multiple, ineffective, simultaneous, uncoordinated "worm-like" atrial contractions; in AF, there is no meaningful systolic activity of the atria. This very fast atrial activity is conducted with a variable AV block, resulting in an "irregularly irregular" ventricular activity: the QRS complexes are irregular, and there is no pattern to this irregularity (unlike, for instance, ventricular bigeminy, where every second beat is a VPB). Importantly, unlike the atria, the ventricles contract normally (albeit irregularly), since the ventricular depolarization is, in and of itself, unaffected. However, the stroke volume is affected by AF, via the Frank-Starling mechanism; thus, (1) ventricular filling varies from one beat to the next, as the different ventricular beats occur after variable-length diastoles, causing variable activation of the mechanism; (2) the lack of a mechanically significant atrial systole deprives the ventricles from the late filling wave (abolished A wave), decreasing ventricular filling and causing underactivation of the mechanism.

Underlying Conditions In addition to normal aging, several diseases can cause AF, by a number of mechanisms: conditions directly or indirectly *increasing the LA pressure*: HTN, CAD, HOCM, MS; *sympathetic* *activation* during physiologic or disease-induced stress; *toxic and metabolic* effects on the atria: alcohol, cafeine, amphetamines, cocaine, carbon monoxide; hypoxia, such as in pulmonary disease or embolism; hyperthyroidism; *atrial ischemia and/or inflammation*: CAD, pericarditis; *obesity*, causing LA dilatation; *iatrogenic effects* on the atria (atriotomy, pacemaker malfunction). These conditions cause LA fibrosis and reduced contractility, as well as pulmonary vein dilatation, triggering the cellular mechanisms (disturbances in calcium handling and in sympathetic regulation, connexin downregulation, etc.), responsible for the generation of AF.

Classification of AF There are multiple modalities of AF classification, outlined in Table 6.7; the ESC/AHA guidelines use the simplest, most clinically relevant classification, based on the clinical setting and the time course of AF. Based on data from implantable cardiac devices, the minimal duration of paroxysmal AF that carries a risk for stroke is of 5.5 h. If validated, this observation might change the understanding of stroke risk in AF, and thus the classification of this disorder.

Diagnosis of AF *Clinical presentation*: AF may cause *palpitations*; exacerbation of HF, both by abolishment of the atrial kick, and by decreasing the LV filling period, with fast HR; *exacerbation of ischemia* with fast HR, compounding the systolic LV dysfunction and causing angina pectoris, MI, and/or severe ventricular arrhythmia; *syncope*, by one of the following mechanisms: decreased CO, e.g., in patients with rapid AV node conduction or with an aberrant pathway (especially poorly tolerated in patients with severe AS, which, like AF, is frequent in the elderly); prolonged sinus recovery time, if AF is a component of the SSS; ventricular tachyarrhythmia; *SCD*, in patients with the WPW syndrome; *thromboembolic complications*, typically CVA; *iatrogenic complications*: AAD-related arrhythmia, anticoagulant-related bleeding; *anxiety*.

On physical examination, the hallmark of AF is a chaotic ventricular rate; furthermore, not all QRS complexes

Table 6.7 Classification of atrial fibrillation (AF)[a]

Criterion	Definition	Type of AF
Number of *previously* diagnosed episodes	0	First-detected[b]
	≥1 (i.e., a total of ≥2 documented episodes)	Recurrent
Natural history	AF terminating *spontaneously*[c] ≤7 days[d] after onset	Paroxysmal[c]
	AF not terminating spontaneously ≤7 days after onset	Persistent
	Long-standing[e] AF, and DCC not attempted or has failed to obtain and/or maintain NSR	Permanent[e]
Comorbidity	No acute or chronic cardiopulmonary disease[f] or HTN, age <60 years; no previous stroke	Lone
	Acute cardiopulmonary disease or HTN (excluding acute-on-chronic conditions)	Secondary
	Chronic cardiopulmonary disease or HTN	No particular designation
	None, but age >60	No particular designation

[a]The considerations in this table apply to AF episodes lasting >30 s; shorter episodes may be important in individual patients and are managed as per clinical judgement

[b]This is a purely descriptive entity; there might have existed previous episodes or not, either undiagnosed, or diagnosed as such but not recalled by patient, and/or not documented

[c]The term does not apply if AF was terminated by treatment

[d]Most cases convert to sinus in the first 24 h

[e]There is no strict definition of the minimum duration that warrants these designations, but a considerable length of time is usually assumed., e.g., >1 year

[f]MI, cardiac surgery, myocarditis, pericarditis, hyperthyroidism, acute pulmonary disease; these cases usually terminate at the same time as the underlying disease

Fig. 6.2 Atrial fibrillation

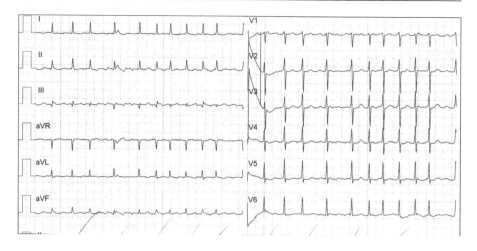

cause a palpable pulse wave, since some of the beats are exceedingly close to the previous beat, with poor ventricular filling and a very low stroke volume. The difference between the number of QRS complexes and the number of palpable pulse beats is called "pulse deficit." If the HR is not too fast, CO is only slightly decreased (due to the loss of the atrial kick), a fact only marginally important in patients with normal LV filling pressures (i.e., no significant systolic or diastolic LV dysfunction). However, (1) AF may trigger or exacerbate HF in patients with LV dysfunction; (2) regardless of the LVEF, AF may cause thromboembolism (due to clot formation in the mechanically inert atria, especially in the LA appendage; these clots can migrate to the LV and hence to the systemic arteries, causing organ infarction – typically, CVA); (3) rapid antegrade conduction over an aberrant pathway, with a very fast HR and/or degeneration to VF may cause syncope or SCD; (4) chronic tachycardia may cause CMP; and finally, 5) palpitations generate considerable anxiety.

The EKG presentation is typical for (1) the presence of f waves, an undulating line replacing the P wave; the undulations may be fine or coarse, grossly similar to the F waves of AF, but lacking the regularity of the latter. Occasionally, coarse f waves may mimic the P waves of MAT, but, unlike MAT, the f waves do not have the clearly-defined morphology of P waves; (2) an "irregularly irregular" ventricular rhythm, at a rate of 120–180 bpm in untreated patients. Additionally, the EKG is important in detecting an anterogradely conducting aberrant pathway, as well as potential AAD toxicity (widened QRS complexes, prolonged QT segment, etc.); these are very important, as they may presage the onset of severe ventricular arrhythmia, the most feared

complication of AAD altogether. Figure 6.2 shows a typical AF tracing.

AF: an EKG diagnosis

While extreme irregularity of the ventricular rate may suggest AF, and a regular ventricular rate decreases the probability of AF, there are important exceptions both ways, as

- Other cardiac rhythms, such as frequent APBs or VPBs, NSR or AT with variable AV block, etc., can mimic AF.
- A regular ventricular rhythm is compatible with AF; this is termed AV dissociation, and occurs with idioventricular or junctional escape rhythms (complete AV block), and with VT. A regular ventricular rhythm in a patient formerly in AF (especially if treated with AAD) mandates obtaining an EKG, to confirm conversion to NSR and to rule out life-threatening ventricular arrhythmia.

Of note, with very rapid HR, it may be impossible to decide, by auscultation, if the rhythm is regular or not; this distinction is easier based on EKG.

Occasionally, EPS and stress test may be required. EPS allows localization and ablation of the ectopic foci, and exercise stress test may elicit AF (when the condition is suspected, but undocumented) and helps assess ventricular rate on exercise and its tolerability. In patients with a CRT device, this can be used for the monitoring of the tendency to paroxysmal AF, using wireless telemetry. AF can then be converted to NSR, using electrical atrial shock.

Other medical tests: *The basic workup* generally includes: CBC, to rule out anemia or systemic inflammation; electrolyte levels; liver function tests; thyroid function tests (hyperthyroidism may manifest exclusively as AF, especially in the elderly); a chest X ray to exclude pulmonary disease; and, if anticoagulation is warranted, baseline coagulation tests. Echo is essential for: (1) identifying cardiac disease underlying AF; (2) assessing the chances for conversion to stable NSR (i.e., termination and nonrecurrence of AF); these chances are low if the antero-posterior LA diameter, viewed from the parasternal long axis, is >4–4.5 cm, or if the LA surface, measured in the apical 4-chamber view, is >16–17 cm^2; (3) assessing the potential importance of conversion to NSR, by identifying atrial kick-dependent conditions, such as severe LV dysfunction, HOCM, severe AS, etc.; (4) identifying AF-associated LA thrombi (LA appendage visualization by TEE); (5) chosing the optimal therapeutic strategy (rate- vs. rhythm control); timing the cardioversion and deciding the duration of anticoagulation therapy, according to the presence or absence of LA thrombus; and assessing the position of the pulmonary veins ostia, an important parameter for RF ablation, as the ectopic foci are usually in the vicinity of these ostia.

AF: Treatment

Treatment strategies: Correctable underlying disorders (e.g., hyperthyroidism) are treated in all patients. ACEI and ARB may have a role in the prevention of AF, although the recent GISSI-AF trial has failed to demonstrate this in patients with recurrent AF. The therapeutic strategy regarding AF itself depends on the clinical setting, and revolves around several questions: (1) *To treat the arrhythmia or not*? Technically, the question arises only for persistent or permanent AF, since paroxysmal AF reverts spontaneosly to sinus, usually within 24 h. However, it is not practical to await reversal beyond 48 h from AF onset, as precardioversion anticoagulation would then become mandatory (see below). The decision to treat AF, in principle, depends on its hemodynamic tolerability, but in practice, the threshold for therapy of a first episode or of a rare recurrence of AF is quite low. At one end of the spectrum (lone, asymptomatic AF with a reasonable HR), no action is required, while at the other end (AF with a rapid HR and hemodynamic collapse), emergency cardioversion is required. The necessity for chronic therapy is also decided on the basis of AF tolerability. Not all patients in whom AF was terminated necessarily require chronic therapy; (2) *If treatment is necessary, what strategy is preferable*: *rhythm control* (conversion to NSR) or *rate control* (opting for permanent AF, keeping HR at 60–80 bpm at rest, and at 90–115 on exertion)? This must be answered in all AF patients, with the possible exception of lone AF, where neither AAD nor AV-node blockers are strictly indicated, but can be used as needed. All other things being equal, the two strategies are equally effective, and the final decision is based on the answers to two important questions: (a) *What are the chances, and how important is it, to obtain a stable NSR*? The chances are broadly defined by the presence and extent of cardiopulmonary disease, and often, by previous experience with that patient (number of previous AF recurrences after successful cardioversion, duration of NSR between recurrences). The age of the AF is also an important factor: the more recent the AF, the better the chances of cardioversion, with the best chances in cases <7 days old, and the lowest, in cases >1 year old; (b) *If the chances to obtain NSR are good or fair, then will one prefer the risk of adverse effects caused by AAD* (*if rhythm control is elected*) *or of those caused by anticoagulants* (*for the rate-control group*)? Note, however, that the rhythm control strategy is not tantamount to chronic AAD; this can be avoided by several options: "pill-in-the-pocket" therapy (especially with Flecainide or Propafenone); repeated cardioversions (often, electrical), in patients with infrequent, well-tolerated episodes of AF; RF ablation of the AF foci; the maze or mini-maze procedures; the atrial defibrillator. On the other hand, the rate control strategy, whether pharmacological or not (AV node ablation and pacemaker), necessarily requires chronic anticoagulation. The different therapeutic options are not mutually exclusive, and there is ample room for creative solutions. Thus, in some patients in whom AF has been converted to NSR, it is perfectly acceptable to prescribe a limited course of AAD, over the first 1–3 months after conversion, when AF recurrences are most frequent. Therapeutic decisions also change with the course of events; for instance, in a patient in whom two conversion attempts have failed, the policy may be switched to rate-control; (3) *Regardless of the rate-vs.-rhythm control decision, is anticoagulation necessary*? With the exception of

and IC drugs) by accelerating AV conduction; therefore, these drugs must be administered only in conjunction with AV blocking agents. Pre-DCC therapy can be initiated before elective hospitalization, if the drugs being considered are available in oral form and are safe in the specific patient. Often, these drugs are continued for a variable period of time after cardioversion (occasionally, on a chronic basis). An initially failed attempt at cardioversion can at times be successfully repeated after preparatory pharmacological treatment. Pre-DCC pharmacotherapy is reviewed in Table 6.9. The duration of this treatment depends on the pharmacodynamics of each drug (e.g., a few days for Class I drugs, a few weeks for Amiodarone, or immediately before cardioversion, for Ibutilide); *The maze ("Cox maze") and the mini-maze procedures*: The maze procedure uses a set of incisions on the endocardium of both atria; the subsequent healing creates "demarcation lines" preventing the progression of the reentrant electrical wavelets responsible for AF. The maze procedure has been widened in scope to include pulmonary vein isolation, otherwise a mainstay of catheter ablation techniques. This is an open-heart surgical procedure *not* required by most AF patients. It has a very high success rate in curing AF, yet is seldom performed due to its majorly invasive nature, time-intensive character, and possible complications, including death, the need for permanent pacing, impaired atrial contraction, and late atrial arrhythmias. It can, however, be carried out at the time of other open heart surgery. Not surprisingly, there has been much interest in replicating this technique by catheter methods. While the intuitively obvious endocardial approach has not proven successful, an epicardial technique, by a minimally-invasive approach (mini-maze), is successful in specialized centers, especially in patients with recurrent AF and no gross anatomical cardiac lesions. Of note, the term "mini-maze" was coined to describe a simplified open-heart maze technique, and is still occasionally used with this meaning; *Catheter ablation*: The proximity of the responsible ectopic foci to the pulmonary venous ostia allows definitive cure of AF, precluding the need for chronic therapy (AAD, anticoagulants). The ablation procedure is similar to the mini-maze approach, in that a series of strategic lesions are placed in the atrial myocardium, to terminate AF. There are, however, two important points of difference: (a) catheter ablation uses the endocardial, not the epicardial approach; (b)

the lesions are meant to isolate the pulmonary veins from the atrial myocardium, rather than to replicate the "maze" lesions. The main complications are related to intensive pulmonary vein manipulation (pulmonary vein stenosis, systemic thromboembolism, atrio-esophageal fistula), or to the development of scar in the LA (atypical AF). At the present time, RF ablation for AF is considered a rescue procedure, if AAD have failed. In the very rapidly evolving field of interventional cardiology, this may well change in the near future. A novel ablation technique in AF patients uses an epicardial, rather than an endocardial approach.

Maintenance of NSR after conversion of AF: The decision for chronic maintenance therapy has been discussed in the introductory remarks. The dosages are outlined in Table 6.9. Cardiovascular comorbidity influences the preferred type of AAD, as outlined in Table 6.10.

The rate control strategy: Rate control can be achieved either pharmacologically or by device techniques. *Pharmacological rate control*: the recommended drugs and the corresponding dosages are outlined in Table 6.11. *Device techniques*: (a) *Catheter techniques* consist of RF ablation of the AV node and permanent pacemaker implantation. The patients still require chronic anticoagulation, but quality of life is substantially improved, and tachycardia-related LV dysfunction is corrected. However, if the LV dysfunction is not tachycardia-related, using RV apical pacing (the conventional placing of the pacemaker electrode) may actually decrease LVEF, as ventricular depolarization proceeds from the apex upwards, causing suboptimal mechanical activity. In these patients, biventricular pacing may be preferable; (b) *Implantable devices* convert episodes of paroxysmal AF by delivering bursts of overdrive pacing or by providing electrical shock. There are pacemakers possessing AF-termination algorithms, but their clinical role is yet to be defined.

Table 6.10 AF: preferred drug therapy according to comorbidity

Type of comorbidity	First-choice	Second-choice
None, or HTN without LVH	Flecainide	Amiodarone, dofetilide, catheter ablation
HTN with LVH	Amiodarone	Catheter ablation
CAD	Dofetilide, sotalol	Amiodarone, catheter ablation
HF	Amiodarone, dofetilide	Catheter ablation

Table 6.11 Control of ventricular rate in permanent AF

	Agent	Acute setting		Nonacute setting	
		Loading dose	Maintenance dose	Loading dose	Maintenance dose
No accessory pathway	*β-blockers*[a]				
	Esmolol	IV 0.5 mg over 1 min	IV 60–200 µg/kg/min over 1 min	N/A	N/A
	Metoprolol	IV 2.5–5 mg over 1 min; up to three doses	N/A	PO 25–100 mg b.i.d.	PO 25–100 mg b.i.d.
	Propranolol	IV 0.15 mg/kg	N/A	PO 40–120 mg b.i.d.	PO 80–240 mg, divided doses
	CCB[b]				
	Diltiazem	IV 0.25 mg/kg over 2 min	5–15 mg/h	PO 120–360 mg/day, divided doses or slow-release	PO 120–360 mg/day, divided doses or slow-release
	Verapamil	IV 0.075–0.15 mg/kg over 2 min	N/A	PO 120–360 mg/day, divided doses or slow-release	PO 120–360 mg/day, divided doses or slow-release
	Other agents				
	Digoxin[c]	IV 0.25 mg each 2 h, up to 1.5 mg total	IV/PO 0.125–0.375 mg daily	PO 0.5 mg daily	PO 0.125–0.375 mg daily
	Amiodarone[d]	IV 150 mg over 10 min	IV 0.5–1 mg/min	PO daily 800, then 600 mg for a week each, then 400 mg for 4–6 weeks	PO 200 mg/day
Accessory pathway	Amiodarone	IV 150 mg over 10 min	IV 0.5–1 mg/min	PO daily 800, then 600 mg for a week each, then 400 mg for 4–6 weeks	PO 200 mg/day

[a]Action onset: IV, in approximately 2–7 min; PO, 4–6 h for metoprolol, 60–90 min for propranolol; C/I in severe LV dysfunction or HF
[b]Action onset: IV, in approximately 5 min; PO, 2–4 h for diltiazem, 1–2 h for verapamil; contraindicated in severe LV dysfunction or HF
[c]Action onset: IV, ≥60 min; PO, 2 days
[d]Action onset: IV, in a few days; PO, 1–3 weeks; for both IV and PO, some effect may be seen earlier

Beyond the rate vs. rhythm control: Dronedarone. Dronedarone (Multaq, one tablet of 400 mg b.i.d. with morning and evening meals) is an antiarrhythmic related to Amiodarone, but lacking the iodine moiety believed to be responsible for the numerous adverse effects seen with this drug. The landmark ATHENA trial has demonstrated Dronedarone to display both rate- and rhythm-controlling properties. Interestingly, while the latter were somewhat inferior to the ability of amiodarone to maintain NSR, there was a reduction in the rate of hospitalization for cardiovascular reasons even in patients who never achieved NSR on the drug (as compared with placebo). This hints at additional, nonantiarrhythmic effects of Dronedarone. Compared to placebo, there was also an impressive 34%

decline in risk of stroke in the Dronedarone group. The safety of Dronedarone in patients with HF or recent deterioration in LV function is not clear (a previous trial was terminated early after an apparent mortality increase among patients with systolic HF). The most common adverse reactions (≥2%) are diarrhea, nausea, abdominal pain, vomiting, and asthenia.

Anticoagulation: In AF, the atria are mechanically inert, causing blood stasis and thrombus formation, progressing to the LV and producing thromboembolism (typically, CVA). The risk of thromboembolism is minimal with lone AF and highest in patients with a previous episode of thromboembolism. Between these two extremes, the risk is variable, and can be stratified to guide antithrombotic therapy. Tables 6.12 and 6.13 review the clinical scenarios regarding AF-related thromboembolism and the recommended drugs. The pharmacological properties of Heparin, LMWH, and direct thrombin inhibitors are discussed in Chap. 2, while those of oral anticoagulants are outlined in the present section.

The necessity, duration, and antithrombotic drug choice (antiplatelet agents vs. anticoagulants) are guided by the risk of thromboembolism. Risk is classified as: *high*: previous CVA, TIA, or other systemic embolism, mechanical valve prosthesis, biological valve prosthesis in the first 3 months postsurgically, with the highest risk in the first postsurgical month, or MS; *moderate*: age ≥75, HTN, HF, LVEF <35%, diabetes; *low or less validated*: age 65–74, female gender,

coronary artery disease, thyrotoxicosis. A risk score (CHADS$_2$ score) can be established, allocating two points of severity for previous CVA or TIA, and one point each for age >75, HTN, diabetes, and HF. The annual risk of stroke increases from an average of 2% for a score of zero, to as high as 18% for the maximum score (6). The indications include:

- If risk factors are absent or weaker/less validated, and optionally in patients with one moderate risk factor, aspirin, 81–325 mg q.d.; if contraindicated, Clopidogrel 75 mg q.d. In Warfarin-intolerant AF patients, the combination of Clopidogrel and aspirin reduces the incidence of major vascular events, particularly stroke, but increases the rate of major bleeding.

- In patients with ≥1 (optionally, ≥2) moderate or ≥1 severe risk factors, Warfarin, to an INR of 2–3 (target 2.5); in patients with mechanical valvular prosthesis, the target INR may be higher (see Chap. 5).

Note that in individual patients who underwent PCI with stent deployment, the antithrombotic regimen is usually more drastic, and should be used in place of the usual AF-related protocol. The application of these guidelines in specific clinical settings is discussed next.

Peri-DCC antithrombotic therapy (regardless of whether cardioversion is pharmacological or electrical)

- *Emergency cardioversion*: Heparin anticoagulation is started at the time of cardioversion, and subsequently titrated to PTT 1.5–2. Oral anticoagulants are started at the same time, and when target INR is reached, Heparin is discontinued, and oral anticoagulation is continued for additional 4 weeks or chronically, depending on the risk profile. The regimen is the same regardless of whether AF is <48 h (in which case pre-DCC anticoagulation is not necessary) or >48 h (when the emergency setting precludes lengthy

Table 6.12 AF-related thromboembolism: clinical scenarios

Clot formation	Timing	Preemptive measures
Preexisting AF-related clot	Early after DCC	Preconversion anticoagulation; TEE
Clot formed after conversion, in the mechanically inert LA[a]	Within 1 month of conversion	Postconversion temporary antithrombotic therapy
Clot formed at the time of recurrent or persistent AF	At any time	Chronic antithrombotic therapy

[a]The delay between resumption of electrical and mechanical atrial activity can last for a few weeks; during this period of "atrial stunning," the emptying velocity of the LA appendage is decreased <20 cm/s (normal >40 cm/s), and there may exist "spontaneous echo contrast" (SEC, or "smoke") – dynamic, whitish, swirling echoes on the 2D examination of the LA, signifying slow flow

Table 6.13 Antithrombotic therapy in AF

The drug	Mechanism	Use in AF	Usual dosage
UFH	Antithrombin stimulation	(1) At the time of, and immediately after emergency cardioversion (bridging to VKA) or in cardioversion for AF <48 h old; (2) before and after surgery, persistent AF (until VKA action is terminated/renewed); (3) in pregnancy, at least during the first trimester and before childbirth	IV bolus 5,000 U, followed by continuous IV drip, 25,000 U/24 h, adjusted as per PTT
LMWH	Inhibition of activated factor X	As with UFH	See Chap. 2
Oral anticoagulants	VKA inhibit hepatic synthesis of the prothrombin complex (factors II, VII, IX, and X)	Chronic anticoagulation; temporary anticoagulation after cardioversion	Warfarin 2.5–7.5 mg/day, Acenocoumarol 1–8 mg/day, both adjusted as per INR

pre-DCC anticoagulation). LMWH, in the usual dosages, may be used for part or all of the treatment.

- *Elective cardioversion*: (1) *AF* <48 h: There is no need for pre-DCC anticoagulation; oral post-DCC anticoagulation is given for 4 weeks or more, according to the risk profile (target INR 1.5–2); (2) *AF* >48 h *or age unknown*: *effective* anticoagulation for 3 weeks before DCC is recommended. If LA thrombus has been ruled out by TEE, pre-DCC anticoagulation can be restricted to IV heparin until PTT 1.5–2 has been reached (usually reached within <24 h). This infusion is continued post-DCC until effective oral anticoagulation (target INR 1.5–2) has been achieved, and continued as above. If LA thrombus is identified, the entire 3-week pre-DCC course is indicated (repeat TEE to ascertain thrombus resolution is optional); as the thromboembolic risk in this subgroup is high, post-DCC anticoagulation is usually maintained longer than the minimum of 4 weeks.
- LMWH may be acceptable for post-DCC management, if VKA are contraindicated, as long as no intraatrial thrombus has been detected by TEE.

The standard oral anticoagulants are Warfarin and Acenocoumarol. They act by antagonizing the hepatic action of vitamin K, responsible for the synthesis of certain coagulation factors ("vitamin K antagonists" = VKA). With both, there is considerable individual variation in the daily requirements. Loading doses increase the risk of bleeding, and must be used with caution, if at all. Oral anticoagulation regimens achieve full effect in 4–5 days, which is also the usual duration of overlap with UFH or LMWH. In current practice, the weekly requirements of Warfarin and Acenocoumarol are divided over 5–6 days, with an 1–2 day pause, to avoid iatrogenic bleeding. Anticoagulants are preferably taken in the evening, so as to allow factoring in the latest INR results for dosage adjustments (on the days INR is measured, blood is, as usual, harvested in the morning). Both Warfarin and Acenocoumarol may interact with certain types of food or drugs. Their efficacy is diminished by the vitamin K content in leafy vegetables: lettuce, broccoli, okra, spring onions, parsley, spinach, green peas, grapes, kiwi, and possibly cranberries and their juice (see http://www.drgourmet.com/md/relative-Warfarinlist.pdf); interaction with drugs is listed at http://www.drugs.com/pro/coumadin.html. The most important interactions are those with Amiodarone and Aspirin (frequently used in AF patients), with proton-pump inhibitors (used against aspirin-related gastritis); NSAIDs; and Erythromycin and its derivatives. Moderate (≤2 drinks daily) alcohol intake does not interfere with VKA; regular high alcohol intake decreases their efficacy; and binge drinking potentiates VKA and may cause hemorrhage. Acute diarrhea may potentiate VKA, by eradicating the intestinal vitamin K-secreting bacterial flora, a situation compounded if broad-spectrum antibiotics are used. The risk of hemorrhage is highest in the elderly. Additional caveats with VKA include: (1) *a paradoxical procoagulant action* of Warfarin, occurring in the first few days of treatment, due to suppression of the natural anticoagulants, protein C, and protein S. Of no consequence in the normal subject, this action may lead to thrombosis (Warfarin skin necrosis and gangrene of the extremities) in patients with protein C or protein S deficiency. The treatment includes fresh frozen plasma and protein C concentrate infusion, vitamin K, and anticoagulation with unfractioned Heparin or LMWH; however, none of these treatments have been validated in clinical trials; (2) *osteoporosis*, mostly in males; (3) *the blue toe syndrome*, caused by cholesterol microembolism (also occasionally seen after cardiac catheterization), with a generally benign prognosis; (4) *fetal malformations*, if used in the first trimester of pregnancy.

VKA-related bleeding is treated with FFP, prothrombin complex concentrate, and, as needed, RBC infusion. Asymptomatic excessive INR prolongation is managed by VKA discontinuation, close follow-up, and optional vitamin K administration. The latter measure is best avoided if INR is not excessively increased, and if anticoagulation is especially important (e.g., mechanical valve prosthesis associated to AF). The dosage of Vitamin K is PO/SC/IM/IV 2.5–25 mg (rarely up to 50 mg); may repeat as needed, 12–48 h after PO, or 6–8 h after parenteral administration.

Antithrombotic therapy in persistent AF is carried out under the same regimen as outlined under "post-DCC therapy." Due to individual variations in susceptibility to VKA, the INR is initially measured every week, and later, every month. This classical prescription may be substantially altered by the availability of INR self-monitoring kits.

Several special situations may occur in the chronically anticoagulated patient:

- *A thromboembolic event despite stable therapeutic INR*: Increase INR to 3–3.5, or, if this is not feasible, add Aspirin, in the usual dosages.

- *Elective surgery*: Discontine VKA for 1 week. If comorbidities contraindicate this (e.g., mechanical valves), or if >7-day VKA discontinuation is necessary, LMWH can be administered, although there are no definite guidelines in this respect. With *emergency surgery*: reversal of anticoagulation with FFP or prothrombin concentrate; VKA or LMWH reinstitution when surgically acceptable.
- *Postoperative AF*: (a) Prophylaxis is best achieved with β-blockers, or, in high-risk patients, with Amiodarone or Sotalol; (b) treatment with AV nodal blocking agents for rate control as a bridge to spontaneous conversion; with Ibutilide or DCC, if immediate conversion is desired; and with anticoagulants (if surgically acceptable), especially in cases lasting >48 h; (c) secondary prevention with usual AAD may be necessary for recurrent postoperative AF.
- *In pregnancy*, rate-control can be achieved with Digoxin, β-blockers, or nondihydropyridine CCB; cardioversion is best achieved by DCC, but Quinidine or Procainamide may be considered in hemodynamically stable patients. Anticoagulation is carried out with Heparin, at least during the first trimester and the last month of pregnancy, due to the risks of teratogenic VKA effect and of uncontrolled peripartum bleeding, respectively. The doses are 25,000 U/24 h continuous IV infusion, or 10–20,000 U SC q12 h, adjusted as per PTT. LMWH may be considered. Occasionally, this regimen is used throughout pregnancy, although VKA may be preferable in high-risk patients, outside of the high-risk time spans.
- *Hyperthyroidism*: β-blockers, or, if containdicated, CCB, as well as anticoagulation (INR 2–3) must be used, continued as needed after restoration of the euthyroid state.
- *Severe lung disease*: Correction of hypoxemia and acidosis may terminate paroxysmal AF. If AF persists, HR can be controlled with Verapamil or Diltizem, or DCC may be administered. β-blockers, Sotalol, and Propafenone are contraindicated.
- *Acute MI*: Use Amiodarone or DCC.

Beyond the Warfarin era: *Dabigatran*: The oral antithrombin agent, Dabigatran (150 mg b.i.d.), holds promise to revolutionize the entire field of anticoagulation, including that of patients with AF. Dabigatran has a much more predictable pharmacological profile than Warfarin, therefore not requiring monitoring. The interactions of Dabigatran with other drugs and with bioactive components in the food appear negligible. In the RE-LY trial, Dabigatran was administered twice daily. The main adverse effect included dyspepsia. Crucially, the LFT were not affected, an important concern, as LFT disturbances denied clinical use of its predecessor, Ximelgatran. Further postmarketing data regarding this issue are eagerly awaited. It appears that, for the moment, patients on a stable, predictable, long-term Warfarin treatment would benefit little from being switched to Dabigatran, but Warfarin-naïve patients probably should be started on this drug. As always, the economic factor plays a major role: Warfarin is extremely cheap, and thus much more readily available in developing nations; this advantage, however, must be carefully balanced against the added economic burden of coagulation parameters follow-up, which is unnecessary with Dabigatran.

Atrial Flutter

Atrial flutter (Fig. 6.3) is a macroreentrant AT, with the reentrant wave coursing around normal structures (the SVC and IVC orifices, the eustachian ridge, the coronary sinus orifice, and the tricuspid annulus), or around atrial scars, usually after atriotomy. The former is termed "typical," and the latter, "atypical" flutter. With typical flutter, the reentry wave can circle either counterclockwise (usually) or clockwise around the tricuspid annulus, with different EKG manifestations (Table 6.14).

Atrial flutter is quite prevalent, being reported in approximately 0.5–1% of EKG tracings reviewed in-hospital. Atypical flutter is common after atriotomy, especially for correction of CHD (e.g., the Mustard procedure). Atrial flutter is associated with the same types of disease as AF; the two entities are in fact frequently associated, and patients may switch repeatedly between AF and flutter, either spontaneously, or at the time of a conversion attempt. The transitional flutter in the process of AF conversion may paradoxically increase the HR, due to "concealed conduction": even AF wavelets not conducted to the ventricles penetrate the AV node to different degrees, and partly depolarize it, increasing its refractoriness and thus slowing the ventricular rate. Concealed conduction is less pronounced with flutter, hence the occasionally increased HR. Similar to AF, flutter may be conducted over an aberrant pathway, with syncope or SCD; flutter may also cause thromboembolism. The clinical presentation is similar to that of AF, but the palpitations tend to be regular, as are the "cannon

Table 6.14 Atrial Flutter: mechanisms and classification

Flutter type	Mechanism	EP characteristics	Varieties	EKG characteristics
I[a] (typical = classic)	Macroreentry around the TV annulus (cavo-tricuspid isthmus)	Usually, 240–340 bpm (untreated); can be terminated with rapid atrial pacing	Counterclockwise Clockwise	Negative flutter waves LII, LIII, aVF Positive flutter waves in LII, LIII, aVF
II[a] (atypical)	Macroreentry around surgical scars	Usually, 340–440 bpm (untreated); not terminated by rapid atrial pacing; etiology unclear	N/A	Continuously undulating pattern, but not fitting the typical and atypical patterns

[a]Some do not consider the designations, type I/typical, type II/atypical as being respectively synonymous, but rather hold that type I flutter can be either typical or atypical, while type II flutter is an imprecisely defined entity, awaiting further study

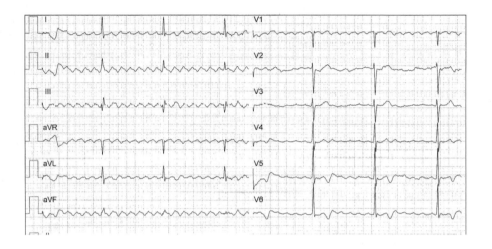

Fig. 6.3 Atrial flutter

'a' waves" seen on inspection of the neck. As opposed to AF, which can last for many years, the typical duration of a flutter episode is of minutes to hours, less commonly days or weeks.

The EKG presentation is reviewed in Table 6.14. Most patients present with some degree of AVB (usually, 2/1), preventing hemodynamic collapse. Occasionally, the AVB is variable, with an ensuing irregular ventricular rhythm. Variations in the degree of AVB may occasionally lead to abrupt increases or decreases of the ventricular rhythm, for instance a decrease from 150 to 75 bpm, when the AVB increases from 2/1 to 4/1. Atrial flutter must not be mistaken for coarse-wave AF or for MAT.

The therapy of atrial flutter is very similar to that of AF, with a few differences. As flutter most often lasts only for a few hours, chronic AAD is mainly guided by the associated AF, if any. Certainly, clinical tolerability

is also very important, but RF ablation, technically simpler and with a higher success rate than in AF, is often preferred to chronic AAD therapy. Atrial flutter is more responsive to electrical cardioversion than AF, and 25–50 J are usually sufficient. Conversely, flutter is *less* responsive than AF to pharmacological agents; therefore, DCC is the preferred therapy for acute cardioversion. In case of DCC failure or contraindication, overdrive pacing is an option. If flutter occurs at the time of cardiac surgery, epicardial pacing is used; otherwise, transesophageal pacing under conscious sedation is used (otherwise, the procedure is quite painful). As opposed to AF, flutter is unresponsive to Adenosine, but this agent can help visualize the flutter waves and establish the correct diagnosis. Less documented than with AF, thromboembolic complications are seen with flutter as well; thus, chronic anticoagulation is carried out as with AF.

6.1.2.2 Supraventricular Arrhythmia Involving the AV Node

The spectrum of junctional arrhythmias is outlined in Table 6.15. With junctional escape beats (JEB) and junctional escape tachycardia, the designation, "arrhythmia," has no pathological connotation; on the contrary, these entities are normal adaptive mechanisms. The last entity in the table, focal junctional tachycardia, is further discussed in the remainder of this section.

Focal ("Automatic") Junctional Tachycardia

Also called "junctional ectopic tachycardia (JET)," this is a relatively infrequent arrhythmia, where the ventricles are activated first, and the atria are activated retrogradely (ventriculo-atrial propagation). The usual HR is 110–250 bpm. This causes "cannon 'a' waves" and may exacerbate HF. *The EKG features* include: absent P waves; a ventricular rate different from the atrial rate ("ventriculo-atrial dissociation"); and narrow QRS complexes, unless BBB is present. The ventricular rhythm is generally regular, but occasionally conducted sinus beats ("captured beats") can create ventricular rhythm irregularities. The onset and termination of JET are gradual ("warm-up," "cool-down"). If very tachycardic, JET may be difficult to differentiate from AT. Adenosine does not terminate JET, but may create transient AVB demonstrating the lack of atrial activity. Occasionally, EPS may be required to establish the diagnosis. *The clinical features* are those of SVT with AV dissociation. Other manifestations depend on the specific underlying condition: *Congenital JET*, usually evident between birth and the age of 4 weeks, manifests as an incessant tachycardia that may cause CMP and death due to HF or to VF. Drug therapy must be used with caution, as it may cause complete AV block. JET

Table 6.15 Junctional arrhythmia

The entity	Mechanism	EKG characteristics	Clinical characteristics	Treatment
Junctional premature beats (JPB)	Automaticity	Retrograde P (negative in LII, V1) before, during, or after QRS; if before QRS, PR is shortened (<0.12 s)	Similar to APBs, but less common. They represent *increased* automaticity, able to supersede the sinus node	β-blockers, if symptomatic
Junctional escape beats (JEB)	Automaticity	As above	Similar to JPB, but due to *normal* nodal automaticity, in the absence of sinus activity	If indicated, treatment of the underlying sinus bradycardia
Junctional escape rhythm	Automaticity	≥3 JEB at normal junctional rate (40–60 bpm). P negative (retrograde atrial depolarization), positive (AV dissociation), or not visible in leads II and V1	As above	As above
Nonparoxysmal junctional tachycardia	Automaticity, delayed afterdepolarizations	As above, but HR 60–120 bpm	Digitalis toxicity, postcardiotomy scar, hypokalemia, ischemia; "reperfusion arrhythmia" after coronary thrombosis; if HR is <100 bpm, occasionally termed "Accelerated Junctional Rhythm"	Treat the underlying condition
Focal ("automatic," "ectopic") junctional tachycardia	Automatic focus in the AV node or the His bundle	Narrow QRS, HR 110–250 bpm; BBB possible; regular or irregular (if AV dissociation); may be mistaken for AF	Rare arrhythmia, mainly seen in young adults; may be chronic and cause CMP	RF ablation, β-blockers, Class IC or Class III AAD
AV node reentrant tachycardia (AVNRT)	See text			

is a major medico-legal pitfall in pediatric cardiology, due to its insidious clinical manifestation, often over-looked EKG characteristics, and severe prognosis; *Idiopathic chronic JET* occurs in patients with a struc-turally normal heart, and may also cause tachycardia-related CMP and HF; *Postoperative JET* is usually transient, and manifests in the first few hours or days after CHD repair. It typically causes hemodynamic compromise; *Nonparoxysmal JET* can be caused by Digoxin toxicity, postcardiotomy scar, hypokalemia, or myocardial ischemia. In itself, it is benign, and, as the HR varies between 70 and 120 bpm, technically, it often does not even qualify as "tachycardia." The overall prognosis is dictated by the underlying disease, as is the treatment. *Treatment*: JET is generally quite resistant to therapy. The therapeutic options include: *AAD*, mainly Amiodarone, Propafenone, Procainamide, Propranolol, or Sotalol; Digoxin must be used with caution, as it may cause VF or accelerate JET. In addition, one must keep in mind that JET can actually be the expression of Digoxin toxicity; *RF ablation* (limited experience in JET); *sequential AV pacing* after rate reduction by phar-macological means can restore the normal AV activa-tion sequence (i.e., antegrade rather than retrograde) and increase CO.

AV Nodal Reentrant Tachycardia (AVNRT)

AVNRT is usually seen in younger, healthy patients; there is a slight preponderance of the female sex. It arises due to the presence of a "fast" and a "slow" pathway within the AV node. Most frequently, the ini-tiating event is an APB occurring at a time when only the slow pathway conducts, the fast pathway still being refractory (the slow pathway has a shorter refractory period). By the time the impulse reaches the distal extremity of the slow pathway, the fast pathway has regained its ability to conduct, and the impulse travels retrogradely up this pathway, with initiation of AVNRT. The above-mentioned mechanism is seen in 85–90% of patients ("slow-fast" = "typical" AVNRT), the rest displaying a "fast-slow" = "atypical" pattern. "Typical" AVNRT is the most frequent SVT overall. Less frequently, the initiating premature beat is ven-tricular, and conducts retrogradely up the fast path-way, then anterogradely down the slow pathway. *The EKG characteristics* of AVNRT include: *initiation* by an APB in case of typical AVNRT, and by either an

APB or a normal sinus beat, in the atypical form. As it depends on one strategically timed beat, the onset of AVNRT is abrupt; *P waves* occur at a rate dictated by the conduction velocity through the slow pathway, since the fast pathway, true to its name, has rapid con-duction velocity. P waves are close to (or hidden within) the QRS complex, and are occasionally misin-terpreted as R' waves in V1. The RP interval is short with typical AVNRT, and long with atypical AVNRT; *the QRS complexes* are narrow (unless aberrant con-duction or BBB are present), and the ventricular rate is identical to the atrial rate, unless AV dissociation is present. Typical AVNRT may present with a variable cycle length at its beginning and termination, reminis-cent of automatic AT; *the termination* is usually abrupt (often due to a conduction block in the slow pathway) and may be followed by a period of sinus bradycardia or asystole, until the sinus node recovers its normal function. *The clinical characteristics* are not different from those seen in other AT. As AVNRT is generally seen in subjects without underlying heart disease, angina or HF are relatively infrequent, but may be seen in patients with preexisting cardiac conditions. Most frequently, there is chest pain in the absence of coronary disease. Although usually paroxysmal, this tachycardia ("atypical AVNRT") may occasionally be chronic ("incessant tachycardia"). *The therapy* of AVNRT depends on the clinical setting, and is out-lined in Tables 6.3–6.5.

6.1.2.3 SVT Involving an Aberrant Pathway

These tachycardias involve the atrial and ventricular myocardium, as well as various stretches of the normal conduction system. The AV connection is made by an aberrant pathway.

"Aberrant pathways" vs. " aberrant conduction"

In both cases, impulse conduction is abnormal ("aberrant"), but in different ways: in the former, the abnormality lies in the anatomic support of conduction (*an extra pathway*), while in the latter, it lies in the (reduced) speed of propagation over *the normal pathways*, with a BBB appearance.

AV Reentrant Tachycardia (AVRT)

Pathophysiology: With AVRT, the AV node represents only one limb of the reentry circuit, the other limb being an aberrant AV pathway, the "Kent bundle." AVRT can also be caused by a connection of one of the atria to the His bundle (atriofascicular pathway, a type of "Mahaim bundle"). Two other types of aberrant pathways have been described, the fasciculoventricular Mahaim bundle, and the "James bundle," bypassing the AV node. Aberrant pathways are most probably congenital, since there is a familial aggregation of cases. Between 7 and 10% of patients have associated Ebstein's anomaly. Approximately 10% of patients with a Kent bundle actually have multiple accessory pathways; this situation is more frequent with associated Ebstein's anomaly. Accessory pathways have a different conduction speed (usually, higher) and refractory period (usually, longer) than the AV node, similar to the slow/fast AV conduction pathways in patients with AVNRT. Similarly, the event initiating AVRT is an APB that blocks in the accessory pathway (due to the longer refractory period), but is conducted through the AV node; by the time this impulse reaches the ventricle, the accessory pathway has regained its conductibility, and can now conduct the impulse retrogradely, generating a reentry arrhythmia. The *EKG presentation* depends on the electrophysiological properties of the aberrant pathway, and is different in NSR vs. AVRT. *The P waves* have a normal morphology in NSR, and are inverted and usually superimposed on the ST segment or on the T wave during AVRT, as in this setting the atria are depolarized after the ventricles. *The PR segment* is normal in NSR without preexcitation, and shortened in case of preexcitation (when the PR segment actually becomes the P-delta segment); *The delta wave* is a deflection seen immediately before the QRS complex, with aberrant pathways capable of antegrade conduction. Patients with an accessory pathway and a delta wave are said to exhibit the "WPW *pattern*"; associated episodes of AVRT (absent in many patients) define the WPW *syndrome*. Importantly, the presence of a delta wave in NSR has no bearing on the QRS morphology during AVRT (see below). In patients with the WPW pattern, the ventricular depolarization occurs both through the normal conduction system and through the accessory pathway, so that the QRS complex is actually a fusion beat, with an initial portion (the delta wave) corresponding to the preexcited ventricular myocardium. The faster the conduction through the accessory pathway,

the greater the contribution of preexcitation to the ventricular depolarization, and the wider the delta wave and the QRS complex will be. Importantly, while the conduction of the impulse over the aberrant pathway is *rapid*, once the impulse reaches the distal end of the pathway, it continues to propagate through the ventricular myocardium – a *slow* propagation similar to that seen in patients with BBB, hence the "slurred" morphology of the delta wave. As mentioned, the delta wave is visible only in patients with antegrade conduction through the aberrant pathway. However, the converse is not true, i.e., not all patients with antegrade conduction through the aberrant pathway display a delta wave, as can occur (1) when the distal end of the aberrant pathway is implanted in the distal lateral ventricular myocardium, leading to the bulk of the ventricular activation during NSR to occur through the AV node, i.e., normally; (2) when the conduction through the Kent bundle is intermittent. The appearance/disappearance of a delta wave on serial EKG tracings is of no predictive value; however, if the delta wave appears and disappears on a beat-to-beat basis (as detected on Holter or stress testing), it suggests a relatively low conduction velocity over the aberrant pathway and a low risk for SCD (see "Clinical Presentation," below). In a patient with an aberrant pathway, the *permanent absence* of a delta wave (if not due to a very laterally placed aberrant pathway, and if it is indeed permanent, a matter of inference based on the available EKG tracings) signifies a concealed pathway, able to conduct only retrogradely, and thus not carrying the threat of SCD. On the other hand, the *permanent presence* of a delta wave is still compatible with a good prognosis, but assessment of the prognosis requires EPS, to induce AF and to assess the rapidity of the resulting ventricular rate. The analysis of the delta wave and QRS morphology allows localization of the aberrant pathway (see below). *The QRS complex* may be either narrow or wide (delta wave), both in NSR and during AVRT. The QRS morphology during NSR depends on the presence and characteristics of the delta wave (discussed above). During AVRT, QRS morphology depends on: (a) *the direction of propagation over the reentry circuit*; the QRS complex will be wide (delta wave present) only if there is antegrade conduction over the accessory pathway, with retrograde conduction through the AV node (antidromic AVRT); the opposite situation produces "orthodromic" AVRT. Orthodromic AVRT accounts for approximately 95% of cases, with the rest being antidromic. It is important to realize that most patients with antegrade conduction over the aberrant pathway in NSR (i.e., delta waves and wide QRS complexes) conduct retrogradely over the same accessory pathway during AVRT (orthodromic AVRT, no delta waves, narrow QRS complexes). As mentioned, the presence of a delta wave in NSR does not allow to predict QRS morphology during AVRT: patients *with a delta wave* in NSR may develop either narrow-complex AVRT (as most pathways capable of antegrade conduction are also capable of retrograde conduction), or wide-complex AVRT. Occasionally, the same patient may present, at different times, with orthodromic or antidromic AVRT. Moreover, *the absence of a delta wave* in NSR is perfectly compatible with the existence of an aberrant pathway able to conduct antegradely (see previous point). Occasionally, however, the absence of a delta wave in patients with an accessory pathway is due to the inability of the pathway to conduct in an antegrade fashion; it conducts only retrogradely ("concealed pathway") both in sinus and during AVRT (orthodromic AVRT only). Generally, the HR of both ortho- and antidromic AVRT is very fast, >200 bpm; (b) *the presence of aberrant conduction*: orthodromic AVRT with aberrant conduction is the most frequent cause of wide-complex tachycardia associated to aberrant pathways; (c) *the presence of BBB*, most frequently left BBB (LBBB); (d) *the presence of an atriofascicular aberrant pathway* (a type of the Mahaim bundle); this connects the atrial myocardium to the right bundle branch, and at the time of AVRT conducts antegradely, with an LBBB morphology. As with preexcitation via a Kent bundle, the impulse conduction beyond the end of the aberrant pathway occurs slowly, through the ventricular myocardium. However, the delta wave per se is absent, being replaced by the LBBB morphology; thus, this antidromic tachycardia is indeed of the wide-complex type, albeit for a (slightly) different reason.

Aberrant pathway localization by EKG

Most frequently, the aberrant pathway is a Kent bundle, connecting either the LA or the RA with the corresponding ventricle. Some patients have more than one aberrant pathway. The WPW pattern can be of two types: A (the most frequent; left-sided pathway) and B (right-sided pathway). The most precise method for pathway localization

Table 6.16 Aberrant pathway localization based on the surface EKG

WPW type	Kent bundle location	EKG		
		P wave during PSVT	QRS complex during NSR	Delta wave during NSR
A	Left-sided	Positive in V1	Tall R in V1	Positive in V1
B	Right-sided	Negative in V1	QS pattern in V1	Negative in V1

is EPS, but important clues can be found on the surface EKG as well. A nonprominent delta wave makes localization difficult, but in itself suggests a left-sided pathway (preexcitation of the posterobasal LV segment, with the bulk of ventricular excitation occurring normally through the AV node). The EKG differentiation criteria are presented in Table 6.16.

Pitfalls of the EKG diagnosis in WPW

- Type A WPW is characterized by tall R waves in lead V1, and may be confused with RBBB, RVH, or posterior wall MI
- Type B WPW is characterized by negative QRS complexes in lead V1, and may be confused with LBBB or anterior wall MI

The EKG manifestations of WPW both in NSR and during SVT are reviewed in Fig. 6.4.

The clinical presentation of AVRT is similar to that of other SVT. In approximately 25% of patients, the disease becomes asymptomatic in time; in fact, patients >40 who have never experienced symptoms often remain asymptomatic for the rest of their lives. The most feared complications are syncope and SCD, due to antegrade conduction over the aberrant pathway, in patients with AF or flutter. The extremely high ventricular rates may degenerate to VF and cause death. The risk factors for SCD in a patient with AVRT include: a shortest RR interval during preexcited AF <250 ms (i.e., a calculated "instantaneous" HR of >240 bpm); a history of symptomatic tachycardia; multiple accessory pathways; and an associated Ebstein's anomaly.

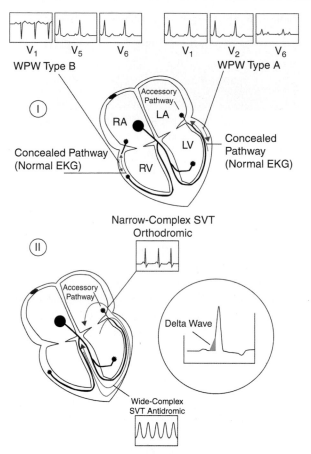

Fig. 6.4 The WPW syndrome. *Upper panel*: antegrade conduction through an accessory pathway is expressed as a delta wave. Retrograde conduction is characteristic of "concealed" accessory pathways. *Lower panel*: regardless of the conduction direction in NSR, the accessory pathways (only LA–LV pathway shown) can be the base of an "endless loop" type of conduction, generating supraventricular tachyarrhythmia (SVT). Antegrade conduction through the accessory pathway (i.e., antidromic, in regard to the normal conduction system) generates wide-complex tachycardia, whereas retrograde (orthodromic) conduction generates a narrow-complex tachycardia

Other Types of Preexcitation

These include:

*   *The permanent form of junctional reentrant tachycardia*: Confusingly, this term has also been used to designate atypical AV nodal reentry and AT; in current usage, AVRT with decremental conduction over the accessory pathway (slower ventriculo-atrial conduction velocities at higher HR) has become the entity thus designated. The decremental retrograde conduction should, in principle, be a beneficial characteristic, since it ensures a slower ventricular rate

during AVRT; the problem, however, is that this arrhythmia tends to be incessant, and, as the HR during AVRT is still quite fast, CMP may ensue.

*   *Preexcitation through a fasciculoventricular Mahaim bundle*, bypassing the distal conduction system by connecting the His-Purkinke fibers to the ventricular myocardium. This arrhythmia is not "supraventricular," but is included here due to its close similarity to the other reentrant tachycardias, and to avoid artificially separating the different preexcitation syndromes.

*   *The LGL syndrome* manifests as a shortened PR, with normal P wave and QRS morphology; this may represent a normal variant (thus redefining the "normal" PR values) or the presence of a peri-AV nodal bypass pathway. It is not clear whether this EKG syndrome has any clinical relevance, i.e., if it ever produces arrhythmia.

A few possibly confusing terms used in the explanations above are summarized in the following glossary.

*   *Antegrade conduction*: Conduction from the atria to the ventricles, either through the AV node, or through an aberrant pathway.
*   *Retrograde conduction*: Conduction from the ventricles to the atria, either through the AV node, or through an aberrant pathway.
*   *Orthodromic AVRT*: AVRT due to antegrade (normal = "straight" = "ortho") conduction through the AV node, and retrograde conduction through the aberrant pathway.
*   *Antidromic AVRT*: AVRT due to antegrade conduction through the aberrant pathway and retrograde conduction through the AV node.
*   *WPW pattern*: Presence of a delta wave.
*   *WPW syndrome*: Presence of a delta wave + episodes of AVRT.
*   *Preexcitation*: Antegrade ventricular or retrograde atrial activation involving an aberrant pathway; of note, with isolated retrograde atrial activation, no preexcitation actually occurs. Initially designating the WPW pattern, the term has expanded in scope, to avoid artificially separated closely related entities.

The interplay of these factors is outlined in Table 6.17.

Table 6.17 Conduction patterns over the aberrant pathway

Rhythm	Conduction		EKG		Remarks
	AV node	Kent bundle[a]	Delta wave	QRS complex	
Sinus	Antegrade	Antegrade	Yes	Wide	"Manifest" aberrant pathway (WPW pattern)
	Antegrade	Retrograde	No	Narrow	"Concealed" pathway
AVRT[b]	Antegrade	Retrograde	No	Narrow	Orthodromic AVRT
	Retrograde[c]	Antegrade	Yes	Wide	Antidromic AVRT[c]

[a]All of the entities in this column, as well as the Mahaim tachycardias and (possibly) the LGL syndrome are defined as "preexcitation"
[b]AVRT + delta wave in NSR = WPW syndrome
[c]Rarely, the retrograde conduction is accomplished through an additional aberrant pathway

The treatment of AVRT is discussed under "general remarks." A few points regarding long-term treatment are discussed below. In asymptomatic patients, preventive therapy is indicated as per the risk factor situation for SCD (see above), with special consideration for professions impacting public safety. Prophylactic therapy consists of RF ablation, successful in approximately 95% of cases, and carrying a ≤1% risk of complete AV block, with the necessity for pacemaker implantation. In symptomatic patients, the therapy of choice is again RF ablation, especially indicated in the presence of previous documented rapid AT antegradely conducted over an accessory pathway. If the patient has rare, well-tolerated episodes of AVRT, the indication for RF ablation is Class II. Pharmacological therapy, if elected, depends on the severity of the clinical manifestations. Thus, (1) with the "WPW syndrome" (especially with a history of atrial anterogradely conducted tachyrrhythmia), as well as with poorly tolerated AVRT, the drugs of choice are Class IC (Flecainide, Propafenone) or Class III agents (Sotalol, Amiodarone), acting both on the AV node and on the aberrant pathway. Despite their inhibitory action on the AV node, β-blockers also appear safe, either as sole therapy or associated to Class IC or Class III agents. CCB and Digoxin are contraindicated; (2) in patients with infrequent, well-tolerated AVRT episodes and no preexcitation (i.e., no evidence of antegrade conduction over the aberrant pathway), on the contrary, CCB and vagal maneuvers are the preferred therapy, with the other drugs being second-choice. Digoxin is contraindicated. The "pill-in-the-pocket" approach using CCB or β-blockers, or simply no chronic therapy at all are also acceptable options.

6.2 Bradyarrhythmia

What is bradycardia?

A HR <60 bpm is considered bradycardia. Several remarks are in order:

- Semantically, the term "bradycardia" has two meanings: (1) an excessively low firing rate of the sinus node; (2) an excessively low ventricular rate. In NSR with normal AV conduction, the two meanings overlap. However, in nonsinus rhythms, the ventricular rate may be excessively low despite a "normal" firing rate, since the active pacemaker normally fires at a slower rate than the sinus node. For instance, the junctional pacemaker has an intrinsic firing rate of 40–60 bpm, and a ventricular pacemaker, a <40 bpm rate. Here, the abnormality is that the prevailing pacemaker is not the sinus node – a situation due to either sinus node dysfunction or to AV block. Therefore, junctional or ventricular rhythms resulting in an excessively low ventricular rate are not termed "junctional bradycardia" or "ventricular bradycardia," but rather "junctional/ventricular rhythm with low ventricular rate." The opposite, however, is not true: an abnormally increased ventricular rate is always designated as "tachycardia," with the mention of the involved pacemaker (sinus/atrial/junctional/ventricular tachycardia).
- Bradycardia is not necessarily pathologic. In highly trained athletes, parasympathetic activation commonly decreases HR to ≤45 bpm, without

any sign of disease. Additionally, the HR can normally decrease during sleep down to 35–40 bpm with marked sinus arrhythmia and even episodes of sinus arrest.

- Conversely, a HR of 60–100 bpm may represent *relative* bradycardia, i.e., a failure to appropriately increase the ventricular rate on exertion.

Thus, *any* bradycardia results from supraventricular pathology, be it sinus node dysfunction or AV block. Therefore, the present section, paralleling "Supraventricular Tachyarrhythmia," is simply titled "Bradyarrhythmia." We shall not deal any further with "appropriate," that is, physiologic bradycardia.

6.2.1 Sinus Node Disease

6.2.1.1 Definition, Etiology, and Entities

Sinus node disease ("sinus node dysfunction," "sick sinus disease") is more aptly termed "sick sinus syndrome (SSS)" to better underscore its multifactorial nature. Widely defined, it refers to abnormal sinus pacemaker activity; a more narrow definition refers to sinus node dysfunction due to loss of anatomic integrity (excluding external influences such as drugs, autonomic innervation, etc.). Anatomic disruption of the sinus node may be acute (e.g., as a complication of acute MI) or chronic (degenerative sclerosis); reversible (e.g., AVB in inferior MI) or irreversible (e.g., AVB in anterior MI). Acute sinus node dysfunction (to be distinguished from the acute *manifestations* of chronic dysfunction) is often multifactorial (e.g., in an MI patient, a combination of ischemia, hypoxia, electrolyte disturbances, drugs, and neurovegetative influences). The main causes of SSS include: *sinus node degeneration and sclerosis*, the most frequent cause (especially prevalent in the elderly, although any age group may be involved); *neurally mediated cardioinhibitory response*, including carotid sinus hypersensitivity; *myocardial disease*: CAD, CMP, hypertensive heart disease, infiltrative heart disease (amyloidosis, sarcoidosis, hemochromatosis, etc.), musculoskeletal dystrophy, or CHD; *iatrogenic*: drugs, atrial surgery (mainly for CHD); *infective or inflammatory heart disease* (myocarditis, Chagas disease, scleroderma, SLE,

etc.); *systemic infection* (sepsis); *electrolyte abnormalities* (hyperkalemia); *endocrine disease* (hypothyroidism); *respiratory failure*; *increased intracranial pressure*; *hypothermia.*

Drug-induced sinus node dysfunction

This is caused mainly by AAD Classes IA, IC, II, III, IV, V; sympathomimetic drugs (Clonidine, Methyldopa, Reserpine); Lithium; Cimetidine; Amitriptyline; and Phenytoin

6.2.1.2 Diagnosis:

SSS is evident on resting EKG in advanced cases, and on Holter EKG or loop recording in milder cases, where the abnormalities are intermittent. Keeping a symptom-log during the Holter test allows rhythm/symptom correlation and helps establish the indication for pacemaker insertion. The role of EPS is controversial, due to the relatively low sensitivity and specificity of the results. EPS is therefore generally reserved for patients in whom suspected SSS has not been demonstrated by EKG monitoring. The most important EPS parameters in this setting are: prolonged sinus node recovery time after overdrive suppression (induced tachycardia suppressing sinus node activity) and abnormally increased sinoatrial conduction time using premature atrial stimuli.

Clinical manifestations: While some patients may be asymptomatic, common complaints include dizziness, presyncope, or syncope, and, with the tachycardia/bradycardia syndrome, palpitations and possible thromboembolic events. Occasionally, the symptoms occur only on exertion (inappropriate sinus bradycardia). The manifestations include fatigue, irritability, memory disturbances, occasionally misattributed in the elderly to the "process of aging." Chronic bradycardia may also cause angina pectoris and HF, up to flash pulmonary edema. The main complication of SSS is SCD, in case of asystole without an effective escape rhythm. The clinical course of the disease is progressive.

Syncope in sinus node dysfunction

SSS-associated syncope most frequently results from excessive bradycardia or asystole (sinus bradycardia or AV block, with a bradycardic or inactive subsidiary pacemaker); excessive tachycardia or ventricular tachyarrhythmia on the background of sinus bradycardia and/or AV block; or prolonged (>3 s) sinus node recovery time after a tachyarrhythmia.

The different entities in the SSS spectrum include:

- *Inappropriate sinus bradycardia (chronotropic incompetence)*, i.e., failure to increase the sinus rate with exercise. The degree of physiological exercise-related tachycardia varies widely among individuals, and the cornerstone for "inappropriateness" definition is the symptomatic status, rather than any precise "cutoff" HR. Thus viewed, the sinus rate is inappropriately bradycardic if it fails to prevent exertional symptoms (excessive fatigue, weakness, presyncope, or full-blown syncope) in the absence of negative chronotropic medication. Pacemaker insertion carries a Class I indication in these patients, and a Class II indication in minimally symptomatic patients with HR <40 bpm. These indications also include chronotropic incompetence resulting from drug therapy for which no alternative exists.
- *Sinoatrial nodal block (SA node exit block)*, characterized by P wave absence in ≥1 cardiac cycle, with the P-P interval following a certain pattern (discussed below). If ≥2 cycles are involved, they need not necessarily be consecutive. Although, by EKG, sinoatrial block manifests as sinus bradycardia, the true sinus node discharge rate is normal, but conduction to the atrial myocardium is defective. Second- and third-degree SA block are identified on the surface EKG. Second-*degree SA block Wenckebach type (Mobitz I)* is characterized by progressive PP shortening, leading to a dropped sinus P wave; the cycle is then repeated. The pause duration is < the sum of the two preceding PP intervals, while the PP interval following the pause is > the PP interval just before the pause. With *second-degree SA block Mobitz II type*, a constant PP interval unexpectedly leads to a dropped P wave, with a pause approximately twice the basic PP interval. (Blocked APBs may mimic this pattern.) With *third degree SA block*, sinus P waves are absent for one or more cycles, and the PP interval bridging the P-less stretch is a multiple of the baseline P-P interval; escape rhythms (occasion-

ally, with nonsinus P waves) are often present. The PP pattern allows distinction from sinus arrest.
- *Sinus arrest*: Absent sinus P waves for ≥1 cycle, with the bridging PP interval generally >3 s, and not a multiple of the baseline P-P interval. This entity is rarely associated with atrial escape rhythms, leading to asystole.
- *Alternating tachycardia/bradycardia*: Atrial or junctional tachycardia on the background of sinus node dysfunction.

6.2.1.3 Treatment

1. *Acute sinus node dysfunction* may be treated pharmacologically or by temporary pacing. Treatment of the underlying condition (e.g., thrombolysis in acute MI) is essential. Pharmacological therapy includes Atropine (1–3 mg IV, bolus) or Isoproterenol (starting at 1 μg/min IV). In the setting of CPR, Isoproterenol is usually not indicated.
2. *Chronic sinus node dysfunction* may require pacemaker insertion, in case of:
   - *Symptomatic bradycardia*, absolute or relative (i.e., inappropriate sinus bradycardia), either spontaneous or caused by drugs for which there is no alternative. (These drugs are often necessary for the tachycardic episodes of SSS itself, but would exacerbate the bradycardic episodes). In principle, pacemaker insertion is not indicated in asymptomatic patients, even in face of dramatic EKG findings. However, there is a Class IIB indication for pacing in "minimally symptomatic" patients with HR <40 bpm, and an abundance of caution often leads to liberal interpretation of the symptomatic status and to pacemaker insertion. The most frequent situation requiring pacing is sinus arrest, as second-degree sino-atrial exit block causes occasional "missed beats," and third-degree sino-atrial exit block usually does not affect normal automaticity of subjacent pacemakers (this automaticity is often compromised in patients with sinus arrest). However, if the subjacent pacemaker is infrahissian, the resulting HR is too bradycardic and too "unstable," that is, may abruptly stop functioning, and pacing is indicated.
   - *Syncope*, either spontaneous or EPS-induced.

The preferred pacing modality is DDD-R, which, as compared with VVI-R pacing, decreases the incidence of AF, and possibly that of stroke, HF, and death (although in these respects the data are conflicting). AAI-R pacing is appropriate if neither AV block, nor atrial tachyarrhythmia is present. (However, there is a 1% per year chance of AVB development in patients with sinus node dysfunction, and thus DDD-R pacing may be preferable in these patients as well). Anti-tachycardia pacing algorithms are useful in the tachy-cardia/bradycardia syndrome.

6.2.2 Electrical Impulse Conduction Disturbances

6.2.2.1 Atrioventricular Block (AVB)

Definition: AVB is defined as disturbed electrical conduction from the atria to the ventricles, due to anatomical or functional disturbances in the AV node or His-Purkinje system (Table 6.18). While any degree of AV block can be caused at any point in the conduction system, first-degree AV block and second-degree Mobitz I AV block are most frequently caused by AVN dysfunction, Mobitz II AV block is generally caused by dysfunction at or below the His bundle, and third-degree AV block is caused by conduction disturbances in the AV node or the His-Purkinje system. The main characteristics of the different types of AV block are reviewed in Table 6.18.

AVB and AV nodal block: two distinct entities

AV block, a derangement of impulse transmission from the atria to the ventricles, can have its anatomical substrate at any level in the conduction system, the AV node being only one (albeit very frequent) such location.

First-degree AVB (PR >20 ms) is common in all age groups, as a normal variant in young subjects without structural cardiac disease, and most often

Table 6.18 AV block: anatomy, EKG, and prognosis

The AV block	Site[a]	PR	P/QRS relationship	QRS morphology	Prognosis[b]
First-degree AVB	Usually, the AV node[c]	>0.20 ms	Each P followed by a QRS complex	Narrow	Benign
Second-degree AVB Mobitz I (Wenckebach)[d]	AV node, above the His bundle	Progressive prolongation, until a P wave is blocked	Each P followed by a QRS complex, except for the blocked P waves (P/QRS ratio 4/3, 3/2, etc.)	Narrow[e]	Benign
Second-degree AVB Mobitz II ("high-degree AVB")	Intra- or infrahisian	Constant	One every 3[f], 4, or more P waves are conducted (3/1, 4/1 block, etc.)	Often, LBBB or RBBB morphology	Potentially severe (high risk of complete AV block)
Third-degree AVB	AV node or His-Purkinje system	N/A[g]	No relationship (AV dissociation[h])	Depends on subsidiary pacemaker	Potentially severe

[a]Any degree of AVB may have its anatomical substrate at any level in the conduction system; the most frequent locations are reviewed here
[b]i.e., the usual prognosis
[c]In rare instances, first-degree AVB can be due to a lesion in the His-Purkinje system (the bundle of His and the Purkinje fibers), alone, or associated to the AV node. His-Purkinje involvement is especially probable in case of a first-degree AVB associated to a BBB
[d]Other EKG characteristics of Mobitz I AVB include: progressive RR shortening prior to the nonconducted P wave; the pause after the conducted P wave is less than twice the PP interval of two consecutively conducted beats
[e]Even if there is an associated BBB, Wenckebach type I block is still usually suprahisian
[f]2/1 AVB cannot be reliably classified by surface EKG as being Mobitz type I or type II
[g]As there is no causal connection between the P waves and the QRS complexes, the measured PR values, which vary randomly, are physiologically meaningless
[h]Third-degree AVB is but one of the possible causes of AV dissociation

due to degenerative changes in the elderly. It is usually asymptomatic, and the first heart sound is weakened on auscultation. In some patients with systolic LV dysfunction, it may impair LV filling (by partial compromise of the atrial kick) and precipitate HF, or decrease exercise tolerance. After RF ablation of the fast AV node pathway, conduction through the slow pathway may translate as first-degree AVB and cause symptoms reminiscent of the pacemaker syndrome. Follow-up is not required, except in the presence of BBB, which is a sign of underlying disease in the His-Purkinje network, rather than in the AV node. In opposition to the classical data outlined above, PR interval prolongation has recently been reported to be associated with increased risks of AF, pacemaker implantation, and all-cause mortality.

Second-degree AVB Mobitz Type I (Wenckebach block) manifests as gradual PR prolongation, until occurrence of a "dropped" P, i.e., a P wave not followed by a QRS complex. The pause is shorter than the sum of any two consecutive conducted beats (R–R interval). It is most frequently caused by AVN dysfunction. **Second-degree AVB Mobitz Type II** manifests as nonconduction of one out of 2, 3, etc., P waves. The PR interval is constant. Importantly, for a 2/1 AVB (every other P wave conducted), it is not possible to establish by means of the surface EKG alone whether the block is of the Mobitz I or Mobitz II type. Second-degree AV block is also asymptomatic, unless the HR is excessively slow. On physical examination, there is a gradual softening of the first heart sound and periodical, dropped pulse waves. Mobitz II block may degenerate to third-degree AV block, with the attending complications. *Third-degree AVB* may cause fatigue or syncope, occasionally with seizures ("Adams-Stokes" attacks). The clinical signs include "cannon 'a' waves" (pulse waves in the jugular veins, due to atrial contraction against closed AV valves, as a result of AV dissociation); variable intensity of the first heart sound; and variable intensity of the pulse beats, according to the degree of filling, i.e., to the (incidental) increased or decreased coordination of the atria and the ventricles. The main types of AV block are presented in Fig. 6.5.

Etiology: AVB can be classified as organic (caused by anatomical lesions of the conduction system) or functional (due to extrinsic influences). Often, the etiology is multifactorial (e.g., β-blockers exacerbating occult AV node dysfunction). The most frequent type of *"lesional"* AVB is idiopathic fibrosis of the conduction system, *Lenegre's disease* and *Lev's disease*. These entities more or less overlap, with the latter placing a particular

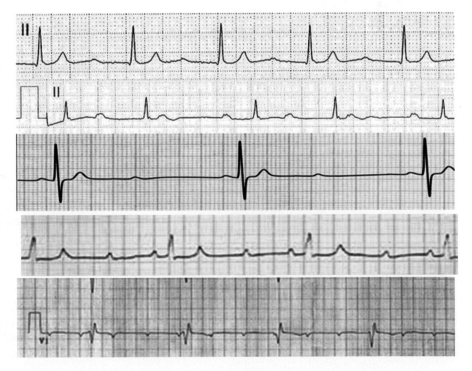

Fig. 6.5 Conduction disorders. (1) First-degree AV block, with a typically prolonged PR segment; (2) second-degree AV block, Wenckebach type, with gradual prolongation of the PR interval, followed by a dropped atrial beat; (3) second-degree AV block 2/1, with every other beat atrial beat not conducted to the ventricle. It is usually not possible to establish whether the block is of the Wenckebach or the Mobitz II type; (4) Mobitz II type block; every third atrial beat is conducted; (5) complete AVB: no connection whatsoever between the atrial and the ventricular electrical activity

emphasis on bundle branch involvement and on coexisting conduction system calcification, occasionally involving the mitral annulus or valve and the AV. Other lesional causes of AVB include *CAD*, chronic or as acute MI (complete AVB with inferior MI is generally due to AV node involvement and is reversible, while with anterior MI, it is often due to lesions to the His and/or bundle branches, indicates extensive damage, and requires permanent pacing); *CHD*, with the AVB either isolated, or associated with septum primum ASD, TGV, or maternal lupus; *calcific valvular disease*, with AV node invasion; and virtually any other cardiac condition, including *CMP*, *myocarditis* (Chagas' disease is frequently involved in South America), *infiltrative disease, AV node involvement as a complication of SBE, collagen vascular diseases, cardiac tumor, or trauma* (mechanical, surgical, catheter- or radiation-related). *Functional AVB* can be due to *excessive parasympathetic activation* (carotid sinus syndrome, vasovagal syncope); electrolyte disorders (hyperkalemia, hypermagnesemia); endocrine disorders (Addison's crisis); or *iatrogenic causes* (β-blockers, CCB, some AAD).

Therapy of AV block: *Medical therapy* is indicated in acute cases, mainly related to acute MI. The agent of choice is Atropine, 0.5–1.0 mg IV, repeated as needed, for a maximum of 2–3 mg in the setting of ischemia, so as to avoid secondary tachycardia with its attending exacerbation of ischemia. In case of AVB due to Digoxin toxicity, specific Fab antibody fragments may be used.

What are the circumstances in which Atropine is ineffective?

These include: infranodal block (therefore, Atropine is more effective in inferior, than in anterior MI-related complete AVB); AVB exclusively caused by ischemia (without a vagal component); postcardiac transplant patients (denervated hearts). Occasionally, Atropine can paradoxically enhance bradycardia: (a) in patients with 2/1 AV block, where it increases atrial rate and the corresponding concealed conduction, increasing AV node refractoriness and converting the patient to Mobitz II AV block; and (b), with doses <0.5 mg, and/or when Atropine is administered slowly; these effects appear to be centrally mediated.

Permanent pacing: The indications and technique of pacing for AVB depend on the degree, etiology, and reversibility of the block. *First-degree AVB* only requires pacing if it is symptomatic and prolonged, or secondary to neuromuscular diseases (where it may unexpectedly evolve to complete AV block; Class IIB indication). *Second-and third-degree AVB* carry a Class I indication for pacing if they are symptomatic. Other indications depend on the etiology, thus: (a) *AVB unrelated to acute MI or to CHD*: pacing is indicated in all patients, with a Class I indication for underlying neuromuscular disease or iatrogenic causes (after RF ablation of the AV node, after valve surgery, etc.), and for associated chronic bi-or trifascicular block. The indication is Class IIA otherwise; (b) *related to acute MI*: if the AVB is persistent (>14 days), or associated with new-onset BBB; (c) *related to CHD*: if there is associated LV dysfunction or if a postoperative Mobitz II or complete AVB persists ≥7 days after cardiac surgery. For third-degree AVB only, the following are also indications for permanent pacing: HR <70 bpm (<50–55 bpm in infants); wide QRS escape rhythm, complex ventricular ectopy, abrupt ventricular pauses >2–3 × basic cycle length, or prolonged QTc; maternal antibodies-mediated block. Optionally, pacing may be indicated even in the absence of the above-mentioned indications, as well as in transient postoperative IIId degree AV block, with residual bifascicular block; (c) *related to cardiac transplantation*: symptomatic bradyarrhythmia 3 weeks after transplantation (Class IIB indication in weeks II or III). The indications for permanent pacing in second- or third-degree AVB are discussed in Table 6.19. Pacemaker type selection is discussed in the relevant section.

Temporary pacing is indicated for Mobitz II or IIId degree AVB with bradycardia causing hypotension or HF; with AV node, Atropine is an alternative. The default modality for temporary pacing is the transvenous approach, but transcutaneous pacing using chest electrodes or transesophageal pacing are available options in emergency situations, if a transvenous pacemaker is difficult to insert. The main shortcomings of these alternatives are patient discomfort and the occasional failure to capture.

Pacemaker terminology: The signification of the different acronyms used for pacemaker designation is reviewed in Table 6.19 (indications for permanent pacing: Tables 6.20 and 6.21).

Table 6.19 Codes for pacemaker characteristics

	I	II	III	IV	V
Function	Chambers paced	Chambers sensed	Response to sensing	Other features	Multisite pacing
Designation[a]	O/A/V/D(A+V)/S	O/A/V/D(A+V)/S	O/T/I/D(T+I)	O/R	O/A/V/D(A+V)

[a]*O* none; *A* atrium; *V* ventricle; *S* single; *D* dual; *T* triggered; *I* inhibited; *R* rate modulation

Table 6.20 Indications[a] for permanent pacing in asymptomatic patients with second- or third-degree AV block

	Etiology		Time course		EKG manifestations		Other
Second-degree AVB	Neuromuscular disease; after RF AV node ablation; or after valve surgery	*or*			Mobitz II block *and* associated with chronic bi-or trifascicular block		
	Associated to MI	*and*	persistent	*and*	Mobitz II *and* associated with BBB of any age		
	Associated to MI	*and*			Mobitz II *and* associated with new-onset BBB		
	Associated to CHD	*and*					ventricular dysfunction
	Associated to surgery for CHD	*and*	persisting ≥7 days postop.	*and*	Mobitz II		
Third-degree AV block[a]	Neuromuscular disease or after RF ablation of the AV node, or after valve surgery	*or*			if associated with chronic bi-or trifascicular block		
	Associated to MI	*and*	persistent	*or*	associated with new-onset BBB		
	Associated to CHD	*and*			wide QRS escape rhythm, complex ventricular ectopy, abrupt ventricular pauses >2–3×basic cycle length, or prolonged QTc	*or*	HR <70 bpm (<50–55 bpm in infants) or LV dysfunction
	Associated to surgery for CHD	*and*	persisting ≥7 days postop.				
	Maternal antibod-ies-mediated block						

[a]There is a Class II indication for permanent pacing in any patient with second-or third-degree AV block; if this strategy is adopted, the present table is redundant

6.2.2.2 Intraventricular Conduction Disturbances

This section groups together conduction disturbances in the His bundle, right and left bundle branches, left hemibranches, and Purkinje network. The etiology is similar to that of AV block. Idiopathic degeneration and acute ischemia are the most frequent causes. The main types of intraventricular conduction disturbances include *LBBB*, *left anterior hemiblock (LAHB)*, *left posterior hemiblock (LPHB)*, *RBBB*, *and Purkinje-type block*. With BBB, the electrical impulse spreads normally only to the nonaffected ventricle; it then spreads abnormally through the myocytes, to the ventricle on the side of the block; this explains the EKG characteristics, including distortions of QRS morphology, duration, and/or axis, as outlined in

Table 6.21, and illustrated in Fig. 6.6. With complete RBBB or LBBB, the T wave axis is normally opposed to that of the QRS complex; a T wave with the same axis as the QRS complex (for instance, a positive T wave in V1–V2, in a patient with RBBB) may signify myocardial ischemia.

Table 6.21 The QRS complex in intraventricular conduction disturbances

	Morphology[a]	Duration	Axis
RBBB			
Complete	rsR′ or rSR′ in V1–V2; qRS in L1, aVL, V5–V6, with a wide terminal S	≥120 ms	Normal
Incomplete	As above	0.100–0.12 ms	Normal
LBBB			
Complete	Broad, monophasic R in L1, aVL, V5–V6; rS or QS in V1–V2	≥120 ms	Usually, left axis deviation
Incomplete	As above	0.100–0.12 ms	Usually, left axis deviation
LAHB	qR in L1, aVL, and rS in LII, III, aVF	Normal (0.06–0.10 ms)	≥ −45° (left axis deviation)
LPHB	qR in LII, III, aVF, and rS in L1, aVL	Normal	+90–120° (right axis deviation)
RBBB+LAHB	rsR′ or rSR′ in V1–V2, and qR in L1, aVL; rS in LII, III, aVF	≥120 ms	−60° to −120° (left axis deviation)
RBBB+LPHB	rsR′ or rSR′ in V1–V2, and qR in LII, III, aVF; rS in L1, aVL	≥120 ms	≥ +120° (right axis deviation)

[a]The EKG diagnosis of BBB requires that the patient be in supraventricular (i.e., sinus or junctional) rhythm, since idioventricular rhythms carry QRS morphology disturbances of their own, which would obscure the characteristic changes of the BBB

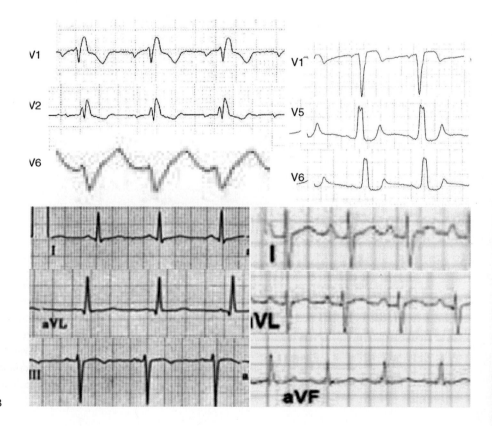

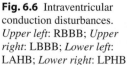

Fig. 6.6 Intraventricular conduction disturbances. *Upper left*: RBBB; *Upper right*: LBBB; *Lower left*: LAHB; *Lower right*: LPHB

"Non-complete" LBBB: two different scenarios

There are two manners in which the conduction through the left bundle branch can be only partly abnormal. Thus,

- *Incomplete* LBBB consists of a partial slowing of conduction through the left bundle before its bifurcation.
- *Left hemiblock* results from selective involvement of one of the two branches of the left bundle, that is, the left anterior or the left posterior hemibranch.

Intraventricular conduction disturbances, if not combined to the extent of producing complete AV block, do not carry symptoms of their own, and the main manifestations are those of underlying disease (e.g., acute MI, where BBB portends a poorer prognosis). In addition to their great pathophysiological similarities, RBBB and LBBB also possess individual characteristics, reviewed below.

RBBB

RBBB is quite common in the general population. However, it may also be associated with chronic lung disease, pulmonary embolism, acute MI (in almost 8% of cases), ASD, and VSD. In the presence of RBBB, these conditions must be ruled out as clinically indicated. In children, RBBB is usually related to CHD or to surgery for CHD. A particular etiology is conduction through a right bundle branch in its partially refractory period, yielding an RBBB morphology (Ashman's phenomenon, rate-dependent RBBB). Rate-dependent LBBB is less common. Clinically, RBBB causes a split S_2, due to delayed closure of the PV, as a result of delayed RV contraction, in the setting of slow electrical conduction to the RV. RBBB is difficult to diagnose in patients with a right accessory pathway, which "compensates" (in its own abnormal manner) the delay in RV activation, blurring or altogether abolishing the RBBB pattern. Conversely, a left accessory pathway conducting antegradely cannot be observed in these patients, as the delta wave is obscured by the RBBB morphology. Notably, RBBB must be distinguished from the Brugada syndrome and WPW syndrome type A. Additional causes of tall R waves in lead V1 include posterior wall MI and RVH.

The only setting when RBBB has a more severe prognosis than LBBB is acute MI.

LBBB

LBBB should generally trigger a more intense work-up for underlying cardiac disease, although it, too, can occasionally be seen in otherwise healthy individuals. Typical causes include CMP (dilated or hypertrophic), HTN, AV disease, and CAD. LBBB must also be distinguished from Type B WPW and anterior wall MI. Notably, LBBB does not prevent diagnosis of LVH. *LBBB in the context of acute MI* represents a complex topic. In this setting, LBBB is slightly more frequent than RBBB (8% of cases). LBBB renders the EKG diagnosis of anterior wall MI difficult, due to the amputated R waves or to the Q waves in V1–V2; however, ST-segment elevation ≥1 mm concordant with the QRS in any lead, or ST depression ≥1 mm in any lead from V1 through V3 suggests an associated MI. This is all the more important, since LBBB is a poor prognostic factor in MI patients. In fact, prognostically, the significance of LBBB in MI patients is a two-faced coin. On one hand, patients with LBBB have a significantly higher mortality; on the other hand, adjusting for co morbidity, mortality is actually *lower* in patients with LBBB, as, in these patients, the conduction disturbance is a marker of better ischemic preconditioning. (In other words, in the already sick population in which LBBB tends to occur, those who actually have the block fare better; however, as compared to the general population, the prognosis is much more severe.) New-onset LBBB, in a context suggestive of acute MI, is an indication for reperfusion within the "window of opportunity." Similar to LBBB, *left hemiblock* generally requires workup for underlying cardiac disease. LAHB is also often associated with anterior MI, and signifies more extensive coronary disease, especially involving the LAD. *Bifascicular block* refers to RBBB+ LAHB (approximately 6% of cases progress to complete AV block), or to RBBB+ LPHB (less frequent, but with an even greater risk of progression to complete AV block). *Trifascicular block* consists of bifascicular block with an associated first-degree AV block.

Purkinje Block

Purkinje block does not reflect as such on the surface EKG. It may cause or contribute to any of the conduction defects reviewed above.

Table 6.22 Indications for permanent pacing in intraventricular conduction disturbances

Etiology		EKG manifestations		EPS manifestations		Other
Neuromuscular disease	*and*	any degree of fascicular block				
Any	*and*	intermittent IIId degree AVB *or* Mobitz II block *or* alternating BBB	*or*	HV interval ≥100 ms[a] *or* or pacing induced infra-His block[b]	*or*	Syncope in the absence of proven AV block, when other causes (mainly VT) have been excluded
Associated to MI	*and*	persistent Mobitz II *and* BBB				
Associated to MI	*and*	transient Mobitz II *and* new-onset BBB				
Associated to MI	*and*	transient IIId degree AVB *and* new-onset BBB				

[a]I.e., markedly prolonged; normal <55 ms[b]Class I indication if symptomatic, Class IIA if asymptomatic

Therapy of Intraventricular Conduction Disturbances
Unifascicular block requires therapy only in the setting of severe HF, where CRT (biventricular pacing) improves both survival and the symptomatic status (Chap. 4). *Bi- and trifascicular block* require pacing if associated to Mobitz II or to IIId-degree AV block; alternating BBB; syncope; neuromuscular disease; or HV interval >100 ms or pacing-induced infra-His block (Table 6.22).

With AVB and with intraventricular conduction defects, ventricular-based pacing and sensing are essential. The possible modalities are VVI, VDD, or DDD. As a rule of thumb, in both sinus and nonsinus rhythms, simple VVI pacing can be used in the absence of chronotropic incompetence, with VVI-R required in its presence. If the patient is in NSR, DDD (no chronotropic incompetence), or DDD-R (with chronotropic incompetence) pacing is an option. DDD pacing can be successfully (and inexpensively) replaced by single-lead VDD pacing. Of note, current pacemakers are capable of automatic mode switch, which avoids conduction of AT to the ventricles, via pacemaker.

The Pacemaker Syndrome

The *pacemaker syndrome* is a complex of symptoms and signs resulting from loss of AV synchrony, as a result of ventricular pacing. It occurs in up to 20% of pacemaker implantees, and is more frequent in those with a higher number of paced ventricular beats, as well as in patients with intact ventriculoatrial conduction. The clinical findings include: exacerbation of HF, due to loss of atrial

kick; cannon "a" waves, due to atrial contraction against a closed AV valve; pulmonary and hepatic congestion, due to an increased pressure in both the LA and the RA; and an increased incidence of AF. As a result of increased LV filling pressures, there is an increase in atrial and brain natriuretic peptide (ANP, BNP) levels. The symptoms include palpitations, exacerbation of HF, hypotension, dizziness, near-syncope, confusion, and nonspecific chest pain. The treatment includes addition of an atrial lead in patients with ventricular pacing only, and pacemaker interrogation and reprogramming in the presence of a DDD pacemaker. *Pacemaker-mediated tachycardia* is a wide-complex rapid heart rhythm that may be mistaken for VT, and is generated by different mechanisms involving the pacemaker itself. One form represents tracking of rapid AT, and is managed by changing the pacemaker settings; another type results from oversensing in the atrial channels (e.g., of myopotentials), and is also managed by pacemaker resetting; finally, endless-loop tachycardia results from sensing of retrograde atrial impulses, and is terminated by placing a magnet over the pacemaker, followed by pacemaker reprogramming.

6.3 Ventricular Arrhythmia

6.3.1 Clinical Entities

6.3.1.1 VPB

VPBs are very frequent in both diseased and healthy individuals, and have causes similar to those of APBs. As they arise in the ventricular myocardium and spread

Table 6.23 Types of VPBs

VPB	Scenarios	Importance
Circumstances of appearance	At rest vs. exercise, with or without coexisting heart disease	Higher risk for SCD in frequent (>10/h) VPBs, especially in patients with underlying cardiac disease
Number	>10 vs. <10/h	See above
Morphology	Single vs. multiple morphologies (uni- vs. multifocal VPBs)	Higher probability of underlying heart disease with multifocal VPBs
Regularity	VPBs may occur at random, or follow a pattern: every second, third, or fourth beat may be a VPB (bi-, tri-, or quadrigeminy)	If frequent, may cause palpitations and/or CMP
Timing	Some VPBs are very precocious, with the QRS complex falling on the previous complex's T wave (R-on-T phenomenon)	An R-on-T VPB may trigger VT or VF; precocious VPBs have a low stroke volume, due to poor filling, and may cause the symptom of "missed beats"
Clustering	Two consecutive PVCs are called a couplet; three are a triplet, termed a "VT run" if HR >100 bpm, and "accelerated idioventricular rhythm" otherwise	Higher risk of significant arrhythmia with couplets and triplets
Effect on the sinus node	Retrograde sinus node depolarization absent (full compensatory pause) or present (incomplete compensatory pause)[a]	Compensatory pauses create the clinical symptom of a "missed beat"

[a]Most commonly, VPBs do not propagate retrogradely to the sinus node, and thus two consecutive sinus P waves fail to activate the ventricles: the first, due to the VPB; and the second, because it reaches the ventricles in their post-VPB refractory period. It is only the third P wave in line that does capture the ventricles; thus, the post-VPB pause is exactly double that of the normal heart cycle (i.e., between the first and the third P). This is a *full compensatory pause*. If the VPB does travel retrogradely and depolarizes the sinus, the latter is reset, and the *compensatory pause is incomplete* (but longer than normal, by the duration of retrograde conduction); these are *interpolated VPBs*

to the contralateral ventricle by nonspecific conduction through the myocytes, their EKG aspect is that of supraventricular beats conducted with a BBB. In patients with a normal-length EKG showing >1 PVC, there are several points of interest, regarding the probability of existing heart disease or the risk for such in the future, as outlined in Table 6.23. VPBs are occasionally used for diagnostic purposes, including analysis of the post-PVC variations in HR (cardiac turbulence), discussed in Chap. 1; of any increase in contractility in a previously hypokinetic ventricular segment after a VPB (*postextrasystolic potentiation*, a sign of myocardial viability); or of increased subaortic or aortic valvular gradients in HOCM or AS that may explain exertional symptoms in patients with otherwise apparently nonsevere disease.

6.3.1.2 Ventricular Escape Beats and Idioventricular Rhythm

Ventricular escape beats and idioventricular rhythm are very similar to VPBs, but result from failure of the sinus node to fire normally, or of the AV node to either normally conduct the impulses to the ventricles or to

generate a pacemaker activity of its own. The average discharge of an idioventricular ectopic focus is of around 40 bpm or less; ≥3 consecutive idioventricular beats are termed an *idioventricular rhythm*. Just like the sinus or junctional rhythms, an idioventricular rhythm can be faster than usual, i.e., "tachycardic." However, for rates <100 bpm, the latter term is avoided, since "tachycardia" is defined by the function of the sinus node (60–100 bpm; tachycardia if >100 bpm). For instance, for an idioventricular pacemaker, a HR of 80 bpm is twice as fast as the usual rate, yet, judging it by "sinus standards," the rhythm is not tachycardic. An idioventricular rate of 40–100 bpm is termed "*accelerated idioventricular rhythm*" (*AIVR*), to allude to the fast HR, while avoiding the confusing term, "tachycardia." Above 100 bpm, an idioventricular rhythm is tachycardic by any standards, and is indeed termed ventricular tachycardia (VT).

AIVR is caused by enhanced automaticity, often combined with depression of the sinus node pacemaker. It was classically considered as an indicator of successful reperfusion after coronary occlusion, although more recent data have challenged this assumption. Other common etiologies of AIVR include ischemia (especially of the inferior wall), digitalis toxicity, and electrolyte imbalance (hypokalemia). The ventricular rate is usually but little in excess of the sinus rate, and thus the pacemaker activity often switches "back and forth" between the sinus node and the ectopic pacemaker. Fusion beats are also frequently seen. The onset and termination of AIVR are usually gradual (nonparoxysmal). The clinical manifestations include cannon "a" waves, loss of the atrial kick, and palpitations. AIVR is generally a benign condition, but it can occasionally exacerbate HF or ischemia. In these cases, treatment is required, and, critically, it is necessary *to avoid* the medications commonly used in VT (e.g., Lidocaine), which may abolish a life-saving replacement pacemaker and precipitate asystole. If treatment is required, it consists of Atropine (0.6–1.2 mg IV), or Isoproterenol (0.5–2.0 µg/min), to increase the sinus rate and allow it to resume its normal pacemaker function. Temporary pacing is effective, but rarely necessary.

6.3.1.3 Ventricular Tachycardia (VT)

Definition and Classification

VT consists in any idioventricular rhythm lasting for ≥3 consecutive beats, at a rate ≥100 bpm (the usual rate is >150 bpm). There are several *classifications* for VT, according to: (a) *its mechanism*: VT can be due to increased automaticity, triggered activity, or reentry; (b) *the underlying condition*: ischemic and nonischemic; (c) *QRS morphology and regularity*: VT can originate in one or more ectopic foci, in either ventricle (monomorphic vs. polymorphic VT). QRS morphology also defines some particular types of VT, i.e., *torsades des pointes*, *bidirectional VT*, and *ventricular flutter* (Table 6.24). Of note, VT originating from a *single ventricular focus* is perfectly compatible with different *QRS morphologies*, as some ventricular complexes are entirely (*captured beats*) or partly (*fusion beats*) due to depolarization initiated in the sinus node and traveling down the normal conduction system. Captures and fusion beats are also seen with polymorphic VT. Monomorphic VT is usually regular (or slightly irregular, due to the idioventricular pacemaker, or to captured sinus beats); (d) *duration*: nonsustained (lasting for ≥3 beats, but <30 s, or requiring termination due to hemodynamic compromise; thus, the designation refers to the net duration of the VT, whatever the modality of termination) vs. sustained VT (≥30 s); (e) *hemodynamic impact*: hemodynamically stable vs. unstable VT. "Hemodynamically unstable" VT associates hypotension and represents a major risk of degeneration

to cardiac arrest; (f) *temporal pattern of repetition*: an increased frequency of VT repetition may represent a clear and immediate vital risk (in ICD implantees, this manifests as an increased number of electrical discharges) and should trigger a reassessment of any precipitating factors (electrolyte disturbance, acute ischemia, etc.), as well as of the therapeutic options (e.g., considering RF ablation in a patient with an ICD). The temporal pattern of VT repetition also defines a number of particular entities that merit a separate discussion: (1) *Torsades des pointes*: see Sect. 6.1.5.6.3; (2) *VT storm* represents the occurrence of >2 (and often, many more) episodes of VT in 24 h, requiring cardioversion. This rare entity is close to incessant VT (discussed below), but differs in that the episodes are unstable, i.e., require immediate cardioversion. VT storm can be monomorphic or polymorphic. Severe underlying heart disease is frequent, but more rarely, VT storm can occur in patients with a structurally normal heart (the Brugada or long QT syndromes (LQTSs), catecholaminergic VT, or drug overdose). In ICD implantees, VT storm may present as frequent (>2 or >3, according to different authors) appropriate shocks within 24 h. If diligent search does not identify correctible causes (acute ischemia, drug toxicity, electrolyte imbalance, suboptimal ICD programming, etc.), the event may simply herald the terminal stage of the underlying cardiac disease, and should prompt reevaluation of the available options (changes in drug therapy, cardiac transplantation, or a conservative approach); (3) *incessant VT* is an infrequent entity, consisting of hemodynamically stable VT lasting for several hours. Severe underlying heart disease is often present, typically acute ischemia; incessant *VT* can be monomorphic or polymorphic; (4) *repetitive monomorphic VT*, characterized by frequent VPBs and NSVT runs, with intervening NSR. It is similar to VT storm (see above), but, unlike that entity, is hemodynamically stable. It typically occurs at rest (although exercise-related cases have been described), and is most frequently idiopathic and self-terminating. Tachycardia-induced CMP is infrequent. The treatment of these entities is discussed in the following sections.

VT: Diagnosis

The clinical manifestations depend on HR and on coexistent organic heart disease. Rates <150 bpm are usually well tolerated (in the absence of severe LV dysfunction, where the loss of the atrial kick may precipitate HF) and can occasionally last for long periods of time. Higher

Table 6.24 VT: EKG manifestations

QRS	
Rate	>100, most often >150 bpm
Width	>0.14 s (RBBB pattern), or >0.16 s (LBBB pattern)[a]
Axis	"superior," i.e., −90 to ±180°, dominant S wave in lead aVF
Morphology	
Monomorphic VT	
RBBB-like pattern[b]	V1: monophasic or biphasic QRS complex; V6: R/S ratio <1; QRS concordance in V1–V6
LBBB-like pattern[b]	V1: LBBB-like pattern; V2: rS, notched complex; QRS concordance in V1–V6[c]; a particular instance is bundle branch-reentrant VT; it involves the His-Purkinje system and usually occurs with CMP.
Ventricular flutter	HR approximately 300 bpm, with no isoelectric interval between the QRS complexes
Polymorphic VT	
Torsade des pointes	Undulating aspect, QRS complexes appear to be twisting around the isoelectric axis. Additional distinctive features: prolonged underlying QTc; typically (but not exclusively), initiation with a short-long-short sequence[d]
Bidirectional VT	Beat-to-beat alternans (electrical axis change) in the frontal axis; usually due to Digitalis toxicity
Other polymorphic VT	Various QRS morphologies, without the characteristics of the other entities
Relationship to sinus node activity	
AV dissociation	No relationship between P waves and QRS complexes
Fusion beats	"Hybrid" beats, generated in part by normal depolarization (initiated by the sinus node), and in part by the ectopic ventricular pacemaker
Captured beats	Occasional normal sinus beats, among the ventricular and the fusion complexes

[a]Some consider 0.14 s the cutoff point for both LBBB and RBBB. VT originating in the proximal His-Purkinje system, however, can have QRS complexes as short as 0.11–0.14 s; at the other end of the spectrum, QRS can be as wide as 0.2 s, mainly with electrolyte abnormalities, severe myocardial disease, or AAD (e.g., Flecainide). The wider the QRS, the higher the probability of VT (rather than SVT with aberrant conduction)

[b]RBBB-pattern VT generally originates in the LV, and LBBB pattern VT, in the RV; an LBBB morphology is also seen with bundle-branch reentrant VT, involving antegrade conduction over the right bundle and retrograde conduction over the left bundle (frequent in DCM patients)

[c]i.e., QRS complexes either uniformly positive, or uniformly negative, throughout the chest leads

[d]A VPB (by definition, at a "short" interval after the previous beat) is followed by a compensatory pause, and finally, after this "long" interval, by a beat with a prolonged QTc; a subsequent VPB ("short" interval) may fall within the QT interval and trigger arrhythmia

HRs are variably tolerated, and symptoms are generally present in all patients at rates >200 bpm. VT may cause sudden death, either by itself (pulseless VT), or (especially with polymorphic VT) by degenerating to VF. *EKG manifestations* – see Table 6.24.

Differentiation of VT from SVT with aberrant intraventricular conduction (*the differential diagnosis of wide-complex tachycardia*) is a task of major importance, as (a) VT is usually substantially more severe (although SVT may also occasionally precipitate acute ischemia or HF), and (b) first-line therapies for SVT, such as β-blockers and CCB may precipitate hemodynamic collapse in VT patients. SVT in a patient with BBB can be identified by the QRS discordance in the chest leads (predominantly positive complexes in V1–V2 only with RBBB, and in V5–V6 only, with LBBB), while pacemaker-dependent tachycardia (for all intents and purposes, a "ventricular" tachycardia) is identified based on the pacemaker spikes and on the presence of the pacemaker generator on clinical and radiological examination. The main problem consists of differentiating VT from SVT with aberrant conduction. Although there exist reliable algorithms, this task is occasionally difficult (especially in the busy ER); in case of doubt, any wide-complex tachycardia should be considered VT and treated as such.

EKG differential diagnosis of wide-complex tachycardia

In a patient *without preexisting BBB or pacemaker rhythm*, a wide-complex tachycardia is considered VT if it has at least one of the following characteristics:

- Absence of an RS complex in all chest leads (a facet of QRS concordance)
- R-to-S interval (measured from the onset of the QRS complex to the nadir of the S wave) >100 ms (a facet of increased QRS width)
- More QRS complexes than P waves (a facet of AV dissociation)
- Morphology criteria of VT in V1 (monophasic R, QR, or RS) or V6 (monophasic R, QR, R:S< 1, or a QS)

Examined in sequence, these elements represent the Brugada algorithm for the differential diagnosis of wide-complex tachycardia, with a reported high sensitivity and specificity, which, however, have been questioned by others. Other algorithms have also been proposed. Any algorithm is useful only *in the absence of hemodynamic compromise*, as the latter mandates emergent therapy (typically, DCC), whatever the underlying nature of the pathologic rhythm. In patients with CAD, HF, past cardiac surgery, or cardiac enlargement, the overwhelming probability is that of VT.

An additional protocol has been developed by Brugada for differentiating VT from antidromic tachycardia, in WPW patients. In these patients, VT is diagnosed if any of the following criteria (also examined in sequence) is positive: (1) predominantly negative complexes in V4–V6; (2) presence of a QR complex in ≥1 lead in V2–V6; or (3) AV relation different than 1:1.

EPS is indicated for assessment of the risk of VT and possible SCD in patients with clinical symptoms (palpitations, presyncope, syncope) and evidence of structural heart disease. The risk is highest in patients with EF <35–40% (Chap. 4), thus ICD implantation is indicated across the board in these patients; paradoxically, then, it is precisely in the lower-risk population, with EF greater than the above-mentioned values, that EPS is most useful. In patients with a structurally normal heart, EPS can be of clear value (e.g., in patients with idiopathic VT), of

debated value (e.g., the Brugada syndrome), or of no value (LQTS). EPS is also helpful in patients with wide-QRS-complex tachycardia of unclear mechanism, as well as for guiding and evaluation of VT ablation.

Other tests: *Echo* is an essential diagnostic tool in assessing the risk of ventricular tachyarrhythmia and SCD, as there is a crucial distinction between the management of patients with or without structural heart disease, respectively. *Holter monitoring*, *event monitors*, or, as a last resource, *implantable recorders* are useful for the evaluation of palpitations, i.e., for assessment of their ventricular vs. supraventricular origin and for further assessment of ventricular arrhythmia complexity and implicit risk of SCD. In patients without structural heart disease, polymorphic VT indicates increased risk. (In patients with structural heart disease, PVCs, NSVT, and VT all portend an increased risk of SCD, but covariate with the degree of LV dysfunction, which is the stronger predictor. In other words, LV dysfunction predicts SCD regardless of demonstrated ventricular arrhythmia, which, however, is frequent in this population.) These diagnostic methods are also useful in patients in whom intermittent QT interval changes, T-wave alternans (TWA), or Brugada-type changes are suspected; *Exercise stress testing* is useful for diagnosis of suspected exercise-induced ventricular arrhythmias (including catecholaminergic VT) and for assessment of the patient's response to the tachycardia or to the treatment (ablation). Frequent PVCs in middle-aged or elderly patients represent another indication for exercise testing. *Signal-averaged EKG (SAECG)*, *HRV*, *baroreflex sensitivity*, and *HR turbulence* can be used to improve the accuracy of SCD risk assessment.

VT: Therapy

General remarks: VT is typically an acute event (the only instance of a subacute course is "incessant VT," i.e., VT lasting for several hours). The therapy consists of termination of the acute event, and, if warranted, of secondary prevention. Avoidance of proarrhythmic drugs or correction of underlying diseases (most notably, revascularization for ischemic VT and correction of electrolyte imbalance) contribute to both these purposes. As an acute event, VT may be hemodynamically stable or unstable the latter, defined as (VT with a palpable pulse, but with BP decrease, or as pulseless VT, a form of cardiac arrest). Hemodynamically unstable VT is a major medical emergency. The different therapeutic modalities and their

Table 6.25 Therapeutic options in VT

Therapy	Acute termination			Secondary prevention
	Unstable VT		Stable VT	
	Cardiac arrest	VT with a pulse		
Electrical	√ (DCC)	√(DCC)	√[1](DCC)	√ (ICD[4])
Pharmacological				
AAD	√	√	√	√
Non-AAD	√[2]	√[2]	–	–
Coronary revascularization	–	(√[3])	√[3]	√
Ablation	–	(√[3])	–	√

[1]Usually, not first-choice therapy
[2]Atropine, adrenaline for cardiac arrest; magnesium sulfate, isoproterenol, for torsades des pointes
[3]Occasionally, VT is not amenable to medical therapy alone, and requires emergency coronary revascularization or RF ablation
[4]ICD may terminate the arrhythmia by DCC or antitachycardia pacing

place in the treatment of VT are reviewed in Table 6.25. Specific considerations regarding the particular types of VT are presented in the following two sections, first by type of VT (hemodynamically stable vs. unstable, monomorphic vs. polymorphic, etc.), and subsequently, by VT etiology.

Pharmacological therapy: The most frequently used AAD for *acute* management of VT and the corresponding dosages are outlined in Table 6.26. As regards chronic maintenance therapy, the only recommended agents are β-blockers and, in certain cases, amiodarone. It must be kept in mind that the procedure of choice in high-risk patients is ICD implantation, *supplemented* as needed by drug therapy.

RF ablation is indicated (a) in patients with hemodynamically stable sustained VT, especially monomorphic (since polymorphic VT is typically generated in multiple foci, making it difficult or impossible to identify and ablate all foci), and who respond poorly to therapy (failure of AAD, multiple ICD shocks despite device reprogramming and adjunctive drug therapy), or who do not wish long-term therapy; (b) in patients with bundle-branch reentrant VT or with VT/VF resulting from antegrade conduction over an aberrant pathway; (c) These indications can be extended (Class IIA recommendation) to patients with lesser degrees of arrhythmia: symptomatic monomorphic nonsustained VT or even frequent monomorphic PVCs, where drug therapy fails or is refused; (d) Additional indications (Class IIB) refer to asymptomatic PVCs, in two different settings: if, by their frequency, they cause or threaten to cause tachycardia-related CMP, or if they cause arrhythmia storm (≥3 episodes of ventricular arrhythmia in a 24-h period); the ectopic focus in this setting is often the Purkinje network.

Electrical therapy: *DCC* is indicated for acute termination of hemodynamically unstable rhythms (VF, pulseless VT), and is an option for stable VT as well.

Table 6.26 The main[a] AAD used for the acute therapy of VT

Drug	Indications	Dosage
Class IA – Procainamide	*Hemodynamically stable VT*: sustained (including repetitive and incessant) monomorphic VT[b]; sustained nontorsade polymorphic VT if recurrent or incessant	IV 20 mg/min for 25–30 min as loading dose, then 2–6 mg/min for maintenance
Class IB – Lidocaine	*VT associated to ACS*, especially in patients with LV dysfunction, as a second-choice alternative to amiodarone; LQT3-associated *torsades des pointes*	IV push 0.5–0.75 mg/kg, then 1–4 mg/min continuous infusion; maximum dose 200–300 mg/h
Class II (β-blockers) – Metoprolol	*VT associated to ACS*, especially if recurrent or incessant, associated to revascularization and followed as needed by Procainamide or Amiodarone	Three boluses of 5 mg at 2 min intervals, then PO 50 mg q8 h for 48 h, then 100 mg b.i.d. maintenance therapy
Class III – Amiodarone	Unstable VT, refractory to DCC and Procainamide; recurrent torsades in the absence of congenital prolonged QT; incessant VT or VT storm, isolated or associated to β-blockers	IV 150 mg over 10 min

[a]Additional AAD labeled for use in VT, but used on a patient-by-patient basis, especially for chronic maintenance therapy, include *Class IA agents*: Quinidine, Disopyramide (oral agents); IV Ajmaline is, used in some European countries as the agent of choice for sustained monomorphic, hemodynamically stable VT and for repetitive monomorphic VT; it is generally not widely available
[b]*Class IB agents*: Mexiletine (especially in LQT3-associated *torsades des pointes*); *Class IC agents*: Flecainide, Propafenone (contraindicated in ischemic VT); *Class III agents*: Sotalol (especially for repetitive monomorphic VT and incessant VT)

For the advantages and disadvantages of DCC in the latter setting, see the relevant section. DCC is possible in pacemaker bearers, but antero-posterior paddle placement is indicated (i.e., as far as possible from the device), and post-DCC pacemaker interrogation is necessary. *The indications for ICD* related to LVEF decreases are presented in Chap. 4, while the other indications are reviewed in Table 6.27. Arrhythmia termination may be achieved by DCC delivery or by antitachycardia pacing. The latter is mainly successful for monomorphic VT, especially in patients without (major) cardiac structural abnormalities. A wearable "ICD vest" has become available, and is recommended in patients with a transient high risk for SCD (for instance, patients with DCM awaiting cardiac transplantation), or in those in whom lead infection has mandated temporary ICD removal.

Occasionally, atrial tachyarrhythmia (most frequently, AF) is misinterpreted by the ICD as ventricular tachyarrhythmia, with inappropriate shock delivery. Occasionally, the situation evolves to an electrical storm, further compromising the cardiac function. Beta-blockade and Amiodarone, or, if necessary,

RF ablation are used to decrease the number of discharges in ICD implantees. Pacing can be used in certain forms of VT, such as bradycardia-dependent and overdrive-suppressible VT.

Surgical therapy for VT: This includes several procedures: (1) *coronary revascularization* (surgical or percutaneous), effective for secondary prevention of SCD in patients with ischemic polymorphic VT or VF, but not in those with sustained monomorphic VT (where RF ablation may be a good option) or with poor LV function (where ICD implantation is indicated; see Chap. 4); (2) *antiarrhythmic surgery*, i.e., surgical resection of arrhythmic foci, in specialized centers; (3) *left cervicothoracic sympathetic ganglionectomy*, involving resection of the lower half of the left stellate ganglion and removal of a number of sympathetic ganglia on the left side. This is indicated for LQTS-associated aborted syncope or cardiac arrest despite combined ICD and β-blocker therapy and surgical therapy; (4) *LV aneurysmectomy* in patients after large anterior infarctions.

Other therapeutic modalities: Spinal cord modulation (impacting the neurovegetative influences on the heart by

Table 6.27 Indications for ICD implantation

Clinical setting		EKG	Class
Secondary prevention			
Survivors of SCD[a]	*and*	VF or sustained VT	I
Syncope of undetermined origin	*and*	significant VT or VF induced at EPS	I
Unexplained syncope and nonischemic DCM (or other advanced structural heart disease)			IIa (IIb)
LQTS	*and/or*	VT under β-blockers	IIa
Brugada syndrome	*or*	VT not causing SCD	IIa
Catecholaminergic polymorphic VT	*and/or*	sustained VT under β-blockers	IIa
Structural heart disease	*and*	spontaneous sustained VT[b]	I
Primary prevention			
HCM with ≥1 risk factor for SCD			IIa
ARVC with ≥1 risk factor for SCD			IIa
Nonhospitalized patients awaiting transplantation			IIa
Cardiac sarcoidosis, giant cell myocarditis, or Chagas disease			IIa
Long-QT syndrome and risk factors for SCD			IIb
Familial cardiomyopathy associated with SCD			IIb
LV noncompaction			IIb

[a]After excluding reversible causes
[b]Regardless of hemodynamic stability

thoracic epidural anesthesia) or general anesthesia may be occasionally required in incessant VT or VT storm.

VT Therapy According to Clinical Manifestations

Pulseless VT

See SCD.

Hemodynamically Unstable VT

"Common" hemodynamically unstable VT: DCC shock is used in all patients with hemodynamically unstable VT; it is recommended to use synchronized DCC in monomorphic VT, whereas with polymorphic VT (as with VF), unsynchronized DCC is used (synchronization is difficult with the former, and impossible with the latter arrhythmia). Exacerbations of HF or of angina pectoris are also typical indications for DCC. With modern biphasic defibrillators, the energy regimen for DCC is of 150-200 J, followed as needed by subsequent shocks of equal or higher intensity. There

Table 6.28 Hemodynamically unstable VT: pharmacological therapy

	Normal EF	Decreased EF
Monomorphic	Amiodarone, Lidocaine,[a] occasionally Sotalol	Amiodarone, Lidocaine,[a] occasionally Sotalol
Polymorphic		
Normal baseline QT[a]	Lidocaine, Amiodarone, Sotalol; β-blockers and revascularization, if ischemic; correction of electrolyte imbalance	Amiodarone, Lidocaine
Prolonged baseline QT (torsades[b])	Mg sulfate, Isoproterenol, β-blockers, Phenytoin, Lidocaine; overdrive pacing[c]	Mg sulfate, Isoproterenol, Phenytoin, Lidocaine; overdrive pacing; use β-blockers cautiously

[a]Procainamide is disfavored, as it can precipitate HF, especially in patients with decreased EF
[b]Typically, runs of torsades are interspersed with stretches of NSR, where QT prolongation may be observed
[c]Procainamide is C/I, as it can prolong the QT interval

remain, however, quite a large number of older, monophasic defibrillators in use, and with these, a maximal energy of 360 J can be used either from the start, or 200 J can be used for the first shock, and 360 J on subsequent shocks, if VT recurs. Importantly, DCC for hemodynamically unstable VT is part of the CPR protocol, and must be optimally combined with thoracic compressions, patient ventilation, and drug therapy (Table 6.30). *The pharmacological treatment* is outlined in Table 6.28. CCB are contraindicated, as they may exacerbate hypotension. Correction of electrolyte imbalance, termination of proarrhythmic drugs, and, occasionally, coronary revascularization and/or RF ablation need to be incorporated in the therapeutic strategy, as VT may be refractory to therapy in the absence of these measures. *Torsade des pointes*: see below. *The treatment of VT storm* mainly involves IV Amiodarone and β-blockers, separately or together. (Paradoxically, however, in some patients it is precisely Amiodarone or Procainamide, given to slow down or abolish VT, that can precipitate VT storm or incessant VT.) Polymorphic VT storm in a patient with CAD strongly suggests acute ischemia and warrants assessment for emergency revascularization. General anesthesia or spinal cord modulation may be considered. Pacing may be tried either for overdrive suppression, or for VT storm due to pause-dependent torsades (triggered by ventricular beats occurring after a pause and displaying a prolonged QT interval). In fact, these cases should be managed altogether as torsades, while keeping in mind a possible ischemic etiology.

Hemodynamically Stable VT

Despite normal blood pressure, *hemodynamically stable VT* remains an emergency, especially with fast ventricular rates and the commonly coexisting structural heart disease (ventricular dysfunction, coronary stenosis, etc.). Early termination of the arrhythmia is warranted due to the tachycardia itself, the loss of the atrial kick, and the potential degeneration into VF and asystole. The classes of therapeutic options are the same as with unstable VT, but with slight departures from that protocol. Thus, *DCC* is more of an elective nature than with unstable VT. The advantages of DCC include a high immediate success rate and the lack of proarrhythmic effect (with the notable exception of Digitalis-related arrhythmias, where DCC can precipitate VT/VF); however, DCC does not prevent VT recurrences and requires deep sedation – two potentially important disadvantages. *Pharmacological therapy* involves, as a preferred agent, IV Procainamide (in some European countries, IV Ajmaline), in the absence of HF and of QT prolongation. Procainamide has better acute conversion rates in this setting than Amiodarone, usually reserved for patients refractory to DCC and Procainamide (a response to Procainamide but not to Amiodarone, although less frequent, is occasionally observed). Lidocaine is very effective in ischemia-related VT, especially when the EF is decreased and Procainamide might be hazardous (close BP monitoring is important). Additionally, it is reasonable to use Amiodarone if it will also be used for maintenance therapy (obviating the need for a loading dose before chronic maintenance therapy); *Ablation* and *overdrive pacing* are useful for patients refractory to cardioversion or with VT recurring despite AAD (or if the latter have unacceptable side effects or are declined by the patient). While CCB are still contraindicated, they (as well as Adenosine) may terminate some cases of idiopathic VT; this approach, however, is acceptable only in the hands of arrhythmia experts. With *repetitive monomorphic VT*, treatment is mainly dictated by the presence of palpitations, and is rarely urgent. If therapy is indicated, this can be carried out pharmacologically (chronic administration of β-blockers, or, atypically in the setting of VT, of CCB; if acute therapy is deemed necessary, it should follow the general lines of stable VT treatment), or by RF ablation. *Incessant VT* can be monomorphic or polymorphic. The former is treated with intravenous Amiodarone or Procainamide, followed, as needed, by VT ablation, while the latter, highly suggestive of ischemia, is treated with IV β-blockers and emergency revascularization, followed, as needed, by IV Procainamide or Amiodarone. Overdrive pacing, general anesthesia, or spinal cord modulation may be occasionally required. In patients with underlying ischemia, emergency revascularization is often required.

VT According to Etiology

Ischemic VT

Acute ischemia causes alteration of action potentials, cell refractoriness, and depolarization propagation, resulting in arrhythmia by increased automatism, reentry, or triggered activity. Acute ischemia may occasionally be caused by coronary spasm, rather than by coronary thrombosis. VT associated with acute ischemia tends to be polymorphic; while ischemia may prolong the QT interval, it does so to a modest extent, and often the QT interval is normal. VT is more frequent in large MI, and a decreased LVEF is by far the most important predictor of severe ventricular arrhythmia after MI. Conversely, early reperfusion after MI decreases the risk of severe arrhythmia. NSVT, T wave alternans, and abnormal SAECG results are additional predictors of ventricular arrhythmia after MI, but their positive predictive value is low, and they are helpful only as auxiliary indicators of risk. Occasionally, sustained monomorphic VT may associate modest cardiac enzyme increases due to increased metabolic demands during tachycardia; a false diagnosis of MI must be avoided by careful assessment (especially as such patients do often suffer from CAD), and the usual treatment protocol should be followed. VT and VF in the first 24–48 h post-MI portend a higher in-hospital mortality only, whereas beyond 48 h, they also carry an increased risk of SCD after discharge. *AIVR* is often seen in MI patients, and differs from VT by its slower rate (<100 bpm). Rarely of clinical concern, this entity was discussed above.

Chronic ischemia may cause ventricular arrhythmia due to reentry circuits around myocardial scars or to the admixture of viable myocytes with the scar tissue; additional possibilities are episodes of acute ischemia (discussed above), pro-arrhythmic drug effects, electrolyte derangements, or non-MI-related mechanisms (e.g., bundle branch reentry). These patients may present with either NSVT, sustained VT (stable or unstable), or cardiac arrest due to pulseless VT or VF. The mortality is high, due to both the arrhythmia and the underlying LV dysfunction. NSVT and sustained monomorphic VT are associated with high late mortality rate in patients with decreased LVEF. Unfortunately, however, there is no evidence that VT suppression prolongs survival. While usually asymptomatic, VT is occasionally very frequently recurrent, causing intolerable palpitations or tachycardia-related CMP; as an extreme, it may manifest as VT storm or incessant VT. If VT does require therapy, the preferred agents are β-blockers, and, in case of failure, Amiodarone or Sotalol. Sustained VT may also carry an indication for ICD (see Table 6.27 and Chap. 4), alone or combined with AAD. VT ablation by catheter or surgical techniques may be required if the VT episodes are more frequent. Catheter ablation is often problematic, as many patients have multiple tachycardia pathways, and only those with one or two circuits may be cured by catheter; additionally, some of these patients may develop de novo circuits, causing VT to recur during follow-up. On the positive side, ablation, even if not curative, may significantly decrease the frequency of VT episodes. Ischemic DCM is similar in many respects to the nonischemic form, discussed below.

VT Associated to Other (Nonischemic) Structural Heart Disease

Valvular heart disease: It is not clear whether VHD per se can cause ventricular arrhythmia, with the possible exception of a flail myxomatous MV. Therefore, treatment should be prescribed according to the guidelines for each individual VHD (with a Class IIB indication for valvular surgery in patients with a flail myxomatous mitral leaflet, severe MR, and severe or frequently recurring ventricular arrhythmia). Of note, the highest frequency of SCD is seen not with mitral, but with AV disease (especially severe AS), but arrhythmia per se does not represent an indication for surgery in these patients.

Congenital heart disease: the most frequent entities associated with SCD include TOF, D- and L-transposition of the great arteries, AS, functional single ventricle, and congenital coronary anomalies, most frequently an anomalous origin of the left coronary artery from the right sinus of Valsalva. The best-studied patients are those with TOF, where a combination of complex ventricular ectopy, ventricular dysfunction, volume overload due to PI, and wide QRS complexes >160 ms are risk factors for SCD. Invasive hemodynamic evaluation and EP studies are indicated in patients with decreased LV function and unexplained syncope; ICD implantation is decided upon based on the EPS results. Some experts also advocate EP studies in patients with NSVT and even with ventricular couplets.

Ventricular arrhythmia caused by *myocarditis, pericarditis, and infiltrative CMP* is treated according to the general principles outlined in the introductory section. ICD implantation is not indicated in the acute phase of myocarditis, but is often necessary in patients with residual LV dysfunction and significant ventricular arrhythmia.

Cardiac involvement in endocrine disease and metabolic disorders may include significant ventricular arrhythmia, by various mechanisms. Thus, hypothyroidism has

been linked to QT prolongation; Addison's disease may cause hyperkalemia; Conn's syndrome may cause hypokalemia; pheochromocytoma may cause excessive catecholamine activity; acromegaly causes increased LV mass. The treatment is that of the underlying endocrinopathy. SCD is several dozen-fold more frequent in the morbidly obese, as well as in patients with anorexia nervosa, due to severe electrolyte disturbances, atherosclerosis (in the obese), and defects in neurovegetative regulation. Diabetes may predispose to severe arrhythmia by promoting atherosclerosis and autonomic neuropathy, or through antidiabetic-associated hypoglycemic episodes, associated with QT prolongation. Other conditions associated to metabolic derangements causing ventricular arrhythmia include: *end-stage renal disease*, where arrhythmia (mainly related to electrolyte abnormalities, myocardial dysfunction, or abnormal BP) may occur due to the disease itself, or as a complication of dialysis (during, and for at least 4–5 h after the procedure); and *PAH*, where SCD is quite frequently seen, and may be due to arrhythmic or nonarrhythmic mechanisms (PA rupture); significant ventricular arrhythmia is especially frequent during cardiac catheterization, which, in PAH patients, must be reserved for absolute indications.

Moderate-to-severe obstructive sleep apnea is associated with an increased risk of all-cause mortality, particularly in middle-aged men. Mortality appears to be driven by a host of cardiovascular and noncardiovascular causes, the former mainly including arrhythmia, ischemia, HTN, and stroke.

A large variety of *recreational substances* (alcohol, nicotine, cocaine) and of *therapeutic agents* (Digitalis, tricyclic antidepressants, phenothiazines, Cisapride, Erythromycin, etc.) have been associated with the genesis of VT.

Other baseline EKG abnormalities of interest in establishing the risk for ventricular tachyarrhythmias comprise novel T wave parameters, including T wave width, principal component analysis, T-wave morphology dispersion, and T-wave residuum. The main arrhythmogenic mechanism investigated by these parameters is myocardial repolarization heterogeneity, an independent predictor of cardiovascular events. According to new data still to be validated, in adults aged ≥30, T-wave markers may be superior to the rate-adjusted QT interval as independent predictors of both all-cause and cardiovascular mortality.

Nonischemic dilated CMP: Just like ischemic DCM, nonischemic DCM can cause SCD. Patients with advanced

longer QT intervals than men (both congenital and acquired); although this difference equalizes by age 50, torsades des pointes remains more frequent in women. In women with congenital LQTS, the highest risk of SCD is in the immediate postpartum period, as during pregnancy the QT segment is (protectively) shortened by tachycardia. Somewhat counterintuitively, it is precisely in this postpartum period that β-blockers are most protective, but in fact, they are also commonly continued during pregnancy (under fetal HR follow-up, as fetal bradycardia may occur). Risk stratification in regard to the possibility of SCD can be carried out on purely *clinical* grounds: high risk in QT >500 ms; aborted SCD in the past; immediate postpartum period (of note, family history of SCD has *not* proved to be a risk factor for SCD), or by *combined clinical, demographic, and genetic analysis* (highest risk in LQT1 and LQT2 patients with a QTc >500 ms and in males with LQT3 irrespective of QT duration). The disease usually presents in childhood, but can be first noted at any age. Genetic testing helps assess the risk profile and establish the optimal therapeutic strategy. The main indicated therapeutic modalities include β-blockers and ICD, alone or in combination, as reviewed in Table 6.29.

Acquired QT segment prolongation is mainly seen in patients with organic heart disease. However, it will be discussed in this section, to avoid artificial separation from the congenital form. *Drugs* frequently causing QT prolongation and ventricular arrhythmia (>1% of patients) include AAD from the Classes IA (Quinidine, Procainamide, Disopyramide, Ajmaline), Ic (Dofetilide, Ibutilide), and III (Sotalol). Other notable drugs potentially causing prolonged QT (albeit with a lesser frequency) include Amiodarone, Erythromycin and some of its newer derivatives (e.g., Clarithromycin); the prokinetic, Cisapride; some antipsychotics (Chlorpromazine, Haloperidol, Thioridazine); some antiemetics (Domperidone, Droperidol); and Methadone, used to treat opioid dependence. An up-to-date list is maintained at www.torsades.org and www.qtdrugs.org. The risk of arrhythmia is higher in the female gender; bradycardia; hypokalemia, hypomagnesemia; recent conversion from AF; HF; and LVH. Most cases of drug-induced torsades des pointes display a "short-long-short" initiation (Table 6.23). The management includes removal of the offending agent; magnesium and potassium repletion; magnesium sulfate for patients with few episodes of torsades des pointes; atrial or ventricular pacing or Isoproterenol with recurrent torsades des pointes. Isoproterenol can also be used to increase HR and abolish postectopic pauses. *CVA*, most notably subarachnoid hemorrhage, may cause QT prolongation and torsades des pointes.

The arrhythmia characteristically arising in patients with a prolonged QT interval is *torsades des pointes*, a form of rapid, generally nonsustained (usually, <20 s) polymorphic VT, which can be self-limiting or degenerate to VF. The triad, LQTS, a polymorphic VT with a typical "undulating" appearance (as if the QRS complexes were twisting around the isoelectric axis), and often, a short-long-short initiation sequence is diagnostic of the condition. Bradycardia is a risk factor for torsades in patients with a prolonged QT interval. The treatment includes DCC, correction of electrolyte disturbances (Magnesium sulfate IV 1–2 g bolus, up to 4 g given over 10–15 min abolishes torsades in most patients), and IV Isoproterenol (IV bolus 0.02–0.06 mg, followed by subsequent

Table 6.29 Long QT syndrome (LQTS): treatment[a]

Type of assessment	Clinical/EKG/genetic parameters	β-blockers	ICD	Indication class
Clinical only	Long QTc interval	√		I
	Long QTc interval and survivor of cardiac arrest (on β-blocker therapy or on no therapy)	√	*and* √	I
Genetic testing available	Normal QTc interval and genetic testing positive for any LQTS	√		IIa
	Normal QTc interval and genetic testing positive for LQT2 and LQT3	√	*and* √	IIb

[a]In all patients, avoidance of the specific triggering situations, including competitive sports; left cardiac sympathetic neural denervation is a Class IIB option in case of β-blocker failure as a primary prevention agent. Several observational studies have found benefit in cardiac pacing for patients with a prolonged QT syndrome, the rationale being that of shortening diastole, and thus reducing the incidence of torsades

boluses of 0.01–0.2 mg and/or by an IV infusion at a rate of 5 μg/min) or pacing to counteract QT-prolonging bradycardia.

The Brugada Syndrome

The Brugada syndrome is a genetic condition carrying a high risk of SCD in the absence of detectable cardiac structural abnormalities; it is characterized by an abnormal EKG, displaying a J-point elevation in leads V1–V3 and an RBBB-like morphology in some patients. These manifestations may be constant or intermittent, spontaneous or provoked by sodium channel blockers, i.e., Class IA AAD. Predisposing factors for SCD in these patients include: male gender (in 90% of patients with a typical EKG); fever; a spontaneous (rather than provoked) EKG pattern; and a history of syncope. As with LQTS, family history does *not* appear to be a risk factor. The role of EP testing and genetic analysis for risk stratification is not clear. Importantly, Holter testing does not reveal premonitory findings such as VPBs or runs of NSVT, but may occasionally demonstrate the typical EKG pattern in patients in whom this finding is intermittent. The associated arrhythmias include rapid polymorphic VT or VF, typically occurring at rest or during sleep. Treatment of the acute arrhythmic episodes is that of cardiac arrest; Isoproterenol or Quinidine can be useful to treat the occasional electrical storm (incessant VT). ICD implantation is mandatory in SCD survivors, and optional after syncope or even in well-tolerated VT; in fact, in real life (and economic considerations allowing), the Brugada syndrome, in any of its clinical or EKG variants, is often managed by ICD implantation.

Catecholaminergic Polymorphic VT (CPVT)

CPVT is a genetically inherited propensity to develop ventricular tachyarrhythmias during physical activity, due to defective calcium handling by the cells. It can be induced by exercise stress test, at a HR of 120–130 bpm. The typical arrhythmia is "bidirectional VT," exhibiting a beat-to-beat alternating QRS axis (rotating by 180°). EPS is not useful, but genetic analysis may identify silent carriers, although it does not help with risk stratification. Beta-blockers are indicated in CPVT patients with spontaneous or documented stress-induced ventricular arrhythmias, as well as in asymptomatic patients with a genetic diagnosis of CPVT. ICD with concomitant use of β-blockers is indicated in survivors of cardiac arrest

and in patients with syncope and/or documented sustained VT under β-blocker therapy.

Idiopathic VT: In the absence of any structural or genetically-identifiable abnormality, VT is termed "idiopathic." The most common form arises from the RV and has a good prognosis (mild symptoms, infrequent syncope). This VT usually has an LBBB, inferior-axis morphology. RVOT VT must be distinguished from ARVC-related VT (discussed above). Less frequently, VT arises in the LVOT; this type of VT may be incessant and is occasionally provoked by exercise. EPS helps establish a precise diagnosis and guides RF ablation. The treatment involves β-blockers and CCB in all patients, and additionally, in RVOT VT (i.e., in most of the cases), Class IC AAD, and catheter ablation.

6.3.1.4 Ventricular Fibrillation (VF)

VF represents a totally chaotic electrical activity of the ventricles, with undistinguishable individual complexes of variable cycle length, morphology, and amplitude, no isoelectric line, and no CO. Together with pulseless electrical activity and asystole, it is a form of cardiac arrest. VF is often preceded by VT, especially of the polymorphic type. Its treatment is one of the great medical emergencies, and will be discussed under "SCD." Virtually, all the causes of VT are also valid for VF patients.

6.3.2 Cardiac Arrest and SCD

Cardiac arrest is defined as the abrupt loss of effective blood flow, sufficient to cause loss of consciousness, leading immediately to death if untreated. If demise occurs shortly after symptom onset (different authors set the timeframe within 1 h or 24 h), the entity is termed "sudden cardiac death" (SCD). As a point of semantics, "arrest" refers to the mechanical activity of the heart, regardless of the presence of electrical activity. Cardiac arrest is most commonly caused by ventricular tachyarrhythmia (most often, VF), but a considerable minority of cases is due to severe bradyarrhythmias, asystole, or pulseless electrical activity. As the latter events also represent the terminal phase of ventricular tachyarrhythmia, it is often difficult to assess the initial event, in out-of-hospital cases. Not surprisingly, survival is best in patients presenting with

VT/VF in the hospital, where very fast intervention is possible. At the other end of the spectrum, patients with out-of-hospital cardiac arrest presenting as pulseless electrical activity or asystole have a dismal prognosis. Overall, >90% of in-hospital, but only around 20% of out-of-hospital cases of cardiac arrest survive to discharge, with many of the latter presenting some form of irreversible neurologic deficit. Up to 80% of patients of any age sustaining cardiac arrest have ischemic heart disease, followed by patients with DCM (10%), and by other causes of lethal arrhythmia: HCM, RV CMP, congenital abnormalities (especially coronary artery anomalies), coronary artery spasm, genetic syndromes such as LQTS, etc. Importantly, the underlying disorder may be of a noncardiac nature, and the "4H/4T" mnemonic for possible causes of cardiac arrest must be kept in mind. 4H= Hypoxia, hypovolemia, hypo/hyperkalemia (metabolic disorders), and hypothermia; 4T= tension pneumothorax, pericardial tamponade, toxins (including drugs), and thrombosis (coronary or PE). While myocardial ischemia remains the main cause for cardiac arrest, it accounts for only part of one of the "T"s in the mnemonic.

As survival is largely dependent on the promptness of initial response, the first priority, in out-of-hospital cases, should be to activate a response team, with CPR started as soon as possible. Basic life support maneuvers should be carried out as usual. If an automated external defibrillator (AED) is available, this should be located and activated at once. In witnessed cases of cardiac arrest, "thumpversion," that is, application of a single strong fist blow to the chest should be considered by health professionals. CPR should be performed in

Table 6.30 Treatment of cardiac arrest[a]

Time (minutes)	0	2	4	6	8	10	12	14[b]
Shock[c]	Ö	√	√	√	√	√	√	√
CPR[d]	√	√	√	√	√	√	√	√
Drugs[e]								
Shockable rhythm	No	No	Epinephrine 1 mg	Consider amiodarone, 300 mg bolus; if isch., consider lidocaine instead, 1–1.5 mg/kg; if torsades, consider loading 1–2 g	Epinephrine 1 mg	No	Epinephrine 1 mg	No
Nonshockable rhythm	Epinephrine 1 mg + atropine 3 mg[f] once	No	Epinephrine 1 mg	No	Epinephrine 1 mg	No	Epinephrine 1 mg	No

[a]All drugs, IV or IO
[b]The ressuscitation efforts sould be continued as appropriate, repeating the same steps, with pauses every 2 min to recheck for pulse and for electrical activity
[c]Biphasic: 200 J; monophasic: 360 J; AED: device-specific. Appropriate only if initial or subsequent periodic assessment (q2 min) reveals a shockable rhythm. Repetition as per next assessment
[d]Same technique, regardless of underlying arrhythmia; 1 cycle of CPR = (a) before intubation: 30 compressions, at a frequency of 100/min, then pause for two breaths. Compressions should be fast (see text), so that 5 cycles should take about 2 min; (b) after intubation, give 8–10 breaths/min, without pausing compressions
[e]β-blockers (propranolol, 1-mg boluses to a total up to 15–20 mg; metoprolol 5 mg, up to 20 mg) or $MgSO_4$ (1–2 g over 1–2 min) may be used in patients with resistant VT (including torsades) or VF, especially with underlying acute ischemia. Sodium bicarbonate (1 mEq/kg) is mainly recommended in prolonged resuscitation runs. In patients with resistant VF due to underlying acute hyperkalemia, hypocalcemia, or CCB, IV 10% calcium gluconate, 5–20 mL, infused at a rate of 2–4 mL/min, can be tried. While ongoing CPR is not a contraindication to fibrinolysis, fibrinolysis as such is not a component of CPR, with the possible exception of patients in whom cardiac arrest results from PE
[f]Only if asystole or HR<60 bpm

cycles (see Table 6.30), with the chest compression components strong and fast (100/min), but allowing for proper chest wall recoil. If the assessed response time of the rescue team is >5 min, a brief (90–180 s) CPR period is recommended prior to attempting defibrillation; otherwise, DCC should be the first maneuver. There are two basic types of defibrillator: monophasic and biphasic. As the former are less effective, they are no longer being maketed, but many still remain in use. The DCC shocks delivered by a monophasic machine for defibrillation purposes are of 369 J. Biphasic defibrillators use different energies, with which the medical staff must be familiarized. In case of doubt whether a defibrillator is monophasic or biphasic, and , what the defibrillation energy is, a 200 J shock should be used, as this value falls within the effective range, whatever device is being used. Synchronized cardioversion is used for monomorphic VT only, as synchronization is not possible in VF and problematic in polymorphic VT, where it may cause degeneration to VF. The algorithm of ressuscitation is reviewed in Table 6.30. The repetition of IV/IO drugs should occur every 3–5 min; in the table, this has been averaged out to 4 min, to better demonstrate the temporal relationship to CPR and DCC. The algorithm differs in rhythms that are shockable (VT, VF) vs. nonshockable (asystole, PEA). The ressuscitation efforts should be continued as clinically warranted, but are generally halted if they fail to produce a pulse within 20–30 min.

Pulseless electrical activity: a misleading designation

Insofar VT, VF, and occasionally SVT with very fast ventricular rates have typical electrical patterns, yet without a pulse, they qualify, literally, for the designation "PEA." However, by convention the latter refers to asystole, agonal rhythm (isolated, bizarre-shaped complexes seen in terminal cases), or occasionally NSR, not generating a pulse. The alternative designation of these rhythms as "nonshockable" is unfortunately not very intuitive either, since the issue is not that DCC *cannot be administered* in these patients, but rather, that DCC *would not be effective*, as it would not influence NSR and would abolish or degenerate other rhythms.

CPR: newer approaches: Recent protocols deemphasize CPR halting for ventilation. By using just two ventilations for every 50 chest compressions, substantial improvement in success rates has been observed. Therapeutic hypothermia has been shown to significantly improve survival and neurological outcomes in unconscious cardiac-arrest survivors.

Bibliography

Guidelines

Epstein AE, DiMarco JP, Ellenbogen KA, et al. ACC/AHA/HRS 2008 guidelines for device-based therapy of cardiac rhythm abnormalities: a report of the American College of Cardiology/American Heart Association Task Force on Practice Guidelines (Writing Committee to Revise the ACC/AHA/NASPE 2002 Guideline Update for Implantation of Cardiac Pacemakers and Antiarrhythmia Devices). *Circulation*. 2008;117:e350-e408.

Zipes DP, Camm AJ, Borggrefe M, et al. ACC/AHA/ESC 2006 guidelines for management of patients with ventricular arrhythmias and the prevention of sudden cardiac death: a report of the American College of Cardiology/American Heart Association Task Force and the European Society of Cardiology Committee for Practice Guidelines (Writing Committee to Develop Guidelines for Management of Patients With Ventricular Arrhythmias and the Prevention of Sudden Cardiac Death). *Circulation*. 2006;114:e385-e484.

Fuster V, Rydén LE, Cannom DS, et al. ACC/AHA/ESC 2006 guidelines for the management of patients with atrial fibrillation: a report of the American College of Cardiology/American Heart Association Task Force on Practice Guidelines and the European Society of Cardiology Committee for Practice Guidelines (Writing Committee to Revise the 2001 Guidelines for the Management of Patients With Atrial Fibrillation). *Circulation*. 2006;114:e257-e354.

The Task Force for Cardiac Pacing and Cardiac Resynchronization Therapy of the European Society of Cardiology. Developed in collaboration with the European Heart Rhythm Association Guidelines for cardiac pacing and cardiac resynchronization therapy. *Eur Heart J*. 2007;28:2256-2295.

The Task Force for the Diagnosis and Management of Syncope of the European Society of Cardiology (ESC). Guidelines for the diagnosis and management of syncope (version 2009). *Eur Heart J*. 2009; doi: 10.1093/eurheartj/ehp298.

The Task Force on the Prevention, Diagnosis and Treatment of Infective Endocarditis of the European Society of Cardiology (ESC). Guidelines on the prevention, diagnosis and treatment of infective endocarditis. *Eur Heart J*. 2009;30:2369-2413.

The Task Force on the Management of Valvular Heart Disease of the European Society of Cardiology. Guidelines on the management of valvular heart disease. *Eur Heart J*. 2007;28:230-268.

Suggested Reading

Wyse DG, Waldo AL, DiMarco JP, et al. Atrial fibrillation fol-low-up investigation of rhythm management (AFFIRM) investigators. A comparison of rate control and rhythm control in patients with atrial fibrillation. *N Engl J Med.* 2002;347(23):1825-1833.

Antunes E, Brugada J, Steurer G, et al. The differential diagnosis of a regular tachycardia with a wide QRS complex on the 12-lead ECG: ventricular tachycardia, supraventricular tachycardia with aberrant intraventricular conduction, and supraventricular tachycardia with anterograde conduction. *Pacing Clin Electrophysiol.* 1994;17(9):1515-1524.

Julian D, Camm A, Frangin G, et al. Randomized trial of effect of amiodarone on mortality in patients with left ventricular dysfunction after recent myocardial infarction: EMIAT. *Lancet.* 1997;349:667-674.

Hein JJ, Wellens MD. Contemporary management of atrial flutter. *Circulation.* 2002;106:649.

Hohnloser SH, Crijns HJGM, van Eickels M, et al. Effect of dronedarone on cardiovascular events in atrial fibrillation. *N Engl J Med.* 2009;360:668-678.

Garza AG, Gratton MS, Salomone JA, et al. Improved patient survival using a modified resuscitation protocol for out-of-hospital cardiac arrest. *Circulation.* 2009;119(19):2597-2605.

Moss AJ, Hall WJ, Cannom DS, Daubert JP, et al. Improved survival with an implanted defibrillator in patients with coronary disease at high risk for ventricular arrhythmia. *N Engl J Med.* 1996;335:1933-1940.

Moss AJ, Zareba W, Hall WJ. Prophylactic implantation of a defibrillator in patients with myocardial infarction and reduced ejection fraction. *N Engl J Med.* 2002;346:877-883.

The Antiarrhythmics Versus Implantable Defibrillators (AVID) Investigators. A comparison of antiarrhythmic-drug therapy with implantable defibrillators in patients resuscitated from near-fatal ventricular arrhythmias. *N Engl J Med.* 1997; 337(22):1576-1583.

Priori SG, Aliot E, Blømstrom-Lundqvist C, et al. Task force on sudden cardiac death. European Society of Cardiology. *Europace.* 2002;4(1):3-18.

The Atrial Fibrillation Follow-up Investigation of Rhythm Management (AFFIRM) Investigators. A comparison of rate control and rhythm control in patients with atrial fibrillation. *N Engl J Med.* 2002;347(23):1825-1833.

Oral H, Knight BP, Tada H, et al. Pulmonary vein isolation for paroxysmal and persistent atrial fibrillation. *Circulation.* 2002;105(9):1077-1081.

Connolly SJ, Ezekowitz MD, Yusuf S, et al. Dabigatran versus warfarin in patients with atrial fibrillation. *N Engl J Med.* 2009;361:1139-1151.

Holmes DR, Reddy VY, Turi ZG, et al. Percutaneous closure of the left atrial appendage versus warfarin therapy for prevention of stroke in patients with atrial fibrillation: a randomised non-inferiority trial. *Lancet.* 2009;374:534-542.

Pericardial Disease

7

Contents

7.1 Background

The pericardium is a double leaflet wrapped around most of the heart, excepting the LA. The very fine inner layer (epicardium) adheres to the myocardium; the outer layer is thicker, fibrous, and relatively nondistensible. As there is continuity between the two layers, the pericardium is also called "the pericardial sac," containing up to 50 mL of clear fluid. The pericardium *prevents excessive cardiac dilatation* (which would affect ventricular filling, and, indirectly, systolic function); *helps RA filling*, as the "negative" (<1 atmosphere) pericardial pressure suctions blood from the great veins (the extra-pericardic LA does not benefit from this mechanism); *protects the heart* from extension of neighboring infection or malignancy; and *prevents excessive respiratory cardiac motion* in the thorax. The pericardium is not essential to life; indeed, its absence (congenital or iatrogenic) does not have a clear pathophysiologic impact.

7.2 Pericardial Disease

Pericardial disease can cause pain and hemodynamic disturbances due to effusion and/or constriction. *Primary pericardial disease* includes congenital defects; pericarditis; and primary tumor. *Secondary disease* mainly consists in pericardial involvement in systemic conditions (heart failure, hyboalbuminemia, etc.) and in traumatic lesions (occasionally iatrogenic).

G.A. Adelmann, *Cardiology Essentials in Clinical Practice*,
DOI: 10.1007/978-1-84996-305-3_7, © Springer-Verlag London Limited 2011

7.2.1 Congenital Anomalies and Normal Variants

7.2.1.1 Congenital Absence of the Pericardium

Congenital absence of the pericardium is relatively rare, and is more frequent in males. The pericardium may be absent partially (occasionally, only in a very small area), or in its entirety. Most frequently, the absence involves a segment of the pericardium over the LV. The portion of the malformed pericardium can occasionally be found as cysts in the pericardial sac. Congenital absence of the pericardium can be isolated, or associated to other CHD. Patients can be asymptomatic or complain of chest pain, occasionally severe (the mechanism is incompletely understood). Generally, no treatment is required, although rarely the LA appendage can herniate through a small pericardial defect, requiring surgery to either enlarge the defect (preventing strangulation), or to repair (suture) it, often with resection of the LAA. These procedures are also performed in case of relentless chest pain, or even in asymptomatic patients, at the time of other cardiac surgery the patient may require. Pericardial absence and LAA herniation are best diagnosed by MRI.

7.2.1.2 Pericardial Cysts

Pericardial cysts are fluid-filled structures in the pericardial sac, resulting from lack of fusion of the embryological "mesenchymal lacunae." They are diagnosed by contrast CT, MRI, or echo. The clinical picture is nonspecific, including atypical chest pain, dyspnea, cough, and occasionally, compression of the right main bronchus; the latter is a surgical emergency, as it may cause atelectasis of an entire lung. Pericardial cyst may hemorrhage and rupture, causing tamponade by rapid discharge of the content into the pericardial sac. Rarely, a cyst can disappear spontaneously, probably by rupture into the pleural space. The management of small cysts is conservative, while larger cysts can be aspired (by a technique similar to pericardiocentesis), or surgically excised.

7.2.1.3 The Epicardial Fat Pad

The epicardial fat pad is a benign fatty collection on the surface of the epicardium, the internal pericardial layer.

By echo, fat may be mistaken for pericardial effusion, as the echodensities are similar. However, typical effusion is first evident behind the posterior LV wall, while a fat pad is situated anterior to the RV wall. Unless it is loculated, true anterior pericardial effusion usually associates a posterior component as well (behind the LV posterior wall). In case of doubt, CT or MRI are indicated.

7.2.2 Pericardial Effusion

As most cases of pericardial effusion are caused by pericarditis, in clinical practice the etiologies, diagnostic measures, and therapies discussed below are supplemented or replaced by those corresponding to pericardial inflammation. However, as not all effusions signify pericarditis, pericardial effusion is discussed separately, in the present section.

7.2.2.1 Etiology

Pericardial effusion can be inflammatory (pericarditis) or noninflammatory, associated to virtually any type of pericardial involvement.

Inflammatory Effusion

See Sect. 7.2.3.

Noninflammatory Effusion

The main etiologies include: *hypoalbuminemia* (hepatic disorders, nephrotic syndrome, etc.), causing passive plasma filtration; *bleeding (hemopericardium),* in some post-MI patients; in aortic dissection progressing to the pericardium; and in hypocoagulability states (primary or iatrogenic); *lymph accumulation (chylopericardium),* in lymph drainage disturbances due to trauma, tumor, and after radiotherapy (lymph duct fibrosis); *hypothyroidism,* generally severe; the occasionally massive exudate accumulates slowly, and tamponade is relatively rare. *Pericardial effusion associated to malignancy* can be an exudate, a transudate, or hemorrhagic. Constrictive pericarditis (CP) can occasionally evolve. Of note, in up to two-thirds of patients with documented malignancy and a pericardial effusion, the latter is *not* malignant (infective, postradiation pericarditis, etc.). *Drug- and toxin-associated effusion:* in addition to the cases of iatrogenic *pericarditis* (Sect. 7.2.3), pericardial *effusion* can also be caused by Cyclosporine, penicillin, antithrombotic and anticoagulant agents, as well as by blood products, antisera, vaccines, animal venom, etc.; *pericardial effusion associated to pregnancy:* minimal or small pericardial effusions are common by the third trimester, as are mild ST depressions and T wave changes. These manifestations are usually silent and do not require therapy. Occult constriction may first become evident in pregnancy, due to the implicit "fluid challenge." *Fetal pericardial effusion* >2 mm in depth should raise the possibility of hydrops fetalis or other serious conditions.

7.2.2.2 Diagnosis

Pericardial effusion can be clinically silent or present as pericarditis, pericardial tamponade (PT), or CP. *Imaging tests*: *chest X-ray* may demonstrate a water jug-shaped cardiac shadow, the body corresponding to the heart, and the neck, to the aorta; *Echocardiography* is the most useful test for detecting pericardial effusion, PT, or CP; occasionally, the cause of the effusion can be detected as well, e.g., myocardial rupture or aortic dissection. Typically, effusion appears as a hypoechoic band behind the LV. A pericardial fat pad can mimic pericardial effusion (see above). Echo can suggest the approximate volume of the effusion; effusions <300 mL are visualized behind the LV, whereas larger effusions are visualized adjacent to both the posterior and the anterior LV wall. This semi-quantitation is important, as PT is *usually* caused by large effusion. Echo can also help decide whether drainage is possible (loculated effusions can be very difficult to reach) and necessary, as in (pre-) PT or very large effusions. The echo signs of PT and CP are discussed in Sects. 7.2.4 and 7.2.5. *CT and MRI* demonstrate atypically located or loculated effusions and allow assessing pericardial thickness and the nature of the effusion. Bloody effusions are radioopaque (just like the myocardium), and contrast material is required for diagnosis (also see Sects. 7.2.4 and 7.2.5). *Analysis of the effusion fluid* is essential if bacterial or neoplastic pericarditis are suspected. Fluid samples are sent for chemical, bacteriological, cytological, and hematological examination. *Chemical analysis* includes assessment of protein content (<3 g/L, and/or a fluid/serum ratio <0.5 with transudates);

LDH levels (<200, with a serum/fluid ratio <0.6, with transudates); glucose levels (levels significantly lower than in the serum are typical of rheumatoid arthritis-related effusion); and tumor markers. The distinction between exudates and transudates is very important, as pericarditis, the most frequent cause of pericardial effusion, causes accumulation of exudate. *Bacteriological tests* (pericardial fluid culture), may demonstrate infection with common bacteria (purulent pericarditis) or tuberculosis; the relevant tests are discussed under "pericarditis." *Cytological tests* allow detection of malignant cells. Special colorations allow to differentiate reactive mesothelial cells from adenocarcinoma cells. *Hematological tests* demonstrate lymphocytosis >5,000/mm³, in lymphocytic-autoreactive pericarditis, and the presence of antisarcolemmal antibodies, in antibody-mediated autoreactive pericarditis.

7.2.2.3 Therapy

Therapy (also refer to Table 7.1) of small effusions (<10 mm in diastole) is generally conservative, while drainage is indicated for large effusions (>20 mm in diastole); in case of tamponade; and in case of suspected purulent, tuberculous, or neoplastic effusion. The therapy of intermediate-size effusions is individualized. Pericardiocentesis carries a relative contraindication in patients with coagulopathy or thrombocytopenia (platelets <50,000/mm³). *Pericardiocentesis* is performed *in the cath lab*, under fluoroscopic guidance (subxyphoid approach; a needle is inserted at 30–45°, pointing towards the left shoulder), or *at the bedside*, under echo guidance, to identify the shortest route (usually, from the left anterior axillary line, in the seventh or eighth intercostal space). Complications include LV puncture (with intrapericardial bleeding and possible tamponade), arrhythmia, and infection. Pericardiocentesis must be used conservatively, as effusion is often recurrent. With massive effusions, no more than 1,000 mL should be drained at the initial procedure, to avoid acute RV dilatation. With purulent pericarditis or rapid reaccumulation, a pericardial drain may be left in place, until the drained volume decreases to <25 mL/day. If abundant drainage is still noted after a few days, surgery is indicated (see below). For massive, recurrent pericardial effusion, a pericardial window can be created under echo guidance (*percutaneous balloon pericardiotomy*); *Pericardial sclerotherapy* uses instillation of corticosteroids, Tetracycline, or

treatment is of indeterminate duration. Other coexisting indications for anticoagulation (e.g., a prosthetic valve) may supersede, in regard of the target INR, the requirements posed by the thrombus per se. Thus, the target range is 2.5–4.0 for patients with highly thrombogenic prosthetic valves (Chap. 5), for patients at risk of thromboembolism when INR is already 2.0–3.0, and in some patients with antiphospholipid antibody syndrome. Warfarin is usually initiated at 5 mg/day, but lower doses should be considered in the elderly (age >70), the malnourished (wt <45 kg), as well as in the presence of liver disorder or previously documented increased sensitivity to Warfarin. Initially, INR should be measured every 1–3 days (initially daily if on therapeutic heparin) until target INR is obtained twice consecutively. Subsequently, INR is measured every 1–4 weeks. A return to monitoring 2–3 times a week is recommended with intercurrent illnesses or a change in medication or diet. INR is measured in the morning to allow dosage adjustment the same evening, should the need arise.

8.5 Rheumatoid Nodules

Rheumatoid nodules are local firm tissue lumps, almost exclusively associated with rheumatoid arthritis. "Rheumatoid nodulosis" is the very rare occurrence of multiple rheumatoid nodules, in the absence of arthritis. Rheumatic nodules are usually subcutaneous, situated especially over bony prominences, but may involve the internal organs, including the heart. Cardiac rheumatic nodules may be asymptomatic or cause blood flow obstruction, arrhythmia, block, embolism, etc.

8.6 Infective Endocarditis

8.6.1 Definition and Etiology

Infective Endocarditis (IE) is an infection of the heart valves, large intrathoracic vessels, intracardiac foreign bodies (prosthetic valves, vascular or intracardiac conduits or patches, etc.), or other structures, such as the interventricular septum, the chordae tendinae, or the mural endocardium. Blood clots (nonbacterial thrombotic endocarditis) form on the surface of damaged cardiac structures (typically, valves) or of non-

endothelialized intracardiac devices. When exposed to otherwise innocuous bacteremia, these thrombi serve as a culture medium, perpetuating the infective process. The typical lesion of IE is called a *vegetation,* a variably mobile structure consisting of a fibrin scaffolding supporting platelets, microorganisms, and inflammatory cells. Vegetations are not vascularized, and thus the antibiotic therapy must be intravenous and prolonged (several weeks). Other endocarditis-related lesions include valve destruction, endocardial ulceration, and abscess. The most common causative pathogens are reviewed in Table 8.1.

There are several modalities of IE *classification: culture-positive vs. culture-negative; left- vs. right-sided* (the latter, in intravenous drug abusers, and mainly caused by *Staphylococcus aureus*); *nosocomial* (most commonly, *S. aureus*, introduced by way of IV lines) *vs. community-acquired* (most commonly, *Streptococcus viridans*); *native vs. prosthetic valve* IE (in turn, early, i.e., <2 months after surgery, and most often caused by contamination at the time of surgery, or late, >2 months postoperatively, most commonly community-acquired).

Culture-negative endocarditis: scenarios

There are several settings in which bacterial cultures can be sterile in a patient with other evidence of endocarditis. These settings include:

- Nonbacterial (e.g., marantic) IE
- IE with "fastidious" germs, such as *Aspergillus, Brucella, Coxiella burnetii, Chlamydia,* and *HACEK* bacteria; in classical (nonautomated) culture systems, these pathogens have demanding requirements for growth (special media, >6 days incubation time)
- Previous antibiotic treatment, with partial inhibition of germ growth
- False echo diagnosis of vegetation (i.e., Lambl's excrescences)

8.6.2 IE Diagnosis

The clinical suspicion of IE mainly arises in the context of unexplained fever, especially in a patient with predisposing cardiac conditions. Suspicion is particularly high in case of a recent history of medical procedures penetrating the body mucosas (see under "prophylaxis,"

Table 8.1 IE pathogens in different clinical settings

Microorganism	Setting	The treatment[a] must include
α-Hemolytic streptococci	Bacteremia associated to a dental procedure	Gentamicin + Penicillin or + Vancomycin (if allergic to Penicillin) or + Ceftriaxone
HACEK organisms[b]	A frequent cause of "culture-negative" IE[e]	Gentamicin + Amoxicillin or + Ceftriaxone (if allergic to Penicillin)
S. aureus	Percutaneous access of bacteria (iatrogenic, traumatic, or in drug abusers)	Native valves: Gentamycin + Oxacillin (MSSA) or + Vancomycin (MRSA or allergy to Penicillin), or Vancomycin alone; prosthetic valves: add Rifampicin
Enterococcus	Gastrointestinal or urinary tract-associated bacteremia	Gentamicin + Penicillin or + Vancomycin; in case of resistance, early valve replacement should be considered
Pseudomonas	Street drugs contaminated with drinking water; skin punctures (e.g., while walking barefoot in contaminated water)	On a case-by-case basis; culture-directed treatment essential (resistance to multiple antibiotics common). Effective antibiotic classes: aminoglycosides; some quinolones; some cephalosporins; ureido- and carboxypen-icillins; some carbapenems; polymyxins; monobactams
S. bovis[d]	Colon malignancy (colonoscopy recommended)	Penicillin or Vancomycin
Candida albicans	Immunocompromised patients	Amphotericin B
Viruses	Acute myocarditis	On a case-by-case basis[e]

[a]The actual dosages and duration depend on factors such as the degree of susceptibility to antibiotics (quantitated as minimal inhibitory concentration, MIC); allergies; whether the valve is native or prosthetic; and whether there was resistance to initial therapy
[b]Hemophilus (parainfluenzae, aphrophilus, and paraphrophilus); Actinobacillus actinomycetemcomitans; Cardiobacterium hominis; Eikenella corrodens; Kingella; these may also be seen with IV drug abusers who contaminate their needles with saliva
[c]The existence of viral endocarditis is disputed
[d]Alongside Clostridium septicum
[e]Alongside Propionella, Neisseria, Brucella, Abiotrophia, or Campylobacter

below). Additionally, IE is an uncommon, but important cause of "fever of unknown origin" (FUO). Predisposing cardiac conditions include degenerative, congenital, rheumatic, or congenital heart disease (e.g., VSD or PDA), or the presence of prosthetic devices. Disease involving native cardiac structures causes endothelial trauma due to the high velocity of blood flow through the abnormal passages, while cardiac prostheses are a good substrate for bacterial growth due to the lack of natural defenses and to the intrinsically thrombogenic nature of the implanted materials. *The clinical manifestations* of IE are reviewed under "minor criteria," below. IE may also present as new-onset rhythm or conduction disturbances, new-onset or aggravation of preexisting HF. In case of high suspicion of IE, blood cultures and an echocardiogram should be obtained immediately. At least three *blood cultures* (1 culture = 1 bottle for aerobic, and 1 for anerobic organisms, each filled with at least 5, ideally 10 mL of blood in adult patients) should be taken over 24 h. If the patient's condition does not allow this delay, the cultures must be spaced at least an hour apart. In patients under short-term or long-term antibiotics, 3 and 6 days, respectively, of washout are ideal before culture harvesting. These waiting periods are often impractical, and empiric antibiotic therapy is started after briefer waiting periods. *Serology* is useful for the diagnosis of microorganisms such as Bartonella, Legionella, Chlamydia, and *Coxiella burnetii*. PCR analysis is useful in the initial diagnosis of IE, especially for the identification of difficult-to-culture organisms. Positive PCR in an antibiotic-treated patient must be interpreted with caution, since the identified DNA material may simply reflect the presence of dead bacteria. The *echo findings* are described under "major criteria," below. A number of normal or pathologic structures may be mistaken for vegetations. These include: *ruptured chordae tendineae* (or chordae that were severed at mitral valve replacement); *myxomatous degeneration* of heart valves; *Lambl's excrescences; the eustachian valve; the Chiari network;* or *fibrin strands* on prosthetic valves, thrombi, tumors, sutures, etc. These structures are discussed in Sect. 8.1. Generally, transthoracic echocardiography is the initial procedure of choice. TEE is indicated if the TTE images are of suboptimal quality; in patients with intracardiac or intravascular prosthetic material; if TTE does not demonstrate vegetations, in a patient with a strong suspicion for IE, including cases of otherwise unexplained AVB, in a suggestive clinical context (intramyocardial abscess possible). In many medical centers in the Western world, TEE is obtained even in the absence of these indications, to avoid missing or underassessing IE lesions. Figure 8.1 shows two cases of IE, one on a prosthetic valve and one on a native bicuspid aortic valve.

The echo, bacteriological, and clinical data are evaluated globally, using the *Duke criteria*. The diagnosis of IE is made in the presence of two major criteria, or one major and three minor criteria, or five minor criteria.

Major criteria:

- **Blood culture**: (harvested as reviewed above): Obtaining from ≥2 separate blood cultures one of the following: viridans-group streptococci, *S. bovis*, or HACEK organisms; *or* community-acquired *S. aureus* or enterococci, in the absence of a primary focus; *or* other microorganisms typical for IE, obtained from two cultures drawn >12 h apart, or

from three out of three or four separate cultures (with first and last sample drawn 1 h apart)

- **Echo criteria**: oscillating intracardiac mass on valve or supporting structures, in the path of regurgitant jets, or on implanted material, in the absence of an alternative anatomic explanation, *or* abscess, *or* a new partial dehiscence of prosthetic valve or new valvular regurgitation (worsening or change of preexisting regurgitation is usually not sufficient, since it may simply represent the natural evolution of that lesion)

Minor criteria:

- Predisposing factors: known cardiac lesion, IV drug abuse
- Fever >38°C
- Vascular phenomena: major arterial emboli (including pulmonary embolism, manifesting as infiltrates of changing location and size), mycotic aneurysm, intracranial hemorrhage, conjunctival hemorrhages, Janeway lesions (see below), Roth's spots (retinal hemorrhages with white or pale centers, seen on fundoscopy), or conjunctival hemorrhages
- Immunological problems: glomerulonephritis, Janeway lesions (vasculitis manifesting as small, nontender, erythematous, hemorrhagic, or nodular lesions

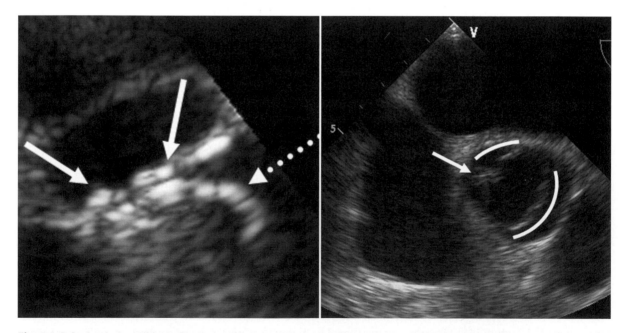

Fig. 8.1 Infective endocarditis. *Left panel:* a large vegetation (*dotted arrow*) on a prosthetic valve (*full arrows*). *Right panel:* a small vegetation (*small arrow*) on a bicuspid aortic valve (*leaflets delineated by curved lines*)

on the palms or soles, with a diameter of a few millimeters), Osler's nodes (similar to the Janeway lesions, but tender)

- Positive blood culture (not meeting a major criterion)
- Positive echocardiogram (not meeting a major criterion)

The significance of IE vegetations: a matter of clinical context

Not all vegetations require antibiotic therapy, as

- Some "chronic" vegetations, generated in a former IE episode, are inactive bacteriologically.
- Patients with rheumatic fever, hypercoagulability, malignancy, or trauma (including that of indwelling catheters) may display nonbacterial thrombotic endocarditis (NBTE). The vegetations have a warty appearance and contain fibrin and thrombocytes, but not microorganisms or inflammatory cells.
- Patients with SLE may present small fibrin strands, interspersed with inflammatory cells, typically seated on the mitral valve, on both the atrial and the ventricular aspect of the valve. This is termed "Libman-Sacks endocarditis" and rarely causes significant valvular dysfunction or embolic phenomena. As SLE may cause fever and other manifestations mimicking IE, the differential diagnosis is very important

---

8.6.3 Therapy of IE

IE prophylaxis has been, for many decades, one of the points of great emphasis in patients with valvular or congenital heart disease, where the presence of nontrivial lesions was. An indication for antibiotic prophylaxis before invasive procedures. Older guidelines for IE management mention these indications in careful detail. However, in-depth analysis of the available evidence has prompted introduction of a simplified, much restricted set of recommendations; in light of the time-honored prophylaxis policy, these changes are nothing short of revolutionary. The changes were predicated on the very low incidence of procedure-related IE (most cases of IE being related to random everyday bacteremia following tooth brushing, bowel movements, etc.), with the risk/benefit ratio of antibiotic therapy no longer justifying the former indications. The indication restrictions concern both the type of procedures and the underlying heart diseases warranting IE prophylaxis. *Procedure-wise,* routine prophylaxis now only addresses (a) *dental procedures* involving manipulation of either gingival tissue or the periapical region of the teeth, or perforation of the oral mucosa (thus, importantly, procedures related to orthodontic appliances do not require prophylaxis) and (b) *procedures on the respiratory tract* involving mucosal incision, such as tonsillectomy. Of note, patients undergoing procedures on infected organs (i.e., for cystitis) often receive antibiotics anyway, but not for the specific purpose of IE prophylaxis. *Underlying condition-wise,* prophylaxis is indicated in patients with prosthetic cardiac valves or prosthetic material used for cardiac valve repair; previous infective endocarditis; unrepaired cyanotic CHD, including palliative shunts and conduits; during the first 6 months post-CHD repair (regardless of the technique, surgical or percutaneous), if patches or prosthetic devices were used; indefinitely post-CHD repair, if there are residual defects at the site of, or adjacent to a prosthetic implant, as these inhibit endothelialization; and in patients after cardiac transplant. While overall embracing the new "conservative" policies in regard to IE prophylaxis, The British Society for Antimicrobial Chemotherapy does continue to recommend prophylaxis for high-risk patients before GI or GU procedures associated with bacteremia. In suitable patients, antibiotics are administered 30–60 min before the procedure, as detailed in Table 8.2.

Pharmacological therapy: patients with IE should be hospitalized for a minimum of 2 weeks; logistics and compliance permitting, uncomplicated patients are then candidates for early discharge and home treatment. The antibiotic treatment for IE caused by the different pathogens is reviewed in Table 8.3.

Therapy for HACEK organisms includes: Ceftriaxone 2 g/24 h IV/IM in 1 dose (may be substituted with Cefotaxime or another third- or fourth-generation cephalosporin) *or* Ampicillin–sulbactam 12 g/24 h IV in 4 doses *or* Ciprofloxacin 1,000 mg/24 h PO or 800 mg/24 h IV in 2 doses, any of these for 4 weeks. Fluoroquinolone therapy is recommended only if cephalosporin and Ampicillin are not tolerated. Ciprofloxacin may be replaced by Levofloxacin, Gatifloxacin, or Moxifloxacin; in case of PVE, the flouroquinolone treatment is of 6 weeks duration.

Surgical therapy is indicated in patients with *HF due to AI or MR; persistent fever and bacteremia* ≥8 days after starting adequate antimicrobial therapy; *local uncontrolled infection,* including abscess, pseudoaneurysm, valve rupture, conduction disturbances, or myocarditis; *microorganisms notoriously resistant* to antibiotics, such as fungi, Brucella, and

Table 8.2 IE prophylaxis

Agent	Indication	Dosage	Remarks
Ampicillin	Default	2 g in adults, 50 mg/kg in children	PO default; IM or IV possible, if unable to take medication PO
Clindamycin	Allergic to Penicillin	600 mg in adults, 20 mg/kg in children	As above
Cephalosporins	Allergic to penicillin and/or unable to take medication PO	Cefazolin or Ceftriaxone IM or IV 1 g in adults or 50 mg/kg in children; Cephalexin PO 2 g in adults or 50 mg/kg in children	
Macrolides		Azithromycin or Clarithromycin 500 g in adults or 15 mg/kg in children	

Table 8.3 Antibiotic regimens in SBE[a]

	Penicillin (for 4 weeks)	Oxacillin (8–12 g/24 h, in 3–4 doses), weeks	Vancomycin (30 mh/kg/24 h in 2 doses), weeks	Gentamicin (3 mg/kg/24 h, in 2–3 doses, maximum 240 mg/24 h), weeks	Rifampicin (900 mg/24 h, in 3 doses)
Streptococcus					
NVE[b], full susceptibility to Penicillin	12–20 m.u.[c] in 4–6 doses[d]			2	
Allergy to penicillin			4		
Lower susceptibility to Penicillin or PVE[e]	20–24 m.u., 4–6 doses[f,g]			2[g]	
			4		
Resistance to Penicillin	As for enterococci				
Enterococcus					
Sensitive to Penicillin[h]	16–20 m.u. in 4–6 doses			4	
Resistant or allergic to Penicillin			6[i]	6	
Staphylococcus					
NVE, MSSA[j], no allergy to Penicillin		≥4		First 3–5 days	
NVE, MSSA, allergy to Penicillin			4–6	First 3–5 days	
NVE, MRSA[k]			6		

Table 8.3 (continued)

	Penicillin (for 4 weeks)	Oxacillin (8–12 g/24 h, in 3–4 doses), weeks	Vancomycin (30 mh/kg/24 h in 2 doses), weeks	Gentamicin (3 mg/kg/24 h, in 2–3 doses, maximum 240 mg/24 h), weeks	Rifampicin (900 mg/24 h, in 3 doses)
PVE, MSSA		6–8		First 2	6–8
PVE, MRSA, CONS[l]			6	6–8	6–8
CNE[m] or urgent empirical therapy					
NVE[n]			4–6	2[o]	
PVE[p]			4–6	2[o]	4–6[q]

[a]Additional therapies are discussed in the text
[b]Native valve endocarditis
[c]Million units
[d]In uncomplicated, responsive cases, may restrict therapy to 2 weeks, without adding Gentamicin, and with ambulatory therapy for the second week; in patients ≥65 or in case of diminished CCT, adjust Penicillin to renal function; in patients allergic to Penicillin, may replace this drug with Ceftriaxone, 2 g/24 h, q.d., for 4 weeks
[e]Prosthetic valve endocarditis
[f]May replace with Ceftriaxone, 2 g/24 h q.d. for 4 weeks
[g]This treatment is followed by Ceftriaxone 2 g/24 h for 2 weeks, whether Penicillin or Ceftriaxone were used in the first part of the treatment
[h]Penicillin MIC ≤8 mg/L, Gentamicin MIC <500 mg/L
[i]In case of resistence to Vancomycin, expert microbiological consult is mandatory, and early valve replacement should be considered. In case of infection with *Enterococcus faecium*, the recommended therapy includes Linezolid 1,200 mg/24 h IV/PO in 2 doses, for ≥8 weeks; *or* Quinupristin–Dalfopristin 22.5 mg/kg/24 h IV in 3 doses ≥8 weeks (This therapy may cause severe myalgia); in case of IE caused by *E faecalis*, the recommended agent is Imipenem/Cilastatin 2 g/24 h IV in four equally divided doses, for ≥8 weeks *plus* Ampicillin 12 g/24 h IV in six equally divided doses ≥8, *or* Ceftriaxone sodium 2 g/24 h IV/IM in 1 dose ≥8 *plus* Ampicillin 12 g/24 h IV in six equally divided doses ≥8weeks
[j]Methicillin-sensitive *S. aureus*
[k]Methicillin-resistant *S. aureus*
[l]Coagulase-negative *S. aureus*
[m]Culture-negative endocarditis
[n]The AHA guidelines recommend adding Ciprofloxacin 1,000 mg/24 h PO or 800 mg/24 h IV in 2 doses and maintaining the Gentamicin therapy for 4–6 weeks. An alternative therapy is with Ampicillin-Sulbactam 12 g/24 h IV in 4 doses *plus* Gentamicin sulfate 3 mg/kg per 24 h IV/IM in three doses, both for 4–6 weeks
[o]This dosage is more precisely calculated as 1.0 mg/kg q8 h
[p]The AHA guidelines recommend adding Cefepime 6 g/24 h IV in three doses
[q]Alternative dose: 450 mg q8 h

Coxiella species, or germs such as *Staphylococcus lugdunensis*, with a strong potential for rapid *destruction* of the cardiac structures; *for MV vegetations* >10 mm, or if they are increasing in size despite antibiotic therapy; or for mitral "kissing" vegetations; *for prosthetic valve endocarditis,* either early (<12 months after surgery) or late, if complicated by serious dysfunction or local uncontrolled infection (see above). Large vegetations, especially if caused by Staphylococcus, should also prompt early surgery. After surgery, a full antibiotic course is mandatory.

8.6.4 IE in Intravenous Drug Abusers

Due to the transcutaneous IV injection of the abused substance, *S. aureus* (most frequently, MRSA) is the most common offender, and the most frequently affected valve (>70% of cases) is the TV (Table 8.3). In Pentazocine addicts, an antipseudomonas agent is required, and if the patient uses brown sugar dissolved in lemon juice, an antifungal must be added (risk of Candida infection); finally, in IVDA with underlying VHD and/or left-sided involvement, treatment against streptococci and enterococci is required.

Bibliography

Guidelines

Nishimura RA, Carabello BA, Faxon DP, et al. ACC/AHA 2008 guideline update on valvular heart disease: focused update on infective endocarditis: a report of the American College of Cardiology/American Heart Association Task Force on Practice Guidelines. *Circulation*. 2008;118:887-896.

Suggested Reading

Lam KY, Dickens P, Chan AC. Tumors of the heart: a 20-year experience with a review of 12,485 consecutive autopsies. *Arch Pathol Lab Med*. 1993;117:1027-1031.

Centofanti P, Di Rosa E, Deorsola L, et al. Primary cardiac tumors: early and late results of surgical treatment in 91 patients. *Ann Thorac Surg*. 1999;68:1236-1241.

Sun JP, Asher CR, Yang XS, et al. Clinical and echocardiographic characteristics of papillary fibroelastomas: a retrospective and prospective study in 162 patients. *Circulation*. 2001;103:2687-2693.

Klug D, Balde M, Pavin D, et al.; for the PEOPLE Study Group. Risk factors related to infections of implanted pacemakers and cardioverter-defibrillators: results of a large prospective study. *Circulation*. 2007;116(12):1349-1355.

Knosalla C, Weng Y, Yankah AC, et al. Surgical treatment of active infective aortic valve endocarditis with associated periannular abscess – 11 year results. *Eur Heart J*. 2000;21:490-497.

Avierinos J-F, Thuny F, Chalvignac V, et al. Surgical treatment of active aortic endocarditis: homografts are not the cornerstone of outcome. *Ann Thorac Surg*. 2007;84:1935-1942.

Strom BL, Abrutyn E, Berlin JA, et al. Risk factors for infective endocarditis: oral hygiene and nondental exposures. *Circulation*. 2000;102(23):2842-2848.

Mylonakis E, Calderwood SB. Infective endocarditis in adults. *N Engl J Med*. 2001;345(18):1318-1330.

Olaison L, Pettersson G. Current best practices and guidelines indications for surgical intervention in infective endocarditis. *Infect Dis Clin North Am*. 2002;16(2):453-475. xi.

Physical Damage to the Heart

9

Contents

9.1 Cardiac Trauma

Cardiac trauma can be *accidental* (in the vast majority of cases, related to motor vehicle accidents, and also, occasionally, caused by falls, aggression, etc.) or *iatrogenic* (mainly CPR, where there is associated trauma to the ribs, lungs, esophagus, etc.). Iatrogenic aortic dissection (after left catheterization), PT (after right catheterization), MR post-PMV, and coronary dissection or rupture after PCI have all been discussed in the corresponding chapters. The present section is dedicated to a discussion of accidental trauma to the heart.

Clinical manifestations: myocardial trauma may cause *arrhythmia and block* (most frequently, first-degree AVB or BBB). The mechanisms include ischemia, commotio cordis, and inflammation resulting from mediator release (interleukin-6, TNF, prostanoids, etc.) by the myocardial cells. These factors also contribute to the onset of respiratory dysfunction. *Commotio cordis* consists in VF in healthy individuals sustaining cardiac trauma during the hyperexcitable period (just before the onset of the T wave). With timely CPR, the prognosis is good; *LV aneurysm* formation; *ischemic injury,* due to coronary damage; and *myocardial rupture.* Rupture can involve a *free wall* (especially of the RA or RV, located anteriorly under the sternum, causing PT), the cardiac *septum* (causing ASD or VSD); or *a papillary muscle* (causing acute MR or TR).

G.A. Adelmann, *Cardiology Essentials in Clinical Practice,*
DOI: 10.1007/978-1-84996-305-3_9, © Springer-Verlag London Limited 2011

Blunt myocardial trauma: a glossary

- Blunt cardiac injury: any nonpenetrating cardiac trauma
- Myocardial contusion: myocardial bruising, with macro- and microscopic changes relatively similar to those caused by ischemia
- Myocardial concussion: cardiac trauma with microscopic pathologic changes only
- Commotio cordis: VF caused by blunt cardiac trauma

Valvular trauma may cause valve laceration or rupture and acute regurgitation. *Coronary trauma* may cause thrombosis, dissection, or rupture, resulting in ischemia and/or PT. Ischemic necrosis usually occurs in the presence of significant coronary atherosclerosis. *Pericardial trauma* may cause PT. Milder pericardial bleeding or posttraumatic effusion may cause constrictive pericarditis many years later. *Vascular trauma* causes dissection or transection of the aorta, pulmonary vein and arteries, SVC, or IVC, causing hemothorax, PT, and/or PE. Lymph duct lesions may cause chylothorax. Pseudoaneurysm formation may be seen in vascular ruptures, contained by a life-saving clot or the serosa; pseudoaneurysms can subsequently rupture, causing sudden death; *Man-made devices* (pacemakers, clips, conduits used in CHD patients) can become *disrupted or thrombosed. Infective complications* may follow open wounds.

The cardiovascular involvement is only a component (often, not the main one) of major trauma, and a comprehensive and speedy assessment of the incurred damage is of the essence. This often involves *emergency thoracotomy*. Serial *EKG tracings and monitoring* are universally obtained. EKG abnormalities may occasionally result not from the current trauma, but from a preexisting condition responsible for the loss of consciousness that *led to* the trauma (e.g., complete AVB in the victim of a motor vehicle accident). If possible, an imaging test is urgently obtained, usually a *chest X-ray* and an *echocardiogram*, the latter also available in the OR. *Routine lab tests* are obtained as a matter of course; troponin and CK-MB levels are also often increased, but their sensitivity and specificity are low. They are, however, of medico-legal importance, as negative levels may be construed to signify the absence of significant cardiac trauma. The

extent of workup is individually tailored. A *CT* or *MRI* inventory of lesions is highly recommended. Often, the patient is hospitalized for a 24-h observation period, to rule out possible late PT, ischemia, etc.

The management of cardiac trauma is dictated by the incurred damage. Overall, >90% of cases do not require surgery for *any* reason, and a minority of those that do, do so for cardiovascular reasons, mostly for myocardial or vascular rupture. Massive PE requires PCI or surgical intervention, thrombolysis being contraindicated. Trauma-related acute MI may require conservative treatment, as thrombolytics are contraindicated, and antithrombotics must be used cautiously, if at all. Cardiopulmonary bypass is strongly advocated for aortic repair, to decrease the incidence of neurological complications. *The prognosis* of cardiovascular trauma varies widely. After blunt trauma, aortic injuries are the second most frequent cause of death, after head trauma.

9.2 High Altitude

High altitude can affect cardiac function, mainly causing ischemia, by a hypoxemic/hypoxic mechanism, as well as by sympathetic-mediated tachycardia (increased oxygen consumption). Severe manifestations are generally seen at altitudes >3,000–3,500 m, higher than those of most settlements (excepting Peru, Nepal, etc.). Cardiac patients traveling to those areas should minimize physical exercise in the first 3–4 days. Exposure to high altitude may also cause noncardiac complications, such as cerebral edema (possibly fatal), retinal hemorrhage, etc. Due to cabin pressurization, *airplane flights* are equivalent to a climb to 1,500–2,500 m, and thus harmless. However, hypoxia resulting from air recirculation contraindicates flight in unstable angina, in severe HF (NYHA III–IV), in severe arrhythmia (in the absence of ICD), in recent MI (2/6 weeks after uncomplicated/complicated MI), and in recent (2–3 weeks) PCI or CABG. Additionally, just like in healthy individuals, long flights can cause DVT and PE. Hydration and active and passive limb motion are essential.

9.3 Radiation

Radiation may affect *the pericardium*, causing effusion, and occasionally, CP or PT. Radiation-related CP has an especially severe prognosis; *the myocardium*, causing dose-dependent DCM. The risk is minimized by the use of mediastinal radiotherapy and increased by concomitant Adriamycin therapy. The usual therapy is recommended; *the endocardium,* causing valvular stenosis or insufficiency; and the *coronary arteries,* classically causing ostial stenosis of the epicardial arteries, both by fibrosis and endothelial damage, favoring the onset of atherosclerosis. As many mediastinal malignancies occur in the young, this form of coronary stenosis has an earlier onset than that caused by atherosclerosis.

9.4 Electrocution

The heart is the organ most susceptible to electrical injury, which mainly causes arrhythmias (especially VF) and structural damage. In order to trigger VF, the current must reach or exceed the fibrillation threshold. Lowering the body impedance and passing a stronger current through the body increase the chances of reaching the threshold. High temperature, humidity, and a large contact surface between the source and the skin, all reduce the impedance. Longer contact and alternative current also increase the risk of VF. *Structural damage* consists in direct myocardial damage; MI due to vasospasm; or in myocardial contusion caused by CPR, by falling, etc. Echo typically shows global LV hypokinesis, transient or permanent.

9.5 Drowning

Drowning represents a unique set of circumstances leading to cardiac arrest. Immersion in cold water (<21°C, or 70°F) triggers the so-called "diving reflex," a set of energy-saving reactions including *bradycardia* up to 50% from basal HR; *peripheral vasoconstriction,* with rerouting of most of the blood to the brain; and, during deeper dives, *blood shifting* to the thoracic cavity to avoid pulmonary collapse under the high external pressure. This reflex may be in part triggered by hypothermia. Ultimately, there ensues cardiac arrest, which may still be amenable to therapy, generally with the usual dismal results seen in out-of-hospital sudden death. With drowning in very cold water (<10°C, or 50°F), hypothermia itself can cause cardiac

arrest. *Secondary drowning* is a form of potentially fatal noncardiogenic pulmonary edema occurring up to 72 h after an episode of near-drowning.

There has been ample debate surrounding the difference between drowning in fresh vs. salty water. Despite evidence that cardiac arrest intervenes sooner in hypoosmotic fresh water (2–3 min, as opposed to 8–10 min for salty water), there is little practical evidence that these findings have any bearing on real-life (primary) drowning. On the other hand, fresh-water near-drowning does associate a distinctly higher risk of secondary drowning. The suspected mechanism is electrolyte disturbance as a result of hypoosmolality-induced hemolysis.

Good prognostic factors in near-drowning:

- Prompt and professional CPR
- Drowning in cold water (see "hypothermia")
- Upper airway spasm (in 10–15% of patients), preventing water from permeating the lungs
- Drowning in salty water (less risk for secondary drowning)

9.6 Thermic Injury to the Heart

9.6.1 Hypothermia

Hypothermia may be accidental or therapeutic. *Accidental* hypothermia occurs in several stages, according to the degree of decrease in core temperature. It is characterized by vasoconstriction, bradypnea, and bradycardia, although lethal ventricular tachyarrhythmia can be noted as well. Patient reheating under constant monitoring is therapeutic (note the high risk of arrhythmia). Due to the protective decrease in metabolism, spectacular recoveries have been reported, and "no patient is dead until warm (i.e., reheated) and dead." *Therapeutic* hypothermia may be induced by a caval catheter, or noninvasively, using chilled water blankets. The latter approach is useful in case of hyperpyrexia, while the former has been proven useful in patients after stroke or after out-of-hospital cardiac arrest. The method is based on the drastic reductions in brain metabolism under hypothermic conditions, allowing neuronal recovery.

9.6.2 Hyperthermia

Hypothermia is also seen in two main settings: heat stroke and malignant hyperthermia. Temperatures >40°C (104°F) are life-threatening, and temperatures ≥45°C (113°F) are almost universally fatal. Dehydration may cause severe hypotension and compensatory tachycardia/tachypnea. Cooling and hydrating the patient are essential. CPR may be required. *Malignant hyperthermia* is a rare life-threatening condition, triggered by exposure to certain gas anesthetics (typically, the now-obsolete Halothane) and to the neuromuscular blocking agent Succinylcholine, during general anesthesia. The susceptibility to this syndrome is genetically inherited, and relatives of an index patient must be tested before exposure (e.g., the Halothane/Caffeine test, where a muscle biopsy sample is exposed to either agent and shows hypercontractility in susceptible patients). The clinical picture includes a drastic increase in skeletal muscle oxidative metabolism, generating rhabdomyolysis, hypoxemia, hypercarbia, hyperthermia, and ultimately circulatory collapse and death, if not promptly treated. Cardiac involvement includes sinus tachycardia, VT, or VF. The muscle relaxant, Dantrolene sodium, is therapeutic.

9.7 Decompression ("Caisson") Disease

Decompression is a rare cause of MI by air embolism. A detailed discussion is beyond the scope of this text.

Bibliography

Suggested Reading

Meredith JW, Hoth JJ. Thoracic trauma: when and how to intervene. *Surg Clin North Am.* 2007;87(1):95-118, vii.

Karmy-Jones R, Jurkovich GJ. Blunt chest injury. *Curr Probl Surg.* 2004;41:223-380.

Ivatury RR. The injured heart. In: Moore EE, Feliciano DV, Mattox KL, eds. *Trauma.* 5th ed. New York: McGraw-Hill; 2004:555-568.

Banning AP, Pillai R. Non-penetrating cardiac and aortic trauma. *Heart.* 1997;78:226-229.

Congenital Heart Disease

10

Contents

10.1 CHD: General Remarks

10.1.1 Background

CHD is heart disease present at birth, as a result of abnormal intrauterine development. Due to the substantial progress in therapy, the number of patients with CHD surviving to adulthood has increased, and it is estimated that, within the next decade, approximately 1 in 150 young adults will suffer from some form of CHD. The risk of CHD in the offspring of affected patients varies widely (2–50%), the highest risk being seen with Marfan's, Noonan's, and Holt-Oram's syndromes, as well as with HOCM. *Risk factors* for CHD include family history and maternal exposure to environmental factors, including chemical, physical, and infectious agents.

10.1.2 Pathophysiology

The different types of structural and functional changes caused by CHD are illustrated in Table 10.1. As can be noted, the adaptive mechanisms ultimately carry complications of their own. The main pathophysiological events caused by CHD include blood shunting, ventricular remodeling, complications of coexisting mechanical deficiencies of the vessels and heart valves, and arrhythmia.

10.1.2.1 Blood Shunting

Blood shunting occurs according to the pressure gradient between the communicating systems, i.e., the PVR/SVR ratio. The systemic pressures are normally higher than the pulmonary ones, and thus the shunt is usually

Table 10.1 Types and mechanisms of CHD

Type of CHD lesion	Example	Disease mechanism	Adaptive mechanism/complications
Pericardium			
Absence	Partial or total	LAA herniation, with possible necrosis; unrestricted cardiac motion in the thorax	N/A
Defective development	Pericardial cyst	Bronchial compression, with atelectasis; rupture in the pericardial sac, with tamponade	N/A
Myocardium			
Partial or total absence of a cardiac wall	ASD or VSD	Intracardiac shunt: L–R, with biventricular volume overload; R–L, with LV volume overload and hypoxemia	Biventricular hypertrophy and dilatation, with ultimate PAH and biventricular failure; atrial dilatation
Defective development of an entire cardiac chamber	Left heart hypoplasia	RV functions both as the pulmonary and as the systemic ventricle and is volume- and pressure-overloaded	RV remodeling (dilatation, hypertrophy) and ultimate failure; polycythemia, cyanosis, CVA
Congenital arrhythmic foci	ARVC	Lethal arrhythmia	N/A
Anomalies of the specialized myocardium	Congenital AVB	Bradycardia, syncope	Ventricular replacement foci, maintaining an acceptable HR
Valves			
Valve absence	Tricuspid atresia	L–R shunt (ASD); R–L shunt (VSD)	See ASD, VSD above
Defective valve development	Bicuspid AV	Increased wear-and-tear causes stenosis and/or insufficiency	LV remodeling, ultimately failure
Defective valve location	Ebstein's anomaly	TR; R–L shunt; arrhythmia, due to the often associated WPW	RV/LV remodeling, ultimately failure
Congenital vascular stenosis	Aortic coarct. (segmental narrowing)	Increased LV afterload	LV remodeling, ultimately failure
Vessels			
Abnormal communication between the great arteries and heart cavities	TGV (LV/PA and RV/aorta connection)	Pulmonary and systemic circulation function in parallel; oxygenated blood does not reach the tissues, venous blood does not reach the lungs	See VSD, above
Abnormal communication between the great vessels	PDA	L–R shunt	See VSD, above
Abnormal position of an artery	TOF	R–L shunt	See ASD, above

left-to-right (*L–R*). In some cases of severe CHD, L–R shunt enables survival. The setting is usually one in which the RV functions as a systemic ventricle, either because it is connected to the "wrong" great artery (i.e., the aorta, in transposition of the great vessel (TGV)), or because there is no functional LV (hypoplastic left heart syndrome- HLHS). However, in the absence of such severe conditions (i.e., in most cases), there are no physiologic benefits to an L–R shunt. L–R shunt (whether "corrective" of an underlying condition or not) leads to biventricular volume overload (of the RV, due to the shunt, and of the LV, due to the increased pulmonary venous return), ultimately causing biventricular dilatation and hypertrophy, PAH, and shunt reversal. PAH adds a component of RV pressure overload. Severe shunt causes high-output, and ultimately low-output HF. Additionally, L–R shunt is responsible for increased pulmonary perfusion, predisposing affected children to recurrent lung infections. *Right-to-left (R–L)* shunt occurs when PVR > SVR, as a result of pathological changes in the RV itself (RVH, RVOT stenosis), in the PV (severe PS or PI), in the PA trunk or large branches (dysplasia, congenital stenosis), or in the small intrapulmonary branches of the PA. The most frequent underlying cause of R–L shunt is an L R shunt that has led to PAH and shunt reversal (*Eisenmenger's syndrome*). R–L shunt unburdens the pressure-overloaded right chambers into the left chambers and is occasionally obligatory for survival; in fact, with some types of CHD (e.g., tricuspid atresia (TA) with intact IVS), a R–L shunt occasionally needs to be created surgically or percutaneously (Rashkind procedure). However, R–L shunt causes complications of its own, notably LV volume overload and arterial desaturation by polycythemia. In turn, polycythemia causes hyperviscosity, cyanosis, and clubbing. *Hyperviscosity* is responsible for headache, visual disturbances, fatigue, tinnitus, muscle weakness and pain, and poor concentration. Patients are at risk for intravascular thrombosis and CVA. *Clubbing* consists in thickening of the last phalanx of the fingers and toes, caused by peripheral vasodilation (to enhance tissue perfusion). *Cyanosis* is generally seen with SatO$_2$ < 80%, due to R–L shunting or to increased O$_2$ extraction in the tissues (with superimposed HF). Cyanosis is associated to a host of medical problems, including reduced platelet counts; prolonged aPTT and INR (minor bleeding is common, major bleeding is uncommon); iron deficiency, mainly due to excessive use of phlebotomy (iron replacement therapy after phlebotomy is necessary); proteinuria and renal failure; acne (a possible source of bacteremia and endocarditis); and fragile gums (soft toothbrushes are recommended). *Paradoxical embolism*, occasionally septic (causing CVA and cerebral abscess), and *hemoptysis* (due to pulmonary vein congestion) may also occur. Stress and pulmonary infection are risk factors for hemoptysis. Decreases in blood volume (dehydration, infection), blood oxygen-carrying capacity (anemia, high altitude, iron deficiency), or systemic resistance (pregnancy, general anesthesia with consequent vasodilation) are especially hazardous. Of note, cyanotic patients need a minimum of 16 g/L of Hb for acceptable oxygenation.

- The absence of cyanosis only implies the absence of *significant R–L shunt*, not the absence of *significant CHD*. Some of the most lethal types of CHD are acyanotic (e.g., TGV without associated ASD).
- Paradoxical embolism may occur even in the absence of Eisenmenger's syndrome, by short-lived shunt reversal, as with exercise or inadvertent Valsalva maneuver.

10.1.2.2 Ventricular Remodeling and Failure

CHD may be responsible for both volume or pressure overload of one or both ventricles, causing ventricular hypertrophy, dilatation, and ultimately, failure. Some frequent scenarios (implicitly alluded to in the previous section) are reviewed again in Table 10.2, with an accent on their impact on ventricular function.

10.1.2.3 Superposition of Additional Defects, as a Result of the Original CHD

Occasionally, the hemodynamic burden, anatomic characteristics, and/or associated or underlying decreased mechanical properties of the heart and vessel tissues, associated to CHD, may cause additional cardiovascular damage. Thus, VSD may close spontaneously by apposition of the anterior tricuspid leaflet, with ensuing TR, or may be the site of aortic leaflet prolapse, with ensuing AI. Similarly, the ascending aorta or PA may dilate excessively, become aneurysmal, and rupture. Such problems are not infrequent with a bicuspid AV and/or coarctation of the aorta, which are associated with abnormalities of the aortic media. Additional CHD

Table 10.2 Abnormal ventricular hemodynamics in CHD patients

	LV[a]	RV[a]
Pressure overload	AS or coarctation; interrupted aortic arch	PS, PA stenosis, or hypoplasia; chronic pulmonary disease; LV failure; MS; cor triatriatum; supramitral membrane
Volume overload	AI or MR; R–L shunt; L–R shunt	PI or TR; L–R shunt

[a]In TGV, the ventricles, as well as their respective physiological challenges, are inverted

diseases causing medial involvement include single ventricle, truncus arteriosus, TGV, and tetralogy of Fallot (TOF).

10.1.2.4 Arrhythmia

Arrhythmia can be due to atrial dilatation or to ventricular dilatation or hypertrophy, to associated aberrant pathways (WPW in Ebstein's patients), and/or appear as a late complication of surgery. Sinus node dysfunction and SVT are the most frequent arrhythmias, most frequently seen after atrial inversion procedures (Mustard, Senning); Fontan procedure; TOF repair; and ASD closure. Ventricular arrhythmias are most frequent in patients with LVOT obstruction and after TOF repair.

10.1.3 Clinical Picture of CHD

The clinical picture of CHD reflects the defect as such, its complications, as well as, frequently, other associated CHD. The anamnesis is extremely important for the assessment of genetic and environmental risk factors for CHD. The main manifestations related to the *cardiac lesions as such* are auscultatory murmurs, due to turbulent flow through either the abnormal intra- or extracardiac connections, or the volume- and/or pressure-overloaded normal cardiac chambers and valves. Thus, the auscultatory murmur of VSD corresponds to blood flow through the abnormal communication, while that of ASD reflects functional stenosis of the normal PV, subjected to abnormally increased blood flow. Palpatory thrills and/or a systolic uplift of the left hemithorax (an expression of increased RV filling) are occasionally associated to the murmurs. Not all types of CHD associate shunt, e.g., bicuspid AV. The variable clinical picture of these conditions is discussed in the appropriate sections. CHD *complications* reflect the main pathophysiological events, i.e., *abnormal loading conditions*, manifesting as left, right, or biventricular remodeling and dysfunction, in turn causing HF; arrhythmia; and abnormally increased or decreased pulmonary or systemic blood pressure; *blood shunting*, manifesting as *arterial hypoxemia* (in turn responsible for cyanosis and hyperviscosity) and *paradoxical embolism. Arrhythmia and heart block* may cause syncope or sudden death; *In children*, CHD may cause failure to thrive and recurrent pulmonary

infection, due to pulmonary congestion (with L–R shunt).

10.1.4 CHD Workup

Echo is the initial, and frequently, the only required imaging procedure to detect CHD and its complications. Due to the extraordinary complexity of some cases of CHD (especially if they were intervened upon), echocardiography may require supplementation by MRI or CT. Additionally, echo is not ideal for imaging the RV, a chamber of paramount importance in many CHD patients. *MRI and ultrafast or multislice CT* are the procedures of choice with complex CHD. They assess RV volume and mass, the pulmonary arteries, artificial conduits, aortic coarctation, etc.; *Nuclear studies* identify wall motion abnormalities and ischemia. *Chest X-ray* may demonstrate dilatation, and occasionally, a distinctive shape of the cardiac shadow (e.g., "boot-shaped heart" in TOF). PA dilatation and PAH are commonly seen as well. *Right heart catheterization* is occasionally necessary for diagnosing the shunt, by demonstrating an "O_2 step-up" in the receiving chambers, and for assessing the vasoreactivity of PAH (see Chap. 11). Absence of PA pressure decrease under IV vasodilators contraindicates certain therapeutic approaches (e.g., ASD closure; CCB treatment for PAH). In patients with R–L shunt, right heart catheterization may cause paradoxical air embolism. *EKG* may demonstrate ventricular and/or atrial hypertrophy, arrhythmia and heart block, cardiac axis deviation, and, with situs inversus, reversal of the QRS complexes in the chest leads. Certain conditions may associate particular EKG waves (epsilon wave with ARVC, "crochetage" with ASD, etc.). *Electrophysiological studies* are important mainly in conditions such as TOF, Ebstein's anomaly (EA), and patients after the Fontan procedure, especially if there are signs of RV failure. *Cardiac biopsy* may be occasionally helpful (ARVC).

10.1.5 Management

10.1.5.1 Medical Therapy

Medical therapy addresses HF, pulmonary infection, hyperviscosity, and IE prophylaxis. The latter is required with unrepaired cyanotic CHD, including palliative shunts and conduits; completely repaired CHD with prosthetic material or device, regardless of the technique that was used (surgical or percutaneous), during the first 6 months after the procedure (after 6 months, the endothelization is complete, and IE prophylaxis becomes redundant); and with repaired CHD with residual defects at or adjacent to the site of a prosthetic patch or prosthetic device. The procedures requiring prophylaxis are discussed in Chap. 8.

10.1.5.2 Interventional Therapy

Interventional therapy can be carried out percutaneously or surgically and is classified as *corrective* or *palliative*, with *cardiac transplant* an option of last resort. Catheter techniques include dilatation and stenting of stenotic native or artificial conduits (e.g., PV or PA, aortic coarctation, surgical conduits); occlusion of native lesions (ASD, PFO, PDA, AV fistulas) or of leaky surgical conduits; and percutaneous valve replacement (e.g., replacement of the PV in TOF).

Corrective Interventions

Corrective interventions aim to establish a "correct" cardiac anatomy and function. Corrective intervention is not necessarily synonymous with surgery (e.g., PDA coiling is, properly speaking, a corrective intervention); however, more complex cases do require surgery. Some complex types of CHD require a staged approach (sequential surgery), while others (e.g., TA) may not be correctible by current techniques. Of note, corrective surgery occasionally requires extensive use of artificial patches or conduits (e.g., the Jatene procedure, in TGV), and thus does not represent creation of a "normal" heart. The only modality of reaching that goal remains cardiac transplant.

> Corrective surgery addresses both structure *and* function. The capacity for functional recovery after anatomic correction is assessed in advance; otherwise, "cosmetic" correction can be lethal (e.g., closing an ASD at the stage of reversed shunt can cause lethal exacerbations of PAH).

Situations where intra- or extracardiac shunt is essential for patient survival include Eisenmenger's complex and types of CHD that, by its very nature, mandates communication between the two circulations for survival. This latter scenario includes

- *Dependence of the right circulation on the left circulation,* such as in TA (where the RA blood can only reach the RV through the byway of the left-sided chambers).
- *Dependence of the left circulation on the right circulation,* e.g., the HLHS, where the RV functions as both a pulmonary and a systemic ventricle, mandating *two* shunts: an ASD (as the LV, the normal final destination of the LA blood, is absent, the blood must be diverted to the RA/RV), and a second shunt, i.e., a PDA, to return some of the blood to the systemic circulation. While corrective surgery is generally not feasible in Eisenmenger's patients (possibly excepting its initial stages), shunt-dependent complex CHD can occasionally be corrected.

Palliative Interventions

Palliative interventions aim to improve pulmonary and systemic perfusion and the loading conditions of the ventricles, by creating a "compensatory anomaly" to correct at least partly the existing abnormalities (e.g., relieving severe PAH by creating an atrial septal communication – the Rashkind procedure). Palliation may be definitive or temporary (as a bridge to complete correction). Some palliative procedures are, by design, intermediary procedures, used (due to their greater technical ease in small children, or to the temporary physiologic improvement that they bring about) as a bridge to subsequent surgery, itself either palliative or corrective. Conversely, the Fontan operation, also a palliative procedure, is meant "to last as much as possible," which usually means a few decades, until failure of the Fontan physiology (passive pulmonary circulation, in the absence of an RV functioning *in the pulmonary circulation*). At this point, a further refinement of the Fontan procedure ("total cavopulmonary circulation, TCPC") is used to buy additional time, or the patient is referred for cardiac transplant. Provocative recent data have cast doubt over the appropriateness of a "Fontan-first" strategy, as this procedure may significantly lower survival after heart transplantation, when the latter finally becomes indicated.

Palliative interventions carry complications of their own. For instance, the Senning and Mustard procedures may cause, among others, severe arrhythmia (see under "TGV"), and the Fontan procedure may cause atrial enlargement and arrhythmia, increased PVR, AV valve regurgitation, and pulmonary arterio-venous malformations. Additionally, the conduits may become occluded. These complications, in turn, require therapeutic intervention (ablation of arrhythmia, replacement of the failing shunt, etc.) (Table 10.3).

10.1.6 CHD Prognosis

CHD prognosis strongly depends on the type and severity of the lesion, the timeliness of therapy, and the associated malformations. Thus, CHD may cause death in utero, immediately after birth, or in early childhood (e.g., HLHS); become symptomatic in adulthood (e.g., bicuspid AV); or go asymptomatic for the whole of a normal life span (e.g., PFO).

Table 10.3 CHD: palliative interventions

Problem	Context	Solution	Shunt[a]	Terminology
Atrium connected to "wrong" ventricle	TGV	Connecting the atria to the "correct" ventricle by artificial conduits	N/A[b]	Atrial inversion procedures (Mustard, Senning)
RA not draining into RV	Tricuspid atresia	Direct RA/PA connection, with a synthetic conduit[c]	R–R	Fontan procedure[d]
Extreme PAH	Tricuspid atresia with intact atrial septum	Reopening or stretching of the PFO	R–L	Rashkind procedure
Decreased pulmonary circulation	Any ductus-dependent CHD[e] with two functional ventricles	Solution 1: Capitalizing on the fact that the pressure in the cavae is higher than that in the PA, by creating a shunt between the PA and the SVC or the IVC (bypassing the RV)	R–R	Blalock-Taussig or Glenn shunt
		Solution 2: Capitalizing on the fact that the pressure in the aorta is higher than in the PA, (a) by reopening the ductus arteriosus[f], or (b) by creating a subclavian-PA anastomosis	L–R	(a) IV Prostaglandin; (b) another variant of BT shunt
Absence of a functional systemic ventricle	Left heart hypoplasia	(a) Connecting the RV to the aorta, by means of the PA, which is separated from its main branches; (b) connecting the PA to the subclavian artery or to the RV	N/A[g]	(a) Norwood procedure; (b) B-T or Sano shunt
Increased pulmonary circulation	Tricuspid atresia w/o PA hypoplasia	Partial ligature of pulmonary arteries, to increase PVR and reduce R–L shunt	N/A[h]	PA banding
Decreased systemic circulation in inferior body	Aortic coarctation	Establishing a connection between the supra- and infracoarctation segment, with supraductal coarctation,[i] by (re)opening the PDA	R–L	IV Prostaglandin

[a]i.e., the type of shunt upon which the palliative procedure is based
[b]Intervention is not a shunt, but reestablishment of "normal" flow
[c]Contraindicated in PAH
[d]Even in the best-case scenario, the Fontan physiology ultimately fails, usually requiring cardiac transplant
[e]Tricuspid or pulmonary atresia with PA hypoplasia; l-TGV; Ebstein's anomaly; TOF; PA stenosis
[f]With severe aortic coarctation or interrupted aortic arch, the pressure in the postcoarctation segment of the aorta is very decreased; ductus reopening in these children aims at creating a R–L shunt
[g]"Left" is absent
[h]In itself not a shunting procedure, the finality of PA banding is strongly related to the concept of shunting, i.e., it creates PAH that diminishes L–R shunt
[i]With infraductal coarctation, the shunting is spontaneous, by way of the intercostal arteries- a form of L–L shunt

10.1.7 CHD and Pregnancy

Maternal risk: Most patients with CHD can tolerate pregnancy well. However, some conditions are considered high-risk. These include: PAH, without or with shunt (Eisenmenger's syndrome); stenotic lesions in the left heart (severe AS, MS, or aortic coarctation); LV dysfunction (LVEF < 35%); mechanical valve prosthesis (mainly due to the concern of Warfarin contraindication in the first and last trimesters, and to the unproven adequacy of LMWH as a replacement); Marfan's syndrome with aortic root dilatation greater than 40 mm; and cyanotic CHD (SatO$_2$ < 85%). Contraception should be achieved by barrier methods or surgical sterilization, as contraceptive pills carry the risk of thrombosis and paradoxical embolism and IUDs may carry the risk of pelvic inflammatory disease (IE prophylaxis is indicated at insertion). As most CHD evolve with age, giving birth in the third decade of life helps avoid pregnancy-related cardiac complications. *Fetal risk*: *Genetic counseling* is available in specialized units. The highest-risk syndromes are reviewed in the introductory section. Teratogenic drugs should be avoided. The risk of some of the main types of CHD in the offspring of patients is reviewed in Table 10.4. *In utero assessment*: Fetal echo is recommended at 16–18 weeks gestation. Chorionic villous sampling and amniocentesis are indicated in selected cases.

10.1.8 CHD and Physical Activity/Sports

With timely and up-to-date therapy, most types of CHD are compatible with a normal or near-normal lifestyle, including physical activity. Contact sports should be avoided after conduit surgery, as well as in Marfan's disease. Strenuous exercise should be avoided in patients with Marfan's disease and unrepaired aortic coarctation. In most other types of CHD, the indications are strongly individualized, but at least recreational sport is permissible in most patients.

10.1.9 CHD and Flying

Concern has been expressed regarding the possible deleterious effect of commercial flight-induced hypoxia, in cyanotic patients, especially those with Eisenmenger's syndrome. While in severe cases oxygen supplementation may be indicated, it appears that most cyanotic CHD patients tolerate this situation well.

10.2 CHD Syndromes

10.2.1 Introduction

CHD is classified based on presence or absence or cyanosis, which indicates R–L shunt, i.e., an abnormal right/left communication and a pulmonary/systemic resistance >1. (In advanced cases, HF may also contribute to cyanosis.) These patients are at risk for additional noncardiac or cardiac abnormalities (the shunt may represent an adaptive mechanism to, or be one the components of CHD), and for any of the complications discussed in Sect. 10.1. In the following classification, the *primary* direction of shunt is taken into account. Thus, the section relative to L–R shunt includes conditions that may, in the late stages, lead to reversed shunt. Aortic coarctation may present with a "left-to-left" shunt (i.e., intercostal anastomoses), in case of infraductal

Table 10.4 Risk of CHD in offspring of patients

Condition	Risk (%)	Remarks
ASD	3	The risk may be greater if ASD is part of a complex syndrome
VSD	Variable	Higher risk in Down patients
AVSD	Variable	Higher risk in Down patients
PS	4	
TOF	1.5–4	The higher risk is seen if the mother is affected; 50% risk in patients with chromosome 22q11 deletion
Coarctation	Variable	
d-TGV	Rare	
l-TGV	4	
Ebstein's	1–6	The higher percentage refers to affected mothers
Marfan's	50	Autosomal dominant transmission

coarctation, or with right-to-left shunt (supraductal coarctation). As the differential cyanosis (i.e., in the lower limbs only) seen in the latter setting is often mild, there is no justification to include coarctation among the cyanotic conditions, and thus this entity is reviewed under "miscellaneous CHD."

10.2.2 Noncyanotic CHD with a L–R Shunt

10.2.2.1 ASD

ASD can be isolated (occasionally manifesting in adulthood only), or associated to other abnormalities (and generally diagnosed in childhood). It accounts for approximately 1/3 of all adult CHD and is twice or three times as frequent in women as in men. Between one third and one half of complex CHD have an associated ASD. *Classification*: *Septum secundum ASD*, the most frequent type, represents up to 75% of all cases; it is situated in the area of the foramen ovale. Up to 20% of patients associate MV prolapse. Symptoms generally appear in early adulthood` and are those of a L–R shunt, with shunt reversal late in the course of the disease, when AF is also frequently associated. *Sinus venosus ASD* (10%) is situated in the area of the venous inflow, at the confluence of the pulmonary veins with the LA. Partial anomalous pulmonary vein drainage is frequently associated (one or more pulmonary veins drain into the RA instead of the LA), causing arterial blood deoxygenation and increased RA/RV preload. *Septum primum ASD* (15%) is situated in the area of the MV and TV, which are often also involved (cleft MV, single AV valve). Technically an ASD, this condition is usually classified as "AV canal," or (referring to its underlying intrauterine origin), as an "endocardial cushion defect." Down's syndrome is often associated. (*Single atrium*, an extreme form of ASD, where the two atria behave as a single chamber, is a cyanotic condition, and is reviewed in the next section.) The different types of ASD are presented in Fig. 10.1, alongside the different types of VSD.

Pathophysiology: Atrial blood admixture volume-overloads the RV, leading to RV hypertrophy and dilatation, with increased RVEDP and CVP. When the RA pressure (CVP) exceeds LA pressure, the flow direction reverses (R–L shunt). Thus, blood admixture first causes an abnormally high O_2 content in the RA, and

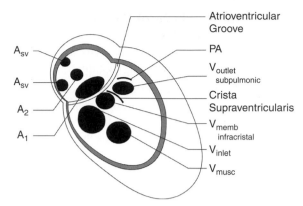

Fig. 10.1 ASD and VSD: A_1, A_2, A_{sv}: septum primum, septum secundum, sinus venosus ASD; *PA* pulmonary artery; V_{memb}: membranous VSD; V_{musc}: muscular VSD. Explanations in the text

later on, an abnormally low O_2 content in the LA. The LV preload is increased by the excess blood volume discharged by the RV into the pulmonary circulation, and thence to the LA. The amount of blood shunted between the two atria depends on the size of the interatrial communication and the LVEDP/RVEDP ratio. Shunt magnitude is expressed by the Qp/Qs ratio, where Qp is the pulmonary blood flow (RV output); Qs is the aortic blood flow (LV output). Normally, the output of the two ventricles is equal (Qp/Qs = 1), but with an intracardiac shunt, the receiving side (in the absence of Eisenmenger's physiology, the right side) handles an excessive volume of blood. With important shunting, Qp/Qs is >1.5–2.5 (i.e., the pulmonary flow is up to 2.5 times higher than the systemic flow).

A low Qp/Qs ratio may signify:

- A very mild problem, i.e., an ASD without hemodynamic significance.
- A very severe problem, i.e., an ASD about to undergo shunt reversal.

Clinical picture: *Symptoms* are mainly those of R–L shunt (Sect. 10.1). ASD is often asymptomatic until the third to fourth decade. *Physical signs*: ASD typically associates a split S_2, due to delayed closure of the PV. (As opposed to healthy subjects, where the aortic valve closes just before the PV, in ASD patients the increased flow through the right heart cavities delays P_2 until well after A_2, hence the split.) Unlike the normal inspiratory S_2 split in children, due to increased venous return in inspiration, the ASD-related split is "fixed," i.e., does not change with respiration. A systolic murmur of functional PS (i.e., disparity between the normal PV opening and the increased blood flow) may be heard over the pulmonic area. AF is often present in adults; sick sinus syndrome is also occasionally noted. Of note, even short-lived shunt reversals, as with exercise, inadvertent Valsalva maneuver, etc., may cause paradoxical embolism.

- With VSD, the typical auscultatory murmur directly reflects flow across the defect.
- With ASD, the auscultatory signs reflect not ASD per se, but the right heart volume overload.

Workup: *Echo* is the diagnostic test of choice, but may miss sinus venosus ASD. Finding an ASD must prompt a search for associated anomalies, occasionally by TEE. Contrast echo can be used (see "PFO"), but in large ASD, contrast is both unnecessary and theoretically hazardous (risk of paradoxical gas embolism); *CT* and *MRI* are occasionally required, in case of suspected associated abnormalities or sinus venosus ASD; *Chest X-ray* may demonstrate RA, RV, and PA dilatation. *Right heart catheterization* demonstrates an "O_2 step-up" between the SVC (normal $SatO_2$) and the RA (abnormally increased $SatO_2$) and assesses PAH and its reversibility under vasodilator therapy. *EKG* may demonstrate: with ostium secundum ASD, IRBBB, and right axis deviation; with ostium primum, left axis deviation and first degree AVB; and with sinus venosus, junctional or low atrial rhythm. RVH and a small positive deflection in V1–V2 ("*crochetage*") may be associated to ASD of any type.

Management: (1) *Medical therapy* involves treatment of HF and atrial arrhythmia, as well as of cyanosis, in patients with reversed shunt; (2) *ASD repair* consists in patching with a piece of synthetic material or pericardial tissue or with a percutaneous device. Repair is *indicated* in defects >10 mm diameter, ideally before first grade, to allow normal adaptation to school. However, even later (age<30) repair generally has good results, provided there is no associated PAH. With complex associated CHD, surgery may be necessary soon after birth. Conservative therapy may be considered in occasional adult asymptomatic patients with an incidentally found small ASD, but many experts advocate defect closure even in this setting, to avoid late RVH and PAH. Repair is *contraindicated* in case of severe irreversible PAH ($PVR > 8$ U/m^2 of body surface, Qp/Qs < 1.5 in the presence of a large defect), as it may precipitate acute RV failure, manifesting as TR and cardiogenic shock. Repair can be carried out surgically or percutaneously. *Surgical repair* is the option of choice for ASDs that are large (stretched diameter >38 mm); close to the MV or TV, and thus not offering sufficient "anchoring" for a percutaneous device; associated to complex CHD, itself requiring surgery; or that occur in children too small for percutaneous device insertion. *Percutaneous repair* uses a "clamshell" device, consisting of two expandable interconnected nitinol disks. The device is introduced transvenously, with expansion of the disks seated on the LA, and then on the RA aspects of the defect. The postintervention evolution is generally good. Physical exercise is restricted only if there is moderate or severe pulmonary vascular disease.

10.2.2.2 PFO

In intrauterine life, the foramen ovale allows blood oxygenation, by routing the venous blood to the left heart and hence to the placenta. At birth, the lungs expand, PVR decreases precipitously, and the foramen seals off. In about 30% of cases, the foramen remains open, allowing minimal L–R shunt, which can be diagnosed by Doppler or B-mode echo (with or without contrast). Normally, the contrast opacifies the RA/RV and appears in the LA only a few beats later (the delay corresponds to the pulmonary circulation); in PFO patients, the LA opacifies soon after the RA, and the abnormal jet can be visualized (Fig. 10.2). While PFO is too small to cause volume overload, it may still cause important complications. Thus, in divers, excessively rapid decompression may cause formation of gas bubbles in the venous blood and paradoxical embolism. Additionally, PFO has been associated to migraine, possibly due to occult episodes of small paradoxical embolism of the brain. While the only available randomized study (the MIST trial) has not found PFO closure helpful in alleviating migraine, this approach may still be warranted in a more rigorously selected patient population (highly symptomatic migraine, moderate-to-large shunts, and neurologic lesions on brain imaging suggestive of an embolic mechanism).

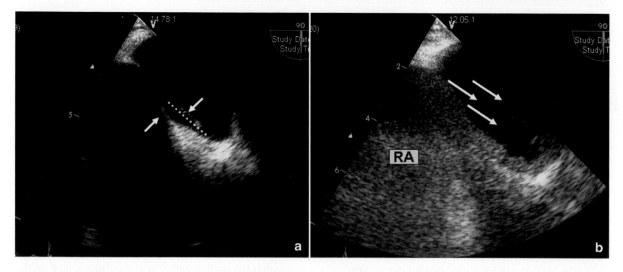

Fig. 10.2 PFO. (**a**) the interatrial communication (*dotted line*) is visible between the two leaflets of the septum primum and the septum secundum (*arrows*); (**b**) contrast study using agitated saline. The air microbubbles opacify the RA and reach the LA, which has a typical "grainy" aspect (*arrows*), by way of a PFO

10.2.2.3 Atrial Septal Aneurysm

Atrial septal aneurysm is a congenital abnormality characterized by bulging and oscillation of atrial septal tissue into either or both atria during the cardiac cycle. Approximately 70% of patients have an associated PFO, placing them at increased risk of cryptogenic stroke.

10.2.2.4 VSD

VSD can be congenital or secondary to MI (Chap. 2). VSD is the most frequent form of CHD, often associated to other cardiac or noncardiac malformations (e.g., Down's syndrome). There are four main types of VSD, with a multitude of synonyms, which only partly convey intuitively the VSD location and its possible impact on valvular function (Table 10.5, Fig. 10.3).

Perimembranous VSD involves the upper part of the IVS. This is the most frequent type of VSD in all age groups, accounting for up to 80% of cases. It may be isolated or associated to other anomalies, such as TOF or PV malformations. Technically a malformation, *interventricular septal aneurysm* is actually a form of spontaneous VSD closure, with what is believed to represent AV valve tissue. Membranous VSD may cause TR, by apposition of a tricuspid leaflet on the septal defect, sealing it off at the cost of severe valvular regurgitation.

Table 10.5 Types of VSD

Designation	Type	Membranous septum inv.	Muscular septum inv.	Location	Valvular problems
Outlet[a]	I	Yes	Occasionally	Just below the PV and the AV	AI
Perimembranous[b]	II	Yes	Yes	Just below the AV	TR
Inlet VSD[c]	III	Yes	Yes	Beneath the septal leaflet of the TV	Single AV valve[d]
Muscular[e]	IV	No	Yes	Muscular septum	N/A

[a]Also termed supracristal, conoseptal, infundibular, subpulmonic, subarterial, subarterial doubly committed, or juxta-arterial
[b]Also termed paramembranous, infracristal, conoventricular, subaortic; subclassified as perimembranous inlet, perimembranous outlet, and perimembranous muscular. These are not to be mistaken for the other classes of VSD, similarly named, but without the qualifier, "perimembranous"
[c]Also termed AV canal
[d]As opposed to the other types of VSD, this is not a complication, but an associated congenital defect
[e]Also termed trabecular

Muscular VSD may be singular and small (of little hemodynamic significance, and closing spontaneously), but occasionally is multiple (with a corresponding cumulative hemodynamic impact); in severe cases, the IVS has a "Swiss cheese" appearance. *Outflow VSD* is situated beneath the AV and PV, occasionally producing AV prolapse and AI. Outflow VSD is more frequent in patients of Asian descent. *Inflow VSD*, a component of the AV septal defect (AVSD) spectrum, is situated close to the AV valves and associates valvular malformations.

VSD pathophysiology: The associated L–R shunt causes increased RV preload, leading to RVH and PAH (the latter, a cause of pressure overload), and increased LV preload, as the shunted blood returns to the LA via the pulmonary veins. The magnitude of shunt depends on the pulmonary and systemic resistances. Hypertrophy of the IVS may increase the resistance to flow in the LVOT or RVOT, influencing the shunt direction and magnitude. A small, restrictive VSD (<5 cm^2), with Qp/Qs <1.5, is termed *maladie de Roger*. Important shunts associate a Qp/Qs >2.

- VSD with an L–R shunt causes biventricular volume overload.
- VSD with a R–L shunt causes LV volume overload and, upon onset of PAH, RV pressure overload.
- RVOT/LVOT hypertrophy may cause RV and/or LV pressure overload, regardless of the direction of shunt.

Clinical picture: *The symptoms* are generally absent with small VSD; with larger VSD, they are those discussed in the introductory section, especially prominent with Eisenmenger's syndrome. *The physical signs* include a split S$_2$ and a continuous murmur spanning both systole and diastole, corresponding to the uninterrupted shunt flow (in the absence of Eisenmenger's, pressure is higher in the LV than in the RV throughout the cardiac cycle). In the absence of Eisenmenger's, the stronger the murmur, the smaller the defect (turbulent flow). The murmur is absent in utero; in the first days after birth, due to high PVR (the murmur appears gradually, paralleling the slow PVR decrease along the first days of extrauterine life); with very large VSDs, when the two ventricles behave as a single chamber; and with increased RVEDP.

Valvular problems associated to VSD

1. Valvular dysfunction caused by VSD:
   - TR, due to RV volume overload or to VSD sealing by tricuspid leaflet apposition
   - AI, due to leaflet prolapse through the VSD
   - MR, due to LV dilatation in the late stages
2. Valvular dysfunction caused by complex CHD that includes VSD.

The workup includes diagnostic imaging and right ventriculography. In addition to demonstrating the VSD and measuring the volume and direction of shunt, catheterization shows O$_2$ step-up in the RV and, with Eisenmenger's, decreased SatO$_2$ in the LV, and directly measures the PA pressure. *EKG* shows LVH and/or RVH, and occasionally, AF.

Natural history: Up to 50% of small VSDs (i.e., with a small shunt not resulting from PAH) and 7% of larger ones may close spontaneously, generally during the first 2 years of life, but occasionally even in adulthood. Spontaneous closure especially involves muscular VSD, but can be seen with membranous VSD as well. Closure is due to myocardial growth, which, in the former case, directly occludes the VSD, and in the latter, "pushes together" the disjunct components of the IVS; the closure is usually incomplete, but sufficient to neutralize any physiological impact of the defect. Spontaneous VSD repair may in turn cause complications, such as severe TR. Large, untreated VSD can lead to PAH and, later on, to Eisenmenger's syndrome.

Management: (1) *General measures* include treatment of HF and of hyperviscosity. IE prophylaxis is indicated in VSD with R–L shunt that was not (or not completely) repaired, as well as in the first 6 months after surgery involving a patch. *VSD closure* is indicated with VSD associating Qp/Qs > 2 in children, and >1.5 in adults. It is generally acceptable to await spontaneous closure until the age of 2 (occasionally, even four, if there are signs of gradual closure), either completely avoiding surgery, or deferring it till the child is more developed. However, in case of PAH, surgery should be carried out before age 2 to avoid the onset of an inoperable R–L shunt. Occasionally, in very young children with severe pulmonary overload, in whom VSD closure cannot to be performed, elastic bands are placed around the pulmonary arteries. This creates reversible PAH, reducing shunt volume. In the second stage (a few years later), the bands are removed and definitive surgery is carried out. This approach is not possible in children with large VSD associating PAH and cyanosis, when surgical repair is indicated as an initial approach. With complex CHD independently requiring surgery, nonmajor VSD may also be closed. VSD closure is *contraindicated* in case of severe irreversible PAH with reversed shunt. Percutaneous closure (with a device similar to that used with ASD) is generally restricted to muscular VSD, as membranous VSD often lacks sufficient tissue around the defect to anchor the device (proper anchoring is not possible on the thin ventricular membrane alone). Surgery may damage the electrical conduction system, which passes close to the area of the defect, and cause AVB.

10.2.2.5 PDA

PDA is one of the most frequent types of CHD. The incidence in the general population is of $1^0/_{00}$ of live births, but it is much more frequent in premature babies and in babies with low weight at birth (<1,500 g) and is twice more frequent in girls. *Pathophysiology*: In utero, the ductus serves to direct most of the pulmonary flow to the aorta, a physiologic R–L shunt driven by the high PA pressure (unexpanded lungs). Accidental intrauterine closure (e.g. in case of maternal ingestion of Indomethacin) can be lethal to the fetus. After birth, physiologic closure of the ductus prevents shunt reversal in face of the very rapid decrease in PVR. Closure usually occurs within the first 15 h of life, but occasionally requires up to 3 months for completion. The fibrotic, closed ductus is known as the *arterial ligament.* Lack of closure beyond age 3 months is termed PDA. The physiological consequences of PDA are the same as with ASD and VSD. *Risk factors* include: *family history* and exposure to *environmental factors*, either chemical (amphetamines, alcohol, Phenytoin, corticosteroids, CCB, chemotherapy, and occasionally, Fluoxetine) or infectious (maternal rubella causes PDA with associated PA stenosis). The *clinical picture* is the same as with isolated ASD or VSD, and some patients are asymptomatic. Auscultation reveals a typical continuous (systolic and diastolic) "machinery" murmur. *Echocardiography* is the main *diagnostic test*, able to visualize PDA and/or the blood flow through it. *Management* includes the same general measures as with

any L–R shunt. *PDA closure* is indicated with significant L–R shunt. Closure can be performed *pharmacologically* (IV Indomethacin or Ibuprofen, which inhibit prostaglandin E, responsible for maintaining the ductus open); *percutaneously* (coiling, to cause ductus thrombosis, and later on, fibrosis. The rare coil migrating into the bloodstream can be retrieved percutaneously or surgically); or *surgically*, usually by ligature and (if the ductus length allows it) division (ductus section between two ligatures). In adults, the ductus is often calcified, posing a risk of rupture at surgery. Therefore, percutaneous closure is the procedure of choice in these patients. Closure is contraindicated in the presence of irreversible PAH or of ductus-dependent CHD, where the ductus makes survival possible (mainly, TA, TGV, HLHS, and severe aortic coarctation).

10.2.2.6 AV Septal Defect (AVSD)

AVSD is a spectrum of entities with a common in utero origin. *Partial AVSD* is synonymous to septum primum ASD, while complete AVSD consists in a primum ASD associating a VSD. Intrauterine echo is diagnostic. Eighty percent of cases associate Down's syndrome, and conversely, approximately 1/3 of Down's patients have AVSD. The clinical signs and the diagnosis are those of the component lesions. Late in the course of the disease, subaortic stenosis may develop. The EKG may show biventricular enlargement, left axis deviation, RBBB, and occasionally, AVB. Generally, these newborns do not require urgent intervention; the preferred strategy is to await the onset of HF symptoms, when the children are older, more developed, and easier to intervene upon. The intervention itself is either surgical or percutaneous.

10.2.2.7 Partial Anomalous Pulmonary Vein Drainage

Partial anomalous pulmonary vein drainage consists in drainage of one or more (but not all) pulmonary veins into the RA and is usually associated to sinus venosus ASD. (The entity, total anomalous pulmonary vein drainage, is a cyanotic condition and is discussed in the corresponding section.) This syndrome may cause RV failure, due to volume overload. The treatment is generally conservative, but severe cases may require surgery.

Occasionally, the abnormal pulmonary vein drainage is not to the RA, but to the SVC. Some patients also have malformations or hypoplasia of the right lung – the so-called "*scimitar syndrome*" (alluding to the X-ray appearance of the pulmonary arteries).

10.2.2.8 The Aorto-Pulmonary Window

The aorto-pulmonary window is a rare form of CHD, consisting in aorta/PA communication of different sizes. Other malformations (VSD, TOF, coronary malformation) are often associated. The symptoms are those of L–R shunt, and the treatment is surgical. The prognosis is essentially that of the associated anomalies.

10.2.2.9 Corrected TGV

Corrected TGV, in principle a noncyanotic CHD, actually often does associate cyanosis, due to coexisting congenital abnormalities. This condition is presented together with TGV, in the following section.

10.2.2.10 Coronary Fistula

Coronary fistula is an abnormal communication between a coronary artery, usually the RCA, and (in order of frequency) the RV, the RA, or the PA. It can occasionally complicate surgery or RF ablation. The clinical picture depends on the site and the magnitude of the abnormality. Auscultation detects a PDA-type murmur ("machinery murmur"). This condition typically causes biventricular volume overload and progressive myocardial ischemia, as the fistula tends to enlarge in time, detracting increasing amounts of blood from the coronary circulation. The treatment consists in surgical or percutaneous closure.

10.2.2.11 Cor Triatriatum

Cor triatriatum consists in LA division into two chambers, by a fibrous or muscular membrane or band. There exist an upper chamber receiving pulmonary blood and a lower chamber leading to the MV. The dividing membrane is intact or perforated ("fenestrated"); the latter situation may considerably alleviate

symptoms. Most frequently, however, the perforations are small and the "restrictive" membrane behaves like tight MS. The mortality is up to 75%, soon after birth. In patients reaching adulthood without symptoms, the clinical condition deteriorates with calcification and occlusion of the fenestrations or with the onset of AF. According to the clinical severity, the treatment may be conservative or surgical (membrane removal).

10.2.3 CHD with R–L Shunt (Cyanotic)

10.2.3.1 Tricuspid Atresia (TA)

TA consists in the total absence of RA/RV communication, due to atresia (complete nondevelopment) of the TV. TA may be isolated or associated with TGV or corrected TGV. All patients have an ASD, allowing R–L shunt and deviation of the blood toward the LV, then back to the RV or the PA through a VSD or a PDA. Frequently associated anomalies include VSD, PS, and persistent left SVC (this vein normally disappears before birth). According to the presence of associated TGV, three types are distinguished: I= no TGV; II= d-TGV; III= l-TGV. According to the degree of PV or pulmonary arteries atresia or stenosis, TA may present with decreased, normal, or increased pulmonary circulation. Other CHD frequently coexists. *Pathophysiology*: *The systemic circulation* is affected by LV volume overload and by the decreased SatO$_2$. The *pulmonary circulation* may be normal or increased, but is most frequently decreased (due to associated PA stenosis or PS). *The clinical picture* depends on PVR, with cyanosis present or not. *Cyanosis*, if present, is evident at birth and associates severe HF; decreased pulmonary circulation; clubbing, occasionally in the first months of life; failure to thrive; and different types of murmurs. Paradoxical embolism and IE may occur. The prognosis depends on the degree of PAH; occasional patients die in the first hours of life. *Acyanotic patients*, i.e., those with unobstructed pulmonary circulation, present with severe (high-output) HF. *Workup* mainly includes *echo, CT, or MRI. Chest* X-ray shows an enlarged cardiac shadow with decreased (80% of cases) or increased pulmonary circulation. *Cardiac catheterization* assesses pulmonary circulation and the degree of closure of the ductus arteriosus; PDA is critical for survival (ductus closure leads to severe aggravation of symptoms). Cardiac catheterization also has a therapeutic application (Rashkind procedure, see below). *EKG* can show "P pulmonale" (tall and peaked P waves, especially in lead II, a sign of RA hypertrophy), as well as left axis deviation and various atrial and ventricular arrhythmias. *Management*: *Pharmacological therapy* most frequently consists in IV prostaglandin to keep (or restore) ductus patency and create an R–L shunt able to increase the pulmonary circulation. In the occasional patient with increased pulmonary circulation, therapy is aimed at correcting biventricular failure and the abnormally *low* PVR.

Invasive therapy: *Percutaneous therapy* consists in the Rashkind procedure, a palliative approach to enlarge or to open the foramen ovale (with a balloon, or in older patients, with a catheter-borne blade). *Surgical therapy* is also palliative, as there still is no available TV reconstruction technique. In patients with *increased pulmonary circulation*, this can be reduced by PA banding. In patients with *decreased pulmonary circulation*, a shunt between the PA and one of the venae cavae is installed (Blalock-Taussig or Glenn shunt), bypassing the RV. This is possible due to the decreased pressure in the PA as compared to the great veins, in the absence of PAH. Unfortunately, as the child grows, the pulmonary-caval conduit may become too narrow. In these cases, a new palliative procedure ("shunt revision") or complex surgical repair is carried out. The latter is a type of Fontan procedure, consisting in direct RA/PA connection, with a synthetic conduit. Fontan surgery cannot be carried out before the age of 4, and PAH represents an absolute contraindication for this procedure. Even in the best-case scenario, Fontan physiology also ultimately fails. The last resort is the replacement of the original anastomoses with an improved type of Fontan circulation (TCPC) or cardiopulmonary transplant. *Prognosis*: Palliative procedures make possible survival to adolescence, and transplant further increases life expectancy.

10.2.3.2 PV Atresia ("Pulmonary Atresia")

PV atresia ("Pulmonary atresia") consists in the absence of a PV, the RV being a blind pouch. It is the extreme form of congenital PS. Pulmonary atresia can present with/without associated VSD. Often, there is associated TA and (in cases associating a VSD), RV hypoplasia as well. Survival depends on the existence of ASD, which channels the RA blood into the LA/LV; subsequently, part of the blood returns to the pulmonary circulation via PDA. The symptoms include cyanosis and LV failure.

The newborn is treated with prostaglandin and stabilized, before undergoing surgery for installation of an aorto-pulmonary shunt, usually within the first days of birth. This is later followed by either complete reparatory surgery (PV opening, or replacement with a donor valve) or (in case of RV hypoplasia) by a Fontan procedure and cardiopulmonary transplant, if the latter fails. IE prophylaxis is indicated. Untreated, this disease is lethal within the first days of life, but with proper treatment the prognosis is fair. Even in the best-case scenario, Fontan physiology ultimately fails. The last resort is the installation of a TCPC shunt or cardiac transplant.

10.2.3.3 Ebstein's Anomaly (EA)

EA is a congenital anomaly of the TV, including abnormal valve implantation, leading to "partial atrialization" of the RV (as the valve is lower than normal, part of the RV is above the TV) and anterior tricuspid leaflet malformation, causing TR. The exact frequency of Ebstein's is unknown, as milder forms may never be diagnosed. EA can associate numerous cardiac malformations, most frequently WPW, PDA (in 50% each), and/or ASD (also very frequent). *Risk factors* include a history of recurrent abortion or of maternal exposure to lithium, benzodiazepines, or synthetic polishes. Rarely, there is a familial pattern of inheritance. *Pathophysiology*: The anterior tricuspid leaflet malformation causes TR, which is amplified by contraction of the "atrialized" RV portion together with the rest of the RV, during atrial diastole. The associated ASD serves to discharge part of the high-pressure RA blood into the LA, leading to cyanosis. In the absence of ASD, the high-pressure RA blood usually reopens the foramen ovale, with ensuing R–L shunt. Arrhythmia is frequent and may be related to associated WPW and/or to RA dilatation. *Clinical picture*: The symptoms generally appear during adolescence. However, they may occasionally appear at birth (severe prognosis) or in adulthood. Symptoms include right or biventricular failure (the combination of LV and PAH may cause severe dyspnea) and palpitations, syncope or sudden death (especially with associated WPW). Patients are at risk for paradoxical embolism and IE. The physical examination reveals gradually evolving cyanosis, a systolic TR murmur and an ASD-related split S_2, and signs of HF and arrhythmia. *Workup*: *The imaging tests* (echo, MRI) demonstrate the presence and severity of the disease; *EKG* shows RA hypertrophy with P pulmonale, delta waves in case of associated WPW, and possible arrhythmia. EPS may be necessary, for identification and ablation of the accessory pathways. Of note, in 50% of Ebstein-associated WPW cases, there are multiple aberrant pathways, which must be carefully investigated by EPS, for complete treatment. *Management*: *Medical therapy* addresses HF, arrhythmia, and IE prophylaxis. *Surgery* is indicated in patients with HF (early on, to avoid irreversible biventricular dysfunction), paradoxical embolism, cyanosis, or intractable arrhythmia. The intervention may be palliative (usually, in very small neonates, by Blalock-Taussig shunt) or corrective, with TV repair; resection of atrialized RV and of the dilated portions of the RA; ASD closure; aberrant pathway resection; and optionally, the maze procedure. Cardiac transplant is the last resort. *The prognosis* depends on the severity of the disease. A severe prognosis is expected in cases diagnosed prenatally or in early childhood, as well as in patients with atrialization of more than 2/3 of the RV.

10.2.3.4 Transposition of the Great Vessels (TGV)

TGV consists in abnormal LV/PA and RV/aorta connections, i.e., *ventriculo-atrial discordance*. To avoid confusion, the systemic RV is referred to as "morphological RV," and the nonsystemic LV, as "morphological LV." TGV is also called d-TGV, to distinguish it from L-TGV, or "corrected TGV." There are several subtypes of TGV, classified by the presence or absence of VSD, LVOT obstruction, and increased PVR (very frequent, the LV contractility being overly strong for the low-pressure pulmonary circulation). About 1/3 of patients associate coronary artery anomalies (e.g., anomalous origin of the LCx from the right coronary sinus). In newborns, TGV is the most frequent cyanotic CHD, occurring in 20–30 out of 100,000 live births. *Pathophysiology*: The main consequence of TGV is that the pulmonary and the systemic circulation do not function "in series" (blood flow first through the lungs, then through the aorta), but "in parallel" (newly oxygenated blood returns to the lungs, and venous blood returns to the RV, both in an "endless loop"). In its pure form, this physiology is equivalent to asphyxia and is incompatible with life (death in utero or soon after birth). Survival is only possible in patients associating

a pulmonary/systemic communication (ASD, VSD, or PDA). The cardiac function of the TGV patient depends on several factors: *Pulmonary vascular reactivity*: if normal, HF develops in the first days after birth, as PVR decreases and RV volume overload evolves; if increased, severe PAH ensues. The pulmonary LV is initially able to counteract the increased PVR, but ultimately decompensates, leading to a decreased LV output (pulmonary hypoperfusion), and a higher volume reaching the RV (increased R–L shunt), as even a dysfunctional LV generates systolic pressures in excess of those of the (systemic) RV. The net result is RV volume overload and failure, with an especially poor prognosis. This rather complex pathophysiology is reviewed in Table 10.6. *The direction of the shunt*: *RV volume overload* occurs both with LV–RV and with RV–LV shunt (via the pulmonary circulation). However, *LV volume overload* only occurs with RV-LV shunt, as excess systemic blood can be stored in the third space. *The degree of restrictiveness of the systemic/pulmonary communication*: As noted, *some* degree of pulmonary/systemic shunt is essential for survival. If the communication is restrictive, cyanosis and HF are evident at birth; if it is large, they become evident over the few hours or days after birth, as the PVR falls, and the short-lived phase of high-output LV failure gives way to low-output failure and increased shunt. An additional important influence on hemodynamics is that of *abnormalities in the aortic media*, frequently associated to TGV and predisposing to AI: aortic aneurysm and rupture; and aortic dissection.

Clinical picture: *Symptoms and signs* include cyanosis and HF (see above). With associated VSD, auscultation detects a systolic murmur, while a continuous systolic and diastolic murmur suggests associated PDA.

Table 10.6 Pathophysiology of transposition of the great vessels (TGVs)

	LV	RV
Pressure overload	In patients with high pulmonary reactivity, and with irreversible PAH	Always, as the RV is not able to counter the increased SVR
Volume overload	With RV-to-LV shunt or with associated AI	Always, as the RV receives an excess of blood from the LV either directly or via the pulmonary circulation

These murmurs indicate the presence of an anatomic basis for immediate survival in TGV patients. Increased blood viscosity may cause neurological signs. As R–L shunt is normal in utero, these newborns are generally well developed, without visible physical malformations or initial cyanosis. *Workup: Imaging tests* (echocardiogram, CT, MRI) are central to the diagnosis. *Echo* typically shows a large, bifurcating artery (the PA), originating from a ventricle with thick muscular striations (trabeculations) – the morphologic LV. Echo can also show the associated coronary anomalies, since in very young patients blood vessel visualization is much better than in adults. *Chest X-ray* may demonstrate changes in pulmonary vascularity, as well as a distinctive "egg-shaped" cardiac shadow. *EKG* can be normal or show signs of RVH. *Catheterization* demonstrates the location and magnitude of shunt, measures the intracardiac pressures, assesses the severity and the reversibility of hypoxemia, and allows performing the Rashkind procedure. The severity of hypoxemia reflects that of the underlying shunt; significant correction of hypoxemia under O_2 administration suggests a pulmonary cause for cyanosis, rather than a cardiac one.

Management: Medical treatment includes therapy of HF and IV prostaglandin, to maintain the ductus arteriosus open. *Interventional treatment includes: The Rashkind procedure* (Table 10.3), performed as soon as the first hours after birth; *the Jatene procedure* (arterial inversion), a definitive repair consisting in reimplantation of the great vessels in the normally corresponding ventricles. The ideal timing is in the second week of life, before the low pulmonary pressures lead to LV "under-use" atrophy and inability to generate systemic pressures. If this deadline is missed, a staged procedure is carried out, involving *Step* 1: PA is banded, to induce PAH and LVH, thus restoring LV capacity for systemic (rather than pulmonary) function; *Step* 2: LV/aorta RV/PA connection. Long-term survival is excellent (>90%), but this procedure is not possible in case of significant coronary abnormalities, which prevent proper mobilization of the aorta. In these patients, the Rastelli procedure is performed; *the Rastelli procedure* consists in inserting an LV/aorta and an RV/PA conduit, with VSD and PV closure (leaving the conduit as the only option for RV emptying). This is performed at 1–2 years of age, after a preparatory Blalock-Taussig procedure (Table 10.3); *atrial inversion procedures* (*Mustard, Senning*), i.e., connecting the atria to the "correct" ventricle by artificial conduits. Only the Mustard procedure is still occasionally used, for TGV

with coronary anomalies, but even then, the Rastelli procedure is preferred. Though rarely (if ever) performed nowadays, these procedures are frequently seen in patients who were operated on as children, in 1965–1975. The reason for their disfavor is the increased incidence of arrhythmia and block (high-risk for sudden death; frequent Holter monitoring required) and of HF, due to the systemic RV function. There may be significant TR and occasional baffle obstruction.

TGV: Prognosis. Untreated, approximately a third of newborns die within the first week, and more than 90% die before their first birthday. In contrast, with proper treatment, survival into adulthood exceeds 90%.

10.2.3.5 Congenitally Corrected TGV

Congenitally corrected TGV involves, in addition to the ventriculo-arterial discordance, an atrio-ventricular discordance, with pumping of oxygenated blood into the aorta and of venous blood into the pulmonary circulation, albeit both by the "wrong" ventricle. The term "corrected" is disputed, as its carries an unjustified connotation of normality, whereas, due to the frequently associated abnormalities, this disease actually has a worse prognosis than the "uncorrected" form. The alternative designation is "l-transposition" for TGV and "d-transposition" for corrected TGV (based on geometrical factors in the intrauterine development; "l"=*levo*=left; "d"=*dextro*=right). In principle noncyanotic, l-TGV may present with cyanosis due to the frequently associated VSD. Additional associated conditions include *third-degree AVB* in up to 30% (risk for SCD); *sinus node disease*, as well as atrial, AV, and ventricular *tachycardia*; coronary artery anomalies; LVOT obstruction; aortic or subaortic stenosis, coarctation, or aortic arch interruption; and TV abnormalities (often insignificant). *Clinical picture: The symptoms and signs* include HF and arrhythmia; with associated PS, prominent cyanosis is present (unto itself, this condition is noncyanotic). In the rare patient without associated anomalies, the diagnosis may be established in adulthood, during workup for TR and HF. *The workup* includes cardiac *imaging* procedures; *catheterization*, which, however, may cause complete AVB; and *EKG*, showing ventricular inversion (right chest leads reflect LV, left leads reflect RV), and arrhythmia and AVB of different degrees. *Management* includes therapy for

HF, arrhythmia, block, and hyperviscosity. *Surgical correction* ("double inversion," i.e., of both the atria and the ventricles) consists in a combination of different procedures, as used with TGV. Immediate and long-term complications are frequent (arrhythmia, AVB, HF, severe TR). Prognosis depends on the degree of hemodynamic disturbance. Additional poor prognostic factors include TR and younger age at surgery.

10.2.3.6 Tetralogy of Fallot (TOF)

TOF accounts for approximately 10% of all cases of CHD and consists in the association of: (1) *PS*, either valvular or subvalvular (infundibular RV stenosis, caused by localized RVH or an elastic band limiting flow toward the PA); (2) *RVH*; (3) *VSD*; and (4) *overriding aorta*: the ascending portion of the aorta is positioned over the VSD-bearing septum, thus draining not only the LV output, but also part of the RV output. Additional malformations can be associated to TOF, such as ASD, left PA stenosis, bicuspid PV, AI, etc. TOF is thought to be due to environmental and/or genetic factors, including maternal exposure to alcohol or anticonvulsive medication (Carbamazepine, Phenytoin) and maternal phenylketonuria. *Pathophysiology* mainly involves R–L shunt, its magnitude dictated by the PVR/SVR ratio, with infundibular RV stenosis importantly influencing PVR. *Clinical picture*: Newborns can display failure to thrive, agitation, and dyspnea. Cyanosis and dyspnea are frequent at all ages and are worsened by exertion (restlessness and crying with newborns, and during play, in older children). These "cyanotic spells" ("tet spells") result from exertional peripheral vasodilation and from sudden RV afterload increase (infundibular spasm). The child instinctively adopts a squatting position, which reduces leg perfusion and improves blood flow to the brain and vital organs. Occasionally, cyanotic spells are seen in patients completely free of cyanosis at rest. Cyanotic spells are a major emergency; left untreated, they may cause syncope, convulsions, CVA, and death. The treatment is discussed below. Cyanosis may be evident immediately after birth or later on. TOF (even after repair) associates *abnormalities of the aortic media*, causing progressive aortic root dilatation which may lead to AI, aneurysmal dilatation and rupture, or aortic dissection. Males and patients associating chromosome 22q11 deletion are at highest risk for this type of complications. Surgery and possibly β-blocker administration should be considered.

> The mechanism of pink tet (acyanotic TOF) involves two extreme manifestations of PS:
>
> - *Minimal PS*, with Qp/Qs >0.8, *or*
> - *Pulmonic atresia*, with right heart flow from a large PDA and/or major aorto-pulmonary collateral vessels

The physical examination additionally reveals prominence of the left hemithorax (caused by RVH); a palpatory thrill and a systolic murmur, due to turbulent flow through the stenotic portion of the RV; clubbing; and occasional paradoxical embolism. The systolic ejection murmur is soft with severe PV obstruction (cyanotic patients) and loud with mild obstruction (pink tet). Arrhythmia (mainly atrial) may be present in older patients with untreated FT.

Workup includes imaging by *echo, CT*, or *MRI* (the latter also very useful for the detection of associated coronary anomalies). *Chest radiography* may reveal a "boot-shaped heart" ("*coeur en sabot*"), reflecting RVH. *Cardiac catheterization* demonstrates the VSD and RV infundibular stenosis, as well as coronary artery anomalies (e.g., origin of all the coronaries from a single trunk). Awareness of these anomalies is very important, to facilitate any catheterization and/or coronary surgery that may be required in the future. *Oxymetry* shows SatO$_2$ decrease, its magnitude corresponding to the severity of the disease; *EKG* may show right axis deviation, RVH, atrial and/or ventricular arrhythmia, and bundle branch block.

Management: *Medical treatment. General measures* include IV prostaglandin, to reopen the ductus arteriosus; treatment of HF, PAH, arrhythmia, etc. *Treatment of cyanotic spells* includes applying the *knee/chest position*, an equivalent of the squatting position; *morphine*, to counteract tachypnea (which increases the venous return to the heart, and, in a vicious circle, further increases arterial desaturation; the vasoconstrictor, *Phenylephrine,* to increase SVR and diminish the shunt; *sodium bicarbonate*, in case of acidosis; in extreme cases, *general anesthesia* and mechanical ventilation, to allow easier

Table 10.7 Double outlet RV (DORV) physiology

Physiology	Type	Blood flow
TOF-like	DORV with a subaortic VSD	RV blood flows mainly to the PA, and LV blood is mostly directed to the aorta, albeit via the VSD and the RV; there is blood admixture in the RV
	DORV associating PS	Blood from both ventricles mainly flows to the aorta, with admixture in the RV[a]
TGV-like	DORV with a subpulmonic VSD[b] and no PS	RV blood flows mainly to the aorta; LV blood flows mainly to the PA
Large VSD-like	All other DORV	Substantial admixture in the RV

[a]RV blood flows mainly to the aorta; LV blood tends to flow through the VSD to the PA, but is halted by PS, and does ultimately reach the aorta
[b]The Taussig-Bing syndrome

pharmacological handling of the pulmonary and peripheral resistance; and *oxygen* therapy, routinely given, though generally ineffective, since the cause of desaturation is blood admixture, not reduced lung oxygenation. Propranolol may be prescribed, to reduce tet spell recurrences. As with other cyanotic CHD, IE prophylaxis is indicated. *Surgical treatment* for TOF is indicated in patients with significant RVOT or PA branch stenosis, usually as a primary operation (VSD closure and RVOT widening), in the first year of life. PAH contraindicates the procedure, and unfavorable PA anatomy may require surgical palliation. If such is the case, the common scenario is to use a Blalock-Taussig shunt, as a bridge to complete corrective surgery or to transplant. The Pott and Waterston shunts are similar to, and have been abandoned in favor of, the Blalock-Taussig procedure. The *postoperative evolution* may be complicated by several problems, some resulting from the surgical procedure and some simply not prevented by it. *Pulmonic insufficiency* most frequently results from surgical relief of RVOT/valvular obstruction and is generally well tolerated. In the occasional patient in whom it does cause HF NYHA class ≥ II, repeat surgery for valve replacement (generally, with a biological prosthesis) is indicated; *RV dilatation and failure*, treated in the usual manner; *residual infundibular stenosis*; and *arrhythmia or heart block*, due to TOF itself or to myocardial surgical scars. These patients have an increased risk of late SCD. *Prognosis*: More than 2/3 of untreated patients die before their tenth birthday, and only a minority survive into adulthood. Therapy improves survival significantly.

10.2.3.7 Double Outlet RV (DORV)

Double outlet RV (DORV) is a form of CHD where both great arteries connect (entirely or partly) to the RV. DORV associates VSD and can associate TGV. The clinical manifestations and therapy depend on the presence, characteristics, and severity of anatomical defects (Table 10.7).

10.2.3.8 Hypoplastic Left Heart Syndrome (HLHS)

HLHS is a rare type of CHD, characterized as marked hypoplasia or absence of the LV and severe hypoplasia of the ascending aorta. The causes are probably genetic. The physiology is that of an RV which must function both in the pulmonary, and in the systemic circulation, leading to severe volume and pressure overload, as well as to ductus-dependence for systemic perfusion. The manifestations include severe cyanosis and HF. Ductus closure causes shock and death, unless treated. *Management*: *Drug therapy* addresses HF and ductus patency (prostaglandin E). *Interventional therapy* involves cardiac transplant or staged palliative surgery. The latter is reviewed in Table 10.8.

10.2.3.9 Hypoplastic Right Heart Syndrome (HRHS)

Hypoplastic right heart syndrome (HRHS) consists in underdevelopment of the RA and RV. It is even less common than HLHS and can associate AS. HRHS

Table 10.8 Hypoplastic left heart syndrome (HLHS): staged palliative surgery

Step	1	2	3
Timing	Within a week of birth	3–6 months of age	18 months–4 years of age
Aim	(a) Relieving the ductus-dependence and allowing RVA to function systemically. (b) Ensuring pulmonary circulation in face of an RV "re-allocated" to the left circulation	Relieving the high PA pressures and some of the blood admixture (i.e., that of venous blood from the upper 1/2 of the body)	Totally relieving arterial desaturation
Mechanism	(a) Separating the main PA from its branches and connecting it to the aorta (b) Connecting the pulmonary circulation to the subclavian artery or to the RV	Replacing the B-T or Sano shunt with an SVC-PA anastomosis	Connect the IVC to the PA as well
Name	(a) *Norwood* procedure; (b) *Blalock-Taussig*, respectively *Sano* shunt	*Bidirectional Glenn*[a] or *Hemi-Fontan*[b] *procedure*	*Fontan* procedure
Physiological challenge	Cyanosis; RV volume and pressure overload; PAH, due to pulmonary circulation being exposed to systemic pressures	Milder cyanosis; RV volume and pressure overload; mild or no PAH	No cyanosis; RV volume and pressure overload; mild or no PAH

[a]The SVC is first separated from the RA
[b]The SVC is not separated from the RA, but a "dam" is installed, to prevent blood flow from the SVC into the RA (as only one of the cavae is involved, this is "half" of a Fontan, or a hemi-Fontan procedure)

manifests as severe cyanosis. Surgical therapy consists in heart transplant or in a staged B-T/Glenn/Fontan procedure.

10.2.3.10 Persistent Truncus Arteriosus

Persistent truncus arteriosus (or simply, *truncus arteriosus*) is a rare form of CHD, caused by genetic disorders and/or environmental factors, and consisting in the absence of division of the truncus arteriosus (the embryological precursor of both the PA and the aorta) into two great vessels. Three types (I, II, and III) are distinguished based on the branching pattern of the pulmonary arteries. Anatomically, there is a single artery arising (by way of an abnormal valve) from the two ventricles, giving rise to both the aorta and the PA. Associated anomalies include a right-sided aortic arch (in approximately 30% of cases); a large VSD; PAH; and cyanosis. *Abnormalities in the aortic media* are frequently associated and predispose to AI; aortic aneurysm and rupture; and aortic dissection. *The clinical picture* includes cyanosis, HF, and hypocalcemia (if associated with the Di George syndrome). On auscultation, there is a systolic ejection murmur along the LSB, a loud S_2, and a widened pulse pressure with bounding arterial pulses. Cardiomegaly and biventricular hypertrophy are detected

by cardiac imaging. Surgery is indicated in the neonatal period and involves patch closure of the VSD and detachment of the pulmonary arteries from the truncus, with connection to the RV by a conduit or tunnel. The truncus itself is left to function as an aorta.

10.2.4 CHD without a Shunt

10.2.4.1 Anomalies of Cardiac Position

The normal position of the body organs is designated as *"situs solitus."* There are several possible anomalies of cardiac positioning. *Dextrocardia* consists in a reversed position of the cardiac apex, which normally points to the left. It can be part of global mirror-image organ positioning (generalized situs inversus) or isolated. *Dextrocardia of generalized situs inversus* is usually unassociated to cardiac or other malformations, with the exception of occasional TGV. The condition's importance mainly resides in the possibility of clinical and EKG misdiagnosis of cardiac or noncardiac conditions with a "reversed presentation" (angina in the right hemithorax; right axis deviation and QRS complex amplitude decrease in the chest leads, from V1 to V6; appendicitis in the

LLQ, etc.). *Isolated dextrocardia* is very often associated to other disorders (frequently, TGV). *Partial situs inversus* (*situs inversus with levocardia*) is the situation where all the organs except for the heart have a reverse position. This is also simply termed "levocardia" and may associate cardiac and noncardiac congenital anomalies. *Situs ambiguus* is characterized by positioning anomalies of a severity intermediate between that of situs solitus (normal) and situs inversus (mirror image); almost all patients have associated CHD, such as TOF, TGV, ASD, VSD, valvular PS, etc.

10.2.4.2 Congenital AVB

Congenital AVB may be isolated (e.g., with maternal autoimmune disease such as lupus) or associated with complex CHD, such as TGV. The mother is most often asymptomatic, while the fetus presents bradycardia, which can be misconstrued as representing fetal distress syndrome. The distinction is important: while fetal distress mandates immediate caesarian section, congenital AVB can be treated with steroids, plasmapheresis (to remove the maternal antibodies), or epinephrine, to accelerate the fetal pulse. After birth, epicardial pacing is used, by a percutaneous or surgical approach, as a bridge to an age when the veins are sufficiently large to allow endocardial electrode positioning. Just like fetal distress (the other prominent cause of fetal bradycardia), *untreated* AVB has a very severe prognosis, with a 30–50% risk of death in utero (hydrops fetalis). Conversely, with correct treatment, life expectancy is virtually unaffected.

10.2.5 Miscellaneous CHD

10.2.5.1 Aortic Coarctation

Aortic coarctation is a congenital stenosis of a segment of the thoracic descending aorta, in the vicinity of the ductus arteriosus, after the subclavian artery takeoff. There are three types of coarctation, according to the situation in relation to the ductus: preductal (a ductus-dependent occasionally encountered in children with Turner's syndrome), ductal (usually occurring at the

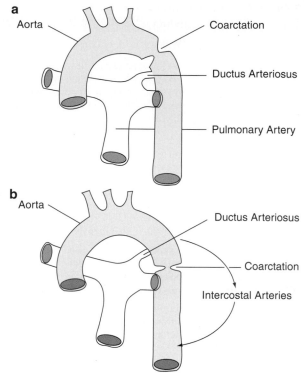

Fig. 10.3 Aortic coarctation: (**a**) preductal coarctation, a ductus-dependent lesion; (**b**) postductal coarctation, the most frequent type in adults. The intercostal arteries serve as anastomotic ducts and are responsible for the typical "rib notching" seen on chest X-ray

time of ductus closure), and postductal, most common in adults, and typically associated to intercostal collaterals (the ductus not being able to bridge between the supra- and infracoarctation segment). The two main types of coarctation, i.e., pre- and postductal, are presented in Fig. 10.3.

Coarctation is believed to result from migration to the aorta and subsequent hypertrophy of a group of muscular cells from the ductus. There is at least some genetic component to the pathogenesis of aortic coarctation, as it is seven times more frequent in Caucasians than in Asians. *Pathophysiology*: Aortic coarctation increases peripheral resistance, i.e., LV afterload, leading to LVH and ventricular dysfunction (diastolic, and later on, combined systolic and diastolic). The hallmark is HTN in the upper half of the body only. In time, arterial bridges between the supra- and infracoarctation segment develop in the postductal variety, most commonly seen in adults. Occasionally, coarctation involves the origin of the left subclavian artery, resulting in defective development of the left upper limb. Approximately 50% of patients associate other forms of CHD, including bicuspid AV (most frequently); VSD; or different degrees of impaired development upstream from the coarctation (aortic arch interruption or even LV hypoplasia). *Noncardiac malformations* include Turner's syndrome and cerebral "berry aneurysms," which can rupture, causing subarachnoid hemorrhage. *Abnormalities in the aortic media* are frequently associated to aortic coarctation and predispose to AI; aortic aneurysm and rupture; and aortic dissection.

The clinical manifestations may reflect the coarctation as such, its complications, and associated malformations. The *coarctation as such* manifests as ischemia in the lower half of the body (cramping, pain, and muscular weakness in the legs); with collateral formation, the symptoms become less frequent (although different degrees of lower body perfusion do persist) and include HTN in the upper half of the body, occasionally associated with epistaxis. In severe cases, the blood pressure in the arm is by >20 mmHg higher than in the leg. (Normally, the blood pressure is higher in the legs than in the arms, due to the effect of gravity.) *Auscultation* reveals a systolic or continuous murmur over the back and a continuous murmur over the dilated arterial intercostal anastomoses. Occasional patients present with underdevelopment of the left arm. *Complications* include HF, especially in severe cases and in very young patients; hypoperfusion of the lower body; and aortic aneurysms associated to the coarctation as such, or as a complication after repair. *Associated anomalies* include AS or AI resulting from associated bicuspid AV; VSD; and occasionally, *Turner's* syndrome (manifesting as short stature, well-developed thorax, small breasts, a characteristic skin fold on both sides of the neck, specific facial characteristics, and certain cognitive deficits). With supraductal coarctation associating a PDA, differential cyanosis (affecting the lower part of the body only), usually mild, may be present. *Workup* includes *echo*, *CT*, and *MRI*, which demonstrate the presence, extent, and severity (length, gradient) of the coarctation; of its complications; and of associated malformations. *Chest X-ray* can demonstrate cardiac dilatation, as well as characteristic indentations on the lower border of the ribs ("rib notching"), corresponding to the supra/infracoarctation anastomoses. On a barium swallow, lateral X-ray images reveal the coarctation "fingerprint" on the esophagus, resembling an "inverted figure of 3."

Cardiac catheterization visualizes the coarctation and assesses the transcoarctation gradient; and the *EKG* typically shows LVH.

Management: *Drug treatment* includes, beside HTN management, IV prostaglandin in the newborn with HF, to open the ductus arteriosus and allow PA/aortic shunt (provided the coarctation is supraductal). This unburdens the pulmonary circulation, while at the same time perfusing the lower half of the body; HTN and HF are treated in the usual manner. Left untreated, coarctation has an 80% mortality before age 50 (due to the complications of HF and HTN). *Interventional therapy* is indicated for supra/infracoarctation BP gradients >30 mmHg; upper limb HTN; and with associated aortic aneurysm. Screening for cerebral berry aneurysms is indicated. *Angioplasty* is the preferred method in adults, both for primary and for recoarctation treatment, but may not be feasible in long coarctations. *Surgical treatment*, best carried out before age 14, may consist in resection and anastomosis, occasionally using a prosthetic tube; coarctation widening by insertion of a synthetic patch; or coarctation bypass using a synthetic tube. *The postsurgical evolution* depends on the age at intervention; the presence of irreversible LV dysfunction (the most frequent postoperative problem) or of HTN; coarctation recurrence; and the presence of surgical complications. The latter include: *lower limb paralysis*, due to intraoperative lesion of the peri-coarctation collaterals, some of which perfuse the spine; this is the most severe complication after coarctation surgery; *severe new-onset HTN in the lower part of the body*, caused by inappropriate persistence of the compensatory mechanisms formerly ensuring adequate perfusion. *Hyperperfusion* especially affects the mesenteric artery and causes severe abdominal pain. Aggressive antihypertensive therapy is recommended. Finally, *aortic dissection* may occur in the segment operated on. During *pregnancy*, the main complication consists in exacerbation of HTN, related to the transcoarctation gradient.

10.2.5.2 Shone's Syndrome

Shone's syndrome associates aortic coarctation to mitral and aortic anomalies. Mitral anomalies mainly include *a supravalvular mitral membrane (SVMM)* and a *parachute MV*, i.e., insertion of the chordae onto one single papillary muscle, with MS-like physiology. (As the leaflets are held in close apposition, the only effective communication between the LA and the LV is through the interchordal spaces.) The aortic anomalies consist in membranous or muscular subaortic stenosis. The treatment is surgical, but LV dysfunction and PAH may persist even after relief of the obstructive lesions.

10.2.5.3   Interrupted Aortic Arch

Interrupted aortic arch is a very rare type of CHD, in which there is a gap between the ascending and descending thoracic aorta. Almost all patients have other associated CHD. Interrupted aortic arch is associated with the DiGeorge Syndrome. This is a ductus-dependent lesion, and IV prostaglandin is used in the preparation for neonatal surgery.

10.2.5.4   CHD Caused by Maternal Exposure to Environmental Factors

CHD caused by maternal exposure to environmental factors includes: *the congenital rubella syndrome*, manifesting as PDA and PA stenosis in 50% of children of mothers exposed within the first 2 months of pregnancy; *exposure to alcohol*, often causing VSD or ASD (alcohol-related birth defects, not representing diagnostic criteria for the fetal alcohol syndrome); *exposure to lithium* (possible EA); *exposure to β-blockers* (fetal bradycardia and hypotension); *exposure to nicotine* might cause increased susceptibility to ischemia in adulthood; *exposure to antidepressants*: Paroxetine can cause multiple heart defects and is contraindicated in pregnancy. MAO inhibitors may cause severe HTN and stroke and are contraindicated. Antidepressants appropriate in the pregnant woman include tricyclics; Bupropion; and the SSRIs, Citalopram, Fluoxetine, and Sertraline (however, these agents may rarely cause a serious condition, "persistent PAH of the newborn"). A recent study has linked early-pregnancy Fluoxetine and Paroxetine treatment to increased fetal risk of CHD.

10.2.5.5   Multisystem Syndromes Associated with CHD

Multisystem syndromes associated with CHD include, among others: *Down's syndrome* (AVSD, VSD, PV abnormalities); *Noonan's syndrome* (aortic coarctation, HCM, ASD, PS); *Turner's syndrome* (coarctation with or without bicuspid PV); *the Williams-Beuren syndrome* (supravalvular AS, occasionally associating multiple stenoses of the pulmonary arteries); and the *Di George syndrome* (*22q11.2 deletion syndrome, velocardiofacial syndrome, conotruncal anomaly face syndrome, congenital thymic aplasia, Strong Syndrome, thymic hypoplasia*), a congenital syndrome with multisystem features, typically including CHD, defects in the palate, mild facial deformity, and recurrent infections (the latter, due to thymus absence or hypoplasia). CHD is seen in 40% of individuals and mainly includes TOF, interrupted aortic arch, VSD, and persistent truncus arteriosus. All these syndromes also involve different degrees of intellectual impairment; *Marfan's syndrome* is an inherited defect of the conjunctive system, and while not a CHD per se, it is a predisposing factor for severe valvular and aortic complications (Chaps. 5 and 11).

10.2.5.6   Persistent Left Superior Vena Cava (PLSVC)

Persistent left superior vena cava (PLSVC) affects 0.3% of the population. The left upper limb, the head, and the neck drain into the RA via the coronary sinus, which is dilated. Isolated PLSVC is benign, but in reality it is very frequently associated with VSD or AVSD, with the corresponding prognosis.

10.2.5.7   Congenital Coronary Anomalies

Congenital coronary anomalies are usually first suspected on coronary angiography carried out for another reason, when a coronary artery appears to be absent and a large myocardial segment appears nonperfused. The most common instance is an *absent left coronary trunk* (with an incidence of 0.47%), where the LAD and the LCx originate from two separate aortic ostia. The other anomalies are, in decreasing order of frequency: *LCx originating from the right sinus of Valsalva*; *RCA originating from the ascending aorta, above the sinus of Valsalva*; *RCA originating from the left sinus of Valsalva*; and the *origin of the left main coronary artery from the right sinus of Valsalva* (in very rare instances, the artery can course between the aorta and the PA, with coronary compression and SCD). An additional form of coronary anomaly is *myocardial bridging*, discussed in Chap. 2.

10.2.5.8 Other CHD

Other CHD, discussed in different chapters of this text, include HOCM, ARVC (Chap. 4); subvalvular, valvular, and supravalvular AS; bicuspid AV; PS (Chap. 5); and pericardial malformations (Chap. 7).

Bibliography

Guidelines

Warnes CA, Williams RG, Bashore TM, et al. ACC/AHA 2008 Guidelines for the management of adults with congenital heart disease: executive summary: a report of the American College of Cardiology/American Heart Association Task Force on Practice Guidelines (Writing Committee to Develop Guidelines for the Management of Adults With Congenital Heart Disease). *Circulation*. 2008;118:2395-2451.

Suggested Reading

Brickner ME, Hillis LD, Lange RA. Congenital heart disease in adults. First of two parts. *N Engl J Med*. 2000;342(4):256-263.

Mas J-L, Arquizan C, Lamy C, et al. Recurrent cerebrovascular events associated with patent foramen ovale, atrial septal aneurysm, or both. *N Engl J Med*. 2001;345:1740-1746.

Webb G, Gatzoulis MA. Atrial septal defects in the adult: recent progress and overview. *Circulation*. 2006;114(15):1645-1653.

Brickner ME, Hillis LD, Lange RA. Congenital heart disease in adults. Second of two parts. *N Engl J Med*. 2000;342:334-342.

Crenshaw BS, Granger CB, Birnbaum Y, et al., for the GUSTO-I (global utilization of streptokinase and TPA for occluded coronary arteries) trial investigators. Risk factors, angiographic patterns, and outcomes in patients with ventricular septal defect complicating acute myocardial infarction. *Circulation*. 2000;101:127.

Dodge-Khatami A, Knirsch W, Tomaske M, et al. Spontaneous closure of small residual ventricular septal defects after surgical repair. *Ann Thorac Surg*. 2007;83(3):902-905.

Hein R, Buscheck F, Fisher E, et al. Atrial and ventricular septal defects can safely be closed by percutaneous intervention. *J Interv Cardiol*. 2005;18:515-522.

Bermúdez-Cañete R, Santoro G, Bialkowsky J, et al. Patent ductus arteriosus occlusion using detachable coils. *Am J Cardiol*. 1998;82(12):1547-1549.

Eerola A, Jokinen E, Boldt T, et al. The influence of percutaneous closure of patent ductus arteriosus on left ventricular size and function: a prospective study using two- and three-dimensional echocardiography and measurements of serum natriuretic peptides. *J Am Coll Cardiol*. 2006;47(5):1060-1066.

Attenhofer Jost CH, Connolly HM, Dearani JA. Ebstein's anomaly. *Circulation*. 2007;115:277-285.

Angiology: Diseases of the Blood Vessels

Contents

11.1 Background

The heart is a modified blood vessel, *embryologically, structurally* (the endothelium, media, and serosa correspond to the endocardium, myocardium, and pericardium, respectively), and *functionally* (both the heart and the blood vessels are composed of an inner cavity for blood flow, and a wall with elastic and muscular cells). Consequently, there is ample similarity between cardiac and vascular diseases.

11.2 Diseases of the Aorta

11.2.1 Aortic Dissection

11.2.1.1 Definition and Prevalence

Aortic dissection (AD) consists in the separation of the aortic intima and media by a thrombus progressing between these layers. The aorta is "skinned" from the interior and has two lumens: *the true (natural)* and *the false lumen* (the trajectory of the thrombus), often substantially larger than the true one. The blood forming the clot usually originates from the lumen and enters between the layers through an endothelial fissure; occasionally, it originates in hemorrhage of the aortic vasa vasorum. Ninety percent of AD involve the first 10 cm of the aorta (i.e., the ascending aorta). Additional entities in the AD spectrum are reviewed below.

G.A. Adelmann, *Cardiology Essentials in Clinical Practice*,
DOI: 10.1007/978-1-84996-305-3_11, © Springer-Verlag London Limited 2011

Aortic dissection: a glossary

- *Dissecting aortic aneurysm:* a synonym of "AD," alluding to the enlarged diameter of the affected segment. Confusion between AD and aortic aneurysm must be avoided.
- *(Total) transection:* a synonym of aortic rupture. Most frequently, traumatic origin; lethal, unless sealed by a clot.
- *Partial transection:* the serosa is initially intact, but subsequently ruptures as well.
- *Intraparietal hematoma:* wall hematoma without an entry point. Mostly caused by trauma-related vasa vasorum hemorrhage.
- *Aortic pseudoaneurysm:* sealed total transection or partial transection of the aorta.

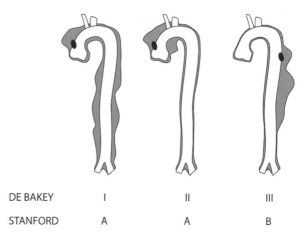

| DE BAKEY | I | II | III |
| STANFORD | A | A | B |

Fig. 11.1 Types and classifications of aortic dissection. The *black dots* indicate the portal of entry

11.2.1.2 Classification

The standard classifications of AD are presented in Table 11.1 and in Fig. 11.1. The Stanford and De Bakey classifications address the site, and the ESC classification addresses the mechanism of AD. As both elements are key in regard to therapy and prognosis, combining the ESC and one of the other classifications offers the most information.

11.2.1.3 Pathophysiology

A major emergency, AD may cause *aortic rupture* with massive internal hemorrhage; *PT,* by progressing to the pericardial sac; *acute AI,* by progression to the AV; carotid artery dissection and CVA; coronary dissection and *myocardial ischemia;* or renal or other *visceral artery dissection,* with acute organ dysfunction (e.g., acute renal failure). These major complications account for the dramatic *mortality* of AD. During the first 2 days, the mortality is of 1–2% for each hour spent without treatment, so that approximately 1/3 of patients die within 24 h (50% within 48 h). By the end of 2 weeks, approximately 75% of untreated patients will have died (90% by 12 months). Mortality in type A dissection is higher than in type B. Survival is accounted for by mechanisms able to arrest the progression of AD, such as *an obstacle* in the aortic wall (e.g., calcification); *a portal of exit,* depressurizing the false lumen; or *hemorrhage-related hypotension,* also depressurizing the false lumen.

Table 11.1 The classifications of AD

Class	Type		
Stanford	A		B
	Ascending aorta involved		Ascending aorta not involved
De Bakey	I	II	III
	60%	10–15%	25–30%
	Origin in the ascending aorta, propagates to arch and often beyond it	Origin in and confined to the ascending aorta	Origin in the descending aorta, rarely extends proximally
ESC	Classical AD (Class 1); intramural hematoma/hemorrhage (Class 2); subtle/discrete AD (Class 3); plaque rupture/ulceration (Class 4); iatrogenic/traumatic AD (Class 5)		

11.2.1.4 Risk Factors and Clinical Picture of AD

Risk factors for AD include: *age:* prevalence peaks at ages 40–70; type B AD is especially prevalent in the elderly; *connective tissue diseases* (Marfan, Ehlers–Danlos, cystic medial necrosis), causing lesions to the vasa vasorum; and the Loeys–Dietz syndrome, a congenital collagen anomaly, clinically similar to Ehlers–Danlos', and with a similarly elevated risk of aortic dissection, but with a better surgical prognosis; *HTN; pregnancy,* especially in the last trimester or early postpartum, due to reduced mechanical resistance in the conjunctive tissue, in preparation for childbirth; *bicuspid AV,* often associated to aortic root dilatation, and occasionally, to aortic coarctation; *aortic aneurysm,* occasionally associated to CHD (e.g., Turner's syndrome); *trauma; aortitis; iatrogenic:* coarctation repair, aortic catheterization or cannulation for cardiopulmonary bypass, etc.

Clinical picture: The main **symptom** is excruciating chest or back *pain,* different from the MI pain by its extreme intensity from the beginning (pain onset is more gradual in MI), and its "tearing" quality ("crushing," in MI). The location of pain onset is suggestive of the affected segment: pain in the anterior thorax corresponds to ascending aorta and/or arch dissection, while back pain suggests dissection of the descending aorta. Spatial progression of pain indicates the direction of AD propagation – e.g., pain irradiated to the neck suggests extension to the carotids (but may equally well be caused by AD-related myocardial ischemia). In approximately 10% of patients (especially with Marfan's disease), AD may be painless, most probably due to damage to the aortic wall sensory terminations. *Syncope* may be due to hemorrhage-related hypotension, PT, vagal activation by the intense pain, etc. **The physical examination** may reveal HTN (functioning both as a risk factor and an aggravating factor), *hypotension* (a poor prognostic sign), *BP asymmetry* between the two upper limbs (differences >20 mmHg, when the aortic take-off of one of the subclavian arteries is involved in dissection or obstructed by the dissecting hematoma); *Signs of complications* (acute AI, PT, organ, or limb ischemia by compression of aortic branches, etc.).

11.2.1.5 Workup

Echocardiography is the default initial procedure. TTE can establish the diagnosis or raise the suspicion of AD, which then requires confirmation by TEE, CT, or MRI. TEE has the great advantage of being available in the OR, while preparations for emergent exploratory thoracotomy are being made. On the other hand, TEE is less specific and sensitive than CT or MRI, and lesions within the 2 cm proximal to the innominate arteries cannot be visualized ("blind spot," corresponding to the superposition of the air-filled trachea on the esophagus). TEE demonstrates the entry portal; the hematoma; the true and the false lumen; and occasionally, an exit portal, or signs of complications (AI, PT, etc.). *CT* and *MRI* are more accurate than TEE, but are more time-consuming and are not available in the OR; *Chest X-ray* demonstrates mediastinal widening >8 cm; an increased distance between the aortic wall and incidental intimal reference points, e.g., calcification (a distance >5 mm suggests AD); and pleural and/or pericardial effusion. *EKG* may show nonspecific tachycardia or, with coronary involvement, signs of acute ischemia. As thrombolytic therapy is strictly contraindicated (lysis of the sealing clot may cause aortic rupture), the possibility of AD must be kept in mind in all MI patients; *Blood tests* may show hypercholesterolemia, anemia, and occasionally, myocardial biomarker elevation. Ongoing research is focusing on blood markers for AD.

11.2.1.6 Therapy

Pharmacological measures (recommended in all patients) include *supportive measures* (blood transfusion, O_2, morphine, etc.) and IV β-blockers (Esmolol, Labetalol), to slow down hematoma progression by decreasing the LV contractility and HR (HR >60 bpm and systolic BP >100 mmHg must be preserved, to avoid organ hypoperfusion). β-blocker therapy is continued after discharge; *Surgery* may be indicated *emergently,* in type A AD, (the great majority of cases), as well as in AD complicating Marfan's disease; or *electively,* in type B AD where AD progression, critical organ ischemia, or intractable pain persist despite conservative therapy. The affected segment is resected under cardiopulmonary bypass, with reconnection of the healthy extremities by a Dacron tube. To avoid brain hypoxia, retrograde cerebral perfusion is used. The procedure consists in pumping blood to the brain through the SVC and is termed "retrograde," as a *vein* is used for *arterial* perfusion. The main complication is paraplegia, mainly seen with type B AD, due to inadvertent surgical lesion of the spinal vessels. *Percutaneous techniques* are indicated in case of ischemia by vascular compression or for unstable type B AD. The techniques include placement of endovascular stent-grafts across the primary entry tears (to seal them off, and thus decompress the false lumen); preliminary data indicate that this approach may also be preferable in stable type B AD, as compared to best medical therapy. Ischemia complicating aortic dissection may be treated in the same manner, or by balloon fenestration, i.e., creation of an exit portal, to decompress the false lumen.

11.2.2 Aortic Aneurysm

11.2.2.1 Definition and Prevalence

Aortic aneurysm (AA) is a dilatation of an aortic segment, involving all three wall layers (intima, media, and serosa), as opposed to a pseudoaneurysm, which is due to rupture of the intima and media, with preservation of the serosa, or to rupture of all three layers, sealed by a clot. The widest diameter of AA is by at least 50% larger than that of the healthy segment preceding it. In the infrarenal aorta, a diameter >3 cm equivalates to AA. AA may be thoracic, abdominal (AAA, or "triple A"), or thoraco-abdominal; 95% of cases involve the infrarenal segment (as opposed to AD, which in 90% of cases involves the *ascending* aorta). The proclivity of the abdominal aorta for aneurysm formation is explained by a *paucity of elastin* in that segment (exposing the aortic wall to trauma during systole) and by the *absence of vasa vasorum,* which, in other aortic segments, increase wall resistance by nutrient supply and by mechanical "anchoring" of the intima to the other wall layers. AA is a form of pathologic vascular remodeling caused by atherosclerosis, at least in its most frequent location, the abdominal aorta; thus, the risk factors for AA coincide with those of atherosclerosis. The role of atherosclerosis in ascending AA is less clear. Additional risk factors include Marfan's disease; bicuspid AV (occasionally associating stress-related aortic root dilatation); severe AI, which increases LV contractility; and aortitis (syphilis, rheumatic disease, etc.). Variants in the chromosomal region 9p21 appear associated to a higher risk of AAA. Finally, the more dilated the aortic

segment, the greater the wall tension, and the greater the tendency toward further dilatation; in this sense, the presence of AA is a "risk factor" for its own progression. The real *incidence* of AA is unknown, as many small AA may go undetected.

11.2.2.2 Diagnosis

AA is most frequently asymptomatic, but may cause nonspecific abdominal pain or compression symptoms (back pain, acute renal failure, renovascular HTN, etc.). The physical examination reveals a pulsatile abdominal mass, occasionally associating a murmur (due to local flow turbulence). The workup includes sonography, CT, or MRI. As TTE only visualizes the first centimeters of the ascending aorta, TEE is required with AA involving the arch or the descending aorta. The main complication is rupture, manifesting as excruciating pain and hemorrhagic shock (hypotension, cold extremities, acute renal failure, clammy skin, etc.). Rarely, a thrombus formed inside the AA may rupture and cause embolism, mainly to the kidneys or to the lower limbs.

11.2.2.3 Therapy

Therapy depends on the site and size of the aneurysm: AA with a diameter <5.5 cm and not compressing the neighboring organs may be treated conservatively (an important option in elderly, high-risk patients). Initial follow-up is carried out every 6 months, and later on annually, if AA enlargement is absent or slow. Surgery is indicated when AA diameter increases by >1 cm/year, or if it reaches 5.5 cm. As with AD, the main complication of surgery is paraplegia. For follow-up, same-technique images should be compared (cross-modality comparison may cause false conclusions as to AA progression). *Pharmacological therapy* includes risk factor management; Doxycillin may be useful for primary or secondary prevention, by inhibition of enzymes that degrade the vessel wall. *Surgical treatment* consists in AA resection and replacing by a synthetic material prosthesis. With AA involving the ascending aorta and/or the arch, surgery requires cardiopulmonary bypass; with AAA, this is not obligatory, but is often used (allowing proper perfusion of the infraaneurysm territory). *Percutaneous treatment* consists in insertion of a synthetic conduit into the affected segment, to reduce wall tension and shearing forces and halt the self-maintained disease progression. Thrombosis and, ultimately, fibrosis occur between the conduit and the AA wall. AA rupture is generally treated surgically, but catheter techniques are emerging in this setting as well.

11.2.3 Aortitis

Aortitis can be infectious, autoimmune, or idiopathic. Aortitis frequently extends to the aortic branches. The typical *manifestations* include weak or absent pulses, often in a nonsymmetrical pattern, and decreased perfusion in the involved territories. Systemic signs reflect the underlying condition. Aortitis is discussed under "vasculitis."

11.2.4 Diseases of the Large Branches of the Aorta

11.2.4.1 Cerebral Vascular Accident

Cerebral vascular accident (CVA) (synonyms: *stroke, ictus*, "*brain attack*," or, underscoring the similarity with cardiac events, "*acute cerebral ischemia*") is defined as sudden, focal interruption of cerebral blood flow, with secondary neurologic deficit. CVA can be ischemic, hemorrhagic, or combined (hemorrhagic transformation of ischemic CVA by bleeding into the necrotic tissue; vessel compression by cerebral hematoma). Occasionally, imaging demonstrates neither ischemia, nor bleeding. This is termed "cryptogenic CVA," believed to be due to a thrombus or embolus that underwent spontaneous fibrinolysis, or to an episode of prolonged cerebral vasoconstriction or hypotension. CVA is the third cause of mortality worldwide.

Ischemic CVA

Etiology and classification: Ischemia accounts for 80% of CVA and is most often due to occlusion of small, deep cortical arteries by microatheroma and lipohyalinosis (lacunar infarction) or to cardiogenic

embolism. Other causes include arterial thrombosis in situ; artery-to-artery embolism (from the carotids or large cerebral arteries); or *other*, less frequent conditions: cerebral artery dissection (local or propagated from the aorta); aortitis; embolization of tumor, vegetation, amniotic fluid, or man-made materials; cerebral vein thrombosis, causing CVA with an especially high tendency to hemorrhagic transformation; and sustained hypotension (shock), especially affecting watershed areas. According to its *evolution time frame*, ischemic CVA is classified as TIA (*spontaneously abating within 24 h*), reversible ischemic neurologic deficit (24–72 h), or full-blown CVA (>72 h). The classical definition of TIA appears completely arbitrary, as in fact, up to 50% of episodes thus classified clinically are actually associated to permanent injury demonstrated by MRI.

Risk factors for ischemic CVA include: *a past personal history of CVA; atherosclerosis* or risk factors for this condition: Systemic atherosclerosis can be a marker for similar lesions in the cerebral arteries, while plaque in the ascending aorta, the aortic arch, or the carotid, or the vertebral arteries may actually function as a source of emboli. Occasionally, the embolic event is precipitated by aortic cannulation, cardiopulmonary bypass, or IABP insertion. Coronary atherosclerosis can cause MI and LV aneurysm formation, a cardiac source of emboli; *low weight at birth; sustained hypotension (shock); coagulation abnormalities* (increased levels of coagulation factor VIII "von Willebrand" might be especially important); *intracardiac masses*, including *tumor* (most frequently, myxoma), *vegetation, mitral annulus calcification* (lower risk) or (most frequently) *thrombus*. Risk factors for cardiac thrombus include: AF or flutter, especially if associated to MS (although, in absolute numbers, most cases of cardiogenic stroke are due to nonvalvular AF); mechanical valve prostheses; LV aneurysm; RA/RV thrombus formed in situ (e.g., on a pacemaker electrode), or migrated from a distance (DVT), in the presence of PFO or ASD; and VSD with Eisenmenger's complex. A lower risk of CVA is associated with PFO in the absence of RA pathology; interatrial septal aneurysm; and LA "smoke" (a whitish hue on the B-mode echocardiogram, corresponding to increased blood viscosity). LA "smoke" is most frequently associated with AF, MS, or LA enlargement. The diagnosis of "smoke" requires meticulous calibration of the echo machine; *other vascular problems:* sickle cell anemia (embolism with RBC aggregates); some types of migraine (migraine may be a risk factor for stroke in women <45, especially in the instance of concurrent cigarette and hormonal contraception use); *toxic effect of drugs:* cocaine, heroin, or amphetamine abuse, causing cerebral and coronary vasoconstriction or vasculitis; alcohol abuse (while 1–2 drinks a day may have a protective effect, ≥3 drinks a day represent a risk factor for CVA), causing direct damage, as well as HTN, AF, and hypercoagulability. *HRT* is a risk factor for CAD, stroke, thrombosis, PE, and breast cancer. The risk applies equally to estrogen/progesterone and to unopposed estrogen preparations. The risk of adverse effects does not apply across the board (see below).

Increased cardiovascular risk with HRT is not definitely proven in

- Women aged 50–59, and possibly within 5 years of menopause onset (HRT may actually decrease the risk)
- Nonequine-derived sources of estrogen (e.g., bioidentical hormone replacement, BHRT)
- Transdermal, rather than oral preparations (the latter undergo hepatic transformation to thrombogenic compounds)

There is an important *connection between CVA and acute MI.* Within 1 month of acute MI, approximately 2–3% of patients sustain an embolic CVA, due to AF or LV aneurysm. Additional patients suffer iatrogenic CVA, either ischemic (plaque dislodgement at aortic cannulation for PCI), or hemorrhagic, due to fibrinolytic and/or antithrombotic medication. Conversely, approximately 3% of CVA patients have concomitant MI, making EKG an integral part of the initial evaluation of a CVA patient. In addition to the signs of ischemia, the EKG may also show AF, possibly responsible for the CVA.

Ischemic CVA: pathogenesis. Ischemic CVA mainly involves the internal carotid and vertebral arteries, and the circle of Willis (carotid/vertebral anastomoses at the base of the brain), or their small branches. The "watershed areas," lying in the "no man's land" between the terminal branches of the carotid and vertebral arteries are especially sensitive to ischemia, in case of hypotension. The "ischemic cascade" is triggered

as early as 60–90 s after ischemia onset. Irreversible brain damage is caused by the release of glutamate from the neurons, by free radical and inflammatory mediator formation, and by blood-brain barrier effraction, allowing further ingress of toxins into the brain tissue. Occasional areas of reversible cerebral damage (similar to myocardial stunning or hibernation) are termed "ischemic penumbra."

Ischemic CVA: Symptoms and signs include manifestations of underlying conditions; neurological signs, focal or global; systemic signs associated to CVA, mainly in its acute phase; and signs of meningeal irritation and cerebral edema. *Underlying conditions* mainly include AF and atherosclerosis, evident as carotid bruits (the longer the bruit, the more severe the stenosis, but bruits are absent with complete occlusion), renal artery bruits, etc.; *Neurological signs* consist in decreased motor and/or sensory function (numbness, diminished tactile, or vibratory perception; vision, hearing, taste, smell, and balance disturbances), as well as severe dizziness, disturbance of behavior and thought, etc. Loss of consciousness and convulsions are more frequent with hemorrhagic CVA. These symptoms have typically a very rapid onset (seconds or minutes).

Nausea, vomiting, headache, and changes in the level of consciousness are more common in hemorrhagic strokes, but the specificity is low. Brain imaging is key for establishing the candidacy to thrombolysis.

The focal signs are contralateral to the cerebral lesion. *Babinski's sign* (extension, rather than flexion of the great toe on the affected side, on mild scratching of the lateral border of the sole with a blunt object) is typically noted. Numerous other neurological signs assess the tactile or vibratory perception, vision, hearing, etc. *Systemic signs* include loss of consciousness, vomiting, behavioral disturbances, etc. *Signs of meningeal irritation and cerebral edema* include: severe headache and nuchal rigidity (*Kernig's sign* and *Brudzinski's signs,* both with a low specificity for meningeal irritation). The *workup of the CVA patient* is reviewed in Table 11.2.

Ischemic CVA: TIA. Typical manifestations include: temporary vision loss *(amaurosis fugax),* aphasia,

Table 11.2 CVA workup: aims and modalities

Stage	Study	Implications
Acute	CT[a] or MRI[b]	Consider thrombolytic therapy in ischemic CVA; evaluate for complications (mainly cerebral edema, compression, or herniation)
	Spinal tap[c]	Bloody fluid confirms the hemorrhagic nature of CVA and contraindicates thrombolysis
Beyond acute	Nuclear techniques (SPECT, PET)	Evaluate brain tissue viability (ischemic penumbra) after the acute phase, to establish candidacy to surgical or percutaneous revascularization
	Arteriography	Assess candidacy for, and carry out intra-arterial thrombolysis or angioplasty
	Carotid duplex[d], transcranial Doppler	Risk stratification for recurrent CVA; decision regarding revascularization for secondary prevention
	Echocardiography[e]	Thrombus and/or potentially thrombogenic lesions (LA dilatation, LA "smoke," MS, PFO, LV aneurysm) mandate anticoagulation
	EKG[f]	AF or flutter mandate anticoagulation
	Hematological evaluation	Treatment of hypercoagulability syndromes

[a]CT does not detect ischemic CVA within the first 6–12 h, and may require as much as 24–48 h for complete visualization of the infarcted area; a small hemorrhagic CVA can occasionally be missed, with possible catastrophic consequences, if thrombolysis is used

[b]MRI has greater sensitivity in the acute phase, but is more time-intensive than CT

[c]Indicated if suspicion of hemorrhagic CVA persists, despite negative CT results

[d]Duplex ultrasonography incorporates two Doppler modalities of vascular investigation, i.e., pulsed-wave and color-Doppler display of hemodynamics. It is applicable to arteries and veins alike. For instance, for the carotid arteries, the peak systolic, end-diastolic, and the ratio between the peak systolic velocities in the internal vs. the common carotid arteries are measured

[e]TEE is required to visualize the most frequent cardiac sources of embolus, i.e., the LA appendage and the aortic arch. An empty LA appendage may still be the culprit, if the clot has completely migrated. Conversely, a clot in the heart cavities may be an unrelated, incidental finding. The probability is higher with "fresh" (inhomogeneous texture, mobile parts on its surface) or freely floating thrombi in the LV or LA

[f]Holter or other monitoring techniques may be used as needed

hemiparesis, paresthesia, etc. On presentation, any stroke is treated as full-blown CVA, since awaiting spontaneous recovery would cause missing the window of opportunity for thrombolysis, in suitable candidates. Thus, some of the stroke episodes treated with thrombolytics might in fact have evolved naturally as TIAs. Practically, however, the risk of superfluous thrombolytic therapy is low, as up to 80% of TIA subside within the first hour; the briefer the episode, the lower the risk of future full-blown CVA; overall, approximately one third of TIA patients will sustain full-blown CVA in the future. The ABCD score can predict likelihood of subsequent stroke and is calculated based on *age* ≥60 years; *BP* ≥140/90 mmHg; the nature of *clinical findings* (muscle weakness, speech disturbances); *diabetes;* attack *duration* ≥60 min. Scores of 1–3, 4–5, and 6–7 are considered low, moderate, and high, respectively. A high risk indicates a probability of CVA of approximately 8% at 2 days, and 12% at 7 days.

Ischemic CVA Management: Primary prevention includes *correction of atherosclerosis risk factors;* administration of *Aspirin* 75–100 mg/q.d. has not been found effective in primary prevention of stroke, but may be considered in high-risk patients; *oral anticoagulation* (Warfarin, Acenocoumarol) is recommended for AF (Chap. 6); mechanical valvular prosthesis (Chap. 5); LA/LV thrombus; and (optionally) in patients with LA "smoke" (Target INR 2.5–3.5, average 3). In all groups, a past history of embolism requires consideration of the higher INR target or addition of low-dose Aspirin. In the absence of AF, carotid stenosis in itself is not an indication for anticoagulation; *proper hydration* in sickle cell anemia patients, to avoid vaso-occlusive episodes; *avoidance of* alcohol in excess, smoking, recreational drugs, and of HRT in women at risk; *treatment of cerebral AV malformations;* interventional management of "significant" (>75%) carotid stenosis, by carotid endarterectomy (surgical removal of the plaque-bearing endothelium), or carotid angioplasty. Either approach uses distal protection devices, to avoid distal plaque embolization.

Therapy: The treatment of ischemic CVA includes *general support measures,* and as indicated, BP management, and revascularization therapy. The JUPITER trial has found a 48% relative risk reduction for total stroke in Rosuvastatin-treated in patients with normal cholesterol levels but elevated CRP. *BP management:* Drastic BP reduction may extend the area of ischemic CVA. BP is kept <180/110 mmHg in thrombolysis candidates and <220/120 mmHg otherwise. *Thrombolysis* with tPA (0.9 mg/kg, not to exceed 100 mg, 10% as a bolus over the first minute; the remainder is given over 1 h) is indicated in CT or MRI-confirmed ischemic CVA, within 4.5 h of onset and associating nontrivial, persistent neurological signs. The contraindications for thrombolytic therapy are similar, but not identical to those observed in the MI patient (Table 11.3 and Chap. 2);

most of the differences simply reflect the design of the clinical trials upon which the indications are based. In patients with acute ischemic stroke lasting ≤6 h and who are either ineligible for or have failed IV thrombolysis, intra-arterial thrombolysis can be considered. Controlled hypothermia (cold saline infusions) and controlled barbiturate coma reduce metabolism and function as *neuroprotective therapy.*

There is increasing evidence that a TIA should be treated with the same aggressiveness as a full-blown CVA, as up to 15% of patients will sustain a stroke within 3 months, with half the cases occurring within the first 48 h.

Primary angioplasty for ischemic stroke via femoral access is an evolving technique. A corkscrew-like device is used to "catch" the clot and remove it, thus avoiding distal embolization. This approach is effective as late as 8 h after symptom onset, substantially expanding the window of opportunity for revascularization.

Table 11.3 Contraindications to IV fibrinolytic therapy: a comparison between MI and CVA

Condition	MI[a]	CVA
CNS conditions		
Ischemic stroke	Past 6 months; TIA within the past 6 months	Past 3 months
Seizure with postictal sequelae; multilobar infarction by CT[b]	Not explicitly mentioned	Contraindicated
Major trauma	Past 3 weeks	Past 3 months
Major surgery	Past 3 weeks	Past 14 days
High risk of hemorrhage		
Active bleeding	Any	Any
Oral anticoagulant therapy	Relative contraindication; no INR values mentioned	INR ≤1.7
Noncompressible vascular punctures	Any	Past 7 days
Gastrointestinal bleeding	Past month	Past 21 days
Heparin	N/A	Normal aPTT
Platelet count	N/A	<100,000 mm^3
Urinary bleeding	N/A	Past 21 days
HTN	Refractory HTN	Systolic <185 mmHg and diastolic <110 mmHg
MI	N/A	Past 3 months
Blood glucose	N/A	<50 mg/dL (2.7 mmol/L)

[a]The contraindications in patients with PE are very similar. Thrombolytic therapy appears safe and effective in catheterization-related stroke
[b]Hypodensity in >1/3 of a cerebral hemisphere

Table 11.4 Secondary prevention of ischemic stroke

Indication	Oral anticoagulants	Antiaggregants
Noncardioembolic stroke/TIA		
	Not recommended	Aspirin 50–100 mg *or* Aspirin 25 mg+ extended-release Dipyridamole (200 mg) *or* Clopidogrel 75 mg
Cardioembolic stroke/TIA and either of the conditions below		
AF	First-line therapy; INR 2.5–3.5, average 3	Aspirin 75–325 mg, if anticoagulants are contraindicated
Aortic atherosclerosis, nonmobile plaque	Not recommended	Aspirin 75–325 mg
Aortic atherosclerosis, mobile plaque in arch	First-line therapy; INR 2.5–3.5, average 3	Aspirin 75–325 mg, if anticoagulants are contraindicated
PFO	Not recommended	Aspirin 75–325 mg
MVP, MV strands	Not recommended	Aspirin 75–325 mg

This technique is also feasible in patients with contraindications for thrombolysis. *Control of hyperglycemia and of fever* (Insulin, Paracetamol) is important in both ischemic and hemorrhagic stroke. Hypoglycemic episodes, often associated with tight glucose control, are poorly tolerated and should be avoided.

Secondary prevention includes pharmacological (Table 11.4) and interventional measures. Surgery and angioplasty are unavailable for the vertebral arteries.

Interventional measures: Carotid endarterectomy is indicated in patients with significant (>75%) carotid stenosis. The procedure is *contraindicated* in patients with total carotid occlusion and/or a history of severe CVA in the affected carotid territory (no viable brain tissue left to rescue from jeopardy). While intracranial plaque extension has classically been a contraindication for angioplasty, PCI is now available in select centers, for symptomatic intracranial stenosis >70%. Endarterectomy is a major intervention, and careful selection of candidates is important. This is especially evident in the numerous patients simultaneously suffering from myocardial ischemia. Patients with >75% carotid stenosis (especially if ≥65 years of age) are at increased risk of CVA after coronary bypass. This mandates a Duplex study before elective CABG. Significant carotid stenosis mandates endarterectomy before bypass (at the same sitting, or more commonly, a few days before). New research indicates the feasibility of carotid artery stenting followed immediately by on-pump CABG. Performing CABG first is not an option. *Technique:* The carotid artery is clamped at both ends, usually with cerebral perfusion by temporary shunt.

The artery is then incised lengthwise, cleaned of plaque, and sutured. The procedure can be carried out under general or local anesthesia, the latter allowing real-time neurological assessment, to detect intraoperative CVA (by atherosclerotic debris embolization or clamping-related hypoxia; the risk is of approximately 3%). The patient's state of consciousness, ability to speak, handgrip strength, etc., are assessed by verbal communication. With general anesthesia, this assessment is performed by EEG or by transcranial Doppler. *The complications* of carotid endarterectomy include CVA; laryngeal compression by a postoperative hematoma, causing asphyxia; lingual nerve damage, with involuntary tongue twitching; and rarely, the *cerebral hyperperfusion syndrome,* manifesting as ipsilateral headache, seizure, and focal neurological symptoms.

Rehabilitation post-CVA is dictated by the type and severity of sequellae and generally includes: physiotherapy, speech therapy, treatment of depression, pain therapy, treatment of urinary and/or fecal incontinence, etc. *Occupational therapy* capitalizes on the physical, psychological, and social value of structured activity and ranges from simply "re-learning the business of living" (walking, personal grooming, etc.) to full vocational retraining, with a strong accent on the person's talents and skills.

Hemorrhagic CVA

Hemorrhagic CVA accounts for 20% of cases of stroke. **Risk factors** include **coagulation defects,** often iatrogenic; *disruption of blood vessel integrity,* acquired (related to age, substance abuse, e.g., amphetamine, cocaine, cranial trauma, etc.) or inborn (AV malformations, aneurysm, or amyloid vasculopathy). *Cerebral AV malformations* are direct connections between the cerebral arteries and veins, bypassing the capillary bed. They are generally congenital and can be limited to the brain or involve additional territories, occasionally as part of complex congenital syndromes. AV malformations may cause hydrocephalus manifesting as headaches, vomiting, nausea, papilledema, sleepiness, coma, gait instability, urinary incontinence, dementia, etc. AV malformations are diagnosed by CT, MRI, or brain angiography ("plate of noodles" aspect). There is no consensus concerning routine investigation in asymptomatic patients at risk (e.g., complex congenital syndromes), as many cases may remain asymptomatic lifelong, and the surgical procedure itself is not free of risk. Moreover, rupture does not always involve the largest malformations. *Cerebral ("berry") aneurysms* are congenital or acquired, localized vascular dilatations, with a very high mortality (70–90%). They are most frequently encountered in patients with aortic coarctation, polycystic renal disease, and in conjunctive tissue diseases (Marfan or Ehlers–Danlos syndrome). HTN is frequently associated. The clinical signs are similar to those of AV malformations, but the tendency to bleed is much higher. Routine investigation for possible cerebral aneurysms is mandatory in patients at risk. *Amyloid vasculopathy* is encountered in several chronic diseases (multiple myeloma, chronic inflammation), as well as in the healthy elderly. It fragilizes the blood vessels and increases their tendency to bleed and might be involved in the genesis of Alzheimer's disease. Unfortunately, there is no effective preventive strategy. *Hemorrhagic transformation* is seen in approximately 25% of patients with ischemic CVA, more frequently in the presence of postictal HTN. It generally occurs within 6–48 h of the initial event, when spontaneous or pharmacological thrombolysis restores blood flow into the necrotic mass. Hemorrhagic transformation is most often asymptomatic.

Hemorrhagic CVA: Pathogenesis. Hemorrhagic CVA damages the brain by the toxic effect of blood, as well as by compression of the cerebral tissue and neighboring vessels by the associated hematoma. Blood diffusion in the cerebral tissue causes meningeal irritation and cerebral edema. According to the site of bleeding, hemorrhagic CVA is classified as *intraaxial* (intraparenchymatous, i.e., involving the brain tissue, or intraventricular), or *extraaxial,* including the following locations: *epidural,* between the skull and the dura mater; *subdural,* between the dura and the pia mater; and *subarachnoid,* between the pia and the brain.

Hemorrhagic CVA: Clinical manifestations: see "Ischemic CVA." *Epidural and subdural hematoma* are most frequently traumatic, but can occur spontaneously, in patients with brain atrophy (the elderly, alcoholics, etc.), and are favored by antithrombotic therapy. Small hematomas may resolve spontaneously. *Subarachnoid hemorrhage* most frequently results from cerebral aneurysm rupture, and less often, from trauma. Symptoms of SAH include rapid onset, excruciating ("thunderclap") headache, vomiting, confusion, fluctuating levels of consciousness, and occasionally seizures. The diagnosis is confirmed by CT, or occasionally by lumbar puncture (yielding bloody fluid).

Hemorrhagic CVA: Management. Primary prevention refers to risk factor correction. Cerebral aneurysms and AV malformations (causing 4% of all hemorrhagic CVA) must be treated. In patients under oral anticoagulation, the INR must be monitored (risk of bleeding with values >5). Amphetamines (recreational or for weight loss) and cocaine must be avoided. *Therapy* includes general life-support measures, as needed; treatment of underlying disorders (HTN crisis, hypocoagulability, etc.); and surgical drainage, in suitable candidates. *Management of HTN crisis* follows more drastic guidelines than those of ischemic CVA. Systolic BP must be kept <180 mmHg, and in case of increased intracranial pressure, ≤160 mmHg. *Iatrogenic hypocoagulability:* See Chap. 2. Of note, as tPA (the only agent approved for CVA) induces little systemic fibrinolysis and has a short half-life (5 min), simply stopping the infusion usually suffices to revert the thrombolytic effect. Thrombolysis reversal is a difficult decision, as symptom escalation may actually represent extension of ischemia. *Noniatrogenic coagulopathy* is treated according to the etiology. AV malformations or aneurysms are resected *surgically* or with a *"gamma knife"* (gamma irradiation of the exact site of the tumor, sparing the healthy tissues). This "radiosurgical" method is generally reserved for inoperable cases, as *complete closure* may evolve over up to 3 years, and fails to occur at all in 10% of cases. Another alternative is embolization of the diseased vessel, usually as an adjunct to radiosurgical therapy. *Intracranial hypertension* manifests as severe headache, vision disturbance, disorientation, vomiting, and cognitive disturbances. It is diagnosed by lumbar puncture, to measure cerebrospinal fluid pressure; by funduscopy, revealing papilledema; and by CT or MRI. *Therapy* includes *elevating the head* end of the bed to 30°, to counteract gravitation and allow drainage of spinal fluid. This measure is indicated in hemorrhagic CVA, but contraindicated in ischemic CVA, where the horizontal position favors blood flow to the brain; *analgesia and sedation*; *osmotic diuretics:* IV Mannitol (0.1 g/kg bolus, followed by 0.25 g/kg q 6 h, with a target serum osmolality of 300–310 mOsm/L; normal 285–295 mOsm/L), to diminish cerebral edema; *spinal fluid drainage* (spinal tap); *neuromuscular blockade,* consisting in anesthesia and mechanical hyperventilation, to decrease blood CO_2 pressure to approximately 25–30 mmHg (normal 35–45mmHg); this induces cerebral vasoconstriction and diminishes edema; and *controlled barbiturate coma,* using large doses of IV barbiturates to decrease brain metabolism and intracranial HTN. Hypotension can further compromise brain perfusion and must be avoided; IV recombinant factor VII might be helpful at ≤4 h after onset of intraaxial hemorrhage (inconclusive data). *Other measures* include aggressive treatment of fever and hyperglycemia (Tylenol, Insulin), since both can aggravate prognosis.

Epidural and subdural hematoma: Small hematomas may resolve spontaneously, while larger, compressive hematomas require surgical drainage. Treatment is surgical or percutaneous ("coiling"). Endovascular coil occlusion is appropriate for both ruptured and at-risk unruptured cerebral aneurysms.

Subarachnoid hemorrhage requires patient stabilization, treatment of cerebral edema, and surgical or percutaneous treatment of bleeding cerebral aneurysm. *Neuroprotective therapy for hemorrhagic CVA:* see Sect. 11.2.4.1.1.

11.2.4.2 The Subclavian Steal Syndrome

The subclavian steal syndrome consists in compensation of decreased subclavian flow, by flow diversion from other arteries, mainly the vertebral, carotid, or LIMA/RIMA. This syndrome is seen in occasional patients with ostial stenosis of the subclavian artery (most often, on the left side) or with a Blalock–Taussig shunt. *The clinical picture* includes *subclavian ischemia* (pain on arm raising) and *ischemia in the blood-deprived territories:* TIA-

like symptoms (mainly dizziness, syncope, dysarthria, and/or vision disturbances); *anginal pain* in patients after CABG using LIMA or RIMA, raising the suspicion of graft occlusion; and a marked (>45 mmHg) BP discordance between the two arms. *Workup:* Duplex, angio-CT/MRI, or invasive angiography show decreased subclavian flow and flow reversal in the vertebral arteries. Most patients are asymptomatic or mildly symptomatic, the only therapy consisting in avoidance of the trigger situations. More severe cases require subclavian endarterectomy; angioplasty and stenting; or (very rarely nowadays) surgical bypass between the carotid artery and the poststenotic subclavian artery.

11.2.4.3 The Thoracic Outlet Syndrome

The thoracic outlet syndrome consists in compression of the brachiocephalic plexus or of the subclavian artery and vein at the level of the thoracic outlet. The compression may be positional (on arm movement, with mobilization of the clavicle) or static (due to muscular hypertrophy). The treatment is conservative (cortisone, occasionally Botox injections), or surgical. DVT and PE are possible. The Paget–von Schroetter syndrome, also termed "effort-induced thrombosis," consists in upper limb DVT after strenuous exercise.

11.2.4.4 Ischemia of the Abdominal Organs

Ischemia of the Liver and Biliary Tract

The dual hepatic blood supply (from the hepatic artery and the portal vein) only allows hepatic ischemia to occur in exceptional circumstances, including *shock; decreased oxygen saturation* of the circulating blood; *increased metabolism* (e.g., sepsis); *vascular trauma* (motor vehicle accidents, surgical trauma, etc.); *portal vein thrombosis,* most frequently complicating sickle cell anemia; or *intrahepatic microvasculopathy* (hepatic graft rejection). The resulting damage is termed *ischemic hepatitis* (a misnomer, since the microscopic aspect of hepatitis is different). This is generally reversible on restoration of hepatic blood flow; however, the prognosis is severe with intractable underlying disorders, as well as in the fulminant form, more frequent with chronic liver disease (especially cirrhosis). *The clinical picture* reflects the underlying disease, as well as the hepatic damage. The latter mainly manifests as nausea, vomiting, and RUQ pain (capsule stretching by the enlarged hepatic parenchyma). *The workup* demonstrates abnormal LFT, both parenchymal and cholestatic; a prolonged INR; and, most frequently, portal vein thrombosis on the imaging tests. *The treatment* is nonspecific and addresses the underlying diseases.

Biliary Duct Ischemia

Biliary duct ischemia may result from surgery, radiotherapy, liver transplant, or arterial thrombosis. Chronic wall edema is followed by duct fibrosis, causing biliary strictures and cholestasis (icterus; pruritus; increased alkaline phosphatase, GGT, and bilirubin levels; stool discoloration; and steatorrhea). *The diagnosis* is established by imaging methods. *The treatment* consists in percutaneous or (rarely today) surgical relief of the stricture.

Splenic Infarction

Splenic infarction is observed in occasional patients with *hematological conditions:* sickle cell anemia, hypercoagulability, leukemia, or lymphoma (insufficient angiogenesis in face of abnormal parenchymal growth); *cardiovascular diseases:* AF, intraventricular thrombus, valvular prosthesis, SBE (septic embolism); *trauma* (road accidents, complications of surgery); or *splenic vein thrombosis.* Approximately one third of patients are asymptomatic, while others may complain of LUQ pain, occasionally irradiated to the left shoulder; fever; chills; and vomiting. Splenomegaly is often associated. The diagnosis is established based on the assessment of the risk factors and the clinical picture and confirmed by imaging tests. Most cases are *treated* conservatively; splenectomy is occasionally necessary and may be complicated by sepsis.

Pancreatic Ischemia

Pancreatic ischemia is seen in rare cases of shock, surgical trauma, or after pancreas transplant (either perioperatively, or with graft rejection). *The symptoms* include extremely severe epigastric pain, nausea, and

vomiting – a picture identical to that of nonischemic pancreatitis and considerably confusing the diagnosis. *The lab tests* mainly show increased levels of pancreatic amylase and lipase. The treatment includes life-sustaining measures (patients are often in shock); NPO orders; occasionally, drainage of stomach fluid by nasogastric tube; and antibiotics. Surgery may be required in intractable cases to remove the necrotic debris of the pancreas.

Mesenteric Ischemia

Mesenteric ischemia (ME) can result from atherosclerosis, embolism, mesenteric vein thrombosis, or non-occlusive ischemia, in patients with shock; after use of vasoconstrictors (e.g., recreational cocaine, Adrenalin for CPR, etc.); and after recent surgery for aortic coarctation or for MI itself. Occlusive ME is relatively infrequent, due to the well-developed anastomotic system between the mesenteric artery branches. *The clinical picture* is different in chronic and acute cases. *Acute cases* manifest as excruciating abdominal pain (e.g., in a patient with AF or recent aortic catheterization), in discordance with the paucity of initial physical signs. Paralytic ileus, peritoneal irritation, and septic shock ensue. *Chronic cases* may manifest as postprandial abdominal pain ("intestinal angina"), or as pain unassociated to meals. Objective signs are scarce initially, but fecal bleeding is possible. *The workup* demonstrates vascular obstructions, with the exception of patients with shock-related ischemia. *Mesenteric arteriography* is the gold-standard test, identifying the culprit lesion. Noninvasive imaging by *CT or MRI* can demonstrate intestinal wall thickening, due to edema; mesenteric thickening; intestinal dilatation; fluid effusion between the mesenteric folds; areas of intestinal necrosis and perforation; atherosclerosis and thrombosis of the large-caliber mesenteric arteries; and, in advanced disease, gas bubbles in the intestinal wall or in the portal vein, due to bacterial activity, a poor prognostic sign; *Duplex* displays arterial anatomy and flow and is mainly useful in chronic cases (acute gas accumulation may prevent optimal ultrasound imaging); *Plain abdominal X-ray* shows nonspecific intestinal dilatation. *Blood tests* are nonspecific and mainly demonstrate increased leukocyte counts and high levels of lactic acid and amylase. Emergency *exploratory laparotomy* may be necessary in acute cases.

The therapy of *occlusive MI* consists in arterial revascularization, usually by a combined surgical and angioplastic approach, the latter considerably shortening the overall procedure time. Surgery is performed in two steps, first to remove the clearly necrotic areas, and 24–48 h later, to assess recovery of areas of borderline viability. *Nonocclusive* MI may respond to therapy of shock and to vasodilators. *The prognosis* of the *acute form* is extremely severe, with 100% mortality if untreated, and >60% mortality if treated. Demise is caused by a combination of septic and hypovolemic shock (caused by fluid storage in the third space), with the severe pain a contributing factor. The paucity of early clinical signs (when therapy has better results) delays the diagnosis and mandates a high index of suspicion. The prognosis is better in the *chronic form,* which may improve spontaneously due to collateral circulation, or require elective surgery.

Renal Ischemia

Renal artery stenosis (RAS) may be caused by *fibrodysplasia* (fibrotic stenosis of one or both renal arteries), mainly in Caucasian females aged 30–40, or by *atherosclerosis,* mainly in patients >50 years of age. Less frequent causes include congenital RAS, radiotherapy, and renal artery graft stenosis. The main pathophysiologic consequences of RAS include renovascular HTN (approximately 1% of all HTN) and chronic renal failure. *The clinical picture* is that of abrupt onset or aggravation of HTN and/or renal failure. Occasionally, the suspicion is raised by onset/aggravation of renal failure under ACEI or ARB treatment (see below). A bruit can be auscultated over the anterior abdomen, lateral of the umbilical area, or in the corresponding area on the back. The bruit corresponds to turbulent renal artery flow; it may be absent in up to 50% of patients, and conversely, a similar bruit may be heard in healthy individuals, especially if young and thin. *Workup: Sonography* is the procedure of choice, showing the stenosis and the turbulent blood flow. Optimal preparation (NPO for 8–12 h preprocedure) is essential, to avoid ultrasound masking by intestinal gas. *(Angio-) CT or MRI* may also demonstrate RAS, although MRI can occasionally miss fibrodysplasia. *Nuclear scan* is used to assess renal function, as reflected by urinary radiotracer elimination. Renal failure manifests as decreased tracer uptake,

due to decreased urinary volume, renal perfusion, or both. Decreased perfusion is seen in many renal diseases, and the usual nuclear scan cannot assess the possible contribution of RAS. This aspect is addressed by demonstrating decreased tracer uptake after Captopril administration. The individual contribution of each kidney to the global renal function and the chance of reversibility of renal failure under treatment are also assessed. *Blood tests* mainly include the "Captopril test", similar in principle to its nuclear correspondent. The element of interest is plasma renin activity, a surrogate for renin levels, very difficult to determine as such. Captopril administration partly counteracts renin effects, and therefore, stimulates renin secretion. A positive test (inordinately high plasma renin activity under Captopril) is an indication for renal angiography. *Renal angiography* has both a diagnostic and a therapeutic application (angioplasty). Renal angiogram (especially angio-CT/MRI) is also justified as a first-choice test, forgoing the other tests.

The medical treatment of RAS consists in management of atherosclerosis risk factors, renal failure, and renovascular HTN. Somewhat paradoxically, ACEI under creatinine follow-up are the treatment of choice for unilateral renovascular HTN (contraindicated in bilateral RAS). Renovascular HTN is usually resistant to medical therapy and requires combined therapy. *Surgical treatment* includes renal artery grafting (with a synthetic conduit) or nephrectomy, in case of irreversible renal damage (as even nonfunctional kidneys may secrete renin and cause HTN, the diseased kidney cannot be simply left in place). *Angioplasty* is mainly used for fibromuscular RAS (suboptimal results have been found in atherosclerotic RAS). The indications for interventional therapy include RAS >80–85%, or 50–80% in the presence of a positive Captopril test or renal failure.

11.2.4.5 Peripheral Vascular Disease

Peripheral vascular disease (PVD) conventionally refers to lower limb ischemia, involving the femoral, deep femoral, popliteal, and the anterior and posterior tibial arteries. The main *cause* of PVD is atherosclerosis. A diagnosis of PVD must prompt workup for systemic atherosclerosis (coronary, carotid, etc.). Rarer causes include vasculitis and embolism (mostly with intracardiac thrombus, typically arrested at points of

Table 11.5 Clinical quantitation of PVD severity

Fontaine	Stage	Stage	Rutherford
N/A	N/A	0	Asymptomatic
Claudication on strong physical exertion, e.g., climbing an abrupt slope	I	1	Mild
Claudication on walking >200 m on a level surface	II	2	Moderate
Claudication on walking <200 m on a level surface; resting pain absent	III	3	Severe
Resting pain[a]	IV	4[b]	Resting pain
N/A	N/A	5[b]	Resting pain and minor tissue loss
N/A	N/A	6[b]	Resting pain and major tissue loss

[a]Pain may be improved by sleeping in a sitting position, as gravity helps perfuse the lower limbs. Skin, nail, and hair changes are frequent
[b]Stages 4, 5, or 6 are also called "critical limb ischemia"; untreated, most cases ultimately require amputation

arterial bifurcation; the most frequent site is the femoral artery bifurcation). *The clinical manifestations* of PVD are designated by the mnemonic, "5P" (Pulse; Paralysis (muscle weakness); Paresthesia; Pallor; Pain). One or more of these symptoms may be absent even in severe disease; for instance, in diabetics, PVD is often painless (due to sensory neuropathy) and peripheral pulses may be normal (microvascular damage). *Claudication* is a deep muscular cramp that subsides at rest, or occasionally, by continuing to walk "through the pain" (opening of collaterals). The peripheral pulses are decreased, and muscle weakness is occasionally associated. The claudication-free stretch (e.g., 200 m on level ground) gives an indication about disease severity, and the site of pain helps localize the stenosis (aortoiliac disease manifests in the thigh and buttock, and disease of the popliteal and tibial arteries affects the calf and the foot). *Gangrene* is a sign of advanced disease. In chronic PVD, *the skin* over the affected area may appear smooth and shiny; cyanotic; ulcerated/gangrenous; or crisscrossed by a network of purple lines ("mottled" skin, or "livedo reticularis," also seen with vasculitis). Hair and nail growth over the affected area may be decreased. In acute PVD, the skin may appear white. *Auscultation* reveals a bruit over the affected artery. *The ankle-brachial index* (normal values >1) decreases to <1 (in severe cases, <0.5). Similarly, the wrist/ankle ratio decreases under stress by 15–20%. The stress may consist in a walk down the hallway or in climbing a flight of stairs. Formal testing is administered on a treadmill, under light exercise (Bruce

stage 1), until the onset of calf pain or completion of 5 min, whichever occurs first. *Allen's test* ascertains the quality of ulnar blood flow, to ensure adequate perfusion of the hand, before radial artery cannulation is undertaken. The utility of this test is not clear. *The workup* for PVD includes Duplex, angio-CT, or angio-MRI. PVD severity can be quantitated by several clinical scales, presented in Table 11.5, alongside their approximate correspondence.

PVD occasionally manifests as distinct syndromes: *Leriche's syndrome* (aortoiliac vascular disease) consists in aortic bifurcation atherosclerosis, commonly with involvement of the iliac arteries. The manifestations include severe claudication, absent femoral pulses, and erectile dysfunction. The treatment is by surgical bypass. *The blue toe syndrome* consists in cholesterol microembolism, generally from aortic plaque, disrupted at cannulation. The toe is purple and tender. The prognosis is very good under conservative treatment. *Buerger's disease* manifests as PVD, but is etiologically a type of vasculitis and discussed in the corresponding section.

PVD: Management Primary and secondary prevention include *management of atherosclerosis risk factors. Smoking cessation* and *physical exercise* to stimulate collateral formation are especially important. The preferred activity is walking, ≥3 times a week, for ≥30–45 min., ideally 1 h. Physical exercise can also be carried out in rehabilitation facilities, on a treadmill set at a speed and incline causing leg cramps (claudication) after 3–5 min, not including the warm-up period.

The patient is then encouraged to continue walking, until the pain becomes moderate; the treadmill is stopped, the patient rests, and when the pain subsides, exercise is resumed. In time, the effort capacity increases and the treadmill is reset accordingly. Strict foot hygiene (to avoid superimposed infection) is key, especially in diabetics.

Pharmacological therapy: Antiaggregants (Aspirin, Plavix) are relatively ineffective for the prevention of PVD progression as such, but are recommended for CVA and IHD prevention, for which the PVD patient is at greatly increased risk. The dosage is established according to the major prevailing risk (70–100 mg daily for IHD, 325 mg q.d. for CVA prevention). Interestingly, a recent metaanalysis has found no prophylactic efficacy to Aspirin in the prevention of coronary disease in PVD patients, administered alone or in association with Dipyridamole; however, Aspirin did appear effective in stroke prevention. *Cilastozol* (100 mg b.i.d.) has vasodilator and anti-aggregant action and is a first-line therapy for PVD. It is contraindicated in HF. Up to 3 months are necessary for effect onset. *Naftydrofuryl* (200 mg tablets t.i.d.) is a vasodilator, having liver toxicity as the main adverse effect. *Pentoxifylline* 400 mg t.i.d. causes vasodilation and reduces blood viscosity; it is a second-line choice in PVD. *Heparin and intra-arterial thrombolytics* are used in acute embolic PVD. Catheter or virus-delivered *angiogenetic factors* are being developed. *Medications of uncertain benefit* include: aminoacids such as L-aginine (a source of NO), carnitine, propionyl-L-carnitine; Gigko biloba extract; and Picotamide (a Dipyridamole-like anti-aggregant). *Ineffective therapies* include vitamin E and prostaglandin. Vasodilators are potentially *harmful,* due to the risk of steal phenomenon. *Interventional therapy* is recommended in patients with symptoms unresponsive to drug therapy and stenosis >70%, or 50–70%, in the presence of positive functional tests (translesional BP gradient >10 mmHg at rest, or >20 mmHg after Papaverine). *Surgical techniques* include aortoiliac, femoral-popliteal, or axillo(bi)femoral bypass, with saphenous or synthetic grafts (GoreTex). The latter technique uses a subcutaneous synthetic conduit, which can be "Y"-shaped in case of bilateral femoral stenosis. Generally, the axillary blood flow is sufficient to avoid upper limb ischemia. In case of unilateral stenosis, a femoral-femoral bypass can be used. *Sympathectomy* to counteract vasoconstriction is rarely used today.

Amputation is indicated in case of extensive necrosis, paresis, intolerable pain, or sepsis. If available, *angioplasty* is used for localized (focal) stenoses <3 cm long. Stents are optionally used in the common or external iliac artery and for "salvage" of suboptimal angioplasty (residual stenosis >50% or arterial dissection). *Other techniques* include *hyperbaric oxygen therapy,* using a chamber with supraatmospheric O_2 pressures to increase the amount of O_2 dissolved in the plasma. This is a last-resort technique, in patients with severe PVD, *spinal stimulation* by a subcutaneous generator delivering small electric impulses to the spine provides analgesia and may stimulate angiogenesis, decreasing amputation rates.

11.3 Venous Disease

11.3.1 Diseases of the Head Veins

11.3.1.1 Cavernous Sinus Thrombosis:

The cavernous sinuses are bilateral intracerebral cavities ensuring the drainage of several cerebral veins. Thrombosis is most often caused by S. aureus infection, ascending from an infected tooth or facial sinus (most often, the sphenoid sinus). *The clinical picture depends on the specific cranial nerve involved and includes, among many other manifestations, proptosis; palpebral ptosis (giving the eye a "half-closed" appearance); chemosis (ocular edema); headache; cranial nerve paralysis, most frequently involving cranial nerve VI (causing strabismus); etc. The clinical course may be slow, rapid, or fulminant. The diagnosis is based on CT or MRI imaging, which visualize both the thrombosis and the causal sinusitis. Invasive angiogram is rarely needed. Uniformly fatal before the antibiotic era, cavernous sinus thrombosis remains fraught with very high mortality (around 20%). Death is caused by extension to the other brain sinuses or to the carotid arteries (causing thrombosis and CVA), cerebral abscess or meningitis, or septic PE (with thrombi reaching the RV). *Therapy* consists in wide-spectrum antibiotics, including an anti-staphylococcal agent, and in sinus drainage (transnasally, for the sphenoid sinus). Anticoagulation is controversial, as are corticosteroids.

11.3.2 Diseases of the Thoracic Veins

The relatively infrequent *SVC syndrome* manifests as abnormal venous drainage in the upper body, due to tumor (e.g., pulmonary), and, less frequently, to intravenous thrombosis. Before the antibiotic era, this syndrome was also seen in late stages of tuberculosis and syphilis infection. The prognosis is that of the underlying disease, thus generally poor (most patients die within 30 months of diagnosis). *The clinical picture* includes headache and dizziness, flushing, dyspnea, cough, and edema and venous distention of the upper limbs and thorax. *The workup* includes CT, MRI, mediastinoscopy, and bronchoscopy with bronchial lavage. The chest X-ray shows mediastinal widening, generally due to tumor and/or lymphadenopathy. *Therapy* includes cortisone, diuretics, and as needed, anticoagulation and chemo- and/or radiotherapy (For diseases of the pulmonary veins, see Chap. 10).

11.3.3 Diseases of the Abdominal Veins

Also refer to 11.2.4.4, for splenic ischemia.

11.3.3.1 The Budd–Chiari Syndrome

The Budd–Chiari syndrome consists in abnormal hepatic vein or IVC drainage, due to thrombosis (hypercoagulation syndromes, polycythemia vera, HRT) or to compression by local tumor. *The clinical picture* (usually of slow onset, but occasionally fulminant) includes an enlarged and tender liver, ascites, and LFT disturbances, ultimately causing *hepatic encephalopathy.* Hepatic vein drainage is achieved by anastomoses in the abdominal and the esophageal wall *(caput medusae,* i.e., tortuous abdominal wall veins, esophageal varices). The diagnosis is established by sonography, CT, and MRI. *Medical therapy* includes salt restriction and anticoagulation (Heparin, Warfarin); catheter-delivered thrombolysis is still experimental. *Interventional therapy* is based on connecting the systemic and functional hepatic circulations (portosystemic shunt). This can be performed surgically or percutaneously, by hepatic vein catheterization (by jugular approach), with intrahepatic needle deployment through the hepatic parenchyma, to reach the portal vein; a plastic stent is subsequently deployed, using the needle as a guide wire. *Hepatic vein angioplasty* is another option. *Liver transplant* is required in fulminant cases or with underlying cirrhosis; recurrences are seen in approximately 10% of transplant patients.

11.3.4 Diseases of the Limb Veins

11.3.4.1 Superficial Phlebitis

Superficial phlebitis is mainly seen with IV administration of irritant substances, venous port infection, or systemic inflammatory disease, such as lupus. The affected vein can be visible as a hot red line, often thickened and tender. Thrombosis is often associated (thrombophlebitis). Despite the lack of risk for PE, superficial phlebitis must not be ignored, as it may be the first sign of serious underlying diseases, such as malignancy (most often, pancreatic), hypercoagulability, or coexisting DVT (in as many as 25% of cases). *The treatment* includes NSAID, cold applications, and occasionally, surgical venectomy.

11.3.4.2 DVT

DVT may be associated to venous insufficiency, vasculitis, trauma, venous compression, or to hypercoagulability states. At 6–7,000,000 cases reported annually (and probably, many more undetected episodes), DVT is an extremely frequent condition. DVT typically affects bedridden or otherwise immobilized subjects (due to blood pooling, dehydration, and systemic inflammation). Orthopedic patients are at very high risk; for instance, DVT appears in up to 80% of patients who underwent knee or hip surgery. Other risk factors include smoking, long periods without exercising the calf muscles (e.g., during a flight), dehydration, hereditary factors (a history of DVT in first-degree relatives), and a history of recurrent abortion (the *lupus anticoagulant syndrome* associates abortion and hypercoagulability). The main importance of lower limb DVT consists in the risk of PE (1–5% of cases of DVT have a fatal outcome). *The clinical picture* includes pain, edema, and occasional erythema in the affected limb. Occasionally, DVT may be completely asymptomatic. Edema may be discreet (measuring the diameter of both legs with a tape measure is recommended). Pain is usually spontaneous, but if absent, it can be elicited by Homans' or Pratt's maneuvers (eliciting pain by extending the patient's toes, to stretch the inflamed vein, or by calf palpation). These signs have low specificity and sensitivity and may even be hazardous, occasionally causing clot dislodgement and PE. There may be superficial vein engorgement, due to reflux from the occluded deep veins, through anastomotic connections (which normally drain blood in the opposite direction, i.e., from the superficial veins into the deep ones). In fact, varices can be the only sign of DVT. Acute and near-complete venous obstruction, with limb cyanosis and pain, is termed *phlegmasia coerulaea dolens*. *Phlegmasia alba dolens* is arterial insufficiency caused by DVT-associated arterial spasm, occasionally in the iliac artery. The lower limb is white and painful. Urgent DVT treatment is essential. *Workup* mainly includes Duplex sonography and angio-CT/MRI, in suspected extension of thrombosis to the iliac vein and/or to the IVC; invasive venography is rarely used today. Blood tests demonstrate increased levels of D-dimers (fragments resulting from fibrin degradation), an indirect indicator of thrombosis. *Management*: Primary and secondary prevention involve risk factor management, avoidance of dehydration, muscular contraction of the legs during long flights, early ambulation after severe disease, and in bedridden and postoperative patients, a strategy as outlined in Table 11.6.

Occasionally, DVT can involve the *upper limbs*, usually caused by pacemaker wires, but occasionally due to effort thrombosis, malignancy, or to the thoracic outlet syndrome. The manifestations, diagnosis, and therapy are similar to those of lower limb DVT; thrombolysis, however, is usually reserved to younger patients with acute-onset DVT.

The management of DVT (Table 11.7) includes prevention of thrombus *extension* (by anticoagulants), to allow spontaneous fibrinolysis of the existing clot, and thrombus lysis, achieved pharmacologically or mechanically (thrombectomy, thrombus fragmentation with or without stenting). The two approaches can be combined (catheter-directed thrombolysis with mechanical thrombus fragmentation). The JUPITER trial has shown that aggressive statin therapy to lower lipids

substantially reduces the risk of DVT, a new aspect of prophylaxis in this disease.

11.3.4.3 Chronic Venous Insufficiency

Chronic venous insufficiency consists in the incapacity of the veins to drain the lower limbs, due to scarring and malcoaptation of the venous valves, mostly as a result of DVT (but only ≤10% of DVT patients develop chronic venous insufficiency). The clinical manifestations include edema and pain in the lower limb, especially at night, and "stasis dermatitis," a brownish, pruriginous discoloration; in its extreme form *(lipodermatosclerosis)*, the skin over the ankle has a "shrunken" aspect, due to subcutaneous scarring. Varicous veins are often associated. The *management* mainly includes venous compression, to increase the venous return and the degree of valve leaflet coaptation. This is achieved with external devices, either passively (with elastic stockings) or actively, with compressive stockings.

11.3.4.4 Lower Limb Varices

Lower limb varices are venous dilatations due to inborn factors (collagen diseases) or secondary to DVT. Risk factors include female gender, pregnancy, old age, obesity, prolonged standing, and DVT. Venous dilatation self-maintains by aggravating valve malcoaptation. The symptoms are very similar to those of CVI, which often coexists. The diagnosis is mainly clinical. The main complication is rupture (mainly due to local trauma, including scratching), with possible massive bleeding. *Management: Noninvasive methods* include: avoiding prolonged standing; sitting with raised feet, as often as possible; strict skin hygiene; and avoiding trauma and scratching. *Medical therapy* involves NSAIDs in usual doses, for acute inflammatory episodes; and Diosmine and Hesperidine, vasoconstrictors stimulating venous blood drainage (no known adverse effects or contraindications). *Surgical therapy* consists in stripping of the great or the small saphenous vein, under general anesthesia (A metal rod is inserted, tied to the vein, and then briskly extracted, to remove the vein). *Other methods* include *sclerotherapy* and intravenous radiofrequency or laser "ablation." The latter methods currently tend to replace

Table 11.6 Primary and secondary DVT prophylaxis

Level of Risk	Prophylaxis[a]	Duration
Low		
Bed rest >3d, prolonged sitting, old age, laparoscopic surgery, antepartum, varicose veins	Early ambulation (where applicable)	Permanent
Moderate		
Nonmajor surgery; arthroscopic knee surgery	LMWH (Enoxaparin 20–40 mg q.d. or b.i.d.[b]) or UFH (SC 5,000 U b.i.d. or t.i.d.) or Fondaparinux (SC 2.5 mg qd, started 6–24 h after surgery)	10 days (assuming normal recovery)
Indwelling CVP catheter; bedridden medical patients; hypercoagulability	As above	Indefinitely or until recovery
Cardiac or respiratory failure; HRT; oral contraceptives; postpartum; cancer	Ambulation, hydration, avoidance of procoagulant medication, etc.	Indefinitely or until recovery
Past DVT[c]	Oral anticoagulation, target INR 2–3, average 2.5; LMWH is preferable in oncological patients	≥3 months, consider indefinite therapy
High		
Hip/knee: arthroplasty or surgery for fractures; major trauma, spinal cord injury; major general surgery	LMWH (as above), Fondaparinux (as above), oral anticoagulants[c] (target INR 2–3, average 2.5; start preoperatively or on the evening of the procedure day)	10–35 days (assuming normal recovery)

[a]In patients intolerant of anticoagulation, mechanical prophylaxis with compressive devices is indicated. The new oral anticoagulant Rivaroxaban holds promise to become the standard of care for thromboembolism prophylaxis after orthopedic surgery. It was shown to be more effective than Enoxaparin for this indication and has the added advantage of oral administration
[b]Started 6 h preoperatively in Europe, 12–24 h postoperatively in the US; LMWH monitoring, usually unnecessary, can be carried out by anti-Xa heparin level monitoring
[c]There is an initial overlap period between LMWH and oral anticoagulants, as the latter have a slow effect (3–5 days for optimal anticoagulation)

Table 11.7 DVT treatment

Treatment	Dosage	Duration	Comments
LMWH	Typically, SC Enoxaparin 1 mg/kg (q.d. or b.i.d.)	5 days on average[a], followed by Warfarin	Monitoring (anti-Factor Xa Heparin levels; target 0.6–1 U/mL for b.i.d., and 1–2 for qd) only in severe RF or pregnancy
UFH	One dose SC 5,000 U, then 17,500 U b.i.d., *or* one dose SC 333 U/kg, then 250 U/kg b.i.d., *or* IV bolus 5,000 U, then 30,000 U/24 h for 1 day, then adjust as per aPTT, or anti-Factor Xa Heparin levels, *or* IV bolus 80 mg/kg, then 18 U/kg/h	As above	aPTT monitoring when using UFH[b]; (target 1.5–2.5)
Fondaparinux	SC 5/7.5/10 mg q.d. for body weight <50/50–100/>100 kg	As above	Unmonitored
Warfarin/ Acenocoumaro[a]	2.5–10 mg q.d., started at the same time as parenteral anticoagulants	≥3 months	INR 2–3

[a]LMWH can be discontinued when INR has been ≥2 for ≥24 h, under Warfarin therapy. LMWH is superior to Warfarin for cancer-associated DVT, when it should be administered at least over the first 3–6 months
[b]Anti-Factor Xa monitoring is optional; if a target level ≥0.35 U/mL has been reached, no dosage increase is needed, even if the aPTT values are subtherapeutic

surgery, due to their good results and the ease of performance (laser ablation only requires local anesthesia, lasts about 1 h, and allows return to daily routine the same day).

11.4 Pulmonary Embolism (PE)

PE most frequently involves a thrombus, but may also be due to fragments of bone marrow (after fractures) or malignant tumors; air bubbles, in the "caisson disease" (high pressures allow more nitrogen to dissolve in the plasma; slow decompression allows gradual transition to small gas bubbles, eliminated through the lungs; with rapid decompression, elimination cannot keep up with bubble production, and embolism ensues); or amniotic fluid and fragments of fetal tissue, an infrequent but very serious complication of pregnancy. Amniotic embolism is a systemic disease, including a first phase, manifesting as dyspnea, hypotension, and cardiac arrest, with a mortality of 50%, and a second phase, affecting roughly half of the survivors of the first phase, manifesting as profuse hemorrhage. Further discussion is beyond the scope of this text. *Risk factors* for PE are classified as *major* (hip or leg fracture or replacement; major or spinal cord surgery or trauma); *moderate* (malignancy or chemotherapy; paralytic stroke; HRT, oral contraceptive therapy; arthroscopic knee surgery; CVP; chronic heart or respiratory failure; postpartum; previous venous thromboembolism; and thrombophilia. The latter mainly includes mutant factor V Leiden, the antiphospholipidic syndrome, protein C or S deficiency, and the MTHFR mutation); or *weak* (bed rest >3 days; immobility due to prolonged sitting, such as in a long car or plane trip; old age; laparoscopic surgery; obesity; antepartum; and varicose veins).

The diagnosis of PE requires a high index of suspicion; indeed, many severe cases are only demonstrated postmortem. *The clinical picture* is nonspecific. Besides the often present *DVT, pulmonary signs* are often noted, including dyspnea, tachypnea, inspiratory pleuritic pain, and cough. Significant tissue necrosis ("pulmonary infarct") may manifest as hemoptysis. *Cardiovascular signs* manifest as tachycardia, hypotension, syncope or sudden death, and right or biventricular dysfunction, leading to shock in severe cases. RV dysfunction *(cor pulmonale)* is due

to increased afterload, of acute or chronic onset (repeated minor or occult PE), while LV dysfunction may result from suboptimal LV filling and/or from IVS dysfunction. Often, there is a feeling of *anxiety ("impending doom"); fever* is occasionally present. The clinical manifestations can be integrated in clinical scores (Table 11.8). These scores are important for prognosis and management. The management is discussed in the corresponding section. *Prognosiswise,* the mortality risk is <1, 3–15, and >15% for patients with a low, intermediate, or high risk of PE, respectively. Basically aimed at establishing the probability of PE, these scores also offer outcome predictions.

Workup for PE is indicated based on the clinical score and on the hemodynamic picture (High-risk PE if hypotension or shock present). The key diagnostic tests are discussed in Table 11.9. Additional tests: *Chest X-ray* demonstrates the *Westermark* sign (an oligemic, i.e., hypoperfused lung area), and *Hampton's hump,* a radioopaque triangle with the base at the pleura and the tip in the hilus, reflecting pulmonary infarction. In current practice, chest radiography is mainly useful for ruling out alternative diagnoses; *Duplex* of the lower limb veins demonstrates DVT, with high sensitivity and specificity. Beside increased D-dimer levels, *blood tests* may demonstrate *increased troponin levels,* reflecting nonischemic myocardial lesions or *hypercoagulability syndromes.* Heart-type fatty acids binding protein (H-FABP) are under research as a marker for myocardial involvement in PE. *The EKG* findings are nonspecific: sinus tachycardia, incomplete RBBB (due to RV pressure overload), and a S1Q3T3 picture. *Blood gas analysis,* with a low sensitivity and specificity, classically demonstrates hypoxia, hypocarbia (decreased CO_2 levels, due to tachypnea), and an increased alveolar-arterial O_2 gradient.

Management of PE: Preventive measures consist in *prevention and treatment of DVT* and in use of an IVC filter, inserted through the femoral vein. A filter is indicated in patients with femoral or iliac DVT and a contraindication to anticoagulation, or with recurrent PE despite optimal anticoagulation. The JUPITER trial has shown that aggressive statin therapy to lower lipids substantially reduces the risk of PE, a new aspect of prophylaxis in this disease.

Therapy is based on the risk scores and on the hemodynamic condition of the patient.

Table 11.8 Clinical probability of PE

Variable	Geneva score	Wells score
Predisposing factors		
Previous DVT or PE	3	1.5
Active malignancy	2	1
Recent surgery or immobilization	2[a]	1.5
Age >65	1	N/A
Symptoms		
Hemoptysis	3	1
Unilateral lower limb pain	3	N/A
Clinical signs		
HR 75–94	3	N/A
HR ≥95	5	N/A
HR ≥100	N/A	1.5
Unilateral edema and pain on palpation of the leg	4	3[b]
Clinical judgment		
Alternative diagnosis less probable	N/A	3
Conclusion: clinical probability	Low, intermediate, or high for scores 0–3, 4–10, and >11, respectively	PE unlikely: 0–4; likely, >4

[a]<1 month
[b]Or any other suggestive clinical sign; the additional "intermediate" category may be used for nonhigh-risk PE only

Table 11.9 Workup for suspected PE

Diagnostic test	High-risk PE	Nonhigh-risk PE	
		High probability ("likely")	Low or interm. prob. ("unlikely")
Pulmonary angiography	If CT is not available, or before embolectomy	If CT not available, or if suspicion persists despite normal CT	No place
Multidetector angio-CT scan	First-choice modality; a positive result mandates therapy; a negative result rules out PE	First-choice modality; a positive result mandates therapy, a negative result is interpreted according to clinical suspicion	If D-dimer assay is positive
Echocardiography	If CT is not available; RV dilatation, hypokinesis[b], or pressure overload are indications for thrombolysis	No place[a]	No place[a]
D-dimers[c]	No place	No place	Negative assay rules out PE
V/Q scan[d]	Negative scan rules out PE; positive scan confirms PE, especially if clinical probability is nonlow		

[a]Echocardiography is in fact indicated in every PE patient, but serves to rule out RA/RV thrombus, PFO, Eisenmenger's syndrome, etc. With acute PE, the RV is unable to generate a peak systolic PAP >50 mmHg; more severe PAH suggests repeated chronic PE, with RV hypertrophy, or non-PE-related PAH
[b]Typically, midfree RV wall hypokinesis, sparing the apex
[c]Less useful in hospitalized patients, since thrombosis of any kind (very frequent in hospitalized patients) may increase D-dimers
[d]As a high percentage of scans are nondiagnostic, this modality is reserved for patients allergic to iodine (in whom CT cannot be performed). A nuclear scan is negative for PE if the perfusion component is normal (no need for the ventilation scan) or if a mismatched ventilation/perfusion defect is noted (abnormal perfusion, normal ventilation). A matched defect suggests other lung diseases (atelectasis, consolidated pneumonia, etc.)

- Unexplained tachypnea, tachycardia, or hypotension (BP<90 mmHg, or a BP decrease ≥40 mmHg for >15 min) raise the clinical suspicion of PE.
- The suspicion is more precisely defined by calculating the clinical risk scores. Note that even a score of zero does not translate as a conclusion of "absent PE," but rather as "PE unlikely"/"low probability of PE."
- Thus, *some* workup will be necessary regardless of the clinical score. The aggressiveness of workup, however, depends on the calculated score and on the hemodynamic status.
- A negative workup for PE rules out the diagnosis, while a positive workup mandates therapy. The aggressiveness of therapy depends on the hemodynamic status.
- If a severity-appropriate work up (nuclear scan, CT, angiography) is not available, the RV is assessed by echo for signs of dysfunction.
- Patients with hemodynamic instability and a positive workup for PE or RV dysfunction are candidates for thrombolysis or embolectomy.

General measures include antithrombotic measures (indicated in all patients), supplemented, in case of shock, with vasopressors and oxygen therapy. *Antithrombotic measures* include *UFH,* (target aPTT 1.5–2.5); in nonhigh-risk patients, *LMWH* represents the first-choice treatment. The agents include Enoxaparin 1 mg/kg b.i.d., or 1.5 mg/kg, q.d., adjusted in renal failure; Tinzaparin 175 U/kg q.d.; or Fondaparinux (5/7.5/10 mg q.d. for body weight <50/50–100/>100 kg). LMWH is continued for ≥5 days and can be discontinued only after obtaining INR values ≥2.5 for ≥2 consecutive days. VKA are contraindicated in the first and third trimesters of pregnancy and should be used cautiously in the second trimester. LMWH are preferred in oncological patients, at least for the first 3–6 months.

Thrombolytic agents are indicated in high-risk patients, as well as in patients with mobile RA/RV thrombi. The contraindications are similar to those of coronary thrombolysis (Table 11.10). The window of opportunity for thrombolysis is much wider than with MI or stroke (up to 2 weeks). However, as these patients usually present in shock, such delays are rare. The thrombolytic regimens are reviewed in Table 11.10.

Table 11.10 Thrombolytic regimens in PE

Regimen	Usual administration	Accelerated administration
Streptokinase	250,000 U loading dose over 30 min, followed by 100,000 U/h, over 12–24 h	1.5 million U over 2 h
Urokinase	4,400 U/kg over 10 min, followed by 4,400 U/kg over 12–24 h	3 million U over 2 h
rtPA	100 mg over 2 h	0.6 mg/kg over 15 min (maximum dose 50 mg)

Thrombolysis is continued by anticoagulant therapy with Warfarin, to a target INR 2–3, average 2.5, for a total duration ≥3 months, and possibly long-term, according to reversibility of risk for recurrent PE. *Interventional management:* Surgical or percutaneous embolectomy is an option in high-risk PE patients in whom thrombolysis is contraindicated or has failed, as well as in patients with an RA/RV thrombus, especially if mobile. *Long-term management* with VKA is indicated for at least 3 months, in patients with a first episode of PE, caused by a reversible condition; for 3–6 months (possibly, long-term), in oncological patients; and long-term, in patients with recurrent PE or with an incurable underlying condition.

11.5 Pulmonary Arterial Hypertension (PAH)

PAH is defined as a *mean* pressure in the main PA of >25 mmHg at rest and >30 mmHg under exertion. The normal pulmonary circulation has a very high functional reserve, and PAH only occurs in severe or advanced disease. PAH occurs as a result of increased *pulmonary vascular resistance (PVR),* measured at catheterization (Chap. 4). Thus, even *mild PAH* signifies *severe pulmonary vascular disease. The prevalence* of PAH is quite high, on a par with that of the underlying diseases. The time-honored and intuitive *classification* of PAH as primary or secondary is not very useful clinically, given several facts: the "secondary" group contains a miscellaneous set of conditions, acting by different mechanisms; some of the "secondary" cases associate pathological abnormalities very similar to those of primary PAH; and there is overlap between the therapy of primary and "secondary" PAH. The current (Venice) classification of PAH, therefore, abandons the term, "secondary PAH," and stresses the different mechanisms involved in the genesis of PAH. This is in part a semantic exercise, since the qualifier, "secondary," is merely replaced with circumlocutions such as "associated with" or "due to." What the Venice classification amounts to is, in brief, a careful classification of the causes of "secondary" PAH. As a result of dispensing with the "secondary" group, the "primary" one (still acknowledged for obvious reasons) is now referred to as "idiopathic PAH." Part of the first class includes idiopathic (primary) PAH (sporadic or familial); the rest of the first class and the totality of the other classes include secondary cases. Thus, class I also includes cases associated to connective tissue disorders; congenital systemic-to-pulmonary shunt; portal hypertension; HIV infection; to drugs or toxins; to sundry etiologies (thyroid disorders, storage disease, etc.); and to pulmonary veno-occlusive disease or pulmonary capillary hemangiomatosis, rarer causes of PAH, with a severe course. Class II includes PAH associated to left heart disease; Class III, PAH associated to hypoxia (of pulmonary or nonpulmonary etiology); Class IV, PAH associated to thrombotic and/or embolic disease; and Class V, PAH associated to miscellaneous diseases.

A few remarks concerning PAH of different etiologies: *Idiopathic PAH* is most frequent in females 20–40 years of age and mainly affects the small pulmonary arteries. Possible mechanisms include thrombosis, endothelial dysfunction, or excessive pulmonary vasoconstriction. *Hypoxia* causes reflex vasoconstriction, and later on, vascular hypertrophy and fibrosis. The main underlying disorders include chronic bronchitis, interstitial lung fibrosis, recurrent PE, and the decreased respiratory drive associated with the Pickwick syndrome. Of note, with acute PE, the RV is unable to generate a systolic pressure >50 mmHg; a higher systolic value suggests a chronic process, with RV hypertrophy. *HIV infection* causes PAH by an unknown mechanism; there is no correlation between either CD4 count or disease stage and the prevalence or severity of PAH. For hypoxia associated to *Eisenmenger's syndrome,* see Chap. 10; *Schistosomiasis* may cause PAH by direct invasion of the PA. The most frequently involved *drugs* causing PAH are cocaine and amphetamine. Some diet pills (the Fenfluramine

in the Fen/Phen combination, as well as the parent compound, Dexfenfluramine) have been found to increase not only the risk of valve disease (Chap. 5), but also that of PAH. *Conjunctive tissue disorders* may cause PAH by interstitial pulmonary fibrosis, isolated PA involvement, or left HF. Yearly echo screening is indicated in scleroderma patients. *Portal HTN* ("portopulmonary HTN") is a pulmonary arterial vasculopathy characterized by vasoconstriction, endothelial and smooth muscle proliferation, plexogenic arteriopathy, and in situ thrombosis and/or fibrosis. The features of this condition are very similar to those of idiopathic PAH. *Pulmonary veno-occlusive disease* and *pulmonary capillary hemangiomatosis* mainly involve venules, but, paradoxically, the PCWP is often normal. The chest X-ray may demonstrate Kerley B lines, patchy pulmonary infiltrates, and pleural effusion. High-resolution CT demonstrates patchy, ground glass-like infiltrates, pleural effusion, mediastinal lymphadenopathy, and thickened septal lines. Bronchoalveolar lavage demonstrates high cell counts and hemosiderin-laden macrophages. *Pediatric PAH* may occur in the neonatal period, when it either resolves spontaneously, or is lethal despite maximal management. The workup and treatment are similar to those in adults; children tend more to be vasoreactive and thus benefit from CCB.

The clinical picture includes dyspnea, fatigue, cough, dizziness and, occasionally, full-blown syncope, due to RV inability to increase output on exertion, and RV or biventricular failure. *The physical signs* reflect the underlying disease, as well as the increased pressures in the PA (loud pulmonic S_2), RV hypertrophy and failure (left parasternal lift, RV S_3; jugular vein distension, hepatomegaly, ascites, peripheral edema, cyanosis), and associated murmurs of TR or PI of various severity.

The workup addresses both the underlying conditions and PAH as such. Diagnosis of underlying diseases is carried out as indicated. *Chest X-ray* demonstrates an enlarged pulmonary trunk (the upper portion of the middle arch, on the left cardiac border), a diameter >17 mm of the right PA (normal <15), and pulmonary vessel "pruning" (rapid tapering and narrowing toward the periphery). Underlying pulmonary or cardiac disease may be noted. *Echo: Imaging signs* demonstrate RV hypertrophy and dilatation, associated dilatation of the RA and of the PA, and flattening of the IVS on the short-axis view ("D-shaped" RV in systole or throughout the cardiac cycle). There may exist a reduced LV diameter, due to underfilling, as well as IVC dilatation and pericardial effusion. Contrast echo (with agitated saline or contrast agents) may demonstrate intracardiac shunt. *Doppler echo* demonstrates a high-velocity TR jet. PA pressure is calculated as $4v^2 + RAP$, where v is the tricuspid jet velocity, and RAP is the right atrial pressure, which can be normal (5 mmHg) or elevated (10/15 mmHg for moderate/ severe elevation, respectively; RA pressure is assessed by jugular vein examination). Additionally, the RV isovolumic relaxation time is increased and the pulmonary acceleration time is decreased. Echocardiography also demonstrates underlying disorders such as left heart disease or intracardiac shunt. *Catheterization* demonstrates a mean PA pressure >25 mmHg at rest, with a resting peak PA pressure >30 mmHg, and a PVR >3 mmHg/l/min (Wood units); the PCWP depends on the underlying condition. *Acute vasodilator testing* allows identification of vasoreactive patients. Under vasodilator therapy (Adenosine, prostaglandin, inhaled NO, etc.) at the time of catheterization, these patients demonstrate a >10 mmHg PA pressure decrease, to an absolute mean PA pressure ≤40 mm Hg, in the presence of an increased or unchanged CO. These patients represent a 10–15% minority of the overall PAH population and warrant a therapeutic CCB trial. *EKG* demonstrates RVH with a strain pattern (inverted T waves), with right axis deviation, increased P-wave amplitude in lead II (RA dilatation), and incomplete RBBB; the findings are specific, but lack sensitivity. *Pulmonary function tests* usually show reduced lung diffusion for CO_2, as well as mild-to-moderate reductions in lung volumes. *Nuclear scan* may demonstrate areas of mismatched ventilation/perfusion (V/Q); if these are in a lobar or segmental distribution, a thromboembolic etiology of PAH is probable. However, smaller, peripheral mismatched areas are also commonly seen in other classes of PAH, as well as in the healthy elderly, and in PAH due to associated veno-occlusive disease. *Arterial blood gases* reveal normal or only slightly decreased PaO_2, and frequently, decreased $PaCO_2$, due to hyperventilation. Severe hypoxemia may reflect secondary opening of a PFO, or other forms of R-L shunt. *CT:* High-resolution CT may be required for the diagnosis of underlying pulmonary or mediastinal disease. Spiral CT is indicated for the identification of cases caused by chronic thromboembolic disease. Invasive pulmonary angiography remains the gold standard in this setting

and is indicated for the selection of candidates for pulmonary endarterectomy. *The exercise capacity* is evaluated by the "6-min walking test", carried out informally over a 30-m level hallway or formally, on a treadmill. Cardiopulmonary exercise testing (to assess $VO_{2\,max}$) is more complex and may occasionally fail to identify subtle changes in the patient's condition.

Therapy improves the symptoms, but might not impact survival. Secondary PAH should not be considered "just a component" of the underlying diseases, as it is a separate (albeit secondary) entity, and its therapy is a key component of patient management. *General measures* include reduced physical exertion, avoiding altitudes >1,500 m, and prevention or termination of pregnancy. Pregnancy and delivery carry a 30–50% mortality in the presence of significant PAH. *Pharmacological treatment:* see Table 11.11. *Invasive measures: Atrial septostomy* (the Rashkind procedure) provides relief of the increased RA/RV pressures, as a bridge to *(heart)-lung transplant,* the last resource in refractory NYHA III-IV patients. *Thrombarterectomy* (surgical extraction of the thrombus) is an additional option, in patients with long-lasting dyspnea and severe PAH, caused by chronic thromboembolic PAH.

Severity and Prognosis: the severity grading of PAH is established based on clinical and work up data. By echo, severe PAH is defined as peak systolic PAP >50 mmHg, corresponding to a mean resting PAP >30–32 mmHg. The prognosis (classically fatal within 2–3 years of diagnosis) has been improved by modern therapy, but remains severe.

11.6 Vasculitis

11.6.1 General Remarks

Although vascular inflammation is seen in numerous conditions (most importantly, atherosclerosis), the term *vasculitis* is generally reserved for autoimmune or (rarely) infectious cases. Vasculitis is generally classified according to the diameter of the affected vessels (small/medium/large vessel vasculitis). An additional classification is based on the ANCA status, a laboratory parameter. *The clinical picture* depends on the affected organs and is thus very variable. Notable manifestations include organ dysfunction (e.g., renal failure), *mononeuritis multiplex* (asymmetrical peripheral nerve

Table 11.11 Pharmacological therapy of PAH

Agent	Agents/dosage	Remarks
Oral anticoagulants	VKA to a target INR of 1.5–2.5 (in the US) or 2–3 (in Europe)	In all patients, except those with porto-pulmonary HTN; caution in HIV patients
Oxygen therapy	Target Sat O_2 >90%	Shunt-dependent hypoxemia is resistant to oxygen therapy
Vasodilators		
CCB	Daily doses (mg): Nifedipine 120–240, Diltiazem 240–720; Amlodipine 2.5–10	In "vasoreactive" patients[a]. Strict BP must not decrease <100 mmHg (RV is preload-dependent)
Prostacyclin and Prostanoid analogs[b]	*Epoprostenol,* 20–40 ng/kg/min by continuous IV infusion	Possible pulmonary edema in pulmonary veno-occlusive disease or capillary hemangiomatosis. Indwelling catheter-related complications possible
	Treprostinil, by continuous IV infusion or SC	SC administration may be very painful
	Iloprost inhalations; 2.5–5 mg q2 h, during waking hours	Pulmonary deposition may reduce systemic effects. May cause flushing, cough, or trismus
	Beraprost PO	
ET (endothelin) receptor antagonists[b]	*Bosentan*[c] 62.5 mg b.i.d., increased to 125 mg b.i.d.	Adverse effects: reversible LFT disturbances (mainly with Bosentan), peripheral edema, URTI, flushing, palpitations, GI manifestations. Sitaxsentan decreases Warfarin metabolism (dose lowering required)
	Sitaxsentan 100 mg q.d.	
	Ambrisentan 5–10 mg t.i.d.	
Phosphodiesterase type 5 inhibitors[b]	*Sildenafil* 20 mg t.i.d.	Pulmonary vasodilators; risk of severe hypotension in patients treated with nitroglycerine. Adverse effects: headache and flushing
	Tadelafil 40 mg q.d.	
Therapy of PAH complications	Diuretics, Digitalis, Dobutamine, for biventricular failure, AF, etc.	Should be always considered, in severe cases, alongside therapy of underlying condition

[a]However, only approximately 50% of these patients will prove to long-term responders (i.e., NYHA I/II with near-normal hemodynamics, under CCB treatment alone)

[b]Indicated in patients not suitable for, or resistant to, CCB; in NYHA III-IV patients, several agents may be required, in combination. Prostanoid analogs also have antiproliferative actions

[c]A recent study has shown that Bosentan may be beneficial for patients with mildly symptomatic PAH

dysfunction, otherwise mainly seen in diabetic patients), and skin manifestations, alongside systemic symptoms.

The workup: Lab tests include inflammatory markers (ESR, CRP, etc.); cryoglobulins, tests for lupus, rheumatoid arthritis, etc.; organ dysfunction tests (e.g., creatinine elevations in renal failure); and ANCA, a group of mainly IgG antibodies against neutrophil and monocyte cytoplasmic antigens. It is not clear whether ANCA are disease markers or actually play a part in pathogenesis. They are increased, among other diseases, in some types of small-vessel systemic vasculitis (ANCA-associated vasculitis), including the Churg–Strauss syndrome, Wegener's granulomatosis, and microscopic polyangiitis (a form of polyarteritis nodosa). There are different types of ANCA; c-ANCA is increased in patients with Wegener's granulomatosis, while p-ANCA is associated with microscopic polyangiitis and with the Churg–Strauss syndrome. *Angiography* (invasive or not), *arterial biopsy,* and *electromyogram* (for peripheral nerve involvement) may be required for diagnosis.

The therapy of vasculitis includes *anti-inflammatory drugs* (Aspirin, steroids, Colchicin); *immunosuppressants* (Cyclophosphamide, Azathioprine, Methotrexate, Mycophenolate, 15-deoxyspergualine); *TNF inhibitors:* Infliximab, Etanercept; *other immunological agents:* monoclonal antibodies against protein CD20 on the surface of B cells: Rituximab; anti-thymocyte globulin, immunoglobulins; immunomodulators (Thalidomide, Dapsone); Interferon; and plasmapheresis. The respective indications and dosages are discussed in the corresponding sections.

11.6.2 Small-Vessel Vasculitis

These vasculitis syndromes occasionally extend to the midsize vessels.

11.6.2.1 Churg–Strauss Arteritis

Churg–Strauss arteritis involves the lungs (asthma, pulmonary infiltrates or hemorrhage), the peripheral nerves, the skin, the mucosas (oral and nasal ulcerations, sinusitis), and other organs (kidney, intestine, etc.). The clinical suspicion is confirmed by lab tests (ANCA, eosiniphilia) and vascular biopsy. The treatment involves Cyclophosphamide and steroids.

11.6.2.2 Microscopic Polyangeitis

Microscopic polyangeitis is an ANCA-positive vasculitis related to Wegener's granulomatosis. Any organ may be affected.

11.6.2.3 Allergic (Hypersensitivity) Vasculitis

Often occurs as a reaction to Penicillin, thiazide diuretics, Sulfa drugs. The manifestations may be limited to the skin (petechiae and purpura) or may involve other organs, most frequently the kidneys. Discontinuation of the offending drug, immunosuppressants, and steroids are therapeutic.

11.6.2.4 Henoch–Schoenlein Purpura

Henoch–Schoenlein purpura is the most frequent pediatric vasculitis, causing joint and abdominal pain and occasionally fecal bleeding. In the absence of renal involvement (cca 1% of cases), this is generally a mild disease, treated with analgetics only. Renal involvement is treated with Cyclophosphamide and steroids. The prognosis is generally favorable; chronic renal failure is rare.

11.6.2.5 Cryoglobulinemic Purpura

Increased levels of cryoglobulins (proteins precipitating at low temperatures) may be associated to hepatitis C, pneumonia, lupus, rheumatoid arthritis, hematologic malignancies, etc. The most common manifestations are purpura, arthralgia, and myalgia. Generally, the treatment addresses the underlying disease.

11.6.2.6 Behçet's Disease

Behçet's disease manifests as oral, genital, and perianal ulcerations (aphthae); occular inflammation, with possible loss of vision; and the phenomenon of *pathergy*, i.e., formation of papulas, 24–48 h after a needle stick. The disease may also cause testicular edema, GI tract lesions, neurological and psychiatric manifestations, arthritis, DVT, or superficial phlebitis. The etiology is unknown, but might be related to food (especially milk), allergy, or to occult infection. There is no specific laboratory test. The prognosis depends on the type and severity of organ involvement. The most serious complication is blindness. *Therapy* includes TNF inhibitors, immunosuppressants, Interferon, immunomodulators, and anti-inflammatory agents (NSAIDs, Colchicine, or steroids).

11.6.2.7 Other Vasculitides

Vasculitis of autoimmune diseases (lupus, rheumatoid arthritis, etc.) involves the small- or mid-sized blood vessels and can range in severity from asymptomatic to fulminant. *Vasculitis associated to viral disease* most frequently involves an immunological reaction triggered by the viral infection, but direct viral involvement is also possible (Hepatitis B or C, Epstein–Barr virus, CMV, HIV, etc.). The manifestations depend on the localization and the severity of the infection. The treatment of severe cases includes organ-specific measures and antiviral therapy, if available.

11.6.3 Mid-Sized Artery Vasculitis

11.6.3.1 Wegener's Granulomatosis

Wegener's granulomatosis may involve the eyes (occasionally causing blindness); the ENT area (flu-like symptoms, epistaxis, nasal septum perforation, deafness); the airways (tracheitis, pneumonia, pulmonary hemorrhage with hemoptysis); the kidneys (renal failure); the joints (arthritis); the nervous system (typically, sensory neuropathy); the skin, including nodules at the elbow, petechiae, purpura, and erythema; and less frequently, other organs. The most frequent complications are renal failure and deafness. *The lab tests* include general inflammatory markers, ANCA ("ANCA-positive vasculitis"), and biopsy (showing vasculitis and granulomas). Untreated, the condition is fatal in a few months. Therapy includes immunosuppressants; steroids; plasmapheresis; SMZ-TMP, useful in localized forms (supporting the infectious hypothesis); monoclonal antibodies against protein CD20 on the surface of B cells *(rituximab)*, or against TNF *(infliximab);* and *antithymocyte globulin.*

11.6.3.2 Polyarteritis Nodoasa (PAN)

PAN involves small or mid-sized vessels and might be caused by the immune response to hepatitis B infection (very frequently associated). The symptoms and signs include general manifestations (fever, weakness, weight loss, muscle pain, diffuse joint pain), and manifestations involving the skin (erythema; ulcerations; areas of localized edema, *livedo reticularis,* or "mottled" skin), the heart (IHD, myocarditis, pericarditis), the kidneys (renal failure, renovascular HTN), the CNS (CVA, convulsions) and peripheral nervous system (paresthesia, burning or pain), the testicles (pain and tenderness), and the intestines (necrosis, perforation). *The work up* is remarkable for increased inflammatory markers and frequently, positive hepatitis B serology; stenosis and/or aneurysms on angiography; and inflammatory findings on vascular biopsy. Untreated, PAN is generally fatal; treatment includes immunosuppressants and steroids and is effective in >90% of cases

11.6.3.3 Kawasaki Disease (Mucocutaneous Node Disease)

Kawasaki disease (mucocutaneous node disease) is a diffuse vasculitis affecting the skin, mucosas, lymph nodes, heart, and vessels. It is most frequent in young (<5 years old) Asian boys and probably involves immunological mechanisms. KD is diagnosed in the presence of ≥3 days of fever and ≥3 out of the following five findings: erythema (typically "strawberry-colored") of the lips or oral cavity or cracking of the lips; rash on the trunk, hands, feet, and genitalia; edema or erythema of the hands or feet; conjunctival

injection; and cervical lymphadenopathy ≥15 mm. There are no specific laboratory tests. The main complication of KD is coronary aneurysm formation (in up to 20% of patients), which can cause MI. Aneurysm formation can be largely prevented by timely therapy (within 7 days of onset), a very important point, since the symptoms (but not the risk for coronary aneurysm) tend to abate spontaneously, even if left untreated. Therapy includes IV immunoglobulins and salycilate (high-dose Aspirin until afebrile, continued at a low dose for approximately 2 months, to prevent thrombosis, should aneurysms have formed). Corticosteroids offer no additional benefit over immune globulin + Aspirin. CABG is an option in children with cardiovascular complications of Kawasaki disease.

11.6.3.4 Isolated CNS Vasculitis

Isolated CNS vasculitis manifests as stroke. The typical angiographic aspect is that of alternating stenoses and aneurysms ("beads on a string"). Meningeal or cerebral biopsy is occasionally required for definitive diagnosis. Cyclophosphamide and steroids have substantially improved an otherwise bleak prognosis.

11.6.4 Large-Artery Vasculitis

11.6.4.1 Takayasu's Disease

Takayasu's disease is an idiopathic vasculitis, causing gradual narrowing and occasional aneurysmal dilatation of the aorta and its branches. Most frequent in young Asian women (ages 15–30), Takayasu's manifests as organ hypoperfusion associated to a systemic inflammatory syndrome (fatigue, fever, nocturnal sweating, anemia, increased ESR). Typically, the lesions first involve the subclavian artery origin, causing decreased or absent radial pulse and left arm weakness/cramping at rest or exertion (arm claudication). Extension of the inflammation to other arteries can cause vision disturbances (optic nerve ischemia), renovascular HTN, neurological signs (dizziness, CVA, convulsions), etc. The PA is affected in 50% of cases. *Therapy* involves steroids, usually at a starting dose of 60 mg Prednisone daily, with gradual weaning, and occasionally, immunosuppressive therapy.

11.6.4.2 Giant Cell Arteritis (GCA)

GCA is a generalized vasculitis, characterized by typical, abnormally enlarged cells. Generally, this disease causes arterial stenosis (due to severe arterial edema), and occasionally, aneurysms. Giant cell arteritis mainly involves elderly Caucasian women and is present in approximately one third of patients with polymyalgia rheumatica (morning stiffness of the neck, shoulders, and thighs). It can affect any arterial territory, but is mainly localized in the head vessels, often involving the temporal artery (which becomes palpable, similar to a tender cord), hence the designation, "temporal arteritis." GCA may cause headache, mandibular pain, especially during chewing (mandibular claudication), scalp pain (typically on combing the hair), and CVA. Definitive *diagnosis* requires temporal artery biopsy (several samples are required, due to patchy involvement); in case of strong suspicion despite negative biopsies, contralateral biopsy is indicated. The major *complication* of GCA is blindness, caused by optical nerve ischemia (by occlusion of the optical nerve vessels, branches of the temporal artery). Vision loss is generally sudden, unilateral, and irreversible. *Therapy* involves Prednisone, and occasionally, Metothrexate, Azathioprine, and/or TNF inhibitors.

11.6.4.3 Infectious Aortitis

Infectious aortitis is mainly caused by *syphilis* in its third (final) stage; vasa vasorum involvement decreases aortic wall resistance and favors AA formation; *gonorrhea; viruses* (herpes, hepatitis or C); *fungal infection; and rickettsial infection.*

11.6.4.4 Buerger's Disease

Buerger's disease *(obliterant thrombangiitis)* is idiopathic vasculitis and thrombosis of the arteries and veins, most frequently seen in young (<45) male smokers. The symptoms include claudication and skin, hair and nail lesions of various severity. The diagnosis is based on exclusion of more frequent causes of PVD (atherosclerosis, autoimmune disease, embolism, etc.). Angiographically, the limb arteries have a "corkscrew" (rather than straight) aspect. The treatment is as for any

PVD, and smoking cessation is imperative. Unfortunately, amputation often becomes necessary.

11.7 Telangectasias

Telangectasias are small vascular dilatations over the face and limbs, but can also involve the internal organs. They may be seen in healthy individuals (e.g., pregnant women) or associated with *cirrhosis* or complex syndromes: *Sturge–Weber* (associating glaucoma and mental retardation); *CREST* (a relatively mild form of scleroderma; "T" stands for telangectasia); *Rendu–Osler–Weber* (hereditary hemorrhagic telangectasia), associating mucosal telangectasia, with occasional epistaxis or GI bleeding, and AV (including cerebral and intrahepatic) malformations causing CVA or severe intrahepatic shunt and high-output HF; *ataxia-telangectasia,* a very severe congenital syndrome manifesting as ataxia, immunological abnormalities, and a tendency to certain malignancies. There is no specific treatment, and the patients are wheelchair-bound by the age of 10 and die by the age of 30; *carcinoid syndrome,* an apudoma, includes benign or malignant secretory GI tumors, causing flushing, diarrhea, bronchoconstriction, and tricuspid or pulmonic valve fibrosis, causing stenosis or insufficiency and ultimately, RV failure. The treatment includes Octreotide (a somatostatin analog), which may decrease the secretory activity of the carcinoid; tumor resection, and occasionally, chemotherapy; *acne rosacea* is a mild form of vasculitis manifesting as chronic facial erythema, mainly in Northern Europeans. *The treatment* of telangiectasia is indicated mainly for cosmetic reasons and involves laser, photo-, or sclerotherapy.

11.8 Vascular Tumor

11.8.1 Benign Tumors

Hemangioma mainly affects *the skin* (manifesting as a "port wine stain" which is a strawberry-like tumorlet or a subcutaneous bluish swelling, both of which may bleed), *the liver* (most often as an incidental sonographic finding, but occasionally causing significant AV shunt and high-output HF), and *the larynx* (which it may obstruct). Hemangioma is more frequent in females, can be evident at birth or a few weeks later, and generally disappears spontaneously, but may persist lifelong. Facial hematoma may be disfiguring. Treatment is indicated in case of complications or for cosmetic reasons and includes steroids, occasionally associated to interferon or vincristine. Surgical or laser resection is also possible.

11.8.2 Malignant Tumors

Malignant hemangioendothelioma is similar to benign hemangioma, but requires, besides surgery, radio- and chemotherapy; *Kaposi's sarcoma* is a herpes virus-related tumor, manifesting as reddish, purple, or brown papulas or nodules, especially on the lower limbs, mouth, face, and genitals. This tumor is usually associated to AIDS and may involve the internal organs; lung involvement manifests as fever, cough, and hemoptysis. In addition to anti-HIV treatment, therapeutic measures include radio- or cryotherapy. Surgical removal is not indicated, due to recurrences at the incision margins. Chemotherapy (especially Anthracycline and Paclitaxel) and interferon are indicated for internal organ involvement.

11.9 Diseases of the Lymphatic Vessels

11.9.1 General Remarks

Diseases of the lymphatic vessels can be *idiopathic* (primary lymphedema) or *secondary* to *surgery* (prostate, colon surgery, or the now infrequent radical mastectomy with axillary lymph node resection); *radiotherapy,* causing lymph vessel fibrosis; *trauma,* causing rupture or stricture; *parasitic infestation* (filariasis); or *medication* (Tamoxifen). The main manifestations include lymphedema and steatorrhea.

11.9.2 Lymphedema

Lymphedema consists in lower limb edema, due to lymphatic duct fibrosis, which may extend to the

veins, causing venous insufficiency. Lymphedema is typically aggravated by long flights, due to the low pressure in the cabin, causing blood retention in the tissues. The diagnosis is based on the clinical picture, in a patient with risk factors. Edema may range from mild to giant *(elephantiasis,* usually seen in the lower limbs, but occasionally involving the upper limb or the face). The edema is "pitting" in the early stages and nonpitting later on, due to fibrosis. *Conservative therapy* includes *compressive stockings* or gloves (15-min sessions of inflation under variable pressure, to increase lymphatic return and rupture the fibrotic strands), followed by *decongestive massage,* in turn followed by the use of *elastic stockings or gloves* or *compressive bandages* facilitating lymph drainage during ambulation. Physical exercise and meticulous hygiene (due to the high susceptibility to infection) and skin humidifying agents are also recommended. The more severe the lymphedema, the lower the prospect of reversibility under treatment. *Surgical therapy* includes lymphatic-lymphatic or lymphatic-venous *bypass; reimplantation* of a portion of the lymphatic-rich large *omentum* to the root of the affected limb, ideally with lymph vessel microsurgical anastomosis; and *fibrotic area excision* followed by skin grafting from other body areas. The cosmetic advantage must be balanced against the risk of further lymph vessel destruction. *Complications* include infection and infrequent malignant transformation (to lymphangiosarcoma, with a severe prognosis).

Bibliography

Guidelines

Hirsch AT, Haskal ZJ, Hertzer NR, et al. ACC/AHA 2005 Practice Guidelines for the management of patients with peripheral arterial disease (lower extremity, renal, mesenteric, and abdominal aortic): executive summary: a collaborative report from the American Association for Vascular Surgery/Society for Vascular Surgery, Society for Cardiovascular Angiography and Interventions, Society for Vascular Medicine and Biology, Society of Interventional Radiology, and the ACC/AHA Task Force on Practice Guidelines (Writing Committee to Develop Guidelines for the Management of Patients With Peripheral Arterial Disease). *Circulation.* 2006;113:1474-1547.

The Task Force for the Diagnosis and Treatment of Pulmonary Hypertension of the European Society Of Cardiology (ESC) and the European Respiratory Society (ERS), endorsed by the International Society Of Heart And Lung Transplantation (ISHLT): Guidelines for the diagnosis and treatment of pulmonary hypertension. *Eur Heart J*. 2009, doi:10.1093/eurheartj/ehp297.

The Task Force for the Diagnosis and Management of Acute Pulmonary Embolism of the European Society of Cardiology (ESC). Guidelines on the diagnosis and management of acute pulmonary embolism. *Eur Heart J*. 2008;29:2276-2315.

Diagnosis and management of aortic dissection. Recommendations of the Task Force on Aortic Dissection, European Society of Cardiology. *Eur Heart J*. 2001; 22:1642-1681.

Suggested Reading

Wells PS, Anderson DR, Bormanis J, et al. Value of assessment of pretest probability of deep-vein thrombosis in clinical management. *Lancet*. 1997;350(9094):1795-1798.

Blum A, Bellou A, Guillemin F, et al. Performance of magnetic resonance angiography in suspected acute pulmonary embolism. *Thromb Haemost*. 2005;93(3):503-511.

Buller HR, Agnelli G, Hull RD, et al. Antithrombotic therapy for venous thromboembolic disease: The Seventh ACCP Conference on Antithrombotic and Thrombolytic therapy. *Chest*. 2004;126(3 suppl):401S-428S.

Goldhaber SZ. Echocardiography in the management of pulmonary embolism. *Ann Intern Med*. 2002;136(9):691-700.

Galiè N, Rubin Lj, Hoeper M, et al. Treatment of patients with mildly symptomatic pulmonary arterial hypertension with bosentan (EARLY study): A double-blind, randomized controlled trial. *Lancet*. 2008;371:2093-2100.

Turpie AG, Lassen MR, Davidson BL, et al.; RECORD4 Investigators. Rivaroxaban versus enoxaparin for thromboprophylaxis after total knee arthroplasty (RECORD4): a randomised trial. *Lancet*. 2009;373(9676):1673-1680.

Glynn RJ, Danielson E, Fonseca FA, et al. A randomized trial of rosuvastatin in the prevention of venous thromboembolism. *N Engl J Med*. 2009;360(18):1851-1861.

Barnett HJ, Taylor DW, Eliasziw M, et al. Benefit of carotid endarterectomy in patients with symptomatic moderate or severe stenosis. North American Symptomatic Carotid Endarterectomy Trial Collaborators. *N Engl J Med*. 1998;339(20):1415-1425.

Diener H-C, Weimar C. Update of secondary stroke prevention. *Nephrol Dial Transplant*. 2009;24(6):1718-1724.

Henderson RD, Eliasziw M, Fox AJ, et al.; for the North American Symptomatic Carotid Endarterectomy Trial (NASCET) Group. Angiographically defined collateral circulation and risk of stroke in patients with severe carotid artery stenosis. *Stroke*. 2000;31:128.

Mohr JP, Thompson JL, Lazar RM, et al., Warfarin-Aspirin Recurrent Stroke Study Group. A comparison of warfarin and aspirin for the prevention of recurrent ischemic stroke. *N Engl J Med*. 2001;345(20):1444-1451.

Nederkoorn PJ, Mali WP, Eikelboom BC, et al. Preoperative diagnosis of carotid artery stenosis: accuracy of noninvasive testing. *Stroke*. 2002;33(8):2003-2008.

SPACE Collaborative Group. 30 Day results from the SPACE trial of stent-protected angioplasty versus carotid endarterectomy in symptomatic patients: a randomised non-inferiority trial. *Lancet*. 2006;368:1239-1247 [Erratum, *Lancet*. 2006;368:1238.].

Yadav JS, Wholey MH, Kuntz RE, et al. Protected carotid-artery stenting versus endarterectomy in high-risk patients. *N Engl J Med*. 2004;351(15):1493-1501.

Blankensteijn JD, de Jong SECA, Prinssen M, et al. Two-year results of a randomized trial comparing conventional and endovascular repair of abdominal aortic aneurysms. *N Engl J Med*. 2005;352:2398-2405.

Cosford PA, Leng GC. Screening for abdominal aortic aneurysm. *Cochrane Database Syst Rev*. 2007; 2. Art. No. CD002945.

Bhatt DL, Fox KA, Hacke W, et al.; CHARISMA Investigators. Clopidogrel and aspirin versus aspirin alone for the prevention of atherothrombotic events. *N Engl J Med*. 2006;354:1706-1717.

Olschewski H. Inhaled iloprost for severe pulmonary hypertension. *N Engl J Med*. 2002;347(5):322-329.

Badesch DB, Champion HC, Gomez Sanchez MA, et al. Diagnosis and assessment of pulmonary arterial hypertension. *J Am Coll Cardiol*. 2009;54(1 suppl):S55-S66.

Heart Disease in Special Populations

12

Contents

12.1 Background

Genetic endowment, the hormonal environment, age, lifestyle (physical exercise, smoking, dietary habits, alcohol consumption, substance abuse, etc.), and coexistent disease (and its treatment), all have their particular effect on each separate individual. There are as many possible variations of disease as there are patients. The list of virtual possibilities is infinite, but some common characteristics emerge in different demographic groups. In the present chapter, we will discuss some of these groups.

12.2 Heart Disease in the Nonpregnant Woman

12.2.1 General Remarks

Despite the fact that more than half the planet's population is of the female gender, most of the clinical trials, especially the less recent ones, were carried out mainly in males, and extrapolation of the results in women may not always be justified. The main influence of female gender is on CAD.

> **As compared to men, women have**
>
> - Higher HDL levels (on average, by 10 mg/dL).
> - Lower LDL and non-HDL levels, before menopause.
> - Higher LDL and non-HDL levels, after menopause, when LDL increases on average by 2 mg/dL each year between ages 40 and 60.
> - A higher incidence of high TG combined with low HDL (metabolic syndrome); TG is a more significant CAD risk factor than in men.

G.A. Adelmann, *Cardiology Essentials in Clinical Practice*,
DOI: 10.1007/978-1-84996-305-3_12, © Springer-Verlag London Limited 2011

Due to *estrogen protection of the coronaries* (by an incompletely understood mechanism involving LDL lowering and increased NO secretion), angina pectoris appears 10–15 years later in women than in men. Unfortunately, prolonging this protection after menopause, by HRT, has not proven effective and has actually increased the incidence of heart disease (as well as that of breast cancer, CVA, and DVT). While there is no cardiological indication for HRT, in certain subpopulations, and under certain formulations and dosages, HRT may still prove beneficial, an issue currently under investigation.

Another particularity of CAD in women is its often *atypical presentation* (stabbing, rather than crushing pain, lasting longer than the few minutes typical in men). Conversely, only about 50% of coronary angiographies in women with clinically suggestive chest pain show angiographically significant stenosis. A normal angiogram in a patient with angina and a positive EKG stress test is characteristic of "the cardiac syndrome X." In women, *ischemic changes on the EKG are often nonspecific* (e.g., T wave flattening). The EKG stress test has low sensitivity and specificity, partly because it especially misses single-vessel disease, the most frequent type of CAD in women. Although major findings on the stress test (marked ST depression, ST elevation) are of diagnostic value, echo stress test or nuclear perfusion scan are the procedures of choice for CAD diagnosis in women. *Cultural factors* play an important role in the underdiagnosis of CAD in women. Some women may be more resilient to pain (and thus seek medical attention later in the course of the disease); additionally, medical caregivers may have a gender-biased approach, with nonspecific symptoms often labeled "psychological." The importance of CAD underdiagnosis in women cannot be overstressed, since MI mortality and recurrence are actually higher than in men. Similarly, the *prognosis* after revascularization is generally poorer, due to the smaller diameter of the coronary arteries. Women also generally have a higher *tendency to postrevascularization complications* (bleeding or pseudoaneurysm).

12.2.2 Syndrome X

Syndrome X (not to be confused with the metabolic syndrome X, currently simply termed "the metabolic syndrome") is an angina-like syndrome mainly seen in women. Syndrome X is attributed to a combination of factors, including small vessel disease, coronary spasm due to endothelial dysfunction, and possibly, a lower pain threshold in affected patients. *The clinical picture* includes typical or atypical pain in the chest and left arm, usually lasting more than just a few minutes (i.e., longer than typical angina). The EKG stress test is positive (possibly, as an expression of the ability of EKG to detect even subtle ischemia). The coronary angiogram is classically described as "normal," but some studies have found a significantly higher prevalence of decreased myocardial blush score in affected patients. Resting EKG often shows nonspecific findings; myocardial perfusion scan is positive in only 30% of cases; and stress echo or stress Dobutamine tests are often negative. *Management* involves the usual CAD medication. Beta-blockers are first-choice therapy; Verapamil or Diltiazem can be prescribed in an attempt to relieve vasospasm. The management of Syndrome X also involves a few agents not otherwise used in CAD. *Aminophyllin* is a nonobvious therapeutic choice, as it antagonizes Adenosine, a natural vasodilator. However, Adenosine may also be responsible for myocardial perfusion imbalance and for angina-like chest pain in the absence of ischemia; in fact, Adenosine accumulation is believed to represent the main mechanism of classical anginal pain as well. *HRT,* by and large removed from the CAD armamentarium, may be tried in Syndrome X patients, in whom it may act as a vasodilator. *Spinal stimulation* achieves analgesia (loss of the "anginal warning mechanism" is acceptable in light of the overall good prognosis) and may stimulate angiogenesis. *The prognosis* of Syndrome X is generally better than that of classical CAD; however, patients with persistent symptoms and severe ischemia on stress testing appear to be at higher risk of MI, stroke, and fatal outcome.

12.2.3 The Takotsubo Syndrome

The Takotsubo syndrome ("transient apical ballooning," "stress CMP") also mainly affects women, especially after a recent major emotional trauma ("broken heart syndrome"). *The clinical picture* includes HF (pulmonary edema is not infrequent); severe angina; EKG changes suggestive of anterior MI; and a typical apical LV dilatation, similar to a Japanese turtle fishing device *(tako tsubo)*. The normal angiogram is in striking discordance to the dramatic clinical picture. Disease mechanisms involve stress-related adrenalin secretion, vasospasm in multiple coronary territories, and abnormal microvascular function. The diagnosis is angiographic and consists in demonstration of the hallmark ballooning in the presence of angiographically normal coronaries. *The treatment* is nonspecific. As in many countries 24/7 angiography is not available, many Takotsubo patients probably do receive, in practice, unwarranted thrombolytic therapy. The importance of not missing the window of opportunity in anterior wall MI overrides the concern of missing the much more infrequent Takotsubo syndrome. *The prognosis* is generally good, but the syndrome may also be fatal, just like "true" anterior MI. Complete recovery from LV dysfunction may require up to 2 months.

12.2.4 Other Clinical Particularities

Other clinical particularities of the cardiovascular system in women include

- *A longer QT interval* than in men (higher risk of torsades).
- In WPW, a higher incidence of *concealed pathways* and *antidromic AV ventricular reciprocating tachycardia*.
- A *smaller heart* (in keeping with the generally smaller stature of women); thus, "high-normal" values may represent cardiac enlargement, and "borderline-low" values may actually be normal. This point is especially important in certain settings: for instance, in women with MR or AI, LV dilatation (and thus, the indication for valve replacement or repair) may be present at technically "normal" LV dimensions. Conversely, some AS patients with borderline indications for valve replacement may in fact be treated conservatively.
- *Severe LVH* in the presence of SVR increases; some elderly women with HTN and/or AS develop subvalvular LVOT stenosis (not dissimilar to that of HOCM), mandating partial resection of the hypertrophic IVS and removal of myocardial calcium deposits at the time of AV replacement. If the patient is too frail for this complex procedure, the indication for surgery should be reconsidered. Another consequence of the increased propensity for LVH is

an increased incidence of HFPEF of women, more easily overlooked than systolic HF.

12.3 Heart Disease in Pregnancy

12.3.1 Physiologic Changes of Pregnancy, Relevant to the Cardiac Function

Physiologic changes of pregnancy, relevant to the cardiac function, mainly include: increased metabolic requirements; the presence of the low-resistance placental circulation and of high levels of vasodilatory estrogen, significantly decreasing LV afterload; increased procoagulant and diminished fibrinolytic activity; and aortic and IVC compression by the pregnant uterus, diminishing the venous return to the heart, especially in the last trimester. *Adaptive mechanisms* in response to these factors include: an increase in blood volume up to 50%; relative tachycardia (HR faster by an average of 10–15 beats/min than before pregnancy); increased CO by up to 50%, with an additional increase during delivery; and BP decrease (especially diastolic) by approximately 10 mmHg. These changes attain a maximum at around 20–24 weeks, i.e., at the end of the second trimester, and last until the end of pregnancy.

12.3.2 Cardiovascular Disease in Pregnancy

Cardiac disease is the most common cause of mortality in pregnancy. Preexisting or de novo maternal heart disease can affect the mother or the fetus. *Cardiovascular complications of preexisting maternal disease* depend, in prevalence and severity, on the type of disease and on the symptomatic status. Asymptomatic patients generally tolerate pregnancy reasonably well. The main conditions involving high risk in pregnancy are reviewed in Table 12.1. *De novo cardiovascular disease* occurs in 1–4% of pregnant women. Whether de novo or as a complication of preexisting heart disease, cardiovascular disease in the pregnant woman presents specifically as HF, arrhythmia, or HTN, or nonspecifically.

Table 12.1 Complications of preexisting cardiovascular disease in pregnancy

Condition	Complication/mechanism	Management
High risk		
Eisenmenger's	Peripheral vasodilatation and low resistance in the placental circulation increase R-L shunt and the degree of cyanosis. The increased blood volume increases RV/LV preload; in addition, LV preload is also increased by the R-L shunt. Associated to the required increase in CO, this ultimately leads to left or biventricular failure. Most deaths occur postpartum	Pregnancy should be prevented or terminated; otherwise, hospitalization is required from Trimester II on, under O_2 and Heparin therapy and fetal monitoring. Vasodilatation should be avoided
Severe PAH	RV or biventricular failure, due to the incapacity of the RV to increase CO and to handle the volume overload	Therapy of PAH (Chap. 11)
Significant LV/RV dysfunction	LV/RV or biventricular failure (see mechanisms, above). Patients with LVEF <40% and/or NYHA class III–IV are at highest risk, with a mortality up to 7%. Pulmonary edema and cardiogenic shock are possible	Therapy of HF (Chap. 4)
Left heart obstruction[a]	LV failure, due to the inability to increase CO and to handle volume overload in face of the fixed stenosis	Rest, β-blockers; C-section and valve replacement (or valvuloplasty as a bridge to surgery) may be required. Percutaneous AVR, in select centers
Severe MS	LA pressure increases due to increased CO. Diastolic filling time decreases with tachycardia	β-blocker therapy; consider valvuloplasty if PAP>50 mmHg despite medical therapy
CVA or TIA	CVA recurrence, due to the procoagulant action of estrogens	Thrombolysis in select patients
Severe arrhythmia	Arrhythmia recurrence, due to increased Adrenalin secretion and myocyte wall tension, under volume overload	As outside pregnancy, but AAD levels must be monitored; DCC is safe to the fetus
Peripartum CMP	Recurrence, by an incompletely understood mechanism	see Chap. 4
Marfan's	Aortic dilatation, dissection, or rupture[b]	Repair of severe root dilatation or severe MR is indicated before pregnancy
Cardiac transplantation	Maternal and fetal risk due to the underlying disease; to anesthetics; and to immunosuppressive therapy	If possible, conservative management
Moderate risk		
Pulmonic stenosis	Pressure overload causing RV failure, arrhythmia, and TR; possible RV failure	Balloon valvuloplasty is rarely needed
Aortic coarctation	Increased blood volume and adrenalin secretion exacerbate HTN and may lead to stroke or aortic dissection	HTN therapy. See Chap. 10 for coarctation repair
After surgery for CHD	Residual defects may lead to late failure and paradoxical embolism. Arrhythmia and heart block can also result from surgical scars	
HCM	Usually well tolerated, but LV diastolic dysfunction may be exacerbated by tachycardia and loss of the atrial kick	HCM treatment as usual (Chap. 4), including β-blocker therapy
Low risk		
Valvular insufficiency	Low risk only if unassociated with LV dysfunction or Marfan's syndrome	Follow-up
L-R shunt	Low risk only if no associated significant PAH	Follow-up

Table 12.1 (continued)

Condition	Complication/mechanism	Management
Nonsevere LVOT/RVOT obstruction	Low risk only if not resulting from a nonlow risk underlying condition	Follow-up
HF NYHA I/II	Low risk only if not resulting from a nonlow risk underlying condition	Follow-up

[a]Severe AS (valve area <1–1.5 cm^2, mean gradient >40 mmHg); moderate MS (valve area <1.5 cm^2)

[b]<1% risk if aortic root diameter <4 cm and if there is no significant AI or MR; 10% risk if the root diameter is ≥4 cm. The majority of valvular problems occur during the first 2–3 days postpartum

12.3.2.1 Heart Failure (HF)

"Normal" fatigue, dyspnea, and peripheral edema starting from the first trimester may actually be the first signs of HF, in which case they gradually increase in severity, reaching their maximum at the end of the second trimester. Delivery is an additional crucial point, due to *increased afterload,* produced by pain-related adrenalin secretion, which also causes tachycardia; and *increased preload,* due to increased venous return (each episode of uterine contraction injects into the circulation 300–500 mL of blood, only partly balanced by delivery-related bleeding). Preload is also increased postpartum, when edema resorbtion and relief of uterine compression on the IVC increase venous return to the heart. Normalization of cardiovascular function requires up to 6–8 weeks after birth.

12.3.2.2 Arrhythmia

Palpitations are common during pregnancy and may be due to either SVT or VT; the latter often occurs in the absence of structural heart disease, and may be β-blocker-sensitive. New-onset VT during the last 6 weeks of pregnancy or in the early postpartum period must raise the possibility of peripartum CMP. The treatment of symptomatic arrhythmia in pregnant women generally does not differ from the usual therapy, including β-blockers and ICD implantation. A notable exception, however, is Amiodarone, which is contraindicated, as it can cause fetal hypothyroidism, growth retardation, and premature birth.

12.3.2.3 HTN in Pregnancy

HTN, whether preexisting or caused by pregnancy, is a risk factor for morbidity both in the mother and in the fetus. BP normally decreases in pregnancy. Pregnancy-related HTN includes gestational (pregnancy-induced) HTN, preeclampsia, and eclampsia (Table 12.2).

Preeclampsia consists in BP >140/90 mmHg on two separate measurements, 4–6 h apart, associated with proteinuria (≥300 mg of protein in a 24-h urine sample). In a patient with preexisting HTN, preeclampsia is diagnosed if systolic BP has increased by 30 mmHg or if diastolic BP has increased by 15 mmHg (in association to proteinuria). Preeclampsia is caused by diffuse endothelial dysfunction and vasospasm and affects up to 5–8% of pregnant women, generally after week 20. Preeclampsia may occur as late as 6 weeks postpartum

Table 12.2 Hypertensive syndromes of pregnancy

BP > 140/90 twice during the same week	Proteinuria	BP > 160/110, signs of organ damage	Convulsions
Eclampsia			
Severe pre-eclampsia			
Mild pre-eclampsia			
Gestational HTN			

and be attributed by the patient to "expected" headache and edema. *Risk factors* include, among others, first pregnancy, pregnancy at the extremes of reproductive age (highest risk in women >35 years), multifetal pregnancy, black race, family history of preeclampsia, diabetes, obesity, chronic HTN, and renal disease. *Mild preeclampsia* may be asymptomatic or manifest as headache and edema. Mild preeclampsia usually remits spontaneously and does not require therapy. *Severe preeclampsia* is defined as BP >160 and/or 110 mmHg diastolic on two occasions 6 h apart, with the patient at bed rest, with proteinuria, usually >5,000 mg in a 24-h collection or > "3+" on two random urine samples collected ≥4 h apart. Severe preeclampsia usually associates signs and symptoms of target-organ or fetal damage: severe headache, visual disturbances, pulmonary edema, oliguria, impaired LFT, mesenteric ischemia, thrombocytopenia, oligohydramnios, decreased fetal growth, or placental abruption. The association of convulsions to this clinical picture defines *eclampsia*. *The HELLP syndrome* (hemolysis, high liver enzymes, low platelet count) is a severe multi-system disease with high fetal and maternal mortality and morbidity. The associated severe HTN must be aggressively treated. Immediate delivery is necessary.

Therapy: severe preeclampsia, gestational HTN, and preexisting HTN persisting during pregnancy are treated with Methyl-dopa and β-blockers. The goal is to maintain systolic BP at 140–155 mmHg and diastolic BP at 90–100 mmHg. Of note, ACEI are contraindicated in pregnancy, and diuretics must be used with care. The therapy of eclampsia includes Nifedipine (5–10 mg IV; repeat q.20 min to maximum of 60 mg), Labetalol (50–100 mg IV; repeat q.30 min to a maximum of 300 mg), and Hydralazine (5–10 mg IV; repeat q.20 min to a maximum of 60 mg). Magnesium sulfate 4–6 g IV over 20 min with a maintenance dose of 1–2 g/h is used against convulsions, as well as prophylactically, in patients with severe preeclampsia. Therapeutic abortion, C-section, or induced delivery are the definitive treatment in otherwise unresponsive preeclampsia and eclampsia.

12.3.2.4 Other Cardiovascular Conditions

Other cardiovascular conditions occasionally affecting the pregnant woman include aortic dissection or rupture (increased risk in Marfan's disease, especially in the third trimester, including labor and delivery), PE (due to the pregnancy-related procoagulant state), and MI by coronary dissection. Pregnancy remains a risk factor for MI, although, in the modern therapeutic era, with a much improved mortality profile.

12.3.3 Workup of Heart Disease in Pregnancy

The default imaging technique in pregnant women is echocardiography, supplemented as necessary with MRI. It is recommended to minimize X-ray studies, especially in the first trimester, when radiation may be teratogenic, mainly to the CNS. However, this danger may have been overestimated in the past, when, additionally, the radiation regimens were higher than in current practice. CT and angio-CT deliver particularly high doses of radiation, and their contraindication in pregnancy is more firmly established. Myocardial perfusion scan is contraindicated (and would in fact rarely be necessary). The EKG may show left axis deviation, especially in the third trimester, due to diaphragm elevation by the pregnant uterus.

12.3.4 Management of Heart Disease in Pregnancy

Drug therapy: *Any* medication must be used only if absolutely necessary, especially in the first trimester; as this is when most unplanned pregnancies are discovered, women with reproductive potential must be vigilant in regard to drug (self)-administration. Unplanned pregnancy is discouraged in women under chronic medical therapy. The official classification of drugs in regard to possible adverse reactions in pregnancy is, unfortunately, of relatively little help to the practitioner, since the vast majority of drugs are classified as "potentially dangerous" (classes B and C), only 2% being considered clearly harmless (class A) and 5% clearly contraindicated (class D). Table 12.3 lists the main cardiologic drugs known to adversely affect the fetus.

Anesthesia in the pregnant woman: anesthesia for nonobsterical surgery or for delivery can be local

Table 12.3 Cardiological drugs in pregnancy

Medication/class	Status	Reason
Antihypertensive medication		
ACEI, ARB, Aliskiren	C/I	Serious malformations, death in utero
β-Blockers	Relative C/I beyond first trimester	Fetal bradycardia, hypoglycemia, impaired intrauterine growth, respiratory distress in the newborn
CCB	Allowed	–
Diuretics[a]	Caution	Excessive dehydration may lead to fetal demise
α-Blockers	Allowed	–
Other anti-HTN drugs Alphametyldopa Hydralazine, Clonidine	Allowed	–
Digitalis	Allowed	–
Antiarrhtyhmic drugs		
Class I	Allowed	–
Class II	See β-blockers, above	
Class III		
Amiodarone	C/I	Possible fetal hypothyroidism[b]
Sotalol	Allowed	–
Ibutilide	Allowed	–
Dofetilide	Allowed	–
Antiaggregants		
Aspirin	C/I	Risk of spontaneous and perinatal complications[c]
Plavix	Allowed	–
Anticoagulants		
Warfarin	Allowed if dose <5 mg/day	Risk of hemorrhage at birth; fetal malformations
Unfractioned heparin	Allowed	–
LMWH	Allowed[d]	–

[a]Furosemide may inhibit lactation
[b]Fetal hypothyroidism may lead to serious malformations and mental retardation. Exceptionally, interruption of Amiodarone is impossible; in these cases, pregnancy termination is suggested, with ICD insertion and planned further pregnancies
[c]Episodic use is probably harmless
[d]LMWH is preferred to Warfarin in first trimester and after week 35; however, LMWH is not always an acceptable replacement for Coumadin (e.g., with mechanical valve prosthesis)

(SC anesthetic in the perineal area), regional, or general. In turn, regional anesthesia can be spinal (delivered into the spinal sac) or epidural (the tip of the needle does not pierce the dura mater). While spinal anesthesia may cause excessive vasodilation and hypotension in patients with HF or valvular stenosis, epidural anesthesia is generally allowed, as it has a lower tendency to cause significant BP changes. General anesthesia allows optimal control of BP and is preferred in the pregnant woman with severe cardiac disease. *SBE prophylaxis:* vaginal delivery associates bacteremia, due to bleeding in a septic territory. Although the indications for SBE prophylaxis are the same as in nonpregnant individuals (Chap. 8), many obstetricians continue to recommend routine prophylaxis in the presence of any valvular or CHD disease.

12.3.5 Fetal Risk

The risk for premature delivery, low birth weight, or death in utero is greatest in fetuses of mothers suffering from HF NYHA III/IV, cyanotic CHD (the risk is highest if $SatO_2 \leq 85\%$), hemodynamic instability, conditions requiring Warfarin dosage >5 mg q.d., or preeclampsia/eclampsia. *The risk for CHD in the fetus:* see Chap. 10.

12.4 Male Gender

Men have a higher incidence of CAD than age-matched premenopausal women. The risk of SCD is higher than in women at any age. WPW syndrome with orthodromic AV reciprocating tachycardia and AF degenerating to VF are more common in men (while concealed pathways and antidromic AV ventricular reciprocating tachycardia are more common in women). NSVT and PVCs are associated with an increased risk of SCD in men, but not in women.

12.5 Heart Disease in Athletes

SCD occurs in 1/200,000 athletes (not necessarily professional) each year; in itself low, the risk is higher than in age-matched individuals. SCD occurs mainly in male athletes, under intense training. HCM (and, less frequently, concentric LVH) accounts for up to 50% of cases. Other risk factors include congenital coronary anomalies (most frequently, LMCA origin from the right coronary sinus; see Chap. 10), critical AS, the Brugada and long QT syndromes, DCM, ARVC, aortic rupture in Marfan's syndrome, doping, and cardiac trauma in contact sports (*commotio cordis*). In about 3%, the cause cannot be identified. The treatment of SCD is reviewed in Chap. 6. There is no consensus as to primary prevention. Ideally, anyone wishing to engage in competitive sports should undergo a routine echocardiogram. However, in view of the low pretest probability of disease, an impractically high number of patients should be screened, in order to obtain just one abnormal result, which, furthermore, would only carry a minute absolute risk of SCD. A possible alternative is routine EKG screening, successfully implemented in Italy, but still not routine elsewhere. It must be kept in mind, however, that approximately 6% of patients with HCM are not picked up by ECG screening. Factoring in the anamnesis (personal and family history of high-risk diseases) and the physical examination (the most frequent underlying disease is HCM, readily diagnosed by its associated systolic murmur) allows appropriate selection of candidates for echo workup. Occasionally, it may be difficult to distinguish between an adaptive response (mild LVH and dilatation, bradycardia) and a pathological impact of strenuous exercise. Even the marked cardiomegaly occasionally seen in athletes is not necessarily pathological, as it may coexist with a perfectly normal function and prognosis. Athletes with non-sustained, asymptomatic exercise-induced ventricular arrhythmias and a structurally normal heart may participate in low-intensity competitive sports. Athletes with more significant rhythm disorders, syncope, or structural cardiac anomalies, and those treated with cardiovascular drugs and devices such as pacemakers and ICDs are generally not allowed to participate in high-grade competition. (In fact, drugs such as β-blockers are forbidden in certain sports, by antidoping regulations.) *Commotio cordis* consists in VF and SCD caused by chest trauma during the ventricular vulnerable period, just before the peak of the T wave. As the responsible mechanism is not cardiac disease, but the unfortunate timing of otherwise benign trauma, no screening or prevention modality is applicable.

12.6 Heart Disease in the Elderly

While the cut-off age for defining a person as "elderly" is debated, the statistics project an explosive increase in the number of senior citizens within the next few decades. Many elderly also have significant noncardiac problems, such as depression (10–15%), cognitive impairment (confusion, dementia in 15–20% of those >85), poor eyesight, and live in precarious material circumstances.

12.6.1 Coronary Artery Disease

In the elderly, CAD is

- *Frequent:* approximately 25% of men and 15% of women ≥75 have clinically manifest CAD, with a high prevalence of asymptomatic atherosclerosis.
- *Severe:* approximately 1/3 of fatal MI are seen in people >80, and angina is often of the unstable variety.
- *Associated to other diseases,* many being risk factors for CAD exacerbation: 50% of those >65 and 2/3 of those >75 suffer from suboptimally treated HTN (typically, isolated systolic HTN).
- *Often, occult:* many elderly are angina-free only because they keep physical activity to a bare minimum. This "strategy" prevents symptoms, but not major complications such as MI and death.
- *Often, atypical in its manifestations,* presenting as dyspnea, due to LV dysfunction or paroxysmal AF, as the LA distends as a result of increased LVEDP. The onset of AF cancels the atrial kick and exacerbates HF.
- *Often, atypical in its response to treatment:* drastic measures are often the most effective (e.g., angioplasty over thrombolysis in the very elderly, bypass over angioplasty), but also carry the highest risk.
- *Often, incompletely treated,* due in part to a feeling of futility, often shared by patients and physicians alike. In fact, the elderly can derive overaverage benefits from certain strategies: for instance, statins save twice as many lives after the age of 65, and smoking cessation yields a 50% reduction in post-MI mortality, half of this percentage in the first year.

12.6.2 VHD

VHD manifestations are often diagnosed late in the elderly, due to a combination of factors: sedentary lifestyle (preventing full symptom expression), depression, and often, logistical and financial challenges. *Calcific AS* is the most frequent VHD in the elderly from developed countries; some elderly women have inordinately severe LVH, often causing subvalvular stenosis, which must be relieved surgically at the time of AV replacement. The elderly with *AI* tend to become symptomatic at lesser degrees of LV dilatation, liable to be missed by echo. *LV dysfunction* caused by MR or AS has a worse prognosis than in younger patients; again, high-risk surgery may offer the only chance of survival.

12.6.3 Arrhythmia

Ventricular arrhythmia often involves preexisting heart disease (MI, CMP, VHD), with a high risk of SCD. However, highly effective therapies are often avoided for fear of side effects (β-blockers), or out of financial constraints (ICD). The main *atrial arrhythmia* is AF, present in approximately 10% of patients >80 and increasing in frequency with further age increases. Paroxysmal AF often manifests atypically (e.g., as dyspnea), and chronic AF is often asymptomatic. AF may be the only manifestation of hyperthyroidism in the elderly, and missing this condition makes antiarrhythmic treatment ineffective. Cautious use of oral anticoagulants is indicated.

12.6.4 HF

Approximately 80% of patients hospitalized for HF are >65. Often, early HF signs (fatigue, dyspnea) are dismissed as "signs of old age" and not further investigated or treated. HFPEF, more liable to be missed by echo, is frequent in the elderly, especially in women. Moreover, even diagnosed HF is often not treated according to guidelines; for instance, many physicians are hesitant to recommend β-blocker or interventional therapy, even in the elderly with clearly established HF. This reluctance is based on the increased frequency and severity of adverse effects in the elderly, which indeed is an important concern. Renal dysfunction is common in this age group and increases the risk of Digitalis toxicity, of hyperkalemia related to the use of Spironolactone, Eplerenone, ACEI, or ARB, and of LMWH accumulation and consequent bleeding. The adverse effects of β-blockers appear at lower doses and are more severe. Finally, diuretic dosage should find the correct balance between relief of pulmonary congestion and excessive preload decrease.

12.6.5 CVA

The elderly are at risk, due to the high frequency of
HTN, diabetes, and amyloid angiopathy, the latter fra-
gilizing the vessels and increasing the risk of hemorrhagic CVA. Women have a relatively greater lifetime
risk of CVA, as their life expectancy is longer, and
CVA is mainly a disease of the elderly. Similarly to
other diseases, nonmajor neurologic manifestations in
the elderly may be ignored by patients and physicians
alike. *Therapy:* initially avoided in patients aged >75,
thrombolysis for ischemic stroke has been ultimately
found effective, with an acceptable risk profile in this
age group. BP management in the elderly with CVA
requires special caution, as cerebral autoregulation is
suboptimal and the risk of hypotensive extension of
ischemia is greater than in younger patients.

12.7 Ethnicity and Heart Disease

The impact of genetic heritage is not always easy to distinguish from that of cultural habits (mainly pertaining
to lifestyle). *African people:* coronary disease is more
severe in African than in Caucasian women; stroke and
HTN are more common in African-Americans than in
other ethnicities, largely related to poor control of
reversible risk factors; response of HTN to ACEI or
β-blockers is generally poor, and that to diuretics very
good; preeclampsia and eclampsia are more frequent in
black women; finally, African people are more susceptible to long QT syndrome and to idiopathic VF. The
complexity of interpretation of such data is vividly
illustrated by the finding that up to 40% of blacks carry
a genetic variant acting like a natural β-blocker, which
might offer protection against HF complications. Thus,
the apparently negative fact of a diminished response to
therapeutic β-blockade may actually express an underlying *protective* mechanism in the black race. *Asian
people* have a greater frequency of Takayasu's,
Kawasaki, and Takotsubo disease, of apical HCM, of
outflow VSD, with its typical complication, AI, and of
congenital coronary aneurysms. In *Indian people,* CAD
is more severe and affects younger ages, probably
largely due to lesser access to medical care. *Roma people* are especially influenced by socioeconomic and cultural factors (poverty, migratory lifestyle, overweight,

smoking, etc.). These result in an often grim risk profile; some studies have found HTN in up to 70%, diabetes in up to 50%, and chronic renal failure in up to 20%
of subjects, with vascular disease prevalence up to 40%
and significantly decreased life expectancy.

12.8 HIV Infection and Heart Disease

Cardiac involvement, classically considered not very
frequent or very important in HIV patients, may in fact
have been underestimated in this population. Recent
research has shown that these patients may in fact face
an almost twofold increase in risk, as compared to HIV
patients. A recent study has found that HIV infection
per se is an independent atherosclerosis risk factor,
of a magnitude possibly similar to smoking and diabetes. Generally a sign of advanced disease, cardiac
involvement can be due to direct HIV invasion; to
viral, bacterial, or parasitic involvement of the heart; to
hypercholesterolemia, possibly related to some anti-
HIV agents; to low LDL levels associated to HIV
infection itself; to decreased efficacy of statins and
fibrates in HIV-positive patients; and/or to low compliance with risk factor management. The main cardiovascular problems include: *endocarditis,* either
infective (opportunistic infection or percutaneous contamination in IV drug users) or noninfective (marantic
endocarditis, a sign of advanced disease); infectious
myocarditis, caused by the HIV virus or by opportunistic agents; early *atherosclerosis* and *MI; cardiac
lymphoma* or *Kaposi's* sarcoma (both occasionally
involving the pericardium); and *RV failure* due to *PAH,*
itself a result of direct HIV invasion or secondary to
lung disease. HIV infection is an important cause of
DCM, due to a combination of factors: accelerated atherosclerosis, suboptimally responsive to therapy; cardiac autoimmune reactions; nutritional deficiencies;
drug toxicity; and opportunistic infections.

12.9 Moderate-to-Severe Obstructive
Sleep Apnea

Moderate-to-severe obstructive sleep apnea is associated with an increased risk of ischemia, arrhythmia,
HTN, and stroke, as well as with noncardiovascular

conditions (daytime sleepiness, restless sleep, and loud snoring; headaches, anxiety and depression; polyuria, nocturia, and G-I reflux). The patient is rarely aware of having difficulty in breathing, the disorder being reported by persons who witnessed the episodes. The formal diagnosis is established by an overnight sleep test (polysomnogram), which demonstrates ≥10 s-long pauses in breathing during sleep, with either an EEG pattern of neurologic arousal or a $SatO_2$ decrease ≥3–4%. The cardiovascular impact of OSA is believed to implicate mechanisms such as sympathetic activation, endothelial dysfunction, as well as increased oxidative stress, inflammation, and platelet aggregability. The therapy includes *weight loss;* use of a *C-PAP* (assisting with inspirium) or *B-PAP mask* (assisting with both inspirium and expirium); use of a *mandibular advancement splint* (MAS), a noninvasive device that gently keeps the mandible in a position slightly forward of the normal and tightens the upper respiratory muscles, while still allowing drinking, speaking, yawning, etc.; and different *surgical approaches,* based on the removal of excess tissue in the throat, such as tonsillectomy, adenoidectomy, or UPPP (uvulopalatopharyngoplasty).

12.10 Heart Disease in Children

Heart disease in children mainly consists in CHD (Chap. 10). MI can be seen in children with Kawasaki's disease, and occasionally, in those with homozygous hypercholesterolemia. In infants, the most common sustained ventricular arrhythmia is accelerated idioventricular rhythm. Ventricular arrhythmias in children >1 with a structurally normal heart have a generally benign prognosis, with the exception of catecholaminergic polymorphic VT. SCD is significantly less frequent than in adults and is mostly seen in patients with CHD (where lethal arrhythmia can result from the CHD itself or from myocardial surgical scars), coronary artery anomalies, cardiomyopathies, genetic disorders such as LQTS, and catecholaminergic polymorphic VT. The role of cardiac arrhythmia in SIDS is under active investigation. The treatment of life-threatening ventricular arrhythmia in children follows the same principles as in other age groups, but the use of ICD in those <10 years of age is technically challenging and requires meticulous patient selection.

Bibliography

Guidelines

The Task Force on the Management of Cardiovascular Diseases During Pregnancy of the European Society of Cardiology. Expert consensus document on management of cardiovascular diseases during pregnancy. *Eur Heart J.* 2003;24:761-781.

Suggested Reading

Shaw L, Bairey Merz C, Pepine C, et al. Insights from the NHLBI-Sponsored Women's Ischemia Syndrome Evaluation (WISE) Study. Part I: gender differences in traditional and novel risk factors, symptom evaluation, and gender-optimized diagnostic strategies. *J Am Coll Cardiol.* 2006;47(3):S4-S20.

Autore C, Conte MR, Piccininno M, et al. Risk associated with pregnancy in hypertrophic cardiomyopathy. *J Am Coll Cardiol.* 2002;40:1864-1869.

Elkayam U, Bitar F. Valvular heart disease and pregnancy. Part I: native valves. *J Am Coll Cardiol.* 2005a;46:223-230.

Elkayam U, Bitar F. Valvular heart disease and pregnancy. Part II: prosthetic valves. *J Am Coll Cardiol.* 2005b;46:403-410.

Elkayam U, Ostrzega E, Shotan A, Mehra A. Cardiovascular problems in pregnant women with the Marfan syndrome. *Ann Intern Med.* 1995;123(2):117-122.

Shepherd J, Blauw G, Murphy M, et al. Pravastatin in elderly individuals at risk of vascular disease (PROSPER): a randomised controlled trial. *Lancet.* 2002;360(9346):1623-1630.

Maron BJ. Sudden death in young athletes. *N Engl J Med.* 2003;34(11):1064-1075.

Grunfeld C, Delaney JAC, Wanke C, et al. Preclinical atherosclerosis due to HIV infection: carotid intima-medial thickness measurements from the FRAM study. *AIDS.* 2009;23(14):1841-1849.

Grinspoon SK, Grunfeld C, Kotler DP, et al. Initiative to decrease cardiovascular risk and increase quality of care for patients living with HIV/AIDS. Executive summary. *Circulation.* 2008;118:198-210.

Silverberg MJ, Leyden W, Hurley L, et al. Response to newly prescribed lipid-lowering therapy in patients with and without HIV infection. *Ann Intern Med.* 2009;150:301-313.

Glossary

aPTT	Activated partial prothrombin time	AVSD	Atrioventricular septal defect
AAD	Antiarrhythmic drugs	BB	Beta blocker
ABI	Ankle-brachial index	BBB	Bundle branch block
ACC	American College of Cardiology	BE	Bacterial endocarditis
ACE	Angiotensin-converting enzyme	BMI	Body mass index
ACEI	Angiotensin-converting enzyme inhibitor	BMS	Bare metal stent
		BNP	Brain natriuretic peptide
ACS	Acute coronary syndrome	BP	Blood pressure
ADP	Adenosine diphosphate	B-T	Blalock-Taussig
AF	Atrial fibrillation	Bpm	Beats per minute
AHA	American heart association	CABG	Aorto-coronary bypass graft surgery
AI	Aortic insufficiency	CAD	Coronary artery disease
AIVR	Accelerated idioventricular rhythm	Cath	catheter, catheterization
ALT	Alanine amino transferase	CCB	Calcium channel blockers
ANCA	Anti-neutrophil cytoplasmic antibody	CHB	Complete heart block
AP	Accessory pathway	CHD	Coronary heart disease
AP	Antero-posterior	CHF	Chronic heart failure
APB	Atrial premature beat	C/I	Contraindicated
ApoA, B	Apolipoprotein A, B	CIN	Contrast-induced nephropathy
AR	Angiotensin receptor blocker	CKD	Chronic kidney disease
ARVC	Arrhythmogenic right ventricular cardiomyopathy	CK	Creatine kinase
		CKMB	Creatine kinase-myocardial band
AS	Aortic stenosis	CMP	Cardiomyopathy
ASD	Atrial septal defect	CO	Cardiac output
AST	Aspartate amino transferase	COPD	Chronic obstructive pulmonary disease
AT	Atrial tachycardia	CP	Constrictive pericarditis
ATP	Adenosine-5`-triphosphate	CrCl	Creatinine clearance
AT	Angiotensin	CPR	Cardiopulmonary resuscitation
AV	Atrioventricular	CRP	C-reactive protein
AV	Aortic valve	CRT	Cardiac resynchronization therapy
AVB	Atrioventricular block	CT	Computed tomography
AVN	Atrio-ventricular node	CTO	Chronic total occlusion
AVNRT	Atrio-ventricular vode reentry tachycardia	CVA	Cerebrovascular accident
		CVP	Central venous pressure
AVR	Aortic valve replacement	CWD	Continuous wave doppler
AVRT	Atrioventricular reciprocating (reentrant) tachycardia	2D	Two-dimensional
		3D	Three dimensional

DBP	Diastolic Blood Pressure	ICD	Implantable cardioverter defibrillator
DCC	Direct current cardioversion	ICH	Intracerebral hemorrhage
DCM	Dilated cardiomyopathy	ICU	Intensive care unit
DDD	Dual chamber pacemaker that senses/paces in the atrium/ventricle and is inhibited/triggered by intrinsic rhythm	IDL	Intermediate-density lipoprotein(s)
		IE	Infectious endocarditis
		ILBBB	Incomplete LBBB
		IMT	Intima-media thickness
DES	Drug-eluting stents	INR	International normalized ratio
DM	Diabetes mellitus	IRBBB	Incomplete RBBB
DORV	Double outlet right ventricle	ISDN	Isosorbide dinitrate
DVT	Deep vein Thrombosis	IVRT	Isovolumic relaxation time
EBCT	Electron beam computed tomography	IVS	Interventricular septum
ECG	Electrocardiogram	IVUS	Intravascular ultrasound
Echo	Echocardiogram/echocardiography	KD	Kawasaki disease
EDV	End diastolic volume	LA	Left atrium
EKG	Electrocardiogram	LAA	Left atrial appendage
EPS	Electrophysiologic study	LAD	Left anterior descending
ER	Emergency room	LBBB	Left bundle branch block
ERO	Effective Regurgitant Orifice	LCx	Left circumflex (coronary artery)
ESC	European Society of Cardiology	LDL	Low-density lipoprotein (cholesterol)
ESD	End systolic diameter		
FDG	Fluoro-deoxy-glucose (fludeoxyglucose)	LIMA	Left internal mammary artery
		LFT	Liver function tests
FFP	Fresh frozen plasma	LMCA	Left main coronary artery
FFR	Fractional flow reserve	LMWH	Low molecular weight heparin
F/U	Follow-up	Lp(a)	Lipoprotein a
HIT	Heparin induced thrombocytopenia	LQTS	Long QT syndrome
HITT	Heparin induced thrombocytopenia and thrombosis	L-R	Left-to-right
		LV	Left ventricle
GI	Gastrointestinal	LVAD	Left ventricular assist device
GPIIb/IIIa	Glycoprotein IIb/IIIa	LVH	Left ventricular hypertrophy
GP	Glycoprotein	LVEDP	Left ventricular end diastolic pressure
GWAS	Genome-wide association scans	LVEF	Left ventricular ejection fraction
HCM	Hypertropic cardiomyopathy	LVOT	Left ventricular outflow tract
HCTZ	Hydrochlorothiazide	MACE	Major adverse cardiac event rates
HDL	High-density lipoprotein(s)	MET	Metabolic equivalent of the task
HbA1c	Glycosylated hemoglobin	MI	Myocardial infarction
HF	Heart failure	MIBG	M-131-Iodobenzylguanidine
HIDA	Hepatobiliary scintigraphy with dimethyliminodiacetic acid	mmHg	Millimeters of mercury
		MR	Mitral regurgitation
HFPEF	Heart failure with preserved ejection fraction	MRI	Magnetic resonance imaging scan
		MRSA	Methicillin resistant S. aureus
HCM	Hypertrophic cardiomyopathy	MSSA	Methicillin-Susceptible S. aureus
HOCM	Hypertrophic obstructive cardiomyopathy	MS	Mitral stenosis
		MUGA	Multigated acquisition nuclear angiography
HR	Heart rate		
HRT	Hormone replacement therapy	MV	Mitral valve
HTN	Hypertension	MVP	Mitral valve prolapse
IABP	Intra – aortic ballon pump	NSAID	Non-steroid anti-inflammatory drug

NSTE-ACS	Non-ST elevation acute coronary syndrome	PVE	Prosthetic valve endocarditis
MV	Mitral valve	PVR	Pulmonary vascular resistance
MVP	Mitral valve prolapse	PWD	Pulsed wave doppler
NO	Nitric oxide	QCA	Quantitative coronary angiography
NPV	Negative predictive value	Qp/Qs	Ratio = pulmonary/aortic blood flow
NSAID	Non-steroid anti-inflammatory drug	RA	Right atrium
NSR	Normal sinus rhythm	RAS	Renal artery stenosis
NSTE-ACS	Non ST-elevation ACS	RAAS	Renin-angiotensin-aldosterone system
NSTEMI	Non ST-elevation myocardial infarction	RBBB	Block + right bundle branch block
		RBC	Red blood cell(s)
NSVT	Nonsustained VT	RCM	Restrictive cardomyopathy
NVE	Native valve endocarditis	RCA	Right coronary artery
NYHA	New York Health Association	RF	Radio frequency
O_2	Oxygen	RFT	Renal function tests
OR	Operating room	RIMA	Right internal mammary artery
PA	Postero-anterior	R–L	Right-to-left
PA	Pulmonary artery	rtPA	Recombined tissue plasminogen activator
PAH	Pulmonary arterial hypertension	RV	Right ventricle
PAN	Panartriitis nodosa	RVEDP	Right ventricular end diastolic pressure
PAP	Pulmonary artery/arterial pressure		
sPAP	Systolic pulmonary artery/arterial pressure	RVEF	Right ventricular ejection fraction
		RVH	Right ventricular hypertrophy
PCI	Percutaneous coronary intervention	RVOT	Right ventricle outflow tract
PCWP	Pulmonary capillary wedge pressure	SAECG	Signal-averaged ECG
PCR	Polymerase chain reaction	SAM	Systolic anterior motion of the mitral valve
PDA	Patent ductus arteriosus		
PE	Pulmonary embolism	SAP	Stable angina pectoris
PEA	Pulseless electrical activity	$SatO_2$	Blood oxygen saturation
PEEP	Positive end-expiratory airway pressure	SBP	Systemic blood pressure
		SCD	Sudden cardiac death
PET	Positron emission tomography	sdLDL	small, dense LDL particles
PFO	Patent foramen ovale	SE	stress echocardiography
PLT	Platelet count	SIDS	Sudden infant death syndrome
PMV	Percutaneous mitral valvuloplasty	SN	Sinus node
pCO_2	Partial pressure of carbon dioxide	SPECT	Single photon emission-computed tomography
POTS	Postural orthostatic tachycardia syndrome		
		SSS	Sick sinus syndrome
PP	Pulse pressure	STEMI	ST-elevation myocardial infarction
PPI	Proton pump inhibitor	SVC	Superior vena cava
PPV	Positive predictive value	SVT	Supraventricular tachyarrhythmia
PS	Pacemaker syndrome	SVT	Supraventricular tachycardia
PTH	Parathyroid hormone	T1/2	The half-life
PSVT	Paroxysmal supraventricular tachycardia	TA	Tricuspid atresia
		TEE	Transesophageal echocardiogram
PT	Pericardial tamponade	TG	Triglyceride
PV	Pulmonic valve	TGV	Transposition of the great vessels
PVB	Premature ventricular	TIA	Transient ischaemic attack
PVD	Peripheral vascular disease	TIMI	Thrombolysis in myocardial infarction

TOF	Tetrology of fallot	VEGF	Vascular endothelial growth factor
t-PA	Tissue plasminogen activator	VF	Ventricular fibrillation
TR	Tricuspid regurgitation	VHD	Valvular heart disease
TS	Tricuspid stenosis	VKA	Vitamin K antagonists
TTE	Transthoracic echocardiogram	VLDL	Very low density lipoprotein
TV	Tricuspid valve	VO$_2$Max	Maximal Oxygen Consumption Capacity
TVI	Time velocity integral		
UA	Unstable angina	VSD	Ventricular septal defect
UFH	Unfractionated heparin	VT	Ventricular tachycardia
URL	Upper reference limit	VTE	Venous thromboembolism
URTI	Upper airway respiratory tract infection	WMA	Wall motion abnormality
		WPW	Wolff–Parkinson–White
VAD	Ventricular assist device		

Index